T0324876

# Skull Base Imaging

# Skull Base Imaging

VINCENT CHONG, MD, MBA, MHPE, FRCR
Department of Diagnostic Imaging
National University Health System
Singapore; Department of Diagnostic Radiology
Yong Loo Lin School of Medicine
National University of Singapore
Singapore

ELSEVIER

# ELSEVIER

3251 Riverport Lane
St. Louis, Missouri 63043

SKULL BASE IMAGING                                    ISBN: 978-0-323-48563-0

---

### Notices

Knowledge and best practice in this field are constantly changing. As new research and experience broaden our understanding, changes in research methods, professional practices, or medical treatment may become necessary.

Practitioners and researchers must always rely on their own experience and knowledge in evaluating and using any information, methods, compounds, or experiments described herein. In using such information or methods they should be mindful of their own safety and the safety of others, including parties for whom they have a professional responsibility.

With respect to any drug or pharmaceutical products identified, readers are advised to check the most current information provided (i) on procedures featured or (ii) by the manufacturer of each product to be administered, to verify the recommended dose or formula, the method and duration of administration, and contraindications. It is the responsibility of practitioners, relying on their own experience and knowledge of their patients, to make diagnoses, to determine dosages and the best treatment for each individual patient, and to take all appropriate safety precautions.

To the fullest extent of the law, neither the Publisher nor the authors, contributors, or editors, assume any liability for any injury and/or damage to persons or property as a matter of products liability, negligence or otherwise, or from any use or operation of any methods, products, instructions, or ideas contained in the material herein.

---

*Content Strategist:* Kayla Wolfe
*Content Development Manager:* Taylor Ball
*Content Development Specialist:* Donald Mumford
*Publishing Services Manager:* Deepthi Unni
*Project Manager:* Janish Ashwin Paul
*Designer:* Renee Deunow

Printed in United States of America

Last digit is the print number:   9   8   7   6   5   4   3   2   1

Working together
to grow libraries in
developing countries

www.elsevier.com • www.bookaid.org

# Contributors

**Abdellatif Bali, MD**
Department of Radiology
Sint-Augustinus Hospital, GZA
Antwerp, Belgium

**Anja Bernaerts, MD**
Department of Radiology
Sint-Augustinus Hospital, GZA
Antwerp, Belgium

**Alexandra R Borges, MD**
Instituto Português de Oncologia de Lisboa Francisco
    Gentil
Champalimaud Foundation
Lisbon, Portugal

**Jan W. Casselman, MD, PhD**
Department of Radiology
AZ Sint-Jan Bruges-Ostend
Bruges, Belgium; Department of Radiology
Sint-Augustinus Hospital, GZA, Antwerp,
Belgium, University of Ghent
Ghent, Belgium

**Margaret N. Chapman, MD**
Assistant Professor
Department of Radiology
Boston Medical Center
Boston University School of Medicine
Boston, MA, United States

**Ya-Fang Chen, MD**
Section of Neuroradiology
Department of Medical Imaging and Radiology
Hospital and Medical College
National Taiwan University
Taipei, Taiwan

**Vincent Chong, MD, MBA, MHPE, FRCR**
Department of Diagnostic Imaging
National University Health System
Singapore; Department of Diagnostic Radiology
Yong Loo Lin School of Medicine
National University of Singapore
Singapore

**Bert De Foer, MD, PhD**
Department of Radiology
Sint-Augustinus Hospital, GZA
Antwerp, Belgium

**Joost van Dinther, MD**
European Institute for ORL - HNS
Department for Otorhinolaryngology - Head & Neck
    Surgery
Sint Augustinus Hospital, GZA
Antwerp, Belgium

**James Thomas Patrick Decourcy Hallinan,
MBChB, BSc, FRCR**
Department of Diagnostic Imaging
National University Health System
Singapore; Department of Diagnostic Radiology
Yong Loo Lin School of Medicine
National University of Singapore
Singapore

**Theresa Kouo, MD**
Assistant Professor
Department of Diagnostic Radiology and Nuclear
    Medicine
University of Maryland School of Medicine
Baltimore, MD, United States

**Ong Yew Kwang, MBBS (Hons), DOHNS,
MRCS, MMed (ORL)**
Assistant Professor
Department of Otolaryngology
National University Health System
Yong Loo Lin School of Medicine
National University of Singapore
Singapore

**Timothy L. Larson, MD**
Swedish Hospital Medical Center
Radia Inc., LLC
Seattle, WA, United States

**Marc Lemmerling, MD, PhD**
Department of Radiology
AZ St. Lucas Hospital Ghent
Belgium; Department of Radiology
Ghent University Hospital
Belgium

**Yen-Heng Lin, MD, MS**
Section of Neuroradiology
Department of Medical Imaging and Radiology
Hospital and Medical College
National Taiwan University
Taipei, Taiwan

**Hon-Man Liu, MD, MBA**
Department of Medical Imaging
Fu Jen Catholic University Hospital
New Taipei City
Taiwan
Section of Neuroradiology
Department of Medical Imaging and Radiology
Hospital and Medical College
National Taiwan University
Taipei, Taiwan

**Robert E. Morales, MD**
Assistant Professor
Department of Diagnostic Radiology and Nuclear
    Medicine
University of Maryland School of Medicine
Baltimore, MD, United States

**Erwin Offeciers, MD, PhD**
European Institute for ORL - HNS
Department for Otorhinolaryngology - Head & Neck
    Surgery
Sint Augustinus Hospital, GZA
Antwerp, Belgium

**Prashant Raghavan, MBBS**
Associate Professor
Department of Diagnostic Radiology and Nuclear
    Medicine
University of Maryland School of Medicine
Baltimore, MD, United States

**Osamu Sakai, MD, PhD, FACR**
Professor
Departments of Radiology, Otolaryngology - Head
    and Neck Surgery, and Radiation Oncology
Boston Medical Center
Boston University School of Medicine
Boston, MA, United States

**Ilona M. Schmalfuss, MD**
Department of Radiology
University of Florida and NF/SG Veterans
    Administration
Gainesville, FL, United States

**Lubdha M. Shah, MD**
Associate Professor of Radiology
Department of Radiology
University of Utah Health Sciences Center
Salt Lake City, UT, United States

**David Soon Yiew Sia, MBBS, FRCR, MMED**
Department of Diagnostic Imaging
National University Health System
Singapore; Department of Diagnostic Radiology
Yong Loo Lin School of Medicine
National University of Singapore
Singapore

**Eric Ting Yuik Sing, MBBS (Hons),
BSc (Medicine), FRANZCR**
Assistant Professor
Department of Diagnostic Imaging
National University Health System
Yong Loo Lin School of Medicine
National University of Singapore
Singapore; Consultant
Department of Diagnostic Imaging
National University Hospital
Singapore

**Chia Ghim Song, MD, FRCR**
Department of Radiology
Singapore General Hospital
Singapore

**Fiona Ting, MBBS (Hons), BSc (Medicine),
MClinEpid, FRACS (OHNS)**
Royal North Shore Hospital
St Leonards, NSW, Australia

**Richard H. Wiggins, III, MD, CIIP, FSIIM**
Professor
Departments of Radiology and Imaging Sciences,
    Otolaryngology, Head and Neck Surgery, and
    BioMedical Informatics
University of Utah Health Sciences Center
Salt Lake City, UT, United States

**Mathew L. Wong, MD**
Washington Otology Neurotology Group
Medina, WA, United States

**Laura Wuyts, MD**
Department of Radiology
GZA Hospitals, campus Sint-Augustinus
Antwerp
Belgium

**Clement Yong, MBBS (Hons), FRANZCR**
Department of Diagnostic Imaging
National University Health System
Singapore; Department of Diagnostic Radiology
Yong Loo Lin School of Medicine
National University of Singapore
Singapore

# Preface

In the last 30 years, skull base surgery has evolved into a subspecialty incorporating multiple disciplines such as neurosurgery, otolaryngology, head and neck surgery, oral maxillofacial surgery, and plastic surgery. Hence (depending on the nature of the pathologic process and disease extent), skull base lesions are often managed by a multidisciplinary team.

During this same period of skull base surgical development, parallel rapid advances in imaging technology have resulted in radiologists playing crucial roles in supporting their clinical colleagues. It is therefore not surprising that imaging specialists have become essential members of the skull base team. In addition, interventional radiologists have started to provide additional support in patient care, thus widening the available treatment options.

In the meantime, clinical evaluation of suspected skull base lesions remains challenging. The anatomy is complex, and the areas of concern are often inaccessible to direct clinical examination. Hence, the diagnosis and assessment of disease extent is frequently impossible without imaging support. In addition, multimodality imaging is often required to provide the crucial information for both diagnosis and prognosis. Finally, it can be appreciated how imaging is indispensable in guiding biopsy, selecting treatment options, planning treatment, and evaluating treatment outcome.

Radiologists supporting the skull base team should have a working knowledge of the relevant anatomy, pathology, and available treatment options along with their indications and contraindications. In this edition of *Skull Base Imaging*, we bring together a team of experts to share their rich experience in evaluating common and not-so-common problems seen in our daily practice. The contributions of these authors range from reviewing diagnostic approaches (that clarify clinical issues) to describing the use of newer imaging techniques (to answer problems that conventional methods have failed to resolve). They have also taken the opportunity to highlight essential imaging anatomy and pertinent surgical pathology. We have also included chapters on posttreatment imaging and neurointerventional approaches as treatment options.

We hope this book will serve as a handy source of reference.

**Vincent Fook-Hin Chong, MBBS, MBA, MHPE, FRCR**
*Department of Diagnostic Imaging*
*National University Health System*
*Singapore*

# Contents

# CHAPTER 1

# Anterior Skull Base

DAVID SY SIA, MBBS, FRCR, MMED •
CLEMENT YONG, MBBS, FRANZCR •
JAMES TPD HALLINAN, MBChB, BSc, FRCR •
VINCENT CHONG, MD, MBA, MHPE

The anterior skull base is a region of interest because it is frequently breached by aggressive disease such as malignancy and infection or even chronic long-standing but progressive lesions such as mucoceles. This resultant transcompartmental spread has a significant impact in prognosis and management. Imaging plays a key role in the assessment of disease extent and management planning.

Most tumors that involve the anterior skull base originate in the sinonasal compartment. Malignant sinonasal tumors are relatively rare, comprising 3% of all head and neck malignancies.[1] These tumors (ranging from the common squamous cell carcinoma [SCC] to the rare sarcomas) are usually aggressive. They generally have a poor prognosis because of extensive disease at presentation and high local recurrence rate.[2] Benign sinonasal tumors are also common, and they include sinonasal polyps, juvenile angiofibroma, and inverted papilloma. These lesions are usually confined to their site of origin and rarely encroach or erode the skull base.

As most sinonasal tumors are amenable to biopsy, the primary role of imaging is in mapping the tumor extent. Information such as osseous erosion, meningeal and brain invasion, or orbital extension is crucial for management planning.[3] Significant advancement in craniofacial surgical approach has enabled safe and reliable resection of sinonasal tumors.[4] The craniofacial approach essentially allows for a wide exposure of the anterior craniofacial structures and can be modified to extend surgical accessibility (depending on the individual case and surgeon preference). The anterior craniofacial approach, as the name suggests, incorporates a combination of transfacial and transcranial procedures. It is important to note that the advances in craniofacial resection techniques are largely contributed by the wealth of information provided by preoperative CT and MRI.

## ANATOMY

The anterior skull base separates the cranial cavity above from the orbit and sinonasal compartments below. This boundary is formed by two bones: the cribriform plate centrally and the orbital plates of the frontal bone laterally (Fig. 1.1). The cribriform plate is the part of the ethmoid bone that consists of two parallel grooves on which the olfactory bulbs sit, separated by a midline triangular process called the crista galli (because of its resemblance to the comb of a rooster). The crista galli serves as an attachment site for the falx cerebri. The floor of each groove has multiple tiny perforations that allow passage of olfactory nerves to the nasal mucosa. The frontal sinuses are located anterior to the cribriform plate.

The thin cribriform plate is well demonstrated on coronal CT images. This structure is also visible on MRI as a linear hypointense signal on T1-weighted and T2-weighted sequences. It is frequently involved by tumors and fractured by trauma or surgery. The orbital plates of the frontal bone constitute a thick and robust barrier to disease spread. The lamina papyracea is the medial orbital wall that separates the orbit from the ethmoid sinus. It is thus named because of its paper-thin appearance and is easily fractured or eroded by tumors. This structure, like the cribriform plate, is easily evaluated on CT. The periorbita is the periosteum lining the walls of the bony orbit to which it is loosely connected. It is continuous with the periosteum of facial bones anteriorly and the dura mater posteriorly through the superior orbital fissure. This structure is indistinguishable from the adjacent orbital wall in normal patients but can be seen as a hypointense line on T1-weighted and T2-weighted MRI when lifted off the underlying bone by tumor, blood, or pus.

## KEY IMAGING CONSIDERATIONS

Intracranial invasion is recognized as the most adverse prognostic factor in sinonasal tumors and is a crucial

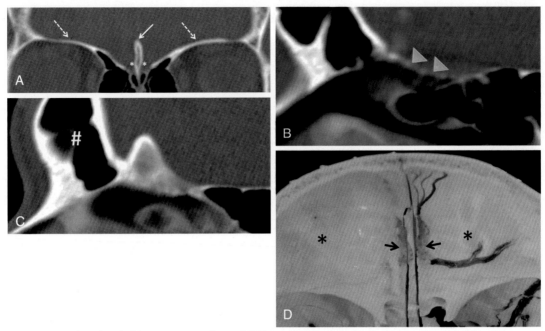

FIG. 1.1 Anterior skull base anatomy. Coronal CT images of the anterior skull base show the thin cribriform plate centrally consisting of olfactory grooves (*asterisks* in **A**) separated by the crista galli in the midline (*solid arrow* in **A**). There are tiny perforations on the floor of each olfactory groove as seen on sagittal CT (*arrowheads* in **B**). The thick orbital plates of the frontal bone form lateral portions of anterior skull base (*dashed arrows* in **A**). The anterior margin of the anterior skull base is formed by the frontal sinuses centrally (*hash* in **C**). Photograph of a dry skull specimen **(D)** shows the anterior skull base seen from above, demonstrating the central cribriform plate with multiple perforations (*arrows*) and the orbital plates laterally (*asterisks*).

feature requiring careful imaging evaluation.[5] Dural invasion alone significantly decreases survival rate from 68% to 25% in a series of adenocarcinomas.[6] On the other hand, orbital invasion by sinonasal malignancy is an independent prognostic factor with a significant impact on survival rates.[7] The incidence of visual involvement is estimated at 50%.[8] This is related to its close proximity to the sinuses and the presence of multiple routes of spread via anatomic foramina, traversing vessels, and nerves, as well as thin bones such as the lamina papyracea. Imaging plays a critical role in determining orbital disease extension (Fig. 1.2).

## Anterior Cranial Fossa Invasion

Intracranial invasion includes breach of the skull base, dural involvement, and brain parenchymal invasion. It is possible that the skull base integrity is compromised by disease without involvement of the adjacent dura mater (Fig. 1.3).

Breach of the anterior skull base is suspected when the cribriform plate is dehiscent on CT or the normal hypointense signal on MRI is lost. Thereafter, the dura should be inspected for evidence of disease such as dural thickening and enhancement. Dural involvement is considered a precursor to brain invasion and is associated with poor recurrence-free survival, disease-specific survival, and overall survival.[9] Although dural spread can be seen on imaging, it may be difficult to differentiate neoplastic involvement from inflammatory change. In general, if the visualized dura appears grossly thickened and has a nodular contour, dural invasion can be assumed. As dural invasion is associated with a high recurrence rate, aggressive resection of potentially involved dura followed by radiotherapy is often undertaken, even though dural infiltration is not evident on MRI.

Tumors may indent the base of the brain without parenchymal invasion. In these cases, a thin cleft of cerebrospinal fluid (CSF) is seen at the interface between the tumor and the brain surface (Fig. 1.4). Apart from

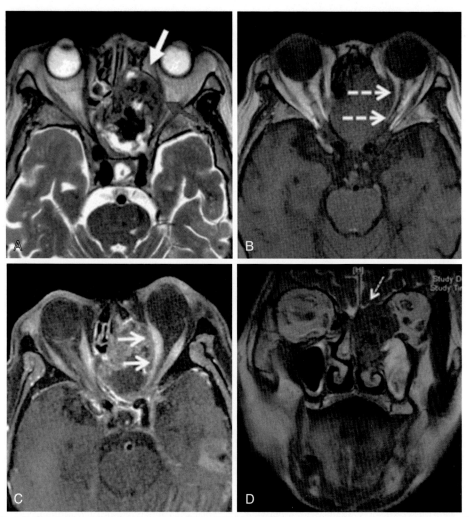

FIG. 1.2 Squamous cell carcinoma. Axial T2 and T1 (**A** and **B**), coronal T2 (**C**), and axial fat-suppressed T1 postcontrast (**D**) images show a necrotic sinonasal tumor invading through the cribriform plate and the medial orbital wall. Note the *black line* representing bowed intact periorbita anteriorly (*white arrow* in **A**), but the posterior aspect of the periorbita is indistinct (*red arrow* in **A**), consistent with orbital invasion. Mass effect on the optic nerve (*dashed arrows* in **B**) and medial rectus muscle (*solid arrows* in **C**) is clearly depicted. Dural invasion in the anterior cranial fossa is also present (*dashed arrow* in **D**) without brain involvement.

the mass effect, the brain demonstrates normal signal characteristics. Aggressive lesions, such as SCC, often invade the frontal lobes, resulting in loss of CSF cleft and presence of brain edema and enhancement.

### Orbital Invasion

The periorbita is the periosteum lining the walls of the bony orbit and has traditionally been regarded as the decisive layer that determines the subsequent extent of surgery.

Transgression of the periorbita means orbit evisceration is required.[10] Eisen showed that tumor adjacent to the periorbita was the most sensitive predictor of orbital invasion.[7] When the hypointense line is lost, orbital invasion is considered to be present. However, this structure can be difficult to visualize separately from the orbital wall even in normal cases, making interpretation extremely challenging. Furthermore, a meta-analysis[11] showed no significant difference in 5-year survival rates between patients

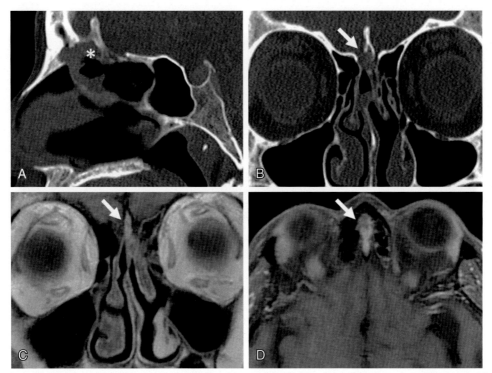

FIG. 1.3 Anterior skull base erosion. Sagittal and coronal CT images (**A** and **B**) show a small lesion that is centered in the roof of the anterior ethmoid sinus and erodes into the frontal sinus and crista galli (*asterisk* in **A**). CT is superior in depicting osseous erosion into the right olfactory groove (*white arrow* in **B**). MRI is excellent in depicting intense postcontrast enhancement of the lesion (*arrows* in **C** and **D**). Note the absence of dural or brain involvement on MRI. This lesion is a histologically proven phosphaturic mesenchymal tumor, a rare tumor that has a tendency to cause oncogenic osteomalacia. (Data from Guglielmi G, Bisceglia M, Schillitani A, et al. Oncogenic osteomalacia due to phosphaturic mesenchymal tumor of the craniofacial sinuses. *Clin Cases Miner Bone Metab.* 2011;8(2):45–49.)

whose orbits were preserved and patients who underwent evisceration. Ianetti[12] described three stages of orbital invasion: grade I, erosion of the medial orbital wall; grade II, extraconal invasion of periorbital fat; and grade III, invasion of the medial rectus muscle, optic nerve, ocular bulb, or skin overlying the eyelid. It is thus perhaps more feasible for the radiologist to use this grading system. Most surgeons now consider grade III invasion as an indication for orbital evisceration. A more conservative approach involves intraoperative microscopic dissection and frozen section of the periorbita before decision for or against evisceration is made.[11,13]

## ANTERIOR SKULL BASE NEOPLASMS
### Squamous Cell Carcinoma

The most common malignant tumor in the sinonasal cavity is SCC, accounting for 60%–75% of all sinonasal cancers.[15] There is a male predominance, with a peak incidence in the fifth to seventh decades. The most frequent location is the maxillary sinus followed by the nasal cavity, ethmoid sinus, and, rarely, frontal or sphenoid sinus.

SCC often shows intermediate signal intensity on T2-weighted sequence, reflecting the hypercellular nature of this tumor. MRI may also show areas of T1-weighted hyperintensity (representing hemorrhage) and areas of T2-weighted hyperintensity (representing necrosis). Bone destruction is characteristic of SCC, but tumor extent is best appreciated on MRI. MRI with contrast agent can demonstrate the enhancing tumor, a feature that helps to distinguish it from benign inflammatory lesions, such as retained secretions, mucoceles, and sinonasal polyps (Fig. 1.5). According to the TNM (tumor, node, and metastasis) classification system, SCC invading the medial orbital wall is classified as T3, whereas involvement of the anterior cranial fossa is T4.

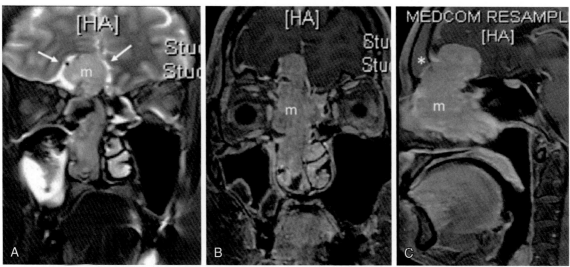

FIG. 1.4 Esthesioneuroblastoma. Coronal T2 **(A)**, coronal and sagittal fat-suppressed T1 with contrast **(B and C)** images show a classic dumbbell-shaped mass (m) with avid enhancement. The tumor involves the anterior cranial fossa but does not invade the brain parenchyma as evidenced by the fluid-filled cleft between the tumor and the brain (*solid arrows*). The frontal lobes are indented but no edema or enhancement is seen. Note the erosion of the frontal sinus and resultant nonenhancing retained secretion (*asterisk* in **C**).

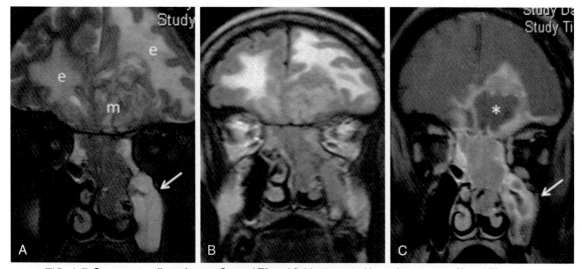

FIG. 1.5 Squamous cell carcinoma. Coronal T2 and fluid-attenuated inversion recovery **(A and B)** and coronal fat-suppressed T1 postcontrast **(C)** images show an aggressive tumor (m) eroding through the cribriform plate and invading the frontal lobes, which show parenchymal edema (e). Note the necrotic appearance of the intraparenchymal component, best seen in postcontrast images (*asterisk* in **C**). Mucosal engorgement of the left maxillary sinus as a result of outlet obstruction is easily distinguished from tumor in the nasal cavity (*arrows* in **A** and **C**).

## Esthesioneuroblastoma

Esthesioneuroblastoma, also known as olfactory neuroblastoma, is rare and accounts for 1%–5% of all sinonasal tumors.[16] This lesion typically affects the adolescent male, with a second peak incidence in the fifth decade. Imaging usually shows a large dumbbell-shaped mass centered at the cribriform plate. The tumor arises from the olfactory epithelium in the superior recess of the nasal cavity and follows the distribution of olfactory nerves through the cribriform plate, hence its characteristic shape and the frequent extension through the anterior skull base (Fig. 1.6). However, the tumor can also spread submucosally in all directions and may present with proptosis and neck node metastasis.[17]

CT can easily identify osteolytic destruction of the skull base and intratumoral speckled calcification

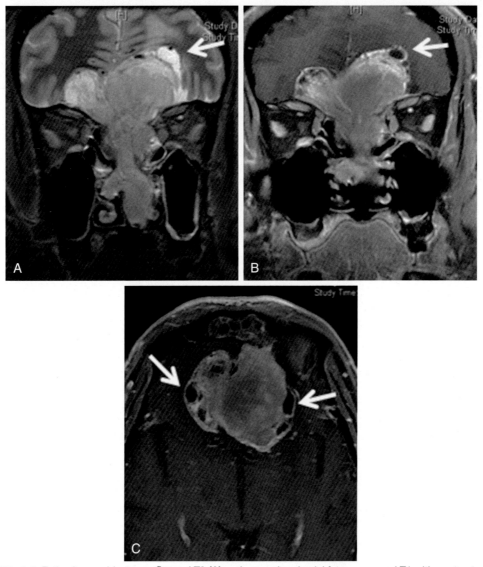

FIG. 1.6 Esthesioneuroblastoma. Coronal T2 **(A)** and coronal and axial fat-suppressed T1 with contrast **(B and C)** images show a large dumbbell-shaped mass in the sinonasal space eroding through the cribriform plate into the anterior cranial fossa. Note the mass effect on the frontal lobes, but no definite parenchymal invasion is evident. Peripheral cystic lesions at the mass-brain interface are a characteristic feature of this tumor (*white arrows*).

(if present). In rare cases, the pattern of bone destruction may be predominantly osteoblastic and has been termed hyperostotic esthesioneuroblastoma. Indeed, the hyperostosis may have a ground-glass appearance, thus mimicking fibrous dysplasia.[18] MRI typically shows nonspecific heterogeneous signals that are indistinguishable from other sinonasal tumors. The presence of cysts at the tumor-brain interface is characteristic of esthesioneuroblastoma and should be actively sought for (Fig. 1.6).[16,19]

### Adenocarcinoma

Sinonasal adenocarcinomas may originate from the respiratory surface epithelium or seromucinous glands and are divided into salivary-type and non-salivary-type adenocarcinomas. The latter are further divided into intestinal and nonintestinal types.[20] These tumors are often seen in males in the sixth decade and, like SCC, are associated with occupational exposure to wood dust and other industrial materials.[21] The imaging features are nonspecific and indistinguishable from those of SCC.

### Adenoid Cystic Carcinoma

Adenoid cystic carcinomas (ACCs) arise in minor salivary gland tissues. They are typically slow growing but often exhibit high recurrence rates. Low-grade ACC may present as an ethmoid polyp that remodels bone and mimics a simple polyp, whereas high-grade ACC may present as a large irregular mass with bone destruction. ACC also demonstrates a high propensity for perineural spread, most commonly involving the trigeminal nerve.[22,23] Up to 60% of tumors show perineural spread.[23] These tumors are able to use peripheral nerves as a direct conduit for tumor growth away from the primary site.[22] The presence of perineural spread indicates a higher risk of local recurrence and metastasis and decreased survival rates.

CT may demonstrate foraminal widening due to tumor spread along the traversing nerve, but this is usually a late finding. Obliteration of fat planes around nerves is the first sign of perineural spread, and this observation is well demonstrated on MRI. In addition, the nerve itself may be enlarged and enhances, and the denervation effects of regional muscles may also be evident on MRI.[24]

### Sinonasal Lymphoma

Sinonasal lymphoma (SNL) is uncommon in the Western population but represents the second most common site of extranodal lymphoma in Asia after the gastrointestinal tract.[25] Reports have documented

that natural killer/T-cell lymphoma is more common than B-cell lymphoma in this location.[26,27] SNL is slow growing and presents with symptoms indistinguishable from those of benign inflammatory disease. In later stages, it causes destruction of the nasal septum and palate (dubbed "lethal midline granuloma syndrome"). Other entities causing similar structural destruction include Wegener granulomatosis and cocaine abuse. On MRI, SNL typically shows increased signals on diffusion-weighted imaging because of hypercellularity and avid contrast enhancement (Fig. 1.7).

### Sinonasal Undifferentiated Carcinoma

Sinonasal undifferentiated carcinoma (SNUC) is a rare tumor arising from the Schneiderian epithelium of the nasal cavity and sinuses. It was originally described by Frierson as a highly aggressive and clinicopathologically distinct carcinoma with rapid growth rate and locally advanced disease at presentation, often involving the orbit and skull base.[28] The imaging features of SNUC are nonspecific. These tumors are frequently large with ill-defined margins and show aggressive bone destruction and hence are indistinguishable from the more common SCC. Studies have confirmed overall poor prognosis, and because of the low incidence of SNUC, there are insufficient data available on the optimal combination of treatment regimen.[29]

### Sarcoma

Sarcomas are a heterogeneous group of malignant tumors arising from mesenchymal tissues. They include soft tissue and bone tumors and are rare compared with the much more common carcinomas of epithelial origin. Sarcomas in the head and neck region represent about 5% of all soft tissue sarcomas.[30] Among the head and neck sarcomas, a significant proportion is found in the sinonasal tract and anterior skull base.[31,32] Several studies show that the most common sarcoma in this region is rhabdomyosarcoma (Fig. 1.8).[33,34] Other reported histologic subtypes include malignant peripheral nerve sheath tumors, fibrosarcomas, and leiomyosarcomas.[35–37] CT and MRI findings are noncharacteristic. The tumors usually show an aggressive mass with necrosis and osseous destruction associated with multicompartmental involvement (Fig. 1.9).

Chondrosarcomas of the skull base are uncommon and typically arise from the basal synchondroses. They are commonly located at the parasellar and clival regions, cerebellopontine angles, and

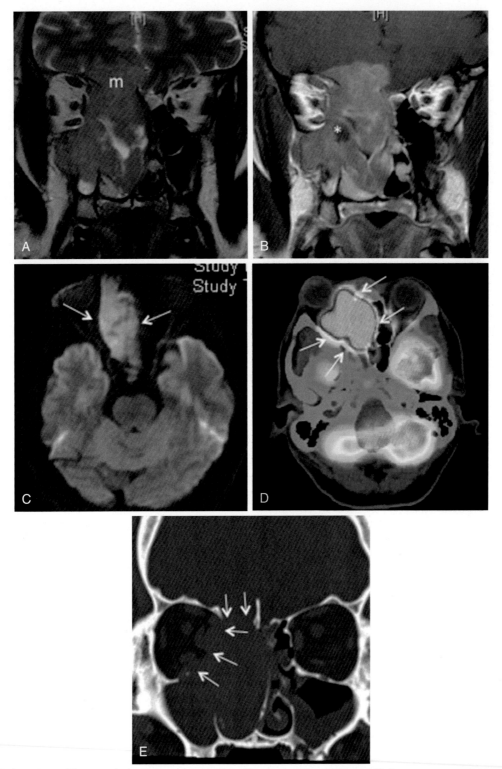

FIG. 1.7 Lymphoma. The mass (m in **A**) shows intermediate T2-weighted signal **(A)** and fairly homogeneous enhancement **(B)** except at areas of necrosis (*asterisk* in **B**). A characteristic feature of lymphoma is decreased diffusivity caused by inherent hypercellularity as reflected by an increased signal on diffusion-weighted imaging (*arrows* in **C**). Intense fluorodeoxyglucose avidity is also evident (*arrows* in **D**). Intracranial and orbital invasion with osseous destruction is well demonstrated on CT (*arrows* in **E**). DWI – diffusion-weighted imaging. FDG – fluorodeoxyglucose.

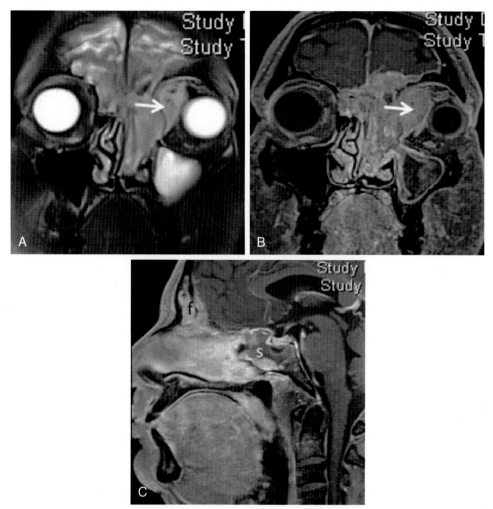

FIG. 1.8 Rhabdomyosarcoma. Coronal T2 and fat-suppressed T1 with contrast images **(A** and **B)** depict an aggressive tumor that has invaded the left orbit and involved the medial rectus muscle (*arrows* in **A** and **B**). Erosion through the anterior skull base is also evident. Sagittal fat-suppressed T1 with contrast image **(C)** shows invasion of the frontal sinus (f) and sphenoid sinus (s).

petrous bone and originate from the falx cerebri and meninges.[38] Chondrosarcoma of the anterior skull base may be seen on CT and MRI as a large aggressive mass causing osseous destruction with internal chondroid pattern of matrix calcification similar to chondrosarcomas elsewhere. By virtue of its location and tumor matrix, the diagnosis can be suggested on imaging.

## Meningioma

Olfactory groove meningiomas comprise 10% of intracranial meningiomas.[39] They may appear as en plaque sessile lesions associated with the underlying skull base hyperostosis. CT appearance may mimic a primary osseous lesion of the skull base if only the hyperostotic component is examined. The majority of meningiomas is benign and slow growing. Extension into ethmoid sinuses occurs in 15% of patients.[40] In such cases, the presence of hyperostosis may prompt the diagnosis of meningioma (Fig. 1.10).

Meningiomas typically appear hyperdense to brain parenchyma on CT and show avid postcontrast enhancement. These lesions often exhibit the characteristic dural tail sign (which is better

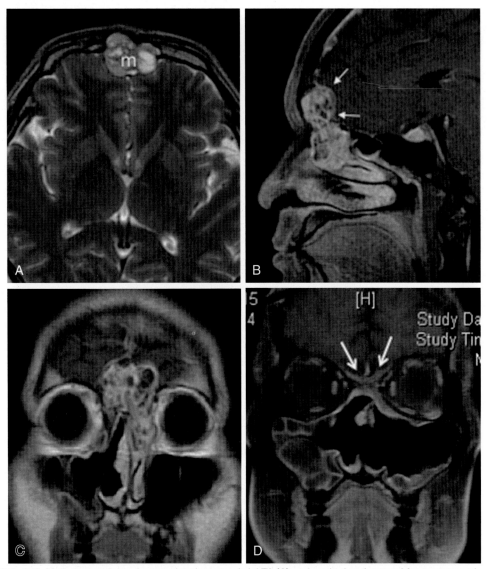

FIG. 1.9 Malignant peripheral nerve sheath tumor. Axial T2 **(A)** and sagittal and coronal fat-suppressed T1 postcontrast **(B and C)** images show an enhancing necrotic/cystic tumor (m in **A**) in the anterior ethmoid sinus invading the frontal sinuses. There is mass effect on the frontal lobes but the enhancing dura, best seen on the sagittal image (*arrows* in **B**), remains thin and intact. Postsurgical dural thickening in the anterior skull base (*arrows* in **D**) remains stable on follow-up scan, thus differentiating it from dural disease involvement.

appreciated on MRI). In addition, MRI may provide better delineation of the tumor with adjacent structures, such as the frontal lobes and optic nerves. In some cases, MR angiography may be useful to evaluate the vascular supply of this mass and provide important information before preoperative catheter embolization.

## NONNEOPLASTIC LESIONS
### Fungal Sinusitis

Fungal sinusitis is broadly classified into invasive and noninvasive types. Invasive fungal sinusitis has been subclassified into three distinct forms: acute fulminant invasive fungal sinusitis, chronic invasive fungal sinusitis, and granulomatous invasive fungal sinusitis.[41]

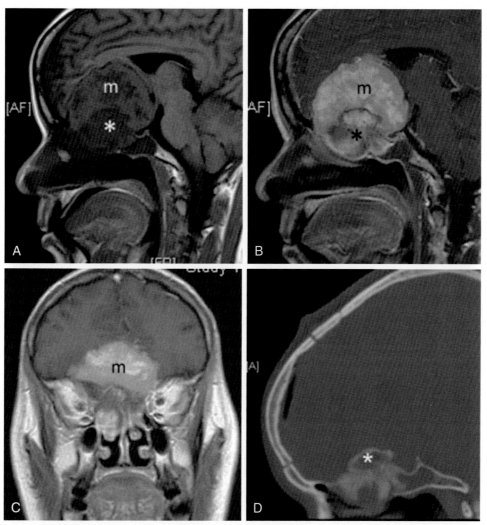

**FIG. 1.10** Olfactory groove meningioma. Sagittal T1 **(A)** and sagittal and coronal T1 fat-suppressed post-contrast **(B** and **C)** images show an extraaxial anterior cranial fossa mass (m in **A–C**) indenting the brain. Extension into the sinonasal space is also seen **(C)**. Note the exuberant hyperostosis at the anterior skull base (*asterisk* in **A, B,** and **D**), better appreciated on the postoperative CT with sagittal reconstruction **(D)**. The presence of hyperostosis and epicenter of tumor being above the skull base should alert the radiologist to the correct diagnosis of meningioma.

Intracranial and orbital invasion is common in acute invasive fungal sinusitis, and mortality tends to be high unless the condition is detected early and treated aggressively (Fig. 1.11).[42] Chronic forms of invasive sinusitis typically have a protracted history of progression and may present a diagnostic challenge because of nonspecific features that overlap with that seen in noninvasive, indolent forms. Hence, in the appropriate clinical context, a high index of suspicion must be maintained.

CT shows partial or complete soft tissue opacification of the affected sinus with, in chronic cases, hyperdense secretions. The invasive type may not demonstrate bone erosion in the early stages. Fungi may spread microscopically along vascular channels through bony walls. MRI helps to depict early perisinus soft tissue infiltration as a sign of invasiveness.[43] Intraorbital or intracranial extensions are well depicted on MRI. Fungal elements may manifest as low T2 signal intensities and thus are misinterpreted as normal

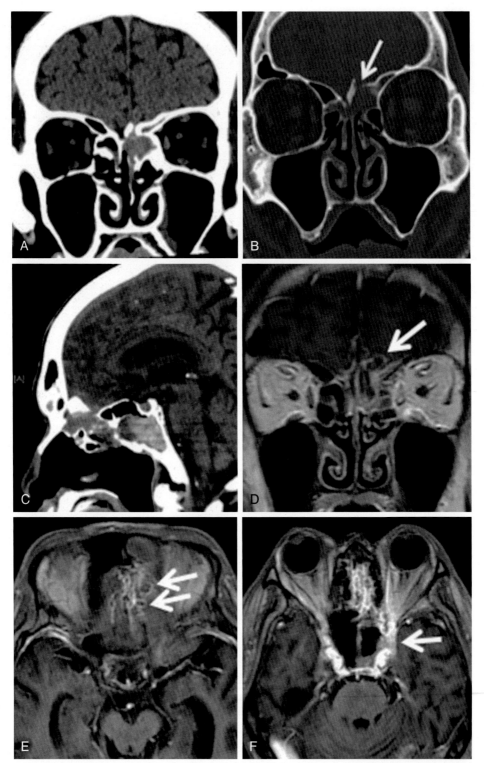

FIG. 1.11 Invasive fungal sinusitis. Opacification of the left ethmoid (e) and sphenoid sinuses (s) is seen in coronal **(A)** and sagittal **(C)** CT images, complicated by erosion of the left cribriform plate, better seen on the coronal bone window (*arrow* in **B**). MRI shows pachymeningeal enhancement at frontal lobe bases with multiple small brain abscesses (*arrows* in **D** and **E**). The left orbital apex and cavernous sinus (*arrow* in **F**) are also involved.

air-filled sinus.[42] Care should be taken to search for other clues of sinusitis, such as mucosal enhancement and perisinus infiltration.

## Mucocele

A mucocele represents the end stage of a chronically obstructed paranasal sinus and occurs secondary to progressive accumulation of secretions and desquamations within an enclosed sinus. It is the most common lesion to cause expansion of a paranasal sinus and is usually seen in adulthood. There is usually a history of chronic nasal polyposis and sinusitis. Mucoceles are most common in the frontal sinus (65%) followed by ethmoid, maxillary, and sphenoid sinuses.[44] A frontal mucocele may be palpable as a mass in the superomedial part of the orbit (Fig. 1.12). It can expand into the orbit and may present with unilateral proptosis, decreased visual acuity, and impaired visual field defect, clinically masquerading as an intraorbital space-occupying mass.[45] In rare cases, it can erode into the subarachnoid space, resulting in CSF leak.[46]

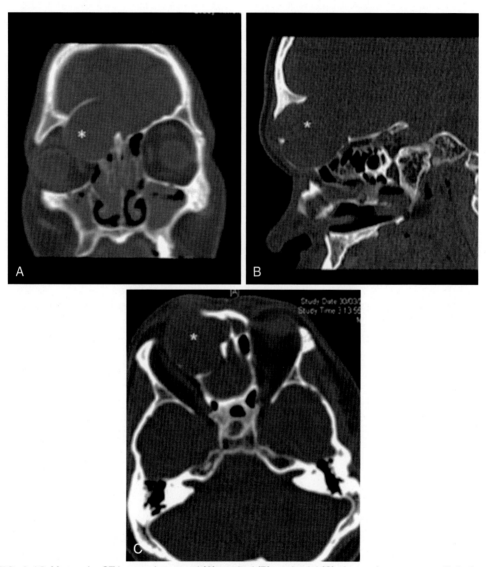

FIG. 1.12 Mucocele. CT images in coronal **(A)**, sagittal **(B)**, and axial **(C)** planes show an expansile lesion (*asterisk*) arising in the right frontal sinus. The osseous walls are remodeled and severely thinned, thus difficult to visualize even on CT. However, the location, shape, and expanded nature of the lesion is consistent with a mucocele. Mass effect on the right orbit is also demonstrated.

Thin-cut CT with coronal and sagittal reformats is the best modality to evaluate the affected sinus and adjacent anatomy and provide vital information for surgical planning. In cases in which the sinus is markedly enlarged causing the wall to be extremely thinned, CT helps to delineate the osseous boundary and may detect focal bony defects. MRI is helpful to portray the high water content of mucus by showing low T1-weighted and high T2-weighted signals. Proteinaceous material is seen as high T1-weighted signal (Fig. 1.13). Mucoceles typically show no central enhancement on postcontrast imaging but may show minimal peripheral enhancement. If thickened peripheral mucosal enhancement is seen, the presence of superimposed infection resulting in mucopyocele needs to be considered. In addition, MRI is excellent at detecting nodular solid enhancement, in which case a neoplastic lesion with secondary mucocele is suspected.

### Fibrous Dysplasia

Fibrous dysplasia (FD) is a congenital disorder with a defect in osteoblastic differentiation and maturation, resulting in the replacement of normal cancellous

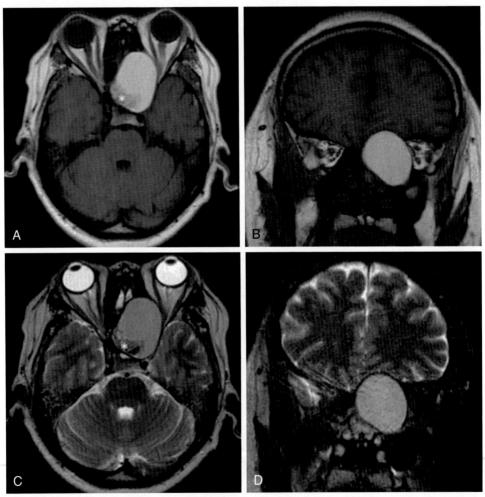

FIG. 1.13 Mucocele. Axial **(A)** and coronal **(B)** MR images show a cystic expanded mass in the posterior left ethmoid sinus with high T1 signal representing proteinaceous content. Inspissated dependent debris is present (*asterisk* in **A** and **C**). Owing to accumulation of inflammatory material, the ethmoid air cell undergoes progressive expansion and remodeling, producing an intact well-defined low-signal osseous border best seen on the T2 images **(C** and **D)**. Note the encroachment into the anterior cranial fossa and left orbit.

bone by fibrous tissue and immature woven bone. It affects the skull and facial bones in 10%–25% of patients with monostotic FD and in 50% of patients with polyostotic FD.[47] Most cases of craniofacial fibrous dysplasia (CFD) are seen in the first three decades of life, and the condition usually stabilizes when the patient reaches skeletal maturity. They commonly lead to otolaryngologic symptoms such as impingement of cranial nerves and the orbit.[48] Most lesions are unilateral. CFD is an example of a primary fibroosseous lesion arising within the skull base as opposed to secondary involvement by soft tissue disease in the adjacent cavity.

The appearance of a ground-glass matrix in an expanded bone lesion on CT is virtually pathognomonic (Fig. 1.14), although pagetoid and cystic variants may demonstrate mixed lucent and sclerotic areas, reflecting the underlying active disease state. MRI features are varied, however, which may present a diagnostic pitfall. The fibrous tissue shows a low to intermediate T1 signal on MRI, depending on the ratio of fibrous tissue to mineralized matrix. Lesions with a high fibrous content have intermediate signals, whereas lesions with a highly mineralized stroma have lower signals. Lesions with a high fibrous content and cystic spaces show high T2 signal intensity.[47] Unlike mature scar tissue, which shows low signal in all pulse sequences, fibrous tissues in FD

are metabolically active, thus accounting for intermediate to high T2 signal intensities. The fibrous tissues are often well vascularized and may enhance intensely after administration of a contrast agent. Correct diagnosis of CFD can be made on MRI if the signals are low on T1 and T2 sequences despite strong enhancement. Confusion arises when CFD shows intermediate signals with enhancement, features that are indistinguishable from neoplastic disease (Fig. 1.15). Under such circumstances, CT should be performed to resolve the problem.[47]

## CONCLUSION

The anterior skull base is an important structure that separates the cranial cavity, the orbits, and the sinonasal compartments. The anatomic construction in this region predisposes itself to risks of transgression by neoplastic and nonneoplastic diseases. It serves as an important landmark that, when breached by disease, has a significant impact on prognosis and management. Cross-sectional imaging modalities such as CT and MRI play vital and complementary roles in the pretreatment evaluation and posttreatment follow-up. Information obtained by imaging studies provides valuable insight into lesion characteristics and helps to direct multidisciplinary treatment strategies.

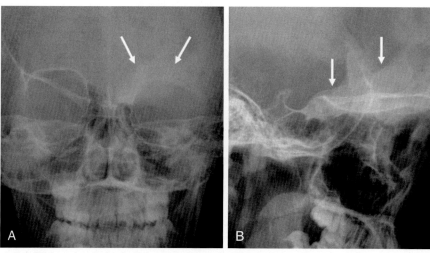

FIG. 1.14 Fibrous dysplasia. An important clue to the diagnosis is unilateral sclerosis and thickening of the left supraorbital rim seen on plain radiographs (*arrows* in **A** and **B**).

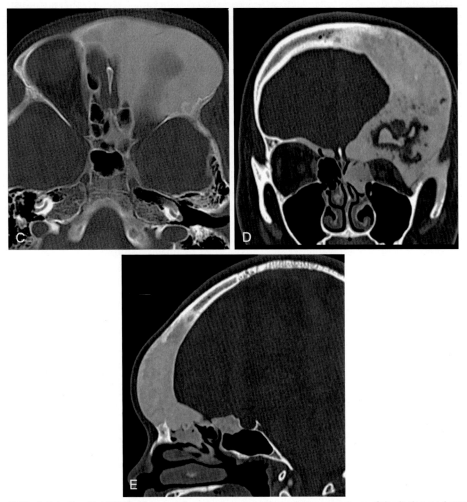

FIG. 1.14, Cont'd CT **(C–E)** is excellent to demonstrate the osseous nature of the lesion and extent of involvement. Note the thickened left anterior skull base encroaching the left orbit. The classic ground-glass appearance is pathognomonic for fibrous dysplasia.

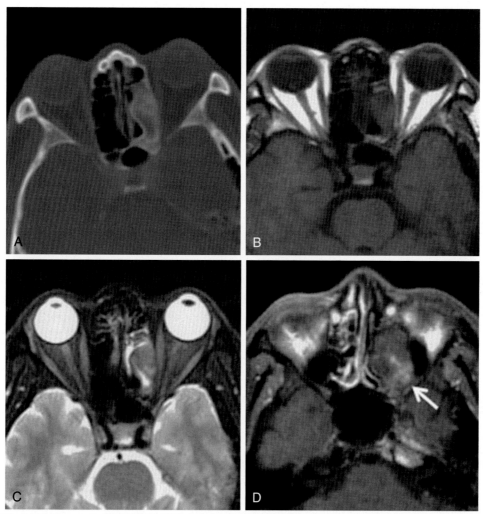

FIG. 1.15 Fibrous dysplasia (FD). FD is localized to the left posterior ethmoid. Note the mixed lucent appearance on CT (*arrows* in **A**) as opposed to the classic ground-glass feature. This lesion shows intermediate T1 **(B)** and T2 signal **(C)** with patchy internal enhancement (*arrow* in **D**), corresponding to a more fibrous content and less mineralized matrix. Without the characteristic appearance of CT, the lesion mimics an aggressive neoplasm on MRI.

## REFERENCES

1. Eggesbo HB. Imaging of sinonasal tumors. *Cancer Imaging*. 2012;12:136–152.
2. McCaffrey TM, Olsen KD, Yohanan JM, Lewis JE, Ebersold MJ, Piepgras DG. Factors affecting survival of pa tients with tumors of the anterior skull base. *Laryngoscope*. 1994;104(8 Pt 1):940–945.
3. Parmar H, Gujar S, Shah G, Mukherji SK. Imaging of the anterior skull base. *Neuroimag Clin N Am*. 2009;19(3):427–439.
4. Varshney S, Bist SS, Gupta N, Singh RK, Bhagat S. Anterior craniofacial resection – for paranasal sinus tumors involving anterior skull base. *Indian J Otolaryngol Head Neck Surg*. 2010;62(2):103–107.
5. Alvarez I, Suarez C, Rodrigo JP, Nunez F, Caminero MJ. Prognostic factors in paranasal sinus cancer. *Am J Otolaryngol*. 1995;16(2):109–114.
6. Roux FX, Brasnu D, Devaux B, et al. Ethmoid sinus carcinomas: results and prognosis after neoadjuvant chemotherapy and combined surgery. A 10-year experience. *Surg Neurol*. 1994;42(2):98–104.
7. Eisen MD, Yousem DM, Loevner LA, Thaler ER, Bilker WB, Goldberg AN. Preoperative imaging to predict orbital invasion by tumor. *Head Neck*. 2000;22(5):456–462.
8. Suarez C, Ferlito A, Lund VJ, et al. Management of the orbit in malignant sinonasal tumors. *Head Neck*. 2008;30(2):242–250.

9. Patel SG, Singh B, Polluri A, et al. Craniofacial surgery for malignant skull base tumors: report of an international collaborative study. *Cancer.* 2003;98(6):1179–1187.

10. Perry C, Levine PA, Williamson BR, Cantrell RW. Preservation of the eye in paranasal sinus cancer surgery. *Arch Otolaryngol Head Neck Surg.* 1988;114(6):632–634.

11. Reyes C, Mason E, Solares CA, Bush C, Carrau R. To preserve or not to preserve the orbit in paranasal sinus neoplasms: a meta-analysis. *J Neurol Surg B Skull Base.* 2015;76(2):122–128.

12. Iannetti G, Valentini V, Rinna C, et al. Ethmoido-orbital tumors: our experience. *J Craniofac Surg.* 2005;16(6):1085–1091.

13. Uyar Y, Kumral TL, Yildirim G, et al. Reconstruction of the orbit with a temporalis muscle flap after orbital exenteration. *Clin Exp Otorhinolaryngol.* 2015;8(1):52–56.

14. Guglielmi G, Bisceglia M, Schillitani A, Folpe A. Oncogenic osteomalacia due to phosphaturic mesenchymal tumor of the craniofacial sinuses. *Clin Cases Miner Bone Metab.* 2011;8(2):45–49.

15. Sanghvi S, Khan MN, Patel NR, Yeldandi S, Baredes S, Eloy JA. Epidemiology of sinonasal squamous cell carcinoma: a comprehensive analysis of 4994 patients. *Laryngoscope.* 2014;124(1):76–83.

16. Som PM, Lidoc M, Brandwein M, Catalano P, Biller HF. Sinonasal esthesioneuroblastoma with intracranial extension: marginal tumor cysts as a diagnostic MR finding. *AJNR Am J Neuroradiol.* 1994;15(7):1259–1262.

17. Aggarwal SK, Kumar R, Shrivastav A, Keshri A, Sharma P. Esthesioneuroblastoma presenting with proptosis and bilateral neck metastasis: an unusual presentation. *J Pediatr Neurosci.* 2011;6(1):78–81.

18. Ahmed M, Knott PD. Hyperostotic esthesioneuroblastoma: rare variant and fibrous dysplasia mimicker. *Korean J Radiol.* 2014;15(1):156–160.

19. Tseng J, Michel MA, Loehrl TA. Peripheral cysts: a distinguishing feature of esthesioneuroblastoma with intracranial extension. *Ear Nose Throat J.* 2009;88(6):E14.

20. Leivo I. Sinonasal adenocarcinoma: update on classification, immunophenotype and molecular features. *Head Neck Pathol.* 2016;10(1):68–74.

21. d'Errico A, Pasian S, Baratti A, et al. A case-control study on occupational risk factors for sino-nasal cancer. *Occup Environ Med.* 2009;66(7):448–455.

22. Paes FM, Singer AD, Checkver AN, Palmquist RA, De La Vega G, Sidani C. Perineural spread in head and neck malignancies: clinical significance and evaluation with 18FDG-PET/CT. *Radiographics.* 2013;33(6):1717–1736.

23. Yousem DM, Gad K, Tufano RP. Resectability issues with head and neck cancer. *AJNR Am J Neuroradiol.* 2006;27(10):2024–2036.

24. Shimamoto H, Chindasombatjaroen J, Kakimoto N, Kishino M, Murakami S, Furukawa S. Perineural spread of adenoid cystic carcinoma in the oral and maxillofacial regions: evaluation with contrast-enhanced CT and MRI. *Dentomaxillofac Radiol.* 2012;41(2):143–151.

25. Woo JS, Kim JM, Lee SH, Chae SW, Hwang SJ, Lee HM. Clinical analysis of extranodal non-Hodgkin's lymphoma in the sinonasal tract. *Eur Arch Otorhinolaryngol.* 2004;261(4):197–201.

26. Kuo TT, Shih LY, Tsang NM. Nasal NK/T cell lymphoma in Taiwan: a clinicopathologic study of 22 cases, with analysis of histologic subtypes, Epstein-Barr virus LMP-1 gene association, and treatment modalities. *Int J Surg Pathol.* 2004;12(4):375–387.

27. Li CC, Tien FF, Tang JL, et al. Treatment outcome and pattern of failure in 77 patients with sinonasal natural killer/T cell or T cell lymphoma. *Cancer.* 2004;100(2):366–375.

28. Frierson Jr HF, Mills SE, Fechner RE, Taxy JB, Levine PA. Sinonasal undifferentiated carcinoma. An aggressive neoplasm derived from Schneiderian epithelium and distinct from olfactory neuroblastoma. *Am J Surg Pathol.* 1986;10(11):771–779.

29. Reiersen DA, Pahilan ME, Devaiah AK. Meta-analysis of treatment outcomes for sinonasal undifferentiated carcinoma. *Otolaryngol Head Neck Surg.* 2012;147(1):7–14.

30. Hoffman HT, Robinson RA, Spiess JL, Buatti J. Update in management of head and neck sarcoma. *Curr Opin Oncol.* 2004;16(4):333–341.

31. Wanebo HJ, Koness RJ, MacFarlane JK, et al. Head and neck sarcoma: report of the head and neck sarcoma registry. *Head Neck.* 1992;14(1):1–7.

32. De Bree R, van der Waal I, de Bree E, Leemans CR. Management of adult soft tissue sarcomas of the head and neck. *Oral Oncol.* 2010;46(11):786–790.

33. Wu AW, Suh JD, Metson R, Wang MB. Prognostic factors in sinonasal sarcomas: analysis of the surveillance, epidemiology and end result database. *Laryngoscope.* 2012;122(10):2137–2142. http://dx.doi.org/10.1002/lary.23442.

34. Szablewski V, Neuville A, Terrier P, et al. Adult sinonasal soft tissue sarcoma: analysis of 48 cases from the French Sarcoma Group database. *Laryngoscope.* 2015;125(3):615–623.

35. Bankaci M, Myers EN, Barnes L, Dubois P. Angiosarcoma of the maxillary sinus: literature review and case report. *Head Neck Surg.* 1979;1(3):274–280.

36. Kuruvilla A, Wenig BM, Humphrey DM, Heffner DK. Leiomyosarcoma of the sinonasal tract. A clinicopathologic study of nine cases. *Arch Otolaryngol Head Neck Surg.* 1990;116(11):1278–1286.

37. Davis EC, Ballo MT, Luna MA, et al. Liposarcoma of the head and neck: the University of Texas M. D. Anderson Cancer Center experience. *Head Neck.* 2009;31(1):28–36.

38. Kan Z, Li H, Zhang J, You C. Intracranial mesenchymal chondrosarcoma: case report and literature review. *Br J Neurosurg.* 2012;26(6):912–914.

39. Hentschel SJ, DeMonte F. Olfactory groove meningiomas. *Neurosurg Focus.* 2003;14(6): Ed4.

40. DeMonte F. Surgical treatment of anterior basal meningiomas. *J Neurooncol.* 1996;29(3):239–248.

41. Epstein VA, Kem RC. Invasive fungal sinusitis and complications of rhinosinusitis. *Otorhinolaryngol Clin N Am.* 2008;41(3):497–524.

42. Aribandi M, McCoy VA, Bazan C. Imaging features of invasive and non-invasive fungal sinusitis: a review. *Radiographics.* 2007;27(5):1283–1296.

43. DelGaudio JM, Swain Jr RE, Kingdom TT, Muller S, Hudgins PA. Computed tomographic findings in patients with invasive fungal sinusitis. *Arch Otolaryngol Head Neck Surg.* 2003;129(2):236–240.

44. Tan CS, Yong VK, Yip LW, Amrith S. An unusual presentation of a giant frontal sinus mucocele manifesting with a subcutaneous forehead mass. *Ann Acad Med Singap.* 2005;34(5):397–398.

45. Aggarwal SK, Bhavana K, Keshri A, Kumar R, Srivastava A. Frontal sinus mucocele with orbital complications: management by varied surgical approaches. *Asian J Neurosurg.* 2012;7(3):135–140.

46. Pizzo LJ, Mishler KE. Frontoethmoid mucocele with CSF leak. *Ear Nose Throat J.* 1984;63(11):571–573.

47. Chong VF, Khoo JBK, Fan YF. Fibrous dysplasia involving the base of skull. *AJR Am J Roentgenol.* 2002;178(3):717–720.

48. Hullar TE, Lustig LR. Paget's disease and fibrous dysplasia. *Otolaryngol Clin N Am.* 2003;36(4):707–732.

# CHAPTER 2

# Imaging of the Paranasal Sinuses and Their Surgical Relevance

CLEMENT YONG, MBBS, FRANZCR •
DAVID SY SIA, MBBS, FRCR, MMED •
JAMES TPD HALLINAN, MBCHB, BSC, FRCR •
VINCENT CHONG, MD, MBA, MHPE, FRCR

One of the earliest computed tomography (CT) evaluations of the paranasal sinuses was published by Hesselink et al. in 1978 as a two-part series: describing both normal and pathologic anatomy.[1] Early CT studies were performed only in the axial and coronal planes, but with the availability of multiplanar high-resolution CT, more complex imaging anatomy and anatomic variations have been documented. As such, preoperative CT has gained favor among ear, nose, and throat surgeons for the planning of functional endoscopic sinus surgery (FESS). Understanding sinus anatomy and its surgical implications will help the radiologist tailor a surgically relevant report, alert the surgeon to critical anatomic variants, and minimize dangerous complications.

The reported incidence of major complications of FESS ranges between 0.0% and 2.25%.[2] Cerebrospinal fluid (CSF) leak is generally accepted as one of the most common and worrisome complication,[3] associated with significant morbidity. Other complications include bleeding, orbital and optic nerve injury, meningitis, and lacrimal duct injury. It is useful to bear these in mind when reviewing the CT study, as they serve as reminders to highlight important structures.

## THE NASAL SEPTUM AND NASAL MUCOSA

The nasal septum is the first structure seen by the endoscopist. Septal deviation is a common deformity, with an incidence of 44.8%, although only 2.1% show obstructive symptoms.[4] It is sometimes associated with a bony spur (Fig. 2.1) and can limit access into the middle meatus or even result in contact point neuralgia as described by Stammberger.[5]

Another common finding is asymmetry of the nasal mucosa and size of the nasal passages. In 1923, Lillie described periodic changes in the nasal mucosa, termed the "nasal cycle."[6] The thickened nasal mucosa seen on CT is a normal cyclical phenomenon and should not be confused with inflammation. These changes are seen in the turbinates, nasal septum, and ethmoid sinuses, sparing the frontal, maxillary, and sphenoid sinuses.[7] The nasal cycle is believed to be controlled by the suprachiasmatic nucleus in the hypothalamus, and this control decreases with age.[8]

## FRONTAL SINUS DRAINAGE PATHWAY

The frontal sinus and the frontal sinus drainage pathway (FSDP) are challenging for both radiologists and surgeons, because of their complex and variable pneumatization patterns. A useful imaging landmark is the frontal beak (FB), a bony ridge formed by the superior extension of the frontal process of the maxillary bone (Fig. 2.2). The frontal ostium is found at the level of the FB, which also serves to separate the fontal sinus superiorly from the FSDP inferiorly (Fig. 2.2).

The FSDP is bordered by the most vulnerable parts of the anterior skull base, sandwiched between the lamina papyracea laterally and the thin lateral lamella of the olfactory fossa medially. Here, the bone can measure as little as 0.05 mm and is easily perforated.[9] Its anterior wall is formed by the FB and agger nasi cell (ANC), whereas the posterior wall of the FSDP is the bulla lamella. The FSDP can be further divided into two compartments:
- Superior compartment: ("frontal recess") is formed by a combination of frontal recess cells that can be classified using standardized criteria developed by Lee et al.[10] Its upper border is the frontal ostium.[11]
- Inferior compartment: ("frontal sinus outflow tract" [FSOT]) is a narrow passageway formed by either the ethmoid infundibulum (38%) or the middle meatus

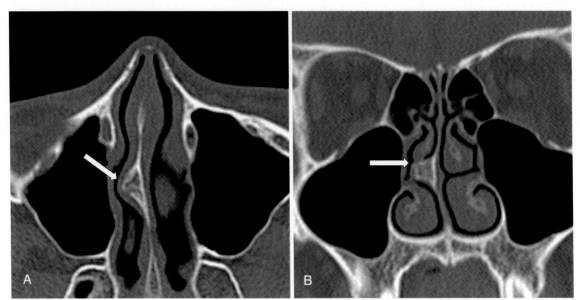

FIG. 2.1 Nasal septum variation. **(A)** Axial and **(B)** coronal CT of a large septal spur (*arrow*) with septal-turbinate contact that can be a cause for contact point headaches.

(62%), depending on the variable anatomic attachment of the uncinate process (Fig. 2.15).[12] The patency of the FSOT is also determined by configuration of the surrounding anterior ethmoid cells.[9]

The superior compartment in particular, shows substantial variation in size, shape, and course. This is due to the unpredictable formation of osseous septations and marginating air cells lining the FSDP. It is not uncommon to find more than a single opening of the frontal sinus into the FSDP (Fig. 2.3).

### Anterior Ethmoid Cells/Frontal Recess Cells

Multiple named air cells are found surrounding the frontal recess. Anatomically, ANCs and frontal cells (FCs) occur along the anterior wall of the frontal recess, whereas suprabullar cells (SBCs), frontal bullar cells (FBCs), and supraorbital ethmoid cells (SOECs) occur posteriorly along the skull base.[10] SBCs do not extend to the frontal sinus unlike the FBCs. Interfrontal sinus septal cells (IFSSCs) occur along the frontal sinus septum. Apart from the ANC, these cells are collectively known as anterior ethmoid cells (AECs) (Fig. 2.4).

### Agger Nasi Cells

The agger nasi cells (Latin for "nasal mound") are the most anterior ethmoidal cells and extend anteriorly into the lacrimal bone (Fig. 2.5), where they are posteromedial to the lacrimal sac. They are anterior to the

anterior attachment of the middle turbinate to the skull base and anteroinferior to the frontal recess, forming the anterior margin of the frontal recess. Because of this intimate relationship, these cells form excellent surgical landmarks[13] and are reliably seen in up to 98.5% of all patients.[14] Opening the ANC usually provides a good view of the frontal recess. The ANC drains into the middle meatus.

Understanding the FSDP is important when evaluating and planning the surgical treatment of frontal sinus disease. At this point, it would also be useful to know that disease within the lateral frontal sinus is difficult to correct endoscopically, often requiring an external approach (Fig. 2.6).[15]

The FSDP is also part of a larger complex known as the ostiomeatal unit (OMU). Its other components comprise the maxillary sinus ostium, ethmoid infundibulum, and hiatus semilunaris (Fig. 2.7). The OMU is the common drainage of the anterior sinuses, and diseased mucosa here impairs ventilation and drainage of the frontal, anterior ethmoid, and maxillary sinuses. FESS is aimed at reestablishing normal ventilation and drainage around the OMU, and the key sinus in FESS is the ethmoid sinus. Its close relationships with the orbit and anterior skull base make these structures vulnerable to trauma during surgery. A good knowledge of the anatomy of the ethmoid bone is essential for understanding the pathologic processes and prevention of surgical complications.

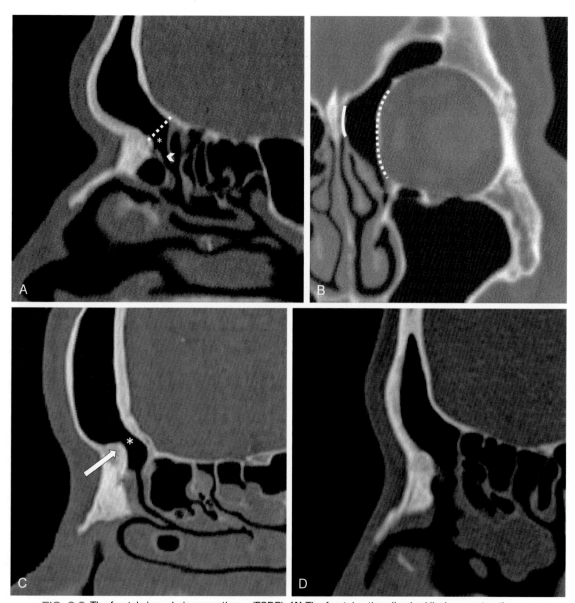

FIG. 2.2 The frontal sinus drainage pathway (FSDP). **(A)** The frontal ostium (*hashed line*) separates the frontal sinus superiorly from the FSDP inferiorly. Note the superior (*asterisk*) and inferior (*arrowhead*) compartments of the FSDP. **(B)** The FSDP is bounded by the lateral lamella medially (*solid line*) and the lamina papyracea laterally (*dotted line*). **(C)** A thick frontal beak (*arrow*) can narrow the frontal ostium (*asterisk*), whereas **(D)** a small frontal beak leaves the frontal ostium widely patent.

## ETHMOID BONE

The word "ethmoid" means "sieve-like" in Greek, largely referring to the porous cribriform plate. It is centrally located within the nasal passage and consists of four parts: the perpendicular plate, the cribriform plate, and two ethmoidal labyrinths (Fig. 2.16).

The key ethmoid structures develop as ethmoturbinal attachments (also known as basal lamellae) along the lateral nasal cavity wall. After a series of regression, at least four basal lamellae remain (Fig. 2.8): the uncinate process, ethmoid bulla, middle turbinate, and superior turbinate.[16] Five, if the supreme turbinate is included.

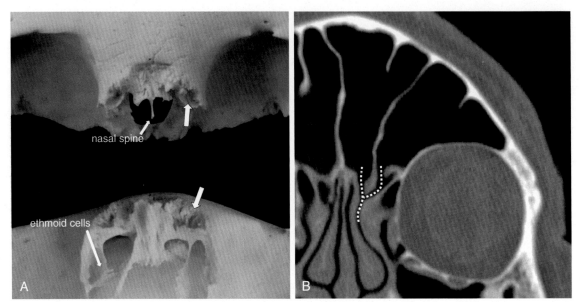

FIG. 2.3 Frontal sinus drainage pathway (FSDP) variation. **(A)** Disarticulated specimen of the anterior skull base showing osseous septations lining the FSDP (*solid arrows*). **(B)** Coronal CT showing a large osseous septation separating the FSDP into two separate channels (*dotted lines*).

This five basal lamellae concept proposed by Killian[17] is perhaps the best way to understand the ethmoid anatomy, with the four main basal lamellae separating the various draining pathways. The frontal and maxillary sinuses drain into the hiatus semilunaris between the first (ANC and uncinate process) and second (ethmoid bulla) basal lamellae. The ethmoid bulla drains via the superior hiatus semilunaris superior (SHS) and sinus lateralis into the middle meatus between the second and third (middle turbinate) lamellae. The third basal lamella (now referred to in various texts as the "basal lamella") separates the anterior and posterior ethmoid air cells, whereas the fourth (superior turbinate) lamella separates the posterior and postreme meatus.[18]

### Middle Turbinate and Basal Lamella

Owing to their embryology, the middle turbinate and basal lamellae are both part of the same structure (the third basal lamella). It divides the ethmoid cells into the anterior and posterior groups, which is important surgically, as the anterior group drains into the middle meatus, whereas the posterior group drains into the superior meatus.

The middle turbinate has attachments to the skull in all three planes (Fig. 2.9): The anterior vertical part attaches superiorly to the cribriform plate (sagittal plane). The middle oblique part loses its connection to the cribriform plate, attaching to the basal lamella or lamina papyracea (coronal plane). The posterior horizontal part forms the roof of the posterior middle meatus. Here, it attaches to the perpendicular plate of the palatine bone/medial wall of the maxillary sinus (axial plane). This three-dimensional orientation, initially sagittal, then coronal followed by an axial plane, gives the middle turbinate remarkable stability. Resection of the posterior portion may lead to anterior instability.[15]

### Middle Turbinate Variants

A concha bullosa is a pneumatized middle turbinate and has a reported prevalence of 34%[19] (Fig. 2.10). A concha bullosa is readily identified on CT, but endoscopic recognition may be difficult. An unremarkable middle turbinate during endoscopy may show extensive pneumatization on CT. Conversely, an endoscopically large middle turbinate may show no pneumatization.

A concha bullosa itself does not necessarily predispose the patient to sinus disease. However, it may obstruct the ethmoid infundibulum. In addition, sinusitis, polyps, and mucoceles may affect the concha bullosa itself. A concha bullosa can be marsupialized, crushed, or excised, but care must be taken to avoid damaging the attachment of the middle turbinate to the skull base. A fracture at this site may lead to an unstable middle turbinate or CSF leakage.[20] A concha bullosa may also occur in the superior turbinate, although this is much less often seen (Fig. 2.11).

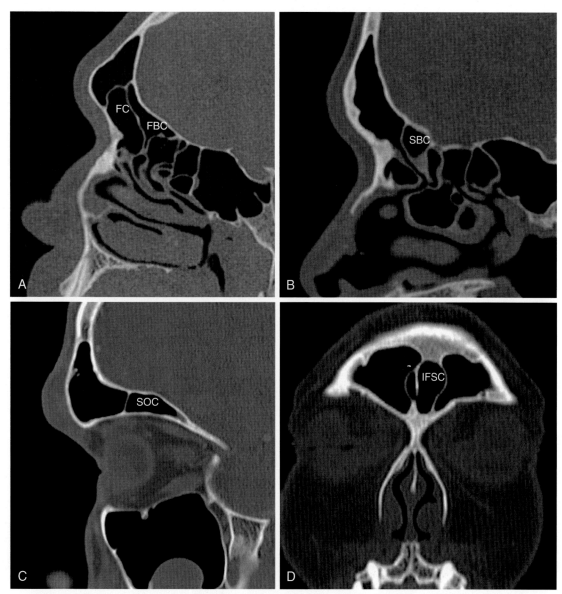

FIG. 2.4 Types of anterior ethmoid cells. **(A)** A frontal cell (FC) and a frontal bullar cell (FBC) extending into the frontal sinus. **(B)** A suprabullar cell (SBC) remaining below the frontal ostium. **(C)** A supraorbital ethmoid cell along the skull base (SOC). **(D)** Coronal CT showing an interfrontal sinus septal cell (IFSC).

Normally, the convexity of the middle turbinate is directed medially. However, in 26% of cases the convexity is directed laterally (Fig. 2.12).[20] This condition is termed paradoxical middle turbinate and is usually of no clinical significance. Turbinate sinus refers to the exaggerated curvature of the middle turbinate, forming an internal concavity (Fig. 2.12).

## Ethmoid Bulla

The ethmoid bulla forms the posterior and superior walls of the ethmoid infundibulum and hiatus semilunaris. The ethmoid bulla is the largest anterior ethmoid air cell. It is also one of the most consistent air cells in the middle meatus and is therefore a reliable anatomic landmark (Fig. 2.13). It often lacks a posterior wall, which is why it is not called a cell but rather a bony lamella with a large airspace behind it.[21] This is in keeping with the second ethmoturbinal attachment in the five basal lamellae concept described earlier in this text.

However, the degree of pneumatization may vary, and failure to pneumatize in 8% of people is termed torus ethmoidalis or torus lateralis (Latin for "lateral bulge").[22] At the other extreme is a giant bulla filling out the entire middle meatus and forcing its way between the uncinate process and the middle turbinate. The lamina papyracea forms its lateral relationship. Superiorly the ethmoid bulla may fuse with the skull base forming the posterior wall of the frontal recess. If it fails to fuse with the skull base, a small suprabullar

recess may connect anteriorly to the frontal recess. Posteriorly it may fuse over a variable distance with the basal lamella. On coronal CT, the ethmoid bulla is only seen superior to the ethmoid infundibulum.

### Sinus Lateralis/Retrobullar Recess/Suprabullar Recess/Lateral Sinus of Grunwald

The sinus lateralis refers to the gap between the ethmoid bulla and the basal lamella, which often drains the ethmoid bulla medially into the middle meatus (Fig. 2.14). The highly variable sinus lateralis is defined by the ethmoid bulla anteriorly, skull base superiorly, basal lamella posteriorly, and the lamina papyracea

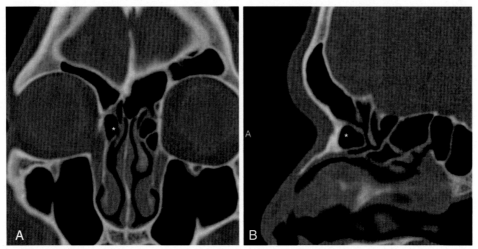

FIG. 2.5 The agger nasi cell. **(A)** Coronal and **(B)** sagittal views of an agger nasi cell (*asterisks*) that is reliably seen on CT in most people.

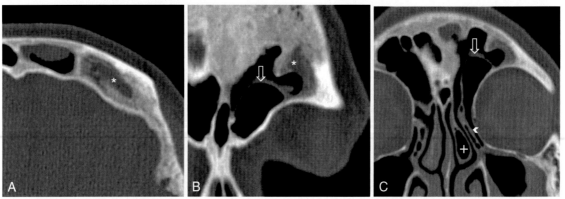

FIG. 2.6 Chronic sinusitis. **(A)** Axial and **(B** and **C)** coronal views of chronic sinusitis within the lateral frontal sinus (*asterisks* in **A** and **B**) caused by drainage obstruction from a type 3 frontal cell (*open arrows* in **B** and **C**). Note the pneumatized uncinate process (*arrow head* in **C**) and concha bullosa (+ in **C**), which often do not obstruct the FSDP.

laterally. If the ethmoid bulla does not fuse with the skull base, the sinus lateralis may extend above the ethmoid bulla and communicate with the frontal sinus. Here, the sinus lateralis is referred to as the suprabullar recess (Fig. 2.14).

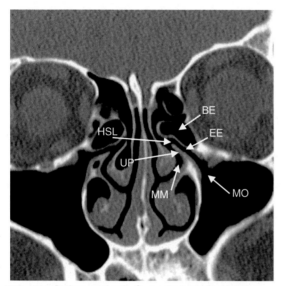

FIG. 2.7 Ostiomeatal unit. Coronal plane showing the components of the ostiomeatal complex. *BE*, bulla ethmoidalis; *EE*, ethmoidal infundibulum; *HSL*, hiatus semilunaris; *MM*, middle meatus; *MO*, maxillary ostium; *UP*, uncinate process.

Endoscopically, the suprabullar recess appears as a cleft above the ethmoid bulla and is equivalent to the SBC and FBC mentioned earlier. The anatomic difference is that SBCs do not protrude into the frontal sinus, whereas FBCs extend into the frontal sinus.

Inflammation in the sinus lateralis may extend anteriorly to the frontal recess and ANCs or posteriorly across a bony dehiscence into the posterior ethmoid air cells. Disease in the sinus lateralis is readily seen radiologically but is difficult to identify endoscopically. Access into the sinus lateralis is through the SHS, which is a "sickle-shaped" cleft. This, however, is often more difficult to identify anatomically than the inferior hiatus semilunaris.

### Ethmoid Infundibulum

It is important to realize that a radiologist sees the ethmoid infundibulum in two dimensions and a surgeon, in three dimensions. Hence the boundaries of the ethmoid infundibulum described in the surgical and radiologic literature may be different. It is part of the anterior ethmoid and opens into the middle meatus through the inferior hiatus semilunaris (Fig. 2.7).

The surgical boundaries of the ethmoid infundibulum are as follows: anteromedially, the uncinate process; posteriorly, the anterior wall of the ethmoid bulla; and laterally, the lamina papyracea. However, the ethmoid bulla appears superior to the ethmoid infundibulum on coronal CT (Fig. 2.13). The ethmoidal infundibulum ends abruptly in an acute angle

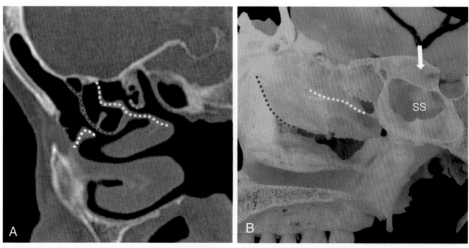

FIG. 2.8 The four basal lamellae. **(A)** Sagittal CT and **(B)** disarticulated specimen in the sagittal plane showing the four ethmoturbinal attachments that develop into (1) the agger nasi cell and uncinate process (*white dotted line* in **A**), (2) ethmoid bulla (*red dotted line* in **A** and **B**), (3) middle turbinate (*yellow dotted line* in **A** and **B**), and (4) superior turbinate (*blue dotted line* in **A** and **B**). The fifth basal lamella, the supreme turbinate, is not shown. Incidentally, an Onodi cell (*arrow* in **B**) is also seen above the sphenoid sinus (SS).

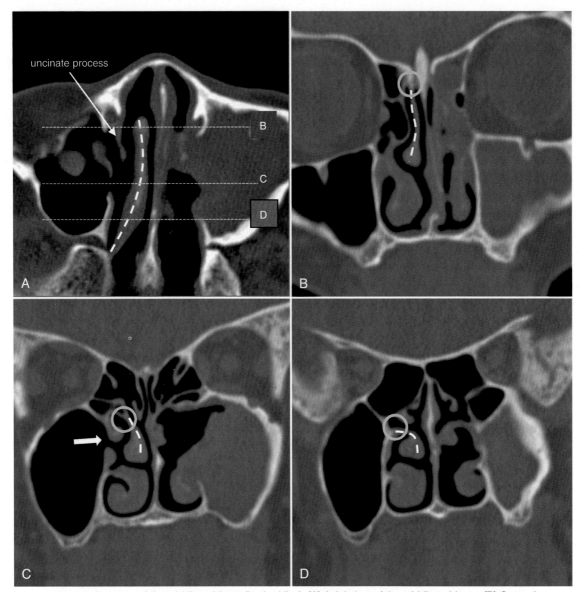

FIG. 2.9 Anatomy of the middle turbinate (*hashed line*). **(A)** Axial view of the middle turbinate. **(B)** Coronal view of the anterior vertical attachment to the cribriform plate (*yellow circle*). **(C)** Middle oblique attachment to the basal lamella (*yellow circle*). **(D)** Posterior horizontal attachment to the medial maxillary sinus wall (*yellow circle*). An accessory maxillary ostium (*arrow* in **C**) is also seen.

anteriorly, where the uncinate process attaches to the lateral nasal wall.

The maxillary sinus ostium opens into the floor of the ethmoid infundibulum (Fig. 2.7). It is not possible to see the maxillary sinus ostium endoscopically without removing the uncinate process. If an ostium is seen endoscopically, it is most likely the anterior or posterior accessory ostium or fontanelle (Fig. 2.9).

## Uncinate Process

The uncinate process is derived from the first basal lamella and is a crescent-shaped bone that forms the boundaries of the ethmoid infundibulum and hiatus semilunaris. It is difficult to completely image in a single CT plane, but viewed through an endoscope, its surgical anatomy becomes much simpler: anteriorly it is attached to the nasolacrimal apparatus (Fig. 2.9),

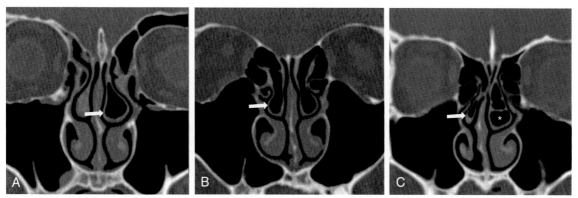

FIG. 2.10 Concha bullosa variation. **(A)** Bulbous type (*arrow*). **(B)** Extensive type (*arrow*). **(C)** Lamellar (*arrow*) and septated type (*asterisk*). Evidently, some of these could be large enough to efface the ethmoid infundibulum and hiatus semilunaris.

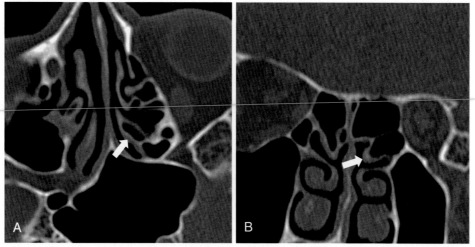

FIG. 2.11 Superior turbinate variation. **(A)** Axial and **(B)** coronal CT of a concha bullosa in the left superior turbinate (*arrows* in **A** and **B**), which is often of little consequence.

inferiorly it is attached to the inferior turbinate, posteriorly it has a free margin, and superiorly the attachment is variable.

On coronal CT, the uncinate process has distinctly different appearances on anterior and posterior sections. In anterior sections, the uncinate process may be seen to attach superiorly to the skull base, laterally to the lamina papyracea or ANCs, or medially to the middle turbinate. Moving posteriorly, it is seen as a thin bone attached inferiorly to the inferior turbinate, with the free edge representing the posterior free margin.

The superior attachment of the uncinate process often deserves particular mention in a radiologic report, as it determines the course of the FSDP. There are three variable attachments (Fig. 2.15):

- If the uncinate process attaches to the middle turbinate (Fig. 2.15A) or skull base (Fig. 2.15B), the frontal sinus opens into the ethmoid infundibulum. Infection in the infundibulum may then affect the frontal sinus. The uncinate process must be removed to gain access to the ethmoid infundibulum and maxillary sinus ostium.
- If the uncinate process inserts into the lamina papyracea or ethmoid bulla (Fig. 2.15C), the ethmoid infundibulum is closed superiorly by a blind pouch called the lamina terminalis or recessus terminalis (Fig. 2.15C). In this situation, the frontal recess and the ethmoid infundibulum are separated and the frontal recess opens into the middle meatus, medial to the ethmoid infundibulum. This explains why

ethmoid infundibular inflammation does not result in frontal sinusitis in some patients. Occasionally, this may also lead to closure of the ethmoid infundibulum, resulting in a hypoplastic maxillary sinus (silent sinus syndrome). This can sometimes be associated with enophthalmos as the orbital floor is retracted downward.[23]

### Uncinate Process Variations

The uncinate process may be medialized, lateralized, pneumatized, or bent. Medialization usually occurs in conjunction with a giant bulla ethmoidalis. Lateralization of the uncinate process may obstruct the infundibulum. The uncinate process may be located just medial to the orbital wall thus endangering the orbit during uncinectomy. Pneumatization of the

uncinate process may be encountered in up to 4% of the population[14] and is thought to represent the extension of the ANC (Fig. 2.6).[23] This variant rarely obstructs the infundibulum.[24] A bent uncinate process may appear as a double middle turbinate on endoscopy.

### Ethmoid Roof

The ethmoid roof is of critical importance for two reasons: First, this thin bony structure partly forms the anterior skull base and is most vulnerable to iatrogenic CSF leaks. Second, the anterior ethmoid artery (AEA) is exposed in the anterior ethmoid as it crosses from the orbit into the anterior skull base and is vulnerable to injury, which can cause devastating bleeding into the orbit.

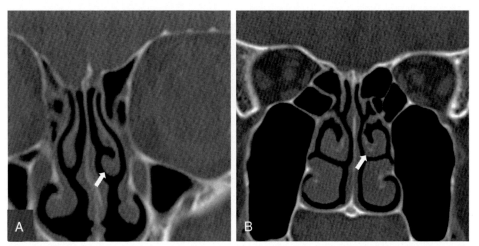

FIG. 2.12 Middle turbinate variation: Sagittal views of **(A)** a paradoxical middle turbinate (*arrow*) and **(B)** turbinate sinus (*arrow*).

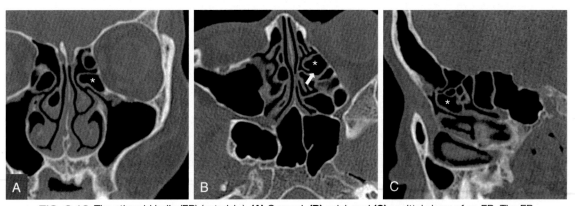

FIG. 2.13 The ethmoid bulla (EB) (*asterisks*). **(A)** Coronal, **(B)** axial, and **(C)** sagittal views of an EB. The EB often lacks a posterior wall (*arrow* in **B**) and is more analogous to a large air space behind the second basal lamella (in keeping with the five basal lamella concept).

Why is it prone to CSF leaks? The paramedian anterior ethmoid roof is a recess of the cribriform plate that houses the olfactory fossa (Fig. 2.16). The bones here are thin, measuring only 0.5 mm and can taper down to a mere 0.05 mm at the ethmoidal sulcus[25] (Fig. 2.17). Unlike the dura in the rest of the skull, the dura within the olfactory fossa is tightly adhered to the

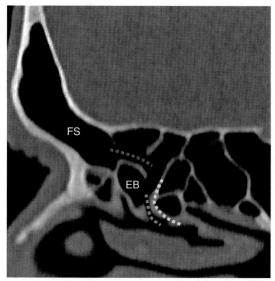

FIG. 2.14 The retrobullar recess. The retrobullar recess/sinus lateralis (*blue dotted line*) is the space between the ethmoid bulla (EB) and the third basal lamella (*yellow dotted line*). If the EB does not fuse with the skull base superiorly, the sinus lateralis can communicate with the frontal sinus (FS) through the suprabullar recess (*red dotted line*).

bone, requiring only minimal trauma to tear it. This is especially true at the entry of the AEA where the artery can already have an intradural course.[25]

The ethmoid roof and lamina papyracea are highly sensitive to pain. In cases that are performed under sedation, increased patient discomfort should warn the operator of the proximity to the ethmoid roof.

The olfactory fossa is divided by the crista galli and bounded laterally by the lateral lamellae. This fragile lamella may be of variable height (up to 16 mm), making it vulnerable to injury. The olfactory fossa merges laterally with the fovea ethmoidalis of the considerably thicker frontal bone, which can be up to 16 mm above the level of the cribriform plate (Fig. 2.16).

The lateral lamella is a critical structure for surgeons, and its depth was classified into three categories according to Keros in 1962.[25,26]

| | | |
|---|---|---|
| Type 1 | Depth of 1–3 mm | 12% of the population |
| Type 2 | Depth of 4–7 mm | 70% of the population |
| Type 3 | Depth of 8–16 mm | 18% of the population |

Type 3 exposes the cribriform plate to trauma. Further dehiscence or defects of the lateral lamella can also result in CSF leak or encephalomeningoceles. Other factors that increase surgical risk include asymmetry or a low-lying ethmoid roof. The foveal angle (between the fovea ethmoidalis and lamina papyracea) is also considered, where a low foveal angle poses increased risk of penetration.

It is also important to remember that the middle turbinate is attached delicately to the cribriform plate anteriorly, and overzealous manipulation of the middle turbinate may disrupt both structures, resulting in

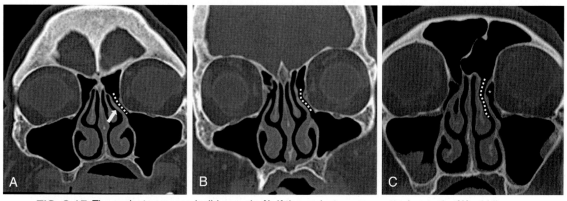

FIG. 2.15 The uncinate process (*solid arrow* in **A**). If the uncinate process attaches to the **(A)** middle turbinate or **(B)** the skull base, then the frontal sinus drainage pathway (FSDP) (*dotted lines*) opens into the ethmoid infundibulum. **(C)** If the uncinate process attaches to the lamina papyracea, the ethmoid infundibulum will be closed superiorly, resulting in a blind pouch called the lamina terminalis (*asterisk*). The FSDP (*dotted line*) then opens into the middle meatus.

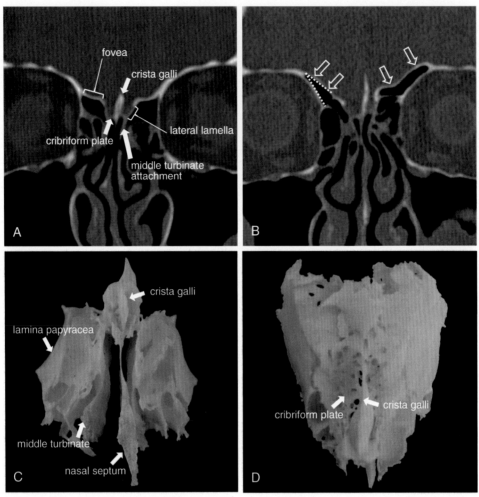

FIG. 2.16 The ethmoid roof. **(A)** The ethmoid roof comprises the fovea, lateral lamella, cribriform plate, and crista galli. The lateral lamella is seen here as the thinnest and most vulnerable part of the roof. **(B)** Asymmetric foveal angle (*dotted lines*), where the ethmoid roof (*open arrows*) is lower on the right. **(C)** Coronal and **(D)** axial disarticulated specimens of the ethmoid sinus.

a floppy middle turbinate and CSF leak.[27] A surgeon avoids completely resecting the middle turbinate, as it is an important surgical landmark during revision surgery. A radiologist reviewing a CT with previous middle turbinectomy should focus on two areas: (1) integrity of the lamina papyracea at the attachment of the basal lamella and (2) integrity of the cribriform plate at the superior attachment of the middle turbinate.

## Anterior Ethmoid Artery

The AEA is a branch of the ophthalmic artery that exits the medial orbital wall at the anterior ethmoidal foramen. This is recognized on CT as a medial notch of the orbit (Fig. 2.17). The AEA then crosses the anterior

ethmoid air cells through a bony canal (the anterior ethmoidal canal) into the anterior cranial fossa at a point in the lateral lamella called the ethmoidal sulcus. The bone here is 10 times thinner than the ethmoid roof and easily perforated by any instrument.

Endoscopically, the AEA can be found by tracing the anterior wall of the ethmoid bulla toward the ethmoid roof, and it is about 1 cm behind the posterior wall of the frontal recess (in the suprabullar recess in up to 85.3% of people).[28] It often hugs the skull base but is not infrequently 1–3 mm below the skull base within a bony mesentery. The anterior ethmoidal canal is approximately 8 mm in length, with 40% of people showing a partial or total bony dehiscence, particularly

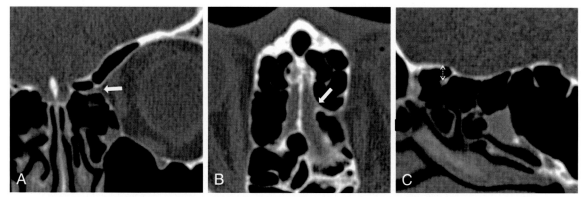

FIG. 2.17 Anterior ethmoid artery (AEA). **(A)** The anterior ethmoidal canal (*solid arrow*) begins as a notch at the medial orbital wall. **(B)** Axial view showing the AEA traversing the anterior ethmoid air cells to reach a point in the lateral lamella called the ethmoidal sulcus (*solid arrow*). **(C)** The AEA is often not fused to the ethmoid roof (*double arrow*) and can appear somewhat partially dehiscent.

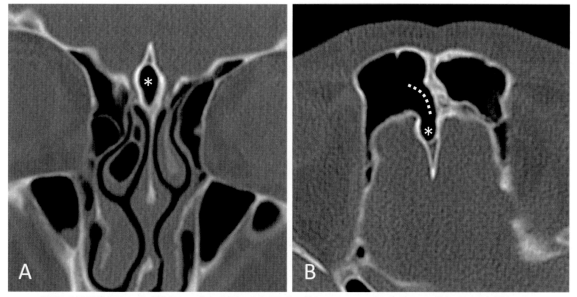

FIG. 2.18 Crista galli. **(A)** Coronal and **(B)** axial CT showing a pneumatized crista galli (*asterisks*). This may reflect communication with the anterior ethmoid cells (*dotted line* in **B**) that increases the risk of breaching the anterior cranial fossa during surgery.

along its inferior margin.[25] The posterior ethmoid artery, located approximately 10 mm posterior to the AEA, is less often injured. Some variations of the AEA do occur, including duplication and replaced arteries.

## Crista Galli

The crista galli (Latin for "rooster's comb") is part of the ethmoid bone. It can also serve as a landmark on coronal CT for identification of ethmoid air cells because being part of the ethmoid bone, it terminates before reaching the sphenoid sinus.[29] A pneumatized

crista galli may indicate communication with the frontal recess (Fig. 2.18). This normal variant is important to highlight in a radiologic report to avoid breach into the anterior cranial fossa during surgery.

## Ethmoid Air Cells

Ethmoid sinus air cells originate from endochondral bone that results in thin bones and variable pneumatization patterns. These air cells are classified into intramural and extramural cells (based on their migration out of the ethmoid bone). Some of these intramural

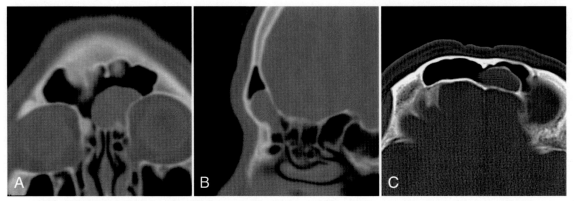

FIG. 2.19 Frontal cell sinusitis. **(A)** Coronal, **(B)** sagittal, and **(C)** axial images showing isolated opacification of a left type 3 frontal cell.

cells have been discussed earlier in the text. Extramural cells include ANCs, Haller cells, FCs, SOECs, IFSSCs, and Onodi cells.

### Extramural Cells

#### Frontal cells

The most widely described of these AECs are the FCs (also known as frontal ethmoidal cells), and they can either narrow the frontal recess (Fig. 2.6) or contain mucosal disease themselves (Fig. 2.19). They are classified into four types according to Bent and Kuhn[11,30] based their relationship with the FB and extension into the frontal sinus (Fig. 2.20).

- Type 1: single cell, not extending into the frontal sinus 24.2%
- Type 2: two or more cells, sometimes extending into the frontal sinus 4.2%
- Type 3: single cell, extending into the frontal sinus 3.1%
- Type 4: isolated cells located in the frontal sinus <<1%

#### Haller cells

The initial description of these cells in 1765 is attributed to Albert von Haller, a 19th century anatomist.[31] There are several definitions for Haller cells, but in general these cells are located below the ethmoid bulla, extending underneath the orbital floor (Fig. 2.21). Reported frequencies range from 10% to 45%.[14,32] The role of Haller cells in sinus disease should be examined in relation to cell size, proximity, and narrowing of the maxillary sinus ostium. Isolated disease of Haller cell is rarely described.

#### Onodi cells (sphenoethmoidal cells)

In 1908, Onodi observed the "frequent intimate relationship of the optic nerve with the last ethmoid cell."[33] The term Onodi cell refers to a posterior ethmoid cell that extends lateral and superior to the sphenoid sinus and is often closely associated with the optic nerve (Fig. 2.22). An Onodi cell can also surround the optic nerve canal and place the nerve at risk during surgery. On coronal section, an Onodi cell can be seen above the sphenoid sinus. Endoscopically, these cells appear as outgrowths of the posterior ethmoid posteriorly and superiorly. They have a pyramidal configuration with the tip of the pyramid pointing away from the endoscopist.

## SPHENOID SINUS

The early development of the carotid arteries and nerves before pneumatization of the paranasal sinuses results in variable appearance of the sphenoid sinus.

### Sphenoethmoidal Recess

The most posterior ethmoid cell and the sphenoid sinus share a common wall laterally. The medial one-third of the anterior sphenoid sinus wall is a free surface in the nasal cavity. This area is called the sphenoethmoidal recess. This recess can be found at the point where the superior turbinate ends posteriorly (Fig. 2.23).

### Sphenoid Sinus Variations

The intersphenoid septum is often deflected to one side, attaching to the bony wall covering the carotid artery. This artery can be injured when the septum is avulsed during surgery (Fig. 2.24). The carotid artery may bulge into the sinus in 65%–72% of patients, and the thin bone separating the artery and sinus may be absent in 4%–8% of cases.[34]

The pterygoid or Vidian canal or the groove of the maxillary nerve may also project into the sphenoid sinus (Fig. 2.24), particularly in cases of hyperpneumatization.

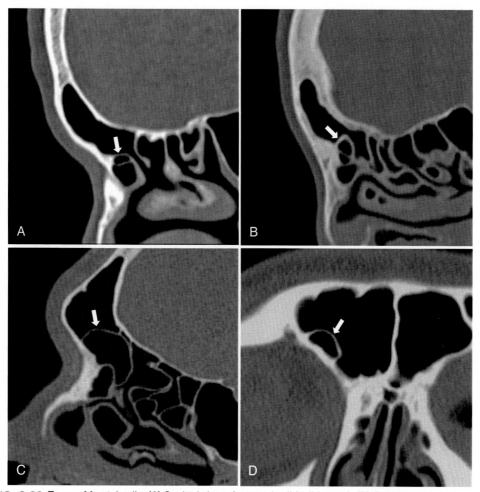

FIG. 2.20 Types of frontal cells: **(A)** Sagittal view of a type 1 cell (*solid arrow*). **(B)** Sagittal view of a type 2 cell (*solid arrow*). **(C)** Sagittal view of a type 3 cell (*solid arrow*). **(D)** Coronal view of a type 4 cell (*solid arrow*).

Sphenoiditis can also, therefore, produce trigeminal neuralgia.

The relationship of the optic nerve with the posterior paranasal sinuses should be reviewed. In addition to the Onodi cell, the course of the optic canal can be divided into four groups according to the classification by Delano et al.[35]

- Type I: the nerve does not indent the sphenoid sinus or contact the posterior ethmoid air cell.
- Type II: the nerve indents the sphenoid sinus without contacting the posterior ethmoid air cell.
- Type III: the nerve courses through the sphenoid sinus with >50% surrounded by air.
- Type IV: the nerve is immediately adjacent to the sphenoid and posterior ethmoid sinus.

Type I configuration is the most common, occurring in 76% of cases. However, in cases of pneumatized anterior clinoid processes, 85% of optic nerves show type II or type III configuration. About 77% of these are also dehiscent,[35] which is significantly higher than the reported overall optic canal dehiscence of between 4% and 24%.[35,36]

## CONCLUSION

In summary, it is important to have a thorough understanding of the paranasal sinus anatomy in relation to FESS. Our contribution as radiologists is to highlight important and dangerous anatomic variants to our surgical colleagues, with the aim of minimizing surgical risk.

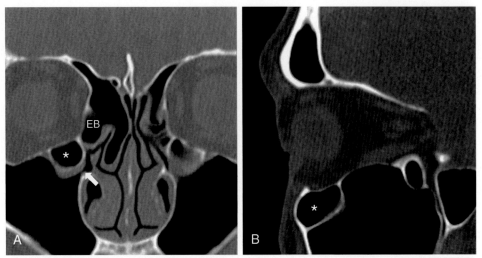

FIG. 2.21 Haller cell. **(A)** Coronal and **(B)** sagittal CT showing a Haller cell (*asterisks*) that is found along the medial floor of the orbit, below the ethmoid bulla (EB in **A**) and adjacent to the maxillary ostium (*arrow* in **A**).

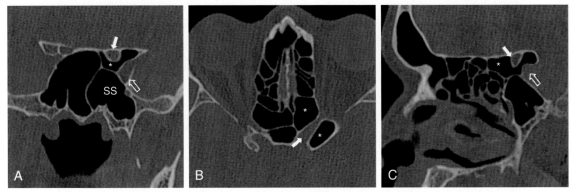

FIG. 2.22 Onodi cell (*asterisks*). **(A)** Coronal, **(B)** axial, and **(C)** sagittal images or an Onodi (sphenoethmoidal cell). This cell reflects the extension of a postreme ethmoid cell above the sphenoid sinus (SS in **A**), lining the optic nerve (*solid arrows*) and internal carotid artery (*open arrows* in **A** and **C**).

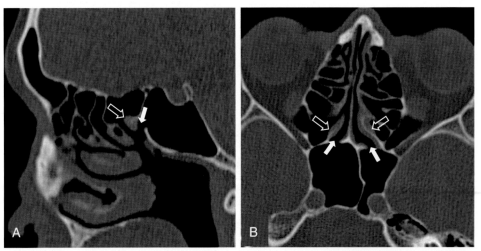

FIG. 2.23 Sphenoethmoidal recess. **(A)** Sagittal and **(B)** axial images of both sphenoethmoidal recesses (*solid arrows*) that are seen consistently medial to the posterior end of the superior turbinates (*open arrows*).

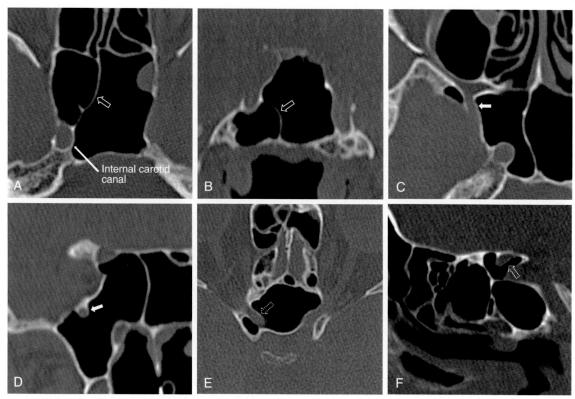

FIG. 2.24 Sphenoid sinus variation. **(A)** Axial and **(B)** coronal CT of an intersphenoid septum (*open arrows*) deflected onto the carotid canal. **(C)** Axial and **(D)** coronal CT showing protrusion of the maxillary nerve groove (*solid arrows*) into the sphenoid sinus. Here, sphenoid sinusitis can sometimes cause trigeminal neuralgia. **(E)** Axial and **(F)** sagittal CT showing a type III course of the optic nerve (*open broken arrows*).

## REFERENCES

1. Hesselink JR, et al. Computed tomography of the paranasal sinuses and face: part I. Normal anatomy. *J Comput Assist Tomogr.* 1978;2(5):559–567.
2. Siedek V, et al. Complications in endonasal sinus surgery: a 5-year retrospective study of 2,596 patients. *Eur Arch Otorhinolaryngol.* 2013;270(1):141–148.
3. Hegazy HM, et al. Transnasal endoscopic repair of cerebrospinal fluid rhinorrhea: a meta-analysis. *Laryngoscope.* 2000;110(7):1166–1172.
4. Ahn JC, et al. Nasal septal deviation with obstructive symptoms: association found with asthma but not with other general health problems. *Am J Rhinol Allergy.* 2016;30(2):17–20.
5. Stammberger H, Wolf G. Headaches and sinus disease: the endoscopic approach. *Ann Otol Rhinol Laryngol Suppl.* 1988;134:3–23.
6. Lillie H. Some practical considerations of the physiology of the upper respiratory tract. *J Iowa State Med Soc.* 1923;13:403–408.
7. Zinreich SJ, et al. MR imaging of normal nasal cycle: comparison with sinus pathology. *J Comput Assist Tomogr.* 1988;12(6):1014–1019.
8. Mirza N, Kroger H, Doty RL. Influence of age on the 'nasal cycle'. *Laryngoscope.* 1997;107(1):62–66.
9. Stammberger H, et al. Special endoscopic anatomy. In: Stammberger H, Hawke M, eds. *Functional Endoscopic Sinus Surgery: The Messerklinger Technique.* Philadelphia, PA: BC Decker Publishers; 1991:61–90.
10. Lee WT, Kuhn FA, Citardi MJ. 3D computed tomographic analysis of frontal recess anatomy in patients without frontal sinusitis. *Otolaryngol Head Neck Surg.* 2004;131(3):164–173.
11. Park SS, et al. Pneumatization pattern of the frontal recess: relationship of the anterior-to-posterior length of frontal isthmus and/or frontal recess with the volume of agger nasi cell. *Clin Exp Otorhinolaryngol.* 2010;3(2):76–83.
12. Kasper KA. Nasofrontal connections. A study based on one hundred consecutive dissections. *Arch Otolaryngol.* 1936;23:21.

13. Wormald PJ. The agger nasi cell: the key to understanding the anatomy of the frontal recess. *Otolaryngol Head Neck Surg.* 2003;129(5):497–507.

14. Bolger WE, Butzin CA, Parsons DS. Paranasal sinus bony anatomic variations and mucosal abnormalities: CT analysis for endoscopic sinus surgery. *Laryngoscope.* 1991;101(1 Pt 1):56–64.

15. Stammberger H, Posawetz W. Functional endoscopic sinus surgery. Concept, indications and results of the Messerklinger technique. *Eur Arch Otorhinolaryngol.* 1990;247(2):63–76.

16. Levine HL, Clemente MP. *Sinus Surgery-Endoscopic and Microscopic Approaches;* 2005.

17. Killian G. Zur anatomie der Nase menschlicher Embryonen. *Arch f Laryngol.* 1895:iii.

18. Hiyama T. The ethmoid bone: clinical imaging anatomy from an embryological point of view. Poster presented at: European Congress of Radiology 2013; March 7-11, 2013; Vienna.

19. Zinreich SJ, et al. Concha bullosa: CT evaluation. *J Comput Assist Tomogr.* 1988;12(5):778–784.

20. Cannon CR. Endoscopic management of concha bullosa. *Otolaryngol Head Neck Surg.* 1994;110(4):449–454.

21. Wright ED, Bolger WE. The bulla ethmoidalis: lamella or a true cell? *J Otolaryngol.* 2001;30(3):162–166.

22. von Kölliker R. Der Lobus olfactorius und die Nervi olfactorii bei jungen menschlichen Embryonen. In: *Sitzungab d Phys-Med Sesellsch zu Würzburg.* 1882: 68–72.

23. Som PM, Curtin HD. *Head and Neck Imaging.* Elsevier Health Sciences; 2011.

24. Zinreich SJ, et al. Paranasal sinuses: CT imaging requirements for endoscopic surgery. *Radiology.* 1987;163(3): 769–775.

25. Kainz J, Stammberger H. The roof of the anterior ethmoid: a place of least resistance in the skull base. *Am J Rhinol.* 1989;3(4):191–199.

26. Keros P. On the practical value of differences in the level of the lamina cribrosa of the ethmoid. *Z Laryngol Rhinol Otol.* 1962;41:809–813.

27. May M, et al. Complications of endoscopic sinus surgery: analysis of 2108 patients–incidence and prevention. *Laryngoscope.* 1994;104(9):1080–1083.

28. Simmen D, et al. The surgeon's view of the anterior ethmoid artery. *Clin Otolaryngol.* 2006;31(3):187–191.

29. Davis WE, Templer J, Parsons DS. Anatomy of the paranasal sinuses. *Otolaryngol Clin N Am.* 1996;29(1):57–74.

30. Bent JP, Cuilty-Siller C, Kuhn FA. The frontal cell as a cause of frontal sinus obstruction. *Am J Rhinol.* 1994;8(4):185–191.

31. Wanamaker HH. Role of Haller's cell in headache and sinus disease: a case report. *Otolaryngol Head Neck Surg.* 1996;114(2):324–327.

32. Kennedy D, Zinreich SJ. Functional endoscopic approach to inflammatory sinus disease: current perspectives and technique modifications. *Am J Rhinol.* 1988;2:89–96.

33. Onodi A. The optic nerve and the accessory cavities of the nose. *Ann Otol Rhinol Laryngol.* 1908;17:1–61.

34. Laine FJ, Smoker WR. The ostiomeatal unit and endoscopic surgery: anatomy, variations, and imaging findings in inflammatory diseases. *AJR Am J Roentgenol.* 1992;159(4): 849–857

35. DeLano MC, Fun FY, Zinreich SJ. Relationship of the optic nerve to the posterior paranasal sinuses: a CT anatomic study. *AJNR Am J Neuroradiol.* 1996;17(4):669–675.

36. Maniscalco JE, Habal MB. Microanatomy of the optic canal. *J Neurosurg.* 1978;48(3):402–406.

# CHAPTER 3

# The Sphenoid Bone

JAMES TPD HALLINAN, MBCHB, BSC, FRCR •
DAVID SY SIA, MBBS, FRCR, MMED •
CLEMENT YONG, MBBS, FRANZCR •
VINCENT CHONG, MD, MBA, MHPE, FRCR

The sphenoid bone is located at the central skull base and is commonly considered the most complex bone in the human body. Although the sphenoid bone is often neglected in relation to the adjacent temporal bone, it forms the major boundary between the intra- and extracranial structures. The various sphenoid foramina to the orbits anteriorly and neck spaces inferiorly are pathways for transmission of disease.

This chapter highlights the normal sphenoid bone anatomy and various disorders affecting the skull base. Understanding the anatomy will enable clinicians to predict intra- and extracranial disease spread and presentation.

## NORMAL ANATOMY

The sphenoid bone forms the central skull base and viewed anteriorly resembles a bird with its wings unfurled. It is a compound bone with a median body and paired lateral greater and lesser wings (Fig. 3.1). At the ventral junction of the body and wings the paired pterygoid processes arise inferiorly, resembling the extended limbs of a bird.[1]

Of interest, the Greek origin of sphenoid (sphen) is likely in reference to a wedge shape seen laterally, with pterygoid (pteron) referring to a fin- or wing-like shape.[2] Another theory for the origin of "sphenoid" is the term os sphecoidale, meaning "bone resembling a wasp." The term is apt given the resemblance to a winged creature. At some point a transcription error to "sphenoidale" may have occurred with loss of the true meaning.[3]

Anteriorly the sphenoid bone articulates with the ethmoid and frontal bones, laterally with the temporal bones, and posteriorly with the basiocciput. Essentially, the sphenoid functions as an attachment site for the majority of the masticator musculature and serves as a key conduit for the passage of nerves and blood vessels of the head and neck. Major foramina and fissures include the optic canal, foramen rotundum, superior orbital fissure, and foramen ovale (Figs. 3.2–3.5).

## SPHENOID BODY

The body of the sphenoid contains the sphenoid sinuses and the pituitary fossa (sella turcica), a deep saddle-shaped depression containing the pituitary gland (hypophysis). The anterior margin of the pituitary fossa (tuberculum sellae) continues anteriorly as the flat superior surface of the sphenoid, termed the planum sphenoidale. This forms the anterior roof of the sphenoid sinuses and articulates with the cribriform plate of the ethmoid bone, which transmits small fibers of the olfactory nerve.[4]

The posterior margin of the pituitary fossa (dorsum sellae) continues inferiorly as the basisphenoid, which articulates with the basiocciput forming the clivus (Latin for "slope"). The clivus continues posteroinferiorly to the foramen magnum, with the petroclival fissures forming the lateral borders. The inferior clivus forms the bony roof of the nasopharynx.

Anteroinferior to the sella turcica are the paired sphenoid sinuses. The thin anterior wall of the sinuses and face of the sphenoid body articulate with the nasal septum at the sphenoidal crest. At either side of the crest are the sphenoid sinus ostia allowing drainage of secretions into the sphenoethmoidal recesses and then into the superior nasal cavity. The lateral borders of the sphenoid bone/sinuses form the medial cavernous sinus walls and are commonly indented by the carotid arteries. The posterior walls of the sinuses are formed by the anterior clivus, which can be of variable thickness, depending on the extent of sinus pneumatization.

## LESSER WING

The lesser wings or orbitosphenoids are paired thin triangular plates that extend laterally from the planum

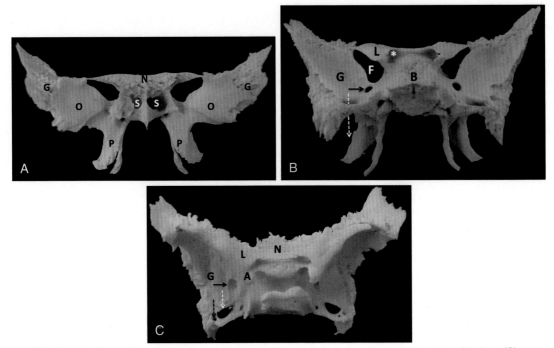

FIG. 3.1 Anatomy of a sphenoid bone specimen. **(A)** Frontal view shows the greater sphenoid wings (G) and pterygoid plates (P) resembling the wings of a bird with extended limbs, respectively. The sphenoid sinus (S), posterior wall of the orbit (O), and planum sphenoidale (N) are also highlighted. **(B)** Posterior view shows the greater wing (G), lesser wing (L), and body (B) of the sphenoid bone. The superior orbital fissure (F), optic canal (*asterisk*), foramen rotundum (*black arrow*), and foramen ovale (*dashed white arrow* through the foramen) are highlighted. **(C)** Superior view shows the lesser wing (L), planum sphenoidale (N), greater wing (G), anterior clinoid process (A), foramen ovale (*dashed white arrow*), foramen spinosum (*dashed black arrow*), and foramen rotundum (*black arrow*).

sphenoidale. Medially they arise from the anterior and superior sphenoid body at two roots. These roots define the optic canal (Figs. 3.2–3.5), which transmits the optic nerve and ophthalmic artery. It is the only canal passing through the lesser wing and is separated from the superior orbital fissure inferolaterally by the optic strut (lower root).[2]

The superior orbital fissure (Figs. 3.2–3.5) is a comma-shaped gap between the lesser and greater wings of the sphenoid bone appearing thin superolaterally and bulbous inferiorly.[5] It transmits cranial nerves (CNs) III, IV and VI (oculomotor, trochlear, and abducens), branches of the ophthalmic division of the trigeminal nerve (CN V1), and several vessels including the ophthalmic veins. In addition, the annulus of Zinn, common tendinous origin of the four rectus muscles, straddles the superior orbital fissure centrally and encircles the optic canal.[6]

The inferior surface of the lesser wing forms the upper boundary of the superior orbital fissure and the posterior orbital roof. The flat superior surface serves as a platform for the basifrontal lobe and posteromedial extensions form the anterior clinoid processes, which are the attachment sites of the tentorium cerebelli.[1]

## GREATER WING

The paired greater sphenoid wings, or alisphenoids, arise from the body of the sphenoid medially and curve superiorly and laterally. The greater wings contribute to the formation of the orbit and middle cranial fossa.

At the orbit, the medial margin of the greater wing forms the inferior margin of the superior orbital fissure and the posterolateral margin of the inferior orbital fissure (Figs. 3.2 and 3.4), which transmits the zygomatic branch of the maxillary nerve (CN V2). The orbital portion of the greater wing also forms the posterolateral wall of the orbit.

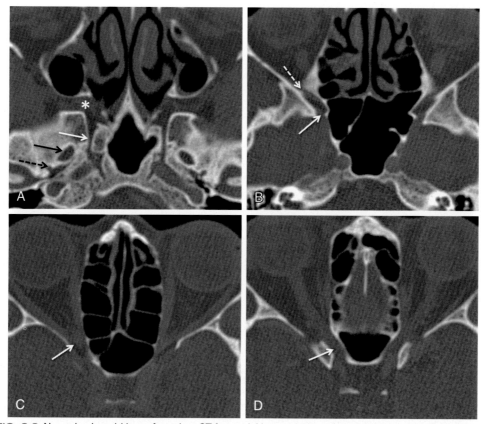

**FIG. 3.2** Normal sphenoid bone foramina. CT face axial bone windows from inferior to superior **(A–D)**. The most inferior section shows the vidian canal (*solid white arrow*), foramen ovale (*solid black arrow* in **A**), and foramen spinosum (*dashed black arrow* in **A**). These foramina are traversed by the vidian nerve, mandibular division of the trigeminal nerve (V3), and the middle meningeal artery, respectively. In **(B)** the foramen rotundum (*solid white arrow*) is seen superior and lateral to the vidian canal and transmits the maxillary division of the trigeminal nerve (V2) into the pterygopalatine fossa (*asterisk* in **A**). The inferior orbital fissure (*dashed white arrow* in **B**) is also seen at the level of the foramen rotundum. In **(C)** the superior orbital fissure is highlighted (*solid white arrow*). This is a major conduit between the cavernous sinus and orbit and transmits cranial nerves III, IV, and VI along with several other vessels and nerves. The most superior section **(D)** shows the optic canal, which transmits the optic nerve and ophthalmic artery.

The cerebral or superior surface of the greater wing forms the majority of the concave middle cranial fossa and has a number of foramina passing through it.

The foramen rotundum is a circular aperture seen at the base of the greater wing anteromedially, just inferior to the superior orbital fissure (Figs. 3.2–3.5). It transmits the maxillary nerve (CN V2) from the middle cranial fossa to the pterygopalatine fossa.

The foramen ovale arises posterolateral to the rotundum and transmits the mandibular nerve (CN V3) from the middle cranial fossa to the masticator space (Figs. 3.2–3.5). The size of the foramina ovale can differ

from side to side.[7] Asymmetry of up to 4 mm can be within normal limits.[8]

The foramen spinosum (Fig. 3.2) is located further posterolateral to the foramen ovale and transmits the middle meningeal artery and a recurrent branch of the mandibular nerve (CN V3). Posterior and medial to the foramen spinosum, each greater wing projects as a triangular process articulating with the squamous and petrous portions of the temporal bone. At the apex of this triangle is the inferiorly projected sphenoid spine (spina angularis). This serves as an attachment site of the tensor veli palatini muscle and the sphenomandibular ligament.

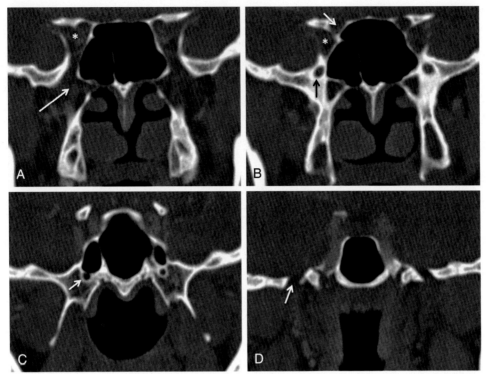

**FIG. 3.3** Normal sphenoid bone foramina. CT face coronal bone windows from anterior to posterior **(A–D)**. The most anterior section **(A)** shows the pterygopalatine fossa (*solid white arrow*) and orbital apex (*asterisk*). More posteriorly **(B)** the separate optic canal (*solid white arrow*), superior orbital fissure (*asterisk*), and foramen rotundum (*solid black arrow*) are noted. The vidian canal is located inferomedial to the foramen rotundum and highlighted more posteriorly in (**C**, *solid white arrow*). The most posterior section shows the vertically oriented foramen ovale (**D**, *solid white arrow*), which transmits the mandibular division of the trigeminal nerve.

Posteromedially the greater wing forms the anterior margin of the foramen lacerum. This represents another potential conduit of disease spread from the nasopharynx. At the lateral temporal surface of the greater wing the muscles of mastication, including the temporalis (superiorly) and lateral pterygoid (inferiorly), attach.

## PTERYGOID PROCESSES

The fin-like pterygoid processes extend inferiorly from the junction between the greater wing and body of the sphenoid. Each pterygoid process is formed of two plates, lateral and medial, which fuse superiorly and anteriorly. The site of fusion serves as the posterior wall of the pterygopalatine fossa, which separates the pterygoid processes from the maxillary sinus anteriorly. The pterygopalatine fossa is an important neurovascular crossroad of the head and neck, communicating with numerous foramina, including the

inferior orbital fissure, foramen rotundum, and the vidian canal (Figs. 3.2–3.5).[9]

The vidian (pterygoid) canal is a communication through the medial plate of the pterygoid between the foramen lacerum posteriorly and the pterygopalatine fossa anteriorly (Figs. 3.2–3.5). The canal lies inferomedial to the foramen rotundum and their intervening distance depends on the degree of sphenoid sinus pneumatization. The vidian artery, vein, and nerve (formed from the greater superficial petrosal nerve and deep petrosal nerve) pass through the canal.[10]

Posteriorly the lateral and medial processes diverge, and enclosed between them is the V-shaped pterygoid fossa. This contains the tensor veli palatini and medial pterygoid muscles. The lateral pterygoid process serves as the site of origin for the medial and lateral pterygoid muscles of mastication. The tensor veil palatini arises superiorly at the base of the medial pterygoid plate at

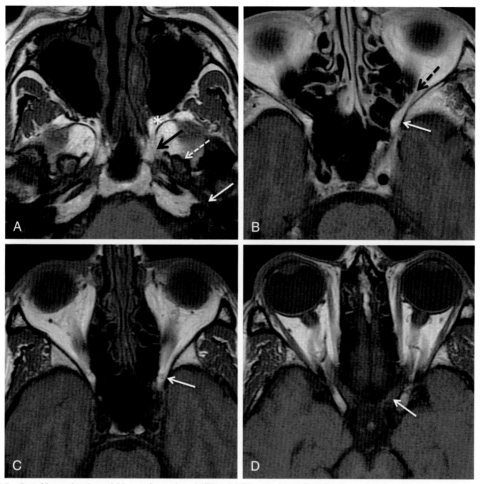

FIG. 3.4 Normal sphenoid bone foramina. MRI axial T1-weighted (T1W) sequences from inferior to superior **(A–D)**. The most inferior section shows the vidian canal (*solid black arrow*) with the greater superficial
petrosal nerve seen more posteriorly arising from the geniculate ganglion of the facial nerve (*solid white arrow*). Foramen ovale transmitting the mandibular division of the trigeminal nerve is also seen (*dashed white
arrow* in **A**). In **(B)** the foramen rotundum (*solid white arrow*) is noted superior and lateral to the vidian canal
and transmits the maxillary division of the trigeminal nerve (V2) into the pterygopalatine fossa (*asterisk* in **A**,
normal appearance with T1W hyperintense fat signal within). The inferior orbital fissure (*dashed black arrow*
in **B**) is also seen at the level of the foramen rotundum. In **(C)** the superior orbital fissure is highlighted (*solid
white arrow*). This is a major conduit between the cavernous sinus and orbit and contains T1W hyperintense fat. The most superior section (*solid white arrow* in **D**) shows the optic canal, which transmits the
optic nerve and ophthalmic artery. On MRI, T1W sequences are useful for assessing for extra- or intracranial spread of disease through the foramina. T1W hyperintense fat signal is seen most prominently at the
pterygopalatine fossa, superior orbital fissure, and orbital apex. If this signal is lost, then underlying disease
may be present and postcontrast sequences should be carefully interrogated.

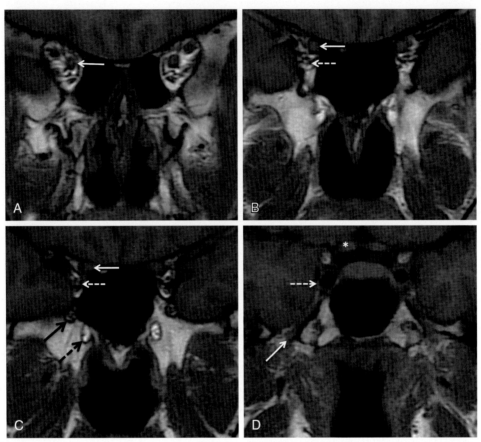

FIG. 3.5 Normal sphenoid bone foramina. MRI face coronal T1-weighted (T1W) sequences from anterior to posterior **(A–D)**. The most anterior section **(A)** shows the optic nerve (*solid white arrow*) at the orbital apex surrounded by the extraocular muscles and T1W hyperintense orbital fat. More posteriorly the optic nerve is seen entering the optic canal (*solid white arrows* in **B** and **C**) with the extraocular muscles and cranial nerves III, IV, and VI converging at the superior orbital fissure (*dashed white arrows* in **B** and **C**). The foramen rotundum containing the maxillary division of the trigeminal nerve (V2, *solid black arrow* in **C**) and the inferomedial vidian canal and internal vidian nerve (*dashed black arrow* in **C**) are noted at the sphenoid body. The most posterior section shows the vertically orientated foramen ovale and mandibular division of the trigeminal nerve (V3, *solid white arrow* in **D**). V3 extends from the Gasserian or semilunar ganglion and does not enter the cavernous sinus (*dashed arrow* in **D**). The prechiasmatic optic nerve is also noted (*asterisk* in **D**).

an oval depression termed the scaphoid fossa. As mentioned previously, the muscle also has an additional attachment site at the scaphoid spine.[6]

## SPHENOID BONE DISORDERS
### Sphenoid Sinus

The paired sphenoid sinuses drain into the nasal cavity through the sphenoethmoidal recesses. The sinuses are lined by the respiratory epithelium, which secretes mucus, serving to protect against infection. Underlying

the epithelium is the capillary-rich lamina propria, which is firmly attached to the periosteum of the adjacent sphenoid bone.[11]

Compared with CT, MRI appearances of sinonasal secretions show a wide variation. In the normal state, the secretions are almost purely water with up to 5% proteinaceous content. These appear as hyperintense on T2-weighted (T2W) and hypointense on T1-weighted (T1W) images. Once a sinus is obstructed, the water content is reabsorbed with a corresponding increase in the protein content. This results in shortening of the

T1W and T2W relaxation times, and at about 25%–30% protein content the secretions may reverse from the normal state, appearing hyperintense on T1W and hypointense on T2W images.[2] At even higher protein contents (35%–40%), the T1W and T2W signals may appear hypointense, similar to any surrounding gas.[12] Knowledge of these appearances is useful in the assessment of mucoceles, which are essentially "mucous tumors" following the same signal characteristics.

Mucoceles are defined as an opacified, expanded sinus resulting from obstruction at the sinus ostium. Mucoceles are most common at the frontal and ethmoid sinuses, with rare occurrences at the sphenoid sinus.[13] They lead to smooth expansion of the bone and when large can impinge on adjacent neurovascular structures. At the sphenoid sinus, the risk of intracranial extension is the greatest, with potential for visual loss and cranial nerve palsies secondary to involvement of the orbital apex and cavernous sinus.

Sphenoid sinusitis is a common condition and mainly results from bacterial infections, although fungal etiologies are also implicated. Fungal infections include aspergillosis, which can produce central hyperdense secretions on CT in the affected sinuses secondary to inspissated mucus and the presence of heavy metals secreted by the fungus.[14] On MRI these hyperdense secretions appear of low signal on T2W images and can mimic air.[15]

In the immunocompromised (e.g., diabetics) an invasive fungal sinusitis can occur with aggressive bony erosion and invasion of the adjacent cavernous sinuses, orbital apex, and the brain (Fig. 3.6).[16] Patients may present with headache or visual symptoms secondary to involvement of the traversing cranial nerves. Life-threatening vascular injury may also occur with cavernous sinus thrombosis and the development of pseudoaneurysms from the adjacent carotid arteries. Overall mortality is in the range of 50%–80%, although reversal of the predisposing condition, e.g., neutropenia, administration of antifungal therapy, and radical surgical debridement, can reduce mortality by up to 18%.[17]

Paranasal sinus malignancies comprise only 0.2% of all malignancies, with 80% occurring in the maxillary sinuses. Primary sphenoid sinus neoplasms are extremely rare, accounting for only 1%–2% of paranasal sinus malignancies.[18] Squamous cell carcinoma, sinonasal undifferentiated carcinoma, and adenoid cystic carcinoma may be encountered. As with infective processes, malignancies commonly present with cranial nerve neuropathies, which is a poor prognostic sign. MRI is useful to delineate the tumor extent from the underlying associated inflammatory changes and to access for intracranial extension. Unfortunately, surgery is rarely curative because of an advanced state of disease at presentation, and aggressive multidisciplinary management, including chemotherapy and radiotherapy, can maximize patient outcomes.[19]

### Foraminal Lesions
#### Orbital apex
The optic canal and superior orbital fissure form the bony orbital apex, which acts as the transition zone for numerous neurovascular structures entering the orbit from the cranium. Lesions at the orbital apex are clinically important, as they can adversely affect vision and lead to ophthalmoplegia.[5] Orbital apex syndrome (Jacod syndrome) is the collective term for cranial nerve deficits associated with a mass lesion at the orbital apex.

A broad range of lesions can occur at this site. Primary tumors are rare and in children include rhabdomyosarcoma. This lesion can be very large at presentation and leads to extensive bony destruction and intracranial involvement. Meningiomas may arise along the optic nerve sheath with classical tram track calcification on CT, although orbital extension of an intracranial meningioma is more common.[20] Optic gliomas (Fig. 3.7) and nerve sheath tumors such as schwannomas may also occur, with the former having a well-documented association with neurofibromatosis type 1.[21] Optic gliomas occur in up to 30% of patients with neurofibromatosis type 1 and most commonly present in childhood.[22] Primary lymphoma has been noted in this region, but is more commonly seen as part of a secondary generalized process.

Malignant spread to the orbital apex from the posterior nasal cavity and nasopharynx is well documented. This most commonly occurs secondary to nasopharyngeal carcinoma (Fig. 3.8) and salivary gland neoplasms, including adenoid cystic carcinoma, which has a high propensity for perineural involvement (31%–96%).[23] Malignant lesions initially gain access to the pterygopalatine fossa from the nasal cavity via the sphenopalatine foramen. Once at this important neurovascular crossroad, spread through the inferior orbital fissure and involvement of the orbit and orbital apex may occur (Fig. 3.8).[24] Obliteration of the normal fat in the pterygopalatine fossa is the earliest sign of malignant infiltration. This may be seen on both CT and MRI but is best demonstrated on MRI using high-resolution precontrasted axial T1W images.[25]

Idiopathic inflammatory pseudotumor (IIP) can also present with acute orbital apex syndrome, most commonly with painful ophthalmoplegia. The condition

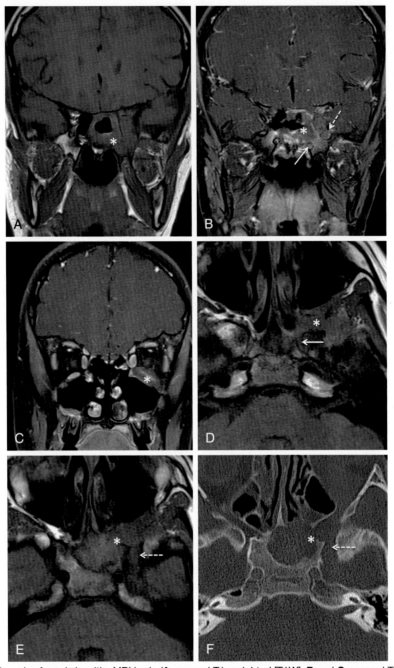

FIG. 3.6 Invasive fungal sinusitis. MRI brain (**A**, coronal T1-weighted [T1W]; **B** and **C**, coronal T1W postcontrast; **D** and **E**, axial T1W; **F**, axial CT bone windows): Heterogeneous T1W iso- to hyperintense opacification and enhancement of the sphenoid sinus is seen with invasion into the left body and greater wing of the sphenoid (*asterisk* in **A** and **B**). There is extension into the inferior orbit (*asterisk* in **C**) and pterygopalatine fossa/sphenopalatine foramen (*asterisk* in **D**) and dehiscence of the left lateral sphenoid sinus wall (*asterisk* in **E** and **F**). The lesion is seen extending into the foramen rotundum and vidian canal because of perineural invasion along the left V2 (*dashed arrows* in **B** and **E**) and vidian nerve (*solid arrows* in **B** and **D**), respectively. There is also extension to the superior orbital fissure and cavernous sinus. The left foramen rotundum is widened on the CT (*dashed arrow* in **F**).

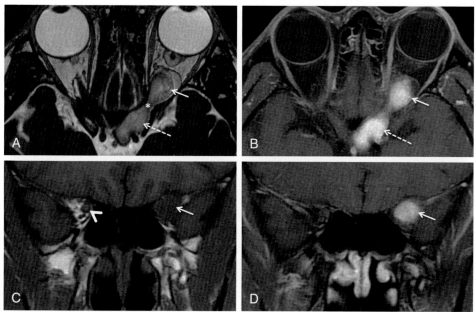

FIG. 3.7 Left optic glioma. MRI brain and orbits (**A**, axial T2-weighted [T2W]; **B**, axial T1-weighted [T1W] postcontrast; **C**, coronal T1W precontrast; and **D**, coronal T1W postcontrast). Fusiform expansion of the left optic nerve is seen from the intraorbital portion (*solid arrows* in **A–D**) extending to the prechiasmatic portion and chiasm (*dashed arrows* in **A** and **B**) with expansion of the left optic canal (*asterisk* in **A**). The nerve shows increased signal on T2W images and hypointense T1W signal with homogeneous enhancement on the postcontrast images. The normal right optic nerve is highlighted (*arrowhead* in **C**).

is a nonspecific, nonneoplastic inflammatory process with no identifiable local or systemic cause. IIP is a diagnosis of exclusion, and biopsy should be performed to exclude neoplastic or infective etiologies. On biopsy, polymorphous lymphoid infiltrate with varying degrees of fibrosis is apparent.[26,27]

On CT and MRI, IIP typically appears as an infiltrative, diffusely enhancing lesion involving the orbit alone. On MRI the lesion appears isointense compared with grey matter on T1W images and iso- to hypointense on T2W images, with greater fibrosis leading to increased hypointensity. Intracranial involvement is unusual, but extension through the superior orbital fissure to the cavernous sinus, middle cranial fossa meninges, and Meckel cave can occur (Fig. 3.9). Differentiation from an en-plaque meningioma (Fig. 3.10) along the middle cranial fossa can be difficult, although IIP rarely shows underlying sphenoid bone erosion or hyperostosis.[28,29]

Other conditions occurring at the orbital apex include optic neuritis (most often associated with multiple sclerosis), metastases (most commonly breast and lung), and inflammatory disease including sarcoidosis.[30] Infection is unusual but typically occurs because

of paranasal sinusitis, either directly from the sphenoid sinus as discussed previously or because of extension of orbital cellulitis.[31]

Bony injury at the orbital apex is not uncommon in the context of major craniofacial trauma. Extensive additional fractures are typically seen involving structures such as the sphenoid sinus, greater and lesser wings, and pterygoid plates.[32,33] Visual loss caused by optic nerve contusion or transection may occur with or without fractures.[34] Injury resulting in a caroticocavernous fistula (CCF) usually presents clinically with headache, pulsatile proptosis, and orbital edema/erythema. Imaging readily demonstrates enlargement of the superior ophthalmic veins and cavernous sinuses. Although CT and MR angiography are suggestive, definitive confirmation of a CCF using digital subtraction angiography is required (Fig. 3.11). This demonstrates early filling of the cavernous sinus and outflow pathways, including retrograde filling of the superior ophthalmic vein, petrosal and sigmoid sinuses, and facial veins. Endovascular treatment of CCF is performed, and options include transarterial-transfistula balloon embolization, stent placement, or internal carotid artery sacrifice.[35]

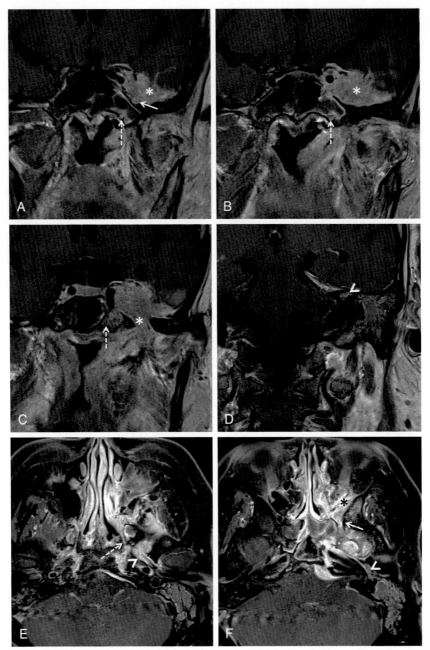

FIG. 3.8 Nasopharyngeal carcinoma with extensive perineural, orbital and intracranial involvement. MRI skull base (a-d: Coronal T1W post-contrast, e&f- Axial T1W post-contrast). There is a left nasopharyngeal carcinoma with enhancing soft tissue compatible with invasion into the sphenoid sinus, left sphenoid body, left pterygopalatine fossa, middle cranial fossa (* in a and b), and cavernous sinus with extension posteriorly along the left tentorium leaflet. There is extensive enhancing perineural invasion at the left foramen rotundum along V2 (solid arrows a and f), left foramen ovale along V3 (* in c) and vidian canal along the vidian nerve (dashed arrows a, b, c and e) extending posteriorly along the greater superficial petrosal nerve (arrowheads in d and e) to the geniculate ganglion of the facial nerve (arrowhead in f). Additional orbital extension through the inferior orbital fissure is apparent (* in f) along with involvement of the posterior fossa.

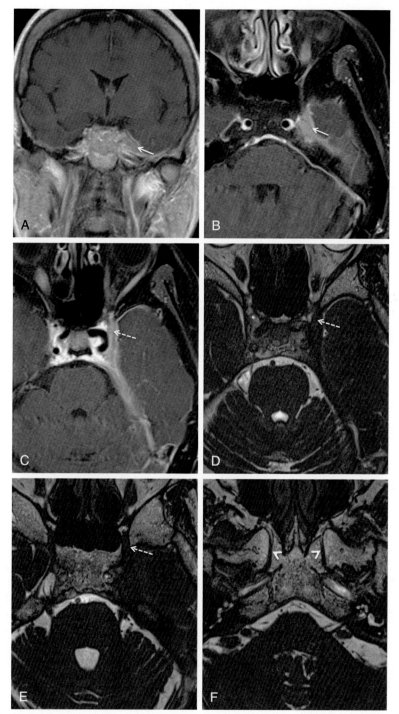

**FIG. 3.9** Idiopathic inflammatory pseudotumor involving the left cavernous sinus, orbital apex, and foramen rotundum/V2 nerve. MRI brain and orbits (**A**, coronal T1-weighted [T1W] postcontrast; **B** and **C**, axial T1W postcontrast; **D–F**, axial T2-weighted constructive interference in steady state [CISS] sequences from superior to inferior). Enhancing soft tissue is seen at the left cavernous sinus/parasellar region (*solid arrows* in **A** and **B**), with extension to the orbital apex, left tentorium, and left foramen rotundum with thickening and enhancement of the left V2 nerve (*dashed arrows* in **C–E**). The left foramen rotundum is expanded. In contrast, the lower vidian canals appear within normal limits (*arrowheads* in **F**). CISS sequences provide high-resolution imaging of the skull base foramina and cranial nerves. Note the normal-caliber left internal carotid artery **(C)**. Considerations in this case include pseudotumor or Tolosa-Hunt syndrome (this patient presented with painful ophthalmoplegia, which is a typical feature of the condition), lymphoma, meningioma (typically narrow the adjacent internal carotid artery), or infection (less likely given the absence of adjacent sinusitis).

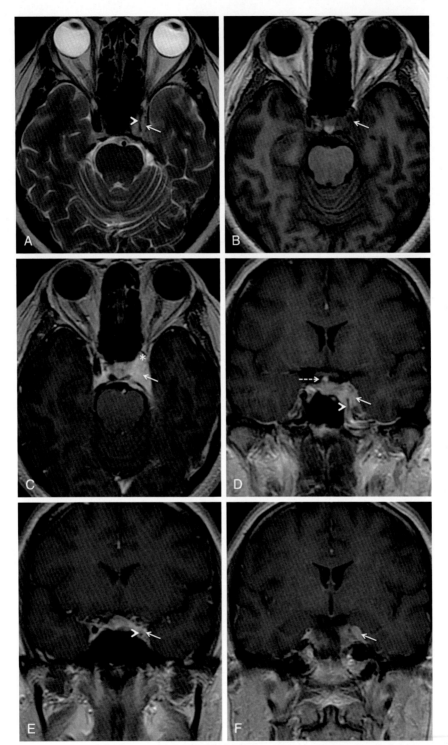

FIG. 3.10 Cavernous sinus and superior orbital fissure lesion. MRI (**A**, axial T2-weighted [T2W]; **B**, axial T1-weighted [T1W] precontrast; **C**, axial T1W postcontrast; **D–F**, coronal postcontrast from anterior to posterior). There is narrowing of the cavernous portion of the left internal carotid artery (*arrowheads* in **A, D,** and **E**) with surrounding T2W hyperintense (*arrow* in **A**), T1W isointense (*arrow* in **B**), and enhancing (*arrows* in **C–F**) soft tissue at the left cavernous sinus, sella (possible enhancement along the infundibulum, *dashed arrow* in **D**), superior orbital fissure (*asterisk* in **C**), and along the left tentorium. Given the narrowing of the left internal carotid artery a meningioma is favored. Other considerations include idiopathic inflammatory pseudotumor (Tolosa-Hunt syndrome) or a neoplastic lesion (e.g., lymphoma). The patient presented with left-sided sixth nerve palsy. The patient did not report any pain, which is a typical feature of Tolosa-Hunt syndrome.

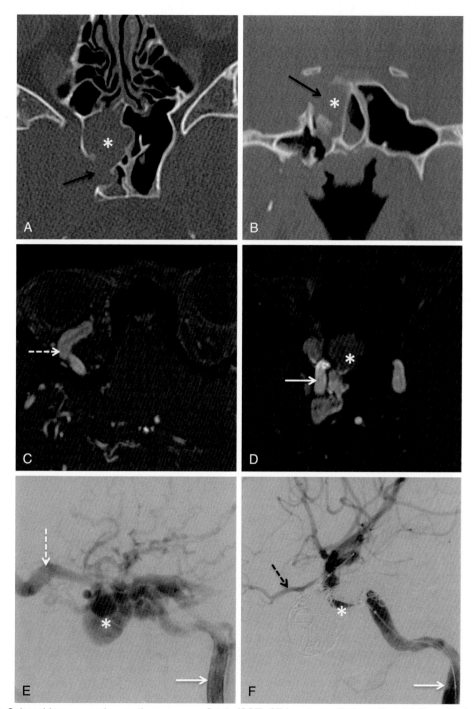

FIG. 3.11 Sphenoid trauma and a caroticocavernous fistula (CCF). CT face bone windows (**A**, axial; **B**, coronal), magnetic resonance angiography (MRA; **C** and **D**, axial), and digital subtraction angiography (DSA) of the right internal carotid artery (ICA; **E**, preintervention; **F**, postembolization). Fractures are seen through the sphenoid body involving the walls of the right sphenoid sinus (*black arrows* in **A** and **B**). Soft tissue opacification of the right sphenoid sinus is seen (*asterisk* in **A** and **B**). MRA shows dilatation of the right superior ophthalmic vein (SOV; *dashed arrow* in **C**) secondary to arterialized flow from a large right ICA (*solid white arrows* **D**–**F**) to cavernous sinus fistula (CCF). A large pseudoaneurysm is seen in the sphenoid sinus corresponding to the soft tissue on CT (*asterisk* in **D**). DSA confirms a large right CCF (*asterisk* in **E**) with flow into a dilated right SOV (*dashed arrow* in **E**). Postembolization image shows no residual flow into the large CCF or SOV (*asterisk* shows coils in the CCF in **F**). Flow into the right ophthalmic artery is preserved (*dashed black arrow* in **F**).

*Foramen ovale, rotundum, and the vidian canal*
The trigeminal nerve (CN V) is the great sensory nerve of the head and neck and also provides innervation to the muscles of mastication. It is the largest cranial nerve and arises from the lateral pons coursing anterosuperiorly through the prepontine cistern to enter the Meckel cave through a dural opening called the porus trigeminus. The Gasserian or trigeminal ganglion is located within the cave and gives rise to three main branches, the ophthalmic (CN V1), maxillary (CN V2), and mandibular (CN V3) nerves. Trigeminal literally means "thrice twinned," referring to the fact that the paired trigeminal nerves give rise to three major branches each.

The ophthalmic (CN V1) and maxillary divisions of the trigeminal nerve (CN V2) pass through the lateral cavernous wall. The ophthalmic branch traverses the superior orbital fissure to enter the orbit and provides sensory innervation to the upper face and globe. The maxillary division of the trigeminal nerve (CN V2) exits the middle cranial fossa through the foramen rotundum. The nerve traverses the roof of the pterygopalatine fossa and continues anteriorly as the infraorbital nerve along the floor of the orbit. It exits the orbit via the infraorbital foramen and provides sensory innervation over the upper teeth and cheek.

The mandibular division of the trigeminal nerve (CN V3) exits Meckel cave directly through the foramen ovale without passing through the cavernous sinus. It enters the masticator space where it divides into several sensory branches (e.g., lingual nerve) and two main motor nerves, the mylohyoid and masticator nerves. Muscles of mastication are innervated by the masticator nerve, whereas the anterior belly of the digastric and mylohyoid muscles at the floor of the mouth are innervated by the mylohyoid nerve.

As discussed at the orbital apex, malignant lesions including nasopharyngeal carcinoma initially gain access to the pterygopalatine fossa from the nasal cavity.[36,37] From this neurovascular crossroads spread through the foramen rotundum along the maxillary nerve can occur (Fig. 3.8).[38] Retrograde extension along the nerve can occur into the cavernous sinus and Meckel cave with infiltration of the trigeminal ganglion and trigeminal nerve proper. It is worth bearing in mind that trigeminal neuralgia may be the first presentation of perineural disease.[39] The vidian nerve is also a target for perineural spread from the pterygopalatine fossa. Once involved the tumor may spread along the vidian nerve to the greater superficial petrosal nerve and facial nerve ganglion (Fig. 3.8).[40]

Perineural spread can also occur along the mandibular nerve through the foramen ovale to Meckel cave and beyond (Fig. 3.12).[41] Tumors that may yield mandibular nerve perineural spread include squamous cell carcinoma arising at the skin, tonsils, and nasopharynx; masticator space malignancies including lymphoma; and parotid tumors.[42] The latter may directly involve the masticator space, although spread along the auriculotemporal nerve (a facial nerve branch) to the mandibular nerve can occur.

MRI is more sensitive than CT for evaluating perineural tumor spread. MRI can show enlargement and enhancement of the nerves with loss of the surrounding fat planes best seen on high-resolution precontrast T1W images (Figs. 3.4 and 3.5).[43] Both antegrade and retrograde involvement of the nerves can be seen, with discontinuous "skip areas" sometimes apparent.[44] On CT the changes are more subtle, and additional smooth widening of the canals and foramina can be visualized (Fig. 3.12). Both modalities may also show masticator muscle denervation secondary to involvement of the mandibular nerve. In acute denervation, there may be swelling and enhancement with increased T2W signal on MRI. In chronic denervation the muscles show atrophy and fatty replacement with corresponding increased T1W signal on MRI.[45]

Fluorodeoxyglucose (FDG)-PET/CT is another modality that plays a key role in the workup and follow-up of many patients with head and neck malignancies. Perineural spread can be detected on this modality with knowledge of abnormal FDG uptake patterns and using the aforementioned CT findings.[46]

On all imaging modalities systematic interrogation of the symmetry and course of the nerves, fat planes, and innervated musculature is key to the detection of perineural disease.[47] Once present, this information is useful in treatment planning, as the entire course of the nerve should be included in the radiation field. In addition, perineural disease signifies a poorer prognosis with an increased risk of local recurrence and metastatic disease.[48]

Other abnormalities occurring along the branches of the trigeminal and facial nerves at the sphenoid bone include inflammatory conditions such as sarcoidosis, schwannomas, and neurofibromas. The last typically occurs in the context of neurofibromatosis. Skull base meningiomas may also infiltrate and extend through the sphenoid foramina, potentially mimicking perineural spread (Fig. 3.13).[46,49]

**Bone**

There are numerous developmental and sporadic abnormalities involving the sphenoid bone.[50] Of these, fibrous dysplasia and neurofibromatosis are the most common.[2]

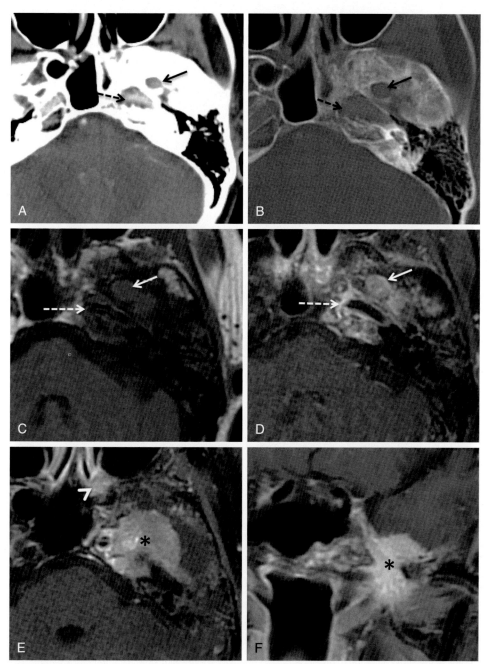

FIG. 3.12 Nasopharyngeal carcinoma with intracranial extension through the foramen ovale (T4 classification). CT brain (**A**, soft tissue postcontrast; **B**, bone windows) and MRI neck/brain (**C**, axial T1-weighted [T1W] precontrast; **D** and **E**, axial T1W postcontrast; **F**, coronal T1W postcontrast). The CT shows patchy sclerosis of the left greater sphenoid wing/body and petrous apex with enhancement within an expanded foramen ovale (*solid black arrows* **A** and **B**) and foramen lacerum (*dashed black arrows* **A** and **B**). Corresponding findings are seen on MRI involving the left greater sphenoid wing with enhancing soft tissue extending through the foramen ovale (likely perineural spread along the left V3 nerve, *solid white arrows* **C** and **D**) and surrounding the petrous portion of the internal carotid artery (likely spread through the foramen lacerum, *dashed arrows* in **C** and **D**). Enhancing soft tissue is also seen along the floor of the middle cranial fossa and close to the left cavernous sinus (*asterisk* in **E**). More anteriorly there is also enhancing soft tissue in the pterygopalatine fossa (*arrowhead* in **E**). The coronal image (**F**) demonstrates the enhancing soft tissue extending from the left parapharyngeal space through the foramen ovale (*asterisk*) into the middle cranial fossa and left cavernous sinus.

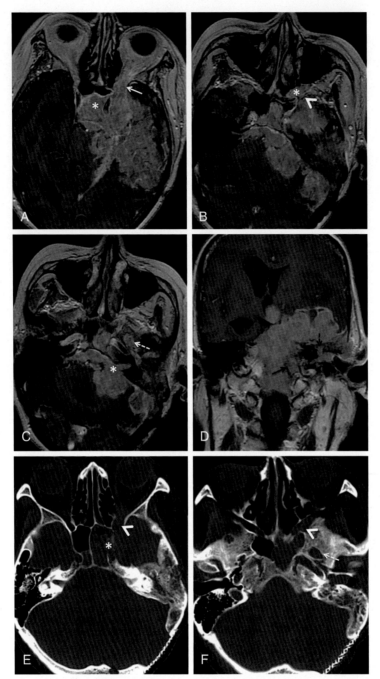

FIG. 3.13 Atypical meningioma at the middle cranial and posterior fossae with extensive perineural extension. MRI brain (**A–C**, axial T1-weighted [T1W] postcontrast sequences from superior to inferior, and **D**, coronal T1W postcontrast) and CT brain (**E** and **F**, bone windows). An extensive extraaxial atypical meningioma is seen along the middle cranial fossa, tentorium, and posterior fossa. There is involvement of the left superior orbital fissure (*arrow* in **A**), cavernous sinus, sella, sphenoid sinus (*asterisk* in **A**), pterygopalatine fossa (*asterisk* in **B**), left V2 nerve with widening of the foramen rotundum (*arrowheads* in **B** and **E**), left V3 nerve with widening of the foramen ovale (*dashed arrows* in **C** and **F**), petrous temporal bone and middle ear (*dashed black arrow* in **D**), prepontine space, and cerebellopontine angle with extension into the left internal auditory canal (*asterisk* in **C**). There is mass effect on the pons and middle cerebellar peduncle. On the coronal image the clivus is involved (*black arrow* in **D**), with enhancing soft tissue also extending into the third ventricle. The corresponding CT bone images show destruction of the left sphenoid sinus wall (*asterisk* in **E**), anterior clivus, and temporal bone/mastoid air cells, with extension into the overlying soft tissues (also seen on the MRI). Widening of the pterygopalatine fossa (*arrowhead* in **F**) is seen on the inferior CT bone windows. Prior unrelated left occipital cranioplasty noted in e&f.

Fibrous dysplasia may affect the skull base, calvarium, and facial bones, leading to the characteristic leontiasis ossea (lions facies) in the most advanced setting. The condition results from a defect in osteoblastic function, leading to progressive fibrous and immature bone replacement. The sphenoid, followed by the frontal bones, is the most commonly involved. The bone is typically expanded with foraminal narrowing best seen on CT, with associated narrowing of traversing vessels identified on CT and MR angiography.

Three patterns of involvement can occur in fibrous dysplasia: cystic (mainly lytic), pagetoid (mixed lytic and sclerotic), and a sclerotic type, which is the most common at the sphenoid and skull base. A classic "ground-glass" appearance has been well described on CT (Fig. 3.14), with more heterogeneous appearances not uncommon, especially on MRI (Fig. 3.15). Higher T2W signal can be seen in cystic areas, compared with lower signal in more ossified or fibrous regions. Variable enhancement is also common, with more intense enhancement seen at areas of greater fibrous tissue content.[51,52]

Neurofibromatosis refers to several hereditary conditions with a propensity for neurogenic tumor development. Up to a third of abnormalities occur in the head and neck, with type 1 neurofibromatosis the most likely etiology.[53] Orbital involvement is uncommon but can include plexiform neurofibromatosis, osseous dysplasia, and neoplasms. As discussed, at the orbital apex, optic nerve gliomas are the most common orbital tumor in neurofibromatosis.[54] Sphenoid and orbital osseous dysplasia typically occurs in association with plexiform neurofibromas, leading to proptosis, buphthalmos, and reduced vision. The greater and lesser wings are typically involved, and smooth enlargement of the sphenoid bone and optic foramina can also be seen as a result of plexiform neurofibroma infiltration of the cranial nerves.[55,56]

Destruction and sclerosis of the sphenoid bone may occur secondary to several neoplasms. The most common lesion is a metastasis, with breast, lung, and prostate tumors the most likely primaries. CT and MRI are complementary in detecting bony erosion and adjacent dural extension, respectively.[57] On MRI, diffusion-weighted imaging is particularly useful for the detection of metastases arising from breast and lung carcinomas but is relatively insensitive for the detection of prostate carcinoma metastases.[58] Radionuclide bone scans are another highly sensitive tool for detecting osseous metastases at the skull base and throughout the whole body in a single sitting.

Meningiomas at the middle cranial fossa can lead to bony erosion, hyperostosis, or permeative sclerosis of the underlying sphenoid bone (Fig. 3.16).[59] These changes may be due to tumor infiltration or a secondary reaction to local factors such as hyperperfusion.[60] Another rare presentation of skull base meningiomas is sphenoid pneumosinus dilatans.[61] Sphenoid bony changes noted on initial CT should be assessed using gadolinium-enhanced MRI. This modality is useful for identifying the extent of sheet-like en plaque meningioma along the middle cranial fossa and any associated extension through the neural foramina.[62,63]

Intense reactive sphenoid bone sclerosis has also been documented in nasopharyngeal carcinoma, both at presentation and secondary to the subsequent post-radiation changes.[64] Erosion of the sphenoid bone may also be seen in nasopharyngeal carcinoma with superior extension into the sphenoid sinus and posterior infiltration into the marrow-rich clivus (Fig. 3.17). On MRI, clival involvement may be suggested because of loss of the normal T1W hyperintense marrow signal.[65]

Primary bone tumors of the sphenoid bone are rare and include chordoma (Fig. 3.18), chondrosarcoma (Fig. 3.19), osteosarcoma (Fig. 3.20), and plasmacytoma. Osteosarcomas may be associated with preexisting lesions such as Paget disease or can be induced after radiation therapy for head and neck tumors.[66] Chordomas typically occur at the clivus in the midline arising from notochordal remnants with underlying bony erosion and internal calcifications. In comparison, chondrosarcomas typically occur off-midline at the petroclival fissure and can show ring and arc calcification on CT in 50% of cases with hyperintense T2W signal on MRI.[67]

## CONCLUSION

The sphenoid bone lies at the central skull base and is a key bridge between the orbit and intra- and extracranial structures. A clear understanding of the sphenoid bone anatomy, including the bony extensions and perforating foramina, is crucial in forming differential diagnoses and assessing for disease extent. Inflammatory and infective processes commonly involve the sphenoid sinus, with risk of life-threatening intracranial spread. Orbital and intracranial malignant perineural spread may also occur through the various foramina and may be easily missed without careful assessment. Bony erosion and sclerosis may occur because of tumors and various hereditary conditions, including neurofibromatosis.

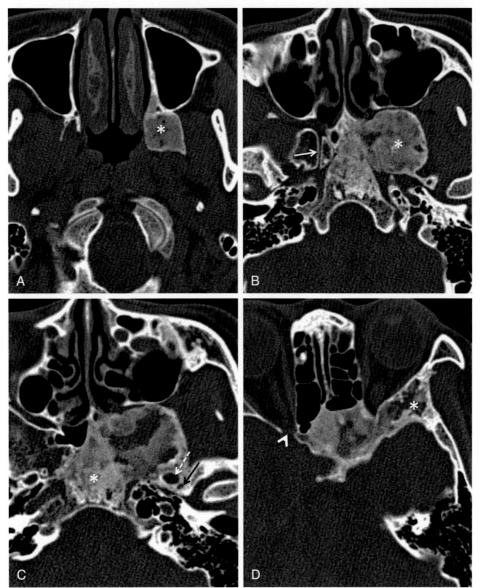

**FIG. 3.14** Fibrous dysplasia of the sphenoid. CT brain (**A–D**, axial bone windows from inferior to superior). There is expansion and predominantly "ground-glass" density of the left pterygoid (*asterisk* in **A**), sphenoid body (*asterisk* in **B**), clivus (*asterisk* in **C**), greater (*asterisk* in **D**), and lesser wings. There is resultant narrowing of the left-sided pterygopalatine fossa, vidian canal (*solid arrow* in **B** shows the unaffected side), and foramen rotundum (not shown). The foramen ovale (*dashed arrow* in **C**) and foramen spinosum (*black arrow* in **C**) are spared. The left superior orbital fissure is also markedly narrowed (*arrowhead* in **D** shows the unaffected side). No focal neurology was noted on history and examination to suggest cranial nerve compression, which is a potential complication of the condition.

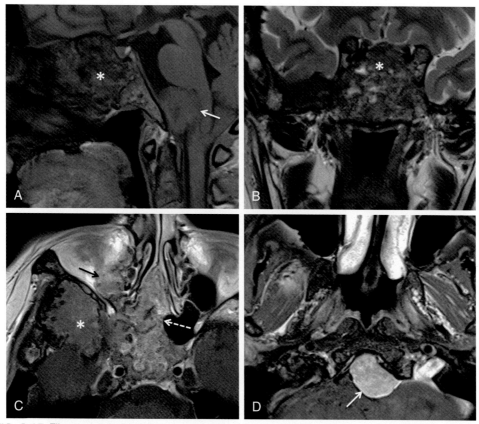

**FIG. 3.15** Fibrous dysplasia of the sphenoid with a clival meningioma. MRI brain (**A**, sagittal T1-weighted [T1W]; **B**, coronal T2-weighted [T2W]; **C** and **D**, axial T1W postcontrast superior to inferior). Bony expansion of the sphenoid is seen mainly involving the body (*asterisk* in **A** and **B**), right greater and lesser wings (*asterisk* in **C**) with encroachment into the right inferior orbit (*black arrow* in **C**), sphenoid sinus, and posterior nasal cavity (*dashed arrow* **C**). The bony involvement shows mixed T1W hypo- to isointensity and T2W hypo- and hyperintense regions with mild heterogeneous enhancement. These findings are suggestive of fibrous dysplasia of the skull base. Fibrous dysplasia has variable appearances on MRI. CT was advised for further assessment of the bony structures. An additional homogeneously enhancing extraaxial meningioma is seen along the clivus with compression and right-sided deviation of the brainstem (*solid arrows* **A** and **D**). No hydrocephalus was apparent.

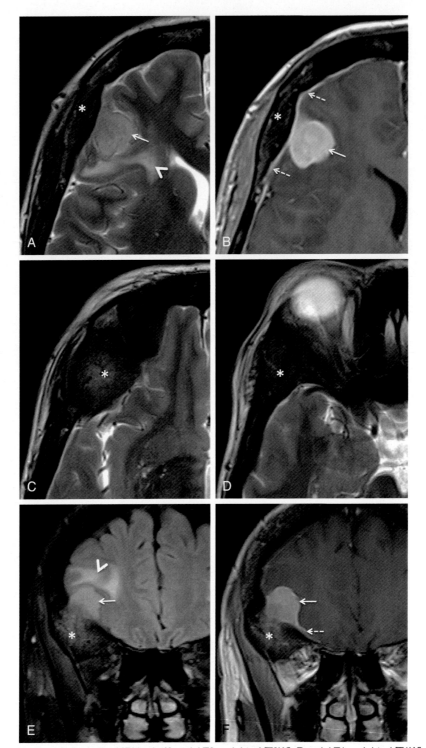

FIG. 3.16 Sphenoid wing meningioma. MRI brain (**A**, axial T2-weighted [T2W]; **B**, axial T1-weighted [T1W] postcontrast; **C** and **D**, axial T2W; **E**, coronal fluid attenuation inversion recovery; **F**, coronal T1W postcontrast). A slightly T2W hyperintense, homogeneously enhancing extraaxial lesion is seen along the right posterior frontal bone and greater sphenoid wing (*solid arrows* in **A**, **B**, **E**, and **F**) with a dural base and enhancing dural tails (*dashed arrows* in **B** and **F**). There is adjacent perilesional vasogenic edema (*arrowheads* in **A** and **E**). The underlying bone is thickened and expanded (*asterisk* in **A–C**) with encroachment into the right orbit (*asterisk* in **D**). There is mild enhancement and hyperintense T2W signal likely because of intraosseous extension of the meningioma and reactive hyperostosis (*asterisk* in **E** and **F**). No enhancing soft tissue was detected in the adjacent orbit.

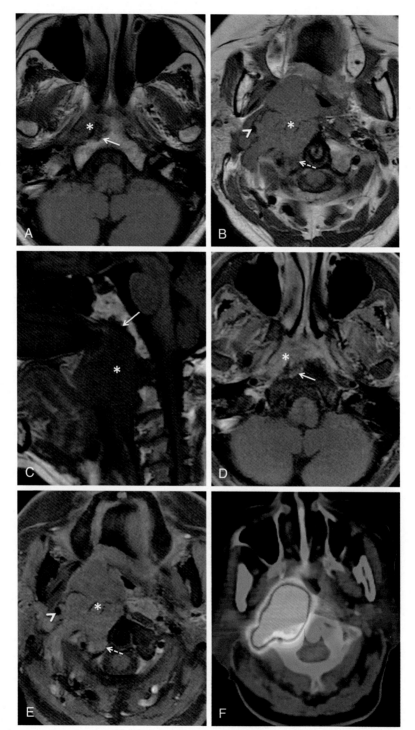

FIG. 3.17 Nasopharyngeal carcinoma with clival and atlas erosion. MRI brain (**A** and **B**, axial T1-weighted [T1W]; **C**, sagittal T1W; **D** and **E**, axial T1W postcontrast) and axial fused 18F-fluorodeoxyglucose (FDG)-PET/CT **(F)**. A large right nasopharyngeal mass is seen showing iso- to hypointensity on T1W images with enhancement (*asterisk* in **A–E**). There is invasion of the clivus (*solid arrows* in **A**, **C**, and **D**) and the right side of the atlas (*dashed arrows* in **B** and **E**). The lesion extends into the right carotid and parapharyngeal spaces and is in close relation to the right internal carotid artery (*arrowheads* in **B** and **E**) and right vertebral artery (lesion erodes into the right foramen transversarium). The nasopharyngeal mass shows marked hypermetabolic FDG uptake on the PET/CT study **(F)**.

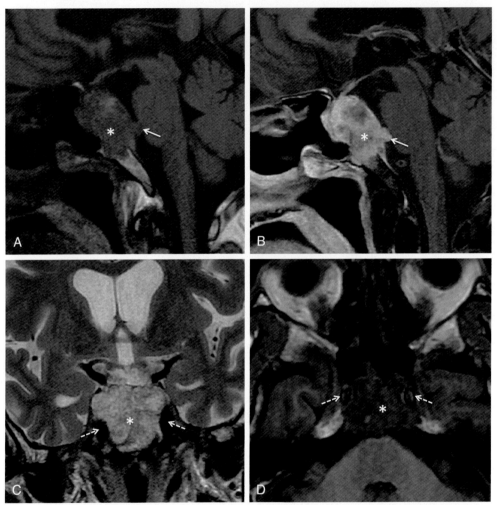

FIG. 3.18 Clival chordoma. MRI brain (**A**, sagittal T1-weighted [T1W] precontrast; **B**, sagittal T1W post-contrast; **C**, coronal T2-weighted [T2W]; and **D**, axial T1W precontrast). An expansile lobulated mass is seen involving the clivus (*asterisk* in **A–D**) with anterior bulging into the sphenoid sinus, involvement of the pituitary fossa, and extension into the prepontine region with abutment of the pons ("thumb" sign, *solid arrows* in **A** and **B**). The lesion shows heterogeneous T2W hyperintensity, T1W hypointensity, and heterogeneous enhancement. The bilateral internal carotid arteries are in close relation to the lesion, with preservation of the normal flow voids (*dashed arrows* in **C** and **D**).

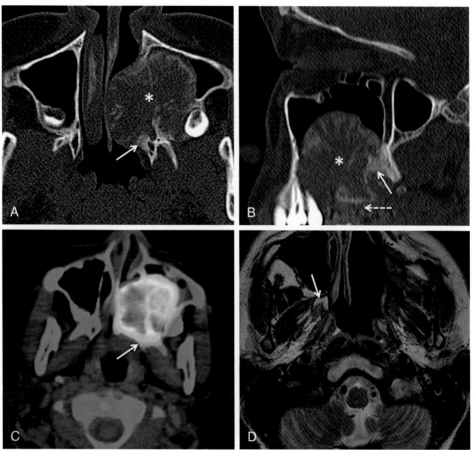

**FIG. 3.19** Chondrosarcoma. CT face (bone windows; **A**, axial; **B**, sagittal), 18F-fluorodeoxyglucose (FDG)-PET/CT (**C**, axial fused image), and MRI sinuses (**D**, axial T2-weighted image). An expansile mass (*asterisk* in **A** and **B**) is centered on the left medial maxillary wall with involvement of the inferior left pterygoid bone (*solid white arrows* in **A–D**, with the normal right pterygoid highlighted in **D**). There is extension into the left maxillary sinus, nasal cavity with abutment of the septum, and destruction of the upper left molars (*dashed arrow* in **B**). Densities noted within are compatible with chondroid calcifications on histology. Intense 18F-FDG PET activity is seen within the lesion compatible with a hypermetabolic, high-grade neoplastic lesion **(C)**. Postsurgical MRI **(D)** shows a wide resection including the left pterygoid.

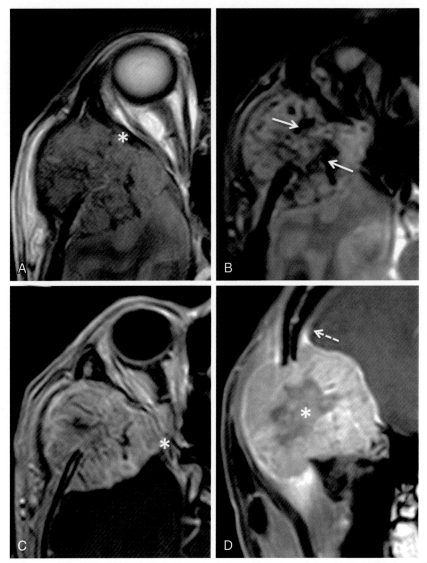

FIG. 3.20 Sphenoid wing osteosarcoma. MRI brain (a: axial T2W, b- axial gradient recalled echo (GRE) T2*, c- axial post-contrast T1W, and d- coronal T1W post contrast). A mixed iso to slightly T2W hyperintense lesion with marked contrast enhancement is seen arising from the right greater wing of the sphenoid with involvement and medial bowing of the right lateral orbital wall (* in a). Central areas of hypointense T2W signal and susceptibility on GRE are likely related to calcification or osteoid matrix (solid arrows in b). There is extension into the right orbit, superior orbital fissure and optic canal (* in c). Relative paucity of central enhancement is likely due to the central calcification (* in d). Dural involvement is seen with an enhancing dural tail (dashed arrow in d). This case shows that dural tails are not unique to meningiomas.

# REFERENCES

1. Mancall EL, Brock DG. Cranial fossae. In: *Gray's Clinical Neuroanatomy*. 1st ed. Philadelphia: WB Saunders; 2011:154.
2. Chong VF, Fan YF, Tng CH. Pictorial review: radiology of the sphenoid bone. *Clin Radiol*. 1998;53:882–893.
3. Schuenke M, Schulte E, Schumacher U, et al. Section 1.12 on sphenoid bone (cranial bones). In: Ross LM, Lamperti ED, Taub E, eds. *Head and Neuroanatomy (Thieme Atlas of Anatomy 1st Edition)*. New York: Thieme; 2011 (Section 1.12).
4. Fehrenbach MJ, Herring SW. Skeletal system. In: *Illustrated Anatomy of the Head and Neck*. Philadelphia: WB Saunders; 2012:52.
5. Daniels DL, Mark LP, Mafee MF, et al. Osseous anatomy of the orbital apex. *AJNR Am J Neuroradiol*. 1995;16:1929–1935.
6. Gray H. The sphenoid bone. In: *Gray's Anatomy of the Human Body*. 41st ed. 1918. Available at: http://www.bartleby.com/107/35.html.
7. Ginsberg LE, Pruett SW, Chen MY, Elster AD. Skull-base foramina of the middle cranial fossa: reassessment of normal variation with high-resolution CT. *AJNR Am J Neuroradiol*. 1994;15:283–291.
8. Sondheimer FK. Basal foramina and canals. In: Newton TH, Potts DG, eds. *Radiology of the Skull Base and Brain*. New York: Mosby; 1971:287–347.
9. Harnsberger HR, Osborn AG, Ross J, et al. *Diagnostic and Surgical Imaging Anatomy*. Salt Lake City, UT: Amirsys; 2006.
10. Osborn AG. Radiology of the pterygoid plates and pterygopalatine fossa. *AJR Am J Roentgenol*. 1979;132:389–394.
11. Dalgorf DM, Harvey RJ. Chapter 1: sinonasal anatomy and function. *Am J Rhinol Allergy*. 2013;27:S3–S6.
12. Som PM, Brandwein M. Sinonasal cavities: inflammatory diseases, tumors, fractures, and postoperative findings. In: Som PM, Curtin HD, eds. *Head and Neck Imaging*. 3rd ed. St Louis: Mosby; 1996:126–315.
13. Eggesbø HB. Radiological imaging of inflammatory lesions in the nasal cavity and paranasal sinuses. *Eur Radiol*. 2006;16:872–888.
14. Zinreich SJ, Kennedy DW, et al. Fungal sinusitis; diagnosis with CT and MR imaging. *Radiology*. 1988;169:439–444.
15. Chong VF, Fan YF. Comparison of CT and MRI features in sinusitis. *Eur J Radiol*. 1998;29:47–54.
16. Mossa-Basha M, Ilica AT, Maluf F, Karakoç Ö, Izbudak I, Aygün N. The many faces of fungal disease of the paranasal sinuses: CT and MRI findings. *Diagn Interv Radiol*. 2013;19:195–200.
17. Aribandi M, McCoy VA, Bazan C. Imaging features of invasive and noninvasive fungal sinusitis: a review. *Radiographics*. 2007;27:1283–1296.
18. DeMonte F, Ginsberg LE, Clayman GL. Primary malignant tumors of the sphenoidal sinus. *Neurosurgery*. 2000;46:1084–1091. Discussion 1091–1092.
19. Vedrine PO, Thariat J, Merrot O, et al. Primary cancer of the sphenoid sinus–a GETTEC study. *Head Neck*. 2009;31:388–397.
20. Hallinan JT, Hegde AN, Lim WE. Dilemmas and diagnostic difficulties in meningioma. *Clin Radiol*. 2013;68:837–844.
21. Goh PS, Gi MT, Charlton A, Tan C, Gangadhara Sundar JK, Amrith S. Review of orbital imaging. *Eur J Radiol*. 2008;66:387–395.
22. Vohra ST, Escott EJ, Stevens D, Branstetter BF. Categorization and characterization of lesions of the orbital apex. *Neuroradiology*. 2011;53:89–107.
23. Barrett AW, Speight PM. Perineural invasion in adenoid cystic carcinoma of the salivary glands: a valid prognostic indicator? *Oral Oncol*. 2009;45:936–940.
24. Daniels DL, Rauschning W, Lovas J, Williams AL, Haughton VM. Pterygopalatine fossa: computed tomographic studies. *Radiology*. 1983;149:511–516.
25. Chong VFH, Fan YF, Khoo JBK, Lim TA. Comparing CT and MRI visualisation of the pterygopalatine fossa. *Ann Acad Med*. 1995;24:436–441.
26. Mangiardi JR, Har-El G. Extraorbital skull base idiopathic pseudotumor. *Laryngoscope*. 2007;117:589–594.
27. Narla LD, Newman B, Spottswood SS, Narla S, Kolli R. Inflammatory pseudotumor. *Radiographics*. 2003;23:719–729.
28. Lee EJ, Jung SL, Kim BS, et al. MR imaging of orbital inflammatory pseudotumors with extraorbital extension. *Korean J Radiol*. 2005;6:82–88.
29. Bencherif B, Zouaoui A, Chedid G, Kujas M, Van Effenterre R, Marsault C. Intracranial extension of an idiopathic orbital inflammatory pseudotumor. *AJNR Am J Neuroradiol*. 1993;14:181–184.
30. Chong VF, Fan YF, Chan LL. Radiology of the orbital apex. *Australas Radiol*. 1999;43:294–302.
31. Sobol SE, Marchand J, Tewfik TL, Manoukian JJ, Schloss MD. Orbital complications of sinusitis in children. *J Otolaryngol*. 2002;31:131–136.
32. Hopper RA, Salemy S, Sze RW. Diagnosis of midface fractures with CT: what the surgeon needs to know. *Radiographics*. 2006;26:783–793.
33. Winegar BA, Murillo H, Tantiwongkosi B. Spectrum of critical imaging findings in complex facial skeletal trauma. *Radiographics*. 2013;33:3–19.
34. Sarkies N. Traumatic optic neuropathy. *Eye*. 2004;18:1122–1125.
35. Chi CT, Nguyen D, Duc VT, Chau HH, Son VT. Direct traumatic carotid cavernous fistula: angiographic classification and treatment strategies. Study of 172 cases. *Interv Neuroradiol*. 2014;20:461–475.
36. Curtin HD, Williams R, Johnson J. CT of perineural tumor extension: pterygopalatine fossa. *Am J Neuroradiol*. 1984;5:731–737.
37. Chong VFH, Fan YF, Khoo JBK. Nasopharyngeal carcinoma with intracranial spread: CT and MRI characteristics. *J Comput Assist Tomogr*. 1996;20:563–639.
38. Chong VFH, Fan YF. Pictorial essay: maxillary nerve involvement in nasopharyngeal carcinoma. *Am J Roentgenol*. 1996;167:1309–1312.
39. Chong VFH. Trigeminal neuralgia in nasopharyngeal carcinoma. *J Laryngol Otol*. 1996;110:394–396.

40. Ginsberg LE, De Monte F, Gillenwater AM. Greater superficial petrosal nerve: anatomy and MR findings in perineural tumor spread. *Am J Neuroradiol.* 1996;17:389–393.

41. Chong VFH. Masticator space in nasopharyngeal carcinoma. *Ann Otol Laryngol.* 1997;106:979–982.

42. Ong CK, Chong VF. Imaging of perineural spread in head and neck tumours. *Cancer Imaging.* 2010;10:S92–S98.

43. Ginsberg LE. MR imaging of perineural tumor spread. *Magn Reson Imaging Clin N Am.* 2002;10:511–525.

44. Nemec SF, Herneth AM, Czerny C. Perineural tumor spread in malignant head and neck tumors. *Top Magn Reson Imaging.* 2007;18:467–471.

45. Fleckenstein JL, Watumull D, Conner KE, et al. Denervated human skeletal muscle: MR imaging evaluation. *Radiology.* 1993;187:213–218.

46. Paes FM, Singer AD, Checkver AN, Palmquist RA, De La Vega G, Sidani C. Perineural spread in head and neck malignancies: clinical significance and evaluation with 18F-FDG PET/CT. *Radiographics.* 2013;33:1717–1736.

47. Maroldi R, Farina D, Borghesi A, Marconi A, Gatti E. Perineural tumor spread. *Neuroimaging Clin N Am.* 2008;18:413–429.

48. Warden KF, Parmar H, Trobe JD. Perineural spread of cancer along the three trigeminal divisions. *J Neuroophthalmol.* 2009;29:300–307.

49. Walton H, Morley S, Alegre-Abarrategui J. A rare case of atypical skull base meningioma with perineural spread. *J Radiol Case Rep.* 2015;9:1–14.

50. Braun IF, Nadel L. The central skull base. In: Som PM, Bergeron RT, eds. *Head and Neck Imaging.* 2nd ed. New York: Mosby; 1991:903–924.

51. Jee WH, Choi KH, Choe BY, Park JM, Shinn KS. Fibrous dysplasia: MR imaging characteristics with radiopathologic correlation. *AJR Am J Roentgenol.* 1996;167:1523–1527.

52. Chong VF, Khoo JB, Fan YF. Fibrous dysplasia involving the base of the skull. *AJR Am J Roentgenol.* 2002;178:717–720.

53. Zimmerman RA, Bilaniuk LT, Mezger RA, et al. Computed tomography of orbitofacial neurofibromatosis. *Radiology.* 1983;146:113–116.

54. Aoki S, Barkovich AJ, Nishimura K, et al. Neurofibromatosis types 1 and 2: cranial MR findings. *Radiology.* 1989;172:527–534.

55. Jacquemin C, Bosley TM, Svedberg H. Orbit deformities in craniofacial neurofibromatosis type 1. *AJNR Am J Neuroradiol.* 2003;24:1678–1682.

56. Jacquemin C, Bosley TM, Liu D, Svedberg H, Buhaliqa A. Reassessment of sphenoid dysplasia associated with neurofibromatosis type 1. *AJNR Am J Neuroradiol.* 2002;23:644–648.

57. Maroldi R, Ambrosi C, Farina D. Metastatic disease of the brain: extra-axial metastases (skull, dura, leptomeningeal) and tumour spread. *Eur Radiol.* 2005;15:617–626.

58. Nemeth AJ, Henson JW, Mullins ME, Gonzalez RG, Schaefer PW. Improved detection of skull metastasis with diffusion-weighted MR imaging. *AJNR Am J Neuroradiol.* 2007;28:1088–1092.

59. Terstegge K, Schörner W, Henkes H, Heye N, Hosten N, Lanksch WR. Hyperostosis in meningiomas: MR findings in patients with recurrent meningioma of the sphenoid wings. *AJNR Am J Neuroradiol.* 1994;15:555–560.

60. Goyal N, Kakkar A, Sarkar C, Agrawal D. Does bony hyperostosis in intracranial meningioma signify tumor invasion? A radio-pathologic study. *Neurol India.* 2012;60:50–54.

61. Miller NR, Golnik KC, Zeidman SM, North RB. Pneumosinus dilatans: a sign of intracranial meningioma. *Surg Neurol.* 1996;46:471–474.

62. Valvassori GE, Buckingham RA. Tumors. In: Valvassori GE, Mafee MF, Carter BL, eds. *Imaging of Head and Neck.* New York: Thieme; 1995:110–131.

63. Li Y, Shi JT, An YZ, et al. Sphenoid wing meningioma en plaque: report of 37 cases. *Chin Med J.* 2009;122:2423–2427.

64. Chong VFH, Fan YF. Pterygopalatine fossa and maxillary nerve infiltration in nasopharyngeal carcinoma. *Head Neck.* 1997;19:121–125.

65. Chong VFH, Fan YF. Skull base erosion in nasopharyngeal carcinoma: detection by CT and MRI. *Clin Radiol.* 1996;51:625–631.

66. Hansen MR, Moffat JC. Osteosarcoma of the skull base after radiation therapy in a patient with McCune-Albright syndrome: case report. *Skull Base.* 2003;13:79–83.

67. Almefty K, Pravdenkova S, Colli BO, Al-Mefty O, Gokden M. Chordoma and chondrosarcoma: similar, but quite different, skull base tumors. *Cancer.* 2007;110:2457–2467.

# CHAPTER 4

# Imaging in Endoscopic Endonasal Skull Base Surgery

DR. ERIC YS TING, MBBS (HONS), BSC (MEDICINE), FRANZCR •
DR. FIONA TING, MBBS (HONS), BSC (MEDICINE), MCLINEPID, FRACS (OHNS) •
DR. GHIM SONG CHIA, MD, FRCR •
YEW KWANG ONG, MBBS (HONS), DOHNS, MRCS, MMED (ORL) •
VINCENT CHONG, MD, MBA, MHPE, FRCR

## INTRODUCTION

The endoscopic endonasal approach has become the preferred surgical approach to many tumors of the ventral skull base, both benign and malignant. Although advances in surgical equipment and technique have played a role in the development, imaging remains one of the cornerstones to the endoscopic endonasal approach, playing an important role in the diagnosis from the preoperative planning stage to intraoperative navigation, postoperative complications, and beyond.

This chapter aims to familiarize radiologists with endoscopic endonasal skull base surgery, including an introduction to the surgical approach, preoperative imaging assessment, postoperative imaging, and follow-up.

## HISTORICAL PERSPECTIVE

In many ways, the endoscopic endonasal approach represents the confluence and continued evolution of surgical technology, drawing influences from a variety of surgical approaches: the transsphenoidal approach, which has for some time been the preferred approach in pituitary surgery; the open craniofacial approach, which has traditionally been the preferred approach to tumors of the ventral skull base; and endoscopic sinus surgery, which opened the door to the endonasal corridor.

The transsphenoidal approach dates back more than a century. Schloffer is generally regarded as the father of modern transsphenoidal surgery, having performed the first transsphenoidal resection of a pituitary tumor in 1907.[1] A number of others, including Oskar Hirsch, Harvey Cushing, and Norman Dott, used the technique; however, it was the French neurosurgeon Gerard Guiot who popularized the technique as the preferred approach to the pituitary in 1956.[2,3] Jules Hardy, a student of Guiot, revolutionized the approach with the introduction of the operating microscope and microsurgical instrumentation in 1967.[2]

The history of anterior skull base surgery dates back to the 1940s, and the first transcranial excisions of orbital tumors were performed by Dandy and Ray and Mclean.[4] In the 1950s and 1960s, the anterior craniofacial approach emerged as the preferred approach for the resection of anterior skull base tumors after it was popularized by Ketcham et al. in 1963.[4,5] Since then, open craniofacial surgery has been the gold standard for surgical management of most tumors of the ventral skull base.

The history of endoscopic sinus surgery dates back to the 1970s, when an Austrian otolaryngologist, Messeklinger, and his protégé, Stammberger, popularized the operation as a treatment for chronic rhinosinusitis.[6,7] In 1996, McCutcheon et al. began using the endoscope to assist in the removal of the extracranial portions of anterior skull base tumors.[8] Thaler et al. expanded on this in 1999, pointing out potential indications for and advantages of using an endoscopic-assisted approach to anterior craniofacial resections.[9] By 2001, the first entirely endoscopic endonasal anterior skull base resections had been described by Casiano et al. for the resection of esthesioneuroblastomas.[10] Since then, the endoscope has become an essential tool in the armamentarium of the skull base surgeon, and its use has extended well beyond the sellar region to tumors primarily arising from the anterior cranial fossa, parasellar region, parts of the middle cranial fossa, paraclival region, and craniovertebral junction.

## PREOPERATIVE PLANNING

All patients planned for endoscopic skull base surgery should undergo complete clinical and radiologic evaluations when decision is made whether or not a certain tumor is suitable for excision via an endoscopic endonasal approach. MRI and CT are often used in concert, providing information that is complementary. For example, CT performs better for the assessment of the bony involvement and anatomic features, such as the extent of pneumatization, whereas MRI is generally better at resolving soft tissue details. Certain skull base lesions, such as the cholesterol granuloma, fibrous dysplasia, or juvenile angiofibroma, have imaging characteristics that can be diagnosed before biopsy, potentially expediting further management decisions. Radiologic evaluation before biopsy is also useful for identifying situations where biopsy is contraindicated, such as in highly vascular lesions or potential "do not touch" lesions, such as arrested pneumatization, aneurysm, or meningoencephalocele (Fig. 4.1). The imaging is also integral to the actual surgery, as volumetric MRI and CT datasets are typically used for intraoperative navigation.

Multislice CT scanners allow the acquisition of high-resolution, thin-slice images within seconds. These images can be viewed as multiplanar and three-dimensional (3D) reformations for preoperative planning and intraoperative navigation. Reconstruction using a bone algorithm allows accurate assessment of the bony architecture. The presence of bony remodeling or bony invasion can help to differentiate an expanding lesion from an invasive process (Fig. 4.2). CT is superior to MR in recognizing important bony anatomic variants that have surgical implications, such as the degree of pneumatization or hyperostosis of the sphenoid sinus, osseous course of the ethmoidal arteries below the skull base, dehiscence or variant septal attachment along the carotid canal, and bony impressions of the internal carotid arteries (ICAs), as well as any dehiscence or variant pneumatization along the optic nerve canals (Onodi cells). Other surgical landmarks that may be useful include identification of any dehiscence of the lamina papyracea, the height of the lateral lamella or depth of the olfactory fossa, and any asymmetry of the skull base, particularly the cribriform plates and fovea ethmoidalis.

High-resolution pre- and post-gadolinium-enhanced MRI sequences are useful for lesion localization, determination of the degree of orbital involvement; assessment of skull base, dural, and intracranial extension; and planning of the surgical approach. A high tissue contrast allows identification of critical neurovascular structures, including the cranial nerves (particularly the optic nerves, chiasm, and tracts), ICAs, circle of Willis, and cavernous sinus in relation to the lesion.

Depending on the nature of the lesion, tumor extent is usually best assessed on contrast-enhanced T1-weighted (T1W) sequences. Tumor enhancement is typically less than that of normal mucosa and can be recognized as an intermediate shade of gray on contrast-enhanced sequences (affectionately known as the "evil gray").[11] The pattern of the enhancement of a mass allows the differentiation of tumor from normal mucoperiosteum, inflammatory polyps, obstructive or inflammatory secretions, and inspissated debris.

Bony invasion should also be recognized preoperatively. In our institution, high-resolution, non-fat-suppressed spin-echo T1W pre- and post-gadolinium-enhanced sequences are employed to provide a detailed anatomy of the skull base and soft tissues. Replacement of the normal hyperintense fat signal in the bone marrow often serves as early evidence of disease involvement, and the enhancement pattern can help the clinician to distinguish between edema and tumor infiltration.

The periorbita is one of the key landmarks in preoperative planning. Not only does the fibrous periorbita represent a relative barrier to the spread of tumor, but it also, when breached, can have grave implications in terms of resectability, morbidity, and prognosis. The interface between tumor and orbit should be carefully assessed and described in the radiology report. The normal periorbita is seen as a thin, hypointense line when viewed perpendicularly on T1W and T2-weighted (T2W) MRI sequences. It is usually best assessed on T2W sequences. Some tumors displace the periorbita without invading it, and these tumors may be safely removed without the need for orbital exenteration. Therefore, it is important to determine whether the periorbita is truly breached or simply displaced. On imaging, the periorbita is considered intact if the linear hypointense signal of the periorbita remains visible at the interface between tumor and orbital fat (Fig. 4.3).[12] The displaced but intact periorbita is typically bowed into the orbit but tapers smoothly toward the point at which it remains attached to the bone.[11] Findings that suggest periorbital invasion include disruption of the hypointense linear signal (Fig. 4.4) or an irregular interface between the tumor and the orbit, with infiltration of the orbital fat (Fig. 4.5). In some cases, particularly at curved or oblique surfaces, doubt will remain. Standard axial and coronal planes may be combined with carefully planned oblique or 3D sequences when a particular interface is in question.

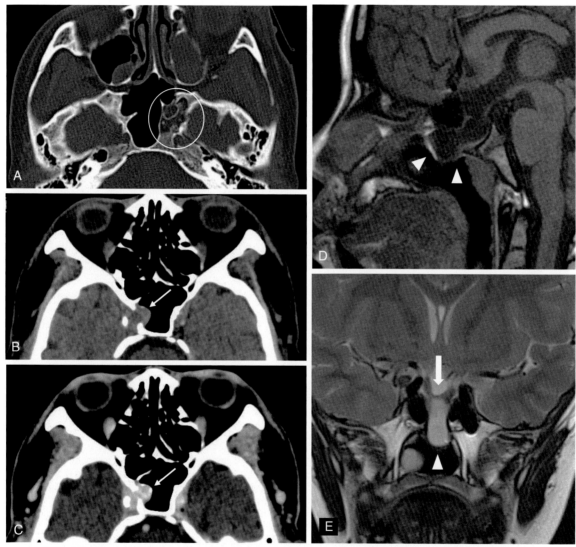

FIG. 4.1 Examples of "do not touch" lesions: Axial CT image **(A)** shows the typical appearance of arrested pneumatization, a nonexpansile lesion with internal curvilinear calcifications, sclerotic margins, and fat density (*circled*). Internal carotid artery pseudoaneurysm **(B and C)**: Axial non-contrast- and contrast-enhanced CT images show a bony defect in the sphenoid sinus wall, with contiguous, enhancing soft tissue protruding through the defect. Note the subtle rim calcification, which should alert the radiologist to the diagnosis (*thin arrows*). In this case, the pseudoaneurysm was related to invasive fungal infection. Sagittal T1-weighted **(D)** and coronal T2-weighted **(E)** images show a transsellar, transsphenoidal encephalocele (*arrowheads* in **D** and **E**) at the location of the craniopharyngeal canal. There is slight prolapse of the optic chiasm inferiorly (*thick arrow* in **E**).

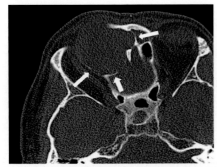

FIG. 4.2 Bony remodeling and expansion. Axial CT (bone algorithm) shows bony remodeling and expansion (*arrows*) in this right frontal mucocele. These are features of a relatively indolent, slowly expansile lesion. Such a process is unlikely to have breached the periorbita despite significant orbital compression.

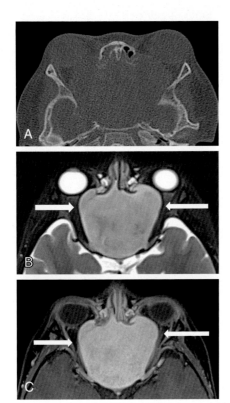

FIG. 4.3 Intact periorbita **(A)**. Axial CT shows dehiscence of the lamina papyracea. Axial fat-suppressed T2-weighted (*arrows* in **B**) and postgadolinium T1-weighted (*arrows* in **C**) images. The low signal of the periorbita is clearly intact, indicating the periorbita has not been breached.

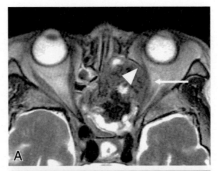

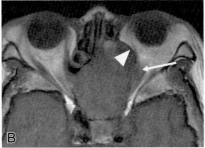

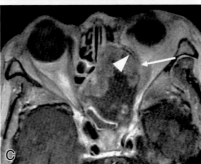

FIG. 4.4 Invasion of the periorbita by squamous cell carcinoma. Axial T2-weighted **(A)**, T1-weighted (T1W) **(B)**, and postgadolinium T1W **(C)** images. The periorbita is partially indistinct (*thin arrows*), indicating invasion. The intact portion of the periorbita remains clearly visible (*arrowheads*).

Another important imaging feature is the extent of intracranial involvement. Sagittal and coronal sequences are generally more useful than axial sequences when assessing intracranial extension in the anterior cranial fossa. CT is useful to determine the extent of bony involvement. Bony erosion is often seen as a sign of periosteal invasion. Again, it is important to distinguish aggressive patterns of bone erosion from more indolent remodeling and demineralization, where the periosteum may remain intact. MRI is the modality of choice for the assessment of intracranial involvement. To enter the intracranial compartment,

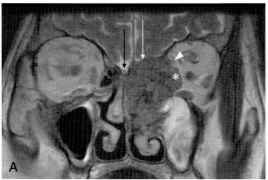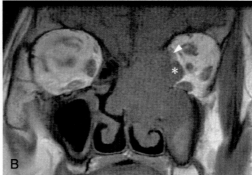

FIG. 4.5 Invasion of the periorbita by squamous cell carcinoma **(A and B)**. Coronal T2-weighted and T1-weighted images show infiltration and loss of fat plane between the tumor and the medial rectus (*asterisk*) and superior oblique muscle bellies (*arrowheads*). Note that there is also intradural extension (*thin white arrow* in **A**). The left olfactory nerve is engulfed by tumor, whereas the right olfactory nerve (*thin black arrow* in **A**) is normal.

tumor must first cross the bone and its double-layered periosteum. From there, tumor must then cross the dura mater and subarachnoid space to reach the pial surface of the brain. The normal dura is seen as a thin, enhancing layer on postgadolinium T1W images, whereas the cerebrospinal fluid (CSF) signal in the subarachnoid space is best assessed on T2W sequences. The bone-periosteum complex is seen as a thin hypointense linear structure on T1W and T2W sequences. When this remains intact, a tumor is considered extracranial.[12,13] Smooth, intact, linear dural thickening and enhancement, less than 5 mm thick, is typically associated with reactive dural changes and is not considered as an indicator of dural invasion.[14] When present, this finding suggests a tumor is intracranial but extradural. If the dural thickening is more focal and nodular and shows the same enhancement pattern as tumor (often an intermediate "evil gray" signal), then the lesion is considered intracranial and intradural (Fig. 4.16). The presence of intradural invasion influences the extent of dural resection and affects the size and complexity of the skull base reconstruction. The extent of pial or brain parenchymal involvement, as demonstrated by enhancement extending along the surface of the brain; vasogenic edema; or frank parenchymal invasion also determine the lesion's resectability.

Perineural spread of tumor is another important feature to recognize. It should be mentioned that when perineural spread is reported radiologically, it refers to the macroscopic spread of tumor away from the primary site of disease, rather than the microscopic finding of perineural infiltration seen on histologic specimens. In these cases, findings that are suggestive of perineural

spread include enlargement and enhancement of major nerves, infiltration of extracranial fat pads, foraminal enlargement, and secondary signs associated with denervation.[15] In our institution, high-spatial-resolution, non-fat-suppressed spin-echo T1W pre- and postgadolinium-enhanced sequences are employed to provide a detailed anatomy of the skull base and soft tissues without the problem of susceptibility artifacts associated with the use of frequency-selective fat-suppression techniques.[16] An alternative approach is to use pre- and postcontrast isotropic high-spatial-resolution volumetric interpolated breath-hold sequences with fat saturation to produce high-spatial-resolution images around the skull base without artifacts.[17]

In addition to standard multiplanar MRI sequences, MR angiogram and CT angiogram may be useful for identifying and assessing the patency of the ICA and the anatomy of the circle of Willis in relation to the tumor. For example, the retropharyngeal course of the ICA is an important surgical consideration in the transodontoid approach for lesions in the craniocervical region and a medial course of the cavernous carotids may narrow the surgical corridor when considering a transsphenoidal approach (Fig. 4.6).

### Surgical Approaches and Anatomic Limitations

Until recently, open surgical approaches dominated as the preferred surgical approach for tumors involving the anterior skull base, including those arising from the sinonasal cavity. Better understanding of endonasal anatomy, technologic advances in surgical equipment such as high-definition camera systems

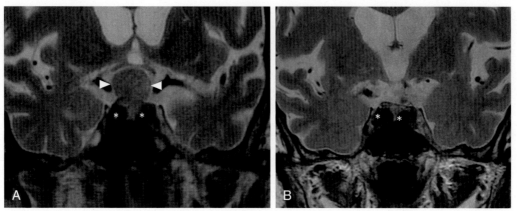

FIG. 4.6 "Kissing" carotids. Coronal T2-weighted images taken before **(A)** and after **(B)** treatment. Bilateral internal carotid arteries (*asterisks*) are shown protruding medially into the sella, narrowing the putative transsphenoidal surgical corridor. Fortunately, the macroprolactinoma (*arrowheads* in **A**) shown in the pretreatment image **(A)** responded to medical therapy **(B)**.

and computer-assisted neuronavigation, and the establishment of multidisciplinary skull base teams have allowed the endonasal approach to become a safe and viable alternative for major anterior skull base surgery. The concept behind the minimally invasive technique is to provide "access and visualization through the narrowest practical corridor," allowing for "maximum effective action at the target with minimal disruption of normal tissues."[18,19] Endoscopic endonasal approaches use the nasal cavity as a surgical corridor to approach anterior skull base lesions, which provides the most direct and least traumatic surgical option while maintaining an acceptable complication rate, of which CSF leak remains the main risk. It is less invasive than open craniofacial surgery and obviates the need for brain retraction while reducing the risk of damage to critical neurovascular structures that would ordinarily be traversed during open surgery.

Various classifications systems have been used to define these approaches. Kassam et al.[19] popularized an anatomically based modular approach to endoscopic endonasal surgery, defining the approach in terms of the "sagittal plane" modules (Fig. 4.7A), roughly limited laterally by the orbits and ICAs, and the "coronal plane" modules (Fig. 4.7B), which describe the lateral limits of the endoscopic endonasal approach. A simplified overview of these approaches is provided in the following sections.

### Sagittal plane
**Transcribriform.** Typical disorders in the anterior cranial fossa accessed via the transcribiform approach include sinonasal tumors such as esthesioneuroblastoma and olfactory groove meningioma.

The endoscopic endonasal surgical access typically involves septectomy, bilateral complete ethmoidectomies, and bilateral frontal sinusotomies with removal of intersinus septum (modified Lothrop or Draf 3). This can be extended laterally with maxillary antrostomies and resection of the lamina papyracea if necessary.

Contraindications to a purely endoscopic endonasal resection include periorbital invasion, superolateral extension of the tumor beyond the mid orbit, invasion through the nasal bone or anterior wall of the frontal sinus, or involvement of the subcutaneous tissues or the skin.

The reporting radiologist should report the presence and extent of intracranial extension and leptomeningeal as well as any cerebral invasion to allow the surgeon to plan the approach with the highest possibility of a complete resection.

**Transplanum.** The transplanum approach to the suprasellar cistern and third ventricle allows the surgeon direct access without having to displace the optic nerves or carotid arteries. It is typically performed as an extension of a transsellar approach.

Typical lesions amenable to the transplanum approach include pituitary adenomas with suprasellar extension or extension into the third ventricle, preinfundibular portion of craniopharyngiomas not extending lateral to the carotid arteries, Rathke cleft cyst, clival chordomas with suprasellar extension, and planum sphenoidale meningiomas.

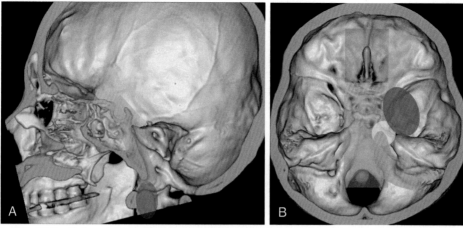

FIG. 4.7 **(A)** Sagittal modules of the extended endoscopic endonasal approach to the ventral skull base. Transcribriform (red), transplanar (light green), transsellar (blue), transclival (pink), transodontoid (purple). **(B)** Coronal modules (simplified): Transorbital (orbit and anterior cranial fossa, orange), suprapetrous (Meckel cave, lateral cavernous and middle cranial fossa, dark green), medial petrous (petrous apex, yellow), and infrapetrous (infratemporal fossa and parapharyngeal space, gray).

The endoscopic endonasal surgical access typically involves bilateral posterior ethmoidectomy, posterior septectomy, and bilateral sphenoidectomies.

Relative contraindications that may preclude complete tumor resection include vascular encasement of the anterior cerebral artery, cavernous sinus invasion, extension lateral or posterior to the carotid arteries, and extension into the orbital apex.

**Transsellar.** The transsellar approach allows access to sellar lesions, such as pituitary adenomas and Rathke cleft cysts (this may be considered as a suprasellar approach), and is combined with the transplant approach for suprasellar lesions, such as craniopharyngiomas and tuberculum sellae meningiomas. The medial cavernous sinus is also accessed through the transsellar approach.

Endoscopic endonasal surgical access typically involves posterior ethmoidectomies, posterior septectomy and bilateral sphenoidectomies, and possible creation of a nasoseptal flap.

Tumor extension lateral to the supraclinoid ICAs or invasion of the lateral cavernous sinus is a contraindication for a pure endoscopic approach.

**Transclival.** The clivus is divided into the upper, middle, and lower thirds anatomically by the neural foramina. The upper third extends from the posterior clinoids to the Dorello canal (containing the abducens nerve, cranial nerve [CN] VI). Endonasally, the middle

clivus lies between the floor of the sella and the floor of the sphenoid sinus, whereas the lower clivus extends from the floor of the sphenoid sinus to the foramen magnum.

The upper transclival approach is seldom used. It requires pituitary transposition to access the interpeduncular cistern, basilar apex, and the posterior third ventricle. The pituitary gland is mobilized onto the planum sphenoidale and the posterior clinoid removed, allowing access to lesions with retroinfundibular extension such as craniopharyngiomas.

The middle transclival approach allows access to the ventral pons, prepontine cistern, basilar trunk, and cisternal portion of CN VI.

The lower transclival approach allows access to the premedullary cistern, vertebrobasilar junction, vertebral arteries, posterior inferior cerebellar arteries, and the cisternal portion of CN IX to XII.

The lateral (transpterygoid) extension of the transclival approach allows access to the jugular fossa.

Typical tumors amenable to the transclival approach include clival chordomas, chondrosarcomas, and petroclival meningiomas.

**Transodontoid.** The transodontoid approach allows access to the inferior clivus, foramen magnum, and C1-C2 vertebrae.

Endoscopically, this extends from the roof of the nasopharynx to the level of the hard palate (corresponding to the level of the C2 vertebra). The fossa of

Rosenmüller, with the parapharyngeal ICA laterally, marks the lateral limit.

Typical disorders accessed through a transodontoid approach include inferior clival chordoma, chondrosarcoma, and foramen magnum or craniocervical junction meningiomas.

The extension of surgery laterally in the coronal plane requires a sound understanding of the course of the parapharyngeal ICA from the neck into the petrous canal. The ICA must be identified, and this often requires exposure of the maxillary sinus, a transpterygoid approach with mobilization of the pterygopalatine contents and Eustachian tube laterally.

### Coronal plane

The coronal modules are complex and can be simplified into transorbital, medial petrous, suprapetrous, and infrapetrous modules. The suprapetrous and infrapetrous modules are accessed via a common transpterygoid approach. It is also important to remember that the coronal plane refers to paramedian access at different depths, moving from superior to inferior in the ventral to dorsal direction, corresponding to the levels of the anterior fossa and orbits, middle fossa and temporal lobe, and the posterior fossa.

**Transorbital (orbital apex/superior orbital fissure/ orbit).** The transorbital approach allows access to orbital lesions, such as orbital hemangioma, schwannoma, and meningioma.

Endonasal access of the orbits is through the lamina papyracea after ethmoidectomy. Care should be taken to avoid the optic nerves and the intraorbital vasculature.

**Medial petrous.** The medial petrous apex is accessed via the medial petrous approach. Typical disorders involving the petrous apex include cholesterol granulomas, whereas petroclival lesions include meningioma, chondrosarcoma, and chordoma, generally involving paramedian extension from the transclival approach.

**Transpterygoid (suprapetrous and infrapetrous modules).** The suprapetrous and infrapetrous modules are both accessed by a common transpterygoid approach.

The transpterygoid approach allows access to lesions that may involve the lateral recess of the sphenoid sinus. The transpterygoid-suprapetrous approach accesses Meckel cave, the lateral compartment of the cavernous sinus (sometimes considered as a separate zone), and the middle cranial fossa. Examples of tumors involving the lateral cavernous sinus include invasive pituitary adenoma, whereas pathologies in the Meckel cave include schwannoma and meningioma.

The transpterygoid-infrapetrous approach gives access to lesions in the infratemporal fossa and parapharyngeal space. Examples of infrapetrous disorders include lateral extension of chondrosarcoma, cholesterol granuloma, cholesteatoma, and chordoma. Disorders in the infratemporal fossa and parapharyngeal space include schwannoma, meningioma, angiofibroma, and CSF leak.

A cavernous ICA aneurysm is an absolute contraindication to endoscopic endonasal surgery. Other contraindications include lesions involving the superolateral region of the cavernous sinus, which contain the cranial nerves.

Preoperative identification of pneumatization of the pterygoid plate, vidian canal, ICA, and optic nerve is important to avoid potential complications.

### Contraindications

It is important to be aware of some of the features on preoperative imaging that represent relative contraindications to a purely endoscopic approach (Box 4.1). Some of these features may preclude a purely endoscopic approach or require a combined approach to achieve optimal local disease control.

Location of the tumor is the most important factor. Direct invasion of the brain or tumors that involve the

---

> **BOX 4.1**
> **Contraindications and Relative Contraindications to a Purely Endoscopic Endonasal Approach With Curative Intent**
>
> Brain invasion
>
> Orbital invasion
>
> Lateral skull base lesion
>
> Lesion in superolateral cavernous sinus
>
> Craniopharyngioma that is isolated to the third ventricle
>
> Lesion with the major component extending over the orbital roof and optic canal and lateral to the foramen ovale
>
> Lesion arising from or extensively involving the frontal sinus
>
> Major vascular encasement
>
> Inability to reconstruct the skull base defect

Data from Learned KO, Lee JYK, Adappa ND, et al. Radiologic evaluation for endoscopic endonasal skull base surgery candidates. *Neurographics.* 2015;5:41–55.

periorbita or skin may require a combined approach. Lesions that encase the ICA or that are lateral to the ICA, lesions within the superolateral cavernous sinus, or lesions involving major vascular structures such as the anterior cerebral arteries or superior sagittal sinus may not be completely resectable. Likewise, tumors with a large component extending into or lateral to the orbital apex or optic canal or lateral to the foramen ovale may not be able to be accessed in their entirety endoscopically. The size and location of a tumor, as well as any previous surgery or radiotherapy, are also important considerations that may affect the ability to reconstruct the skull base after excision.

As a general rule, active sinonasal infection is a contraindication for endonasal skull base surgery and should be adequately treated before surgery.

### Skull Base Reconstruction

Although the goal of the endoscopic endonasal skull base surgeon is to complete a gross total resection of the tumor with clear margins, the surgery is not complete until there has been adequate reconstruction of the anterior skull base to achieve a watertight seal and prevention of CSF leaks. Successful dural closure serves as a barrier between the intracranial and intranasal regions, limiting the risk of infective complications such as meningitis and cerebral abscess. Other considerations include providing a structural support and coverage for neural and vascular structures and restoration of sinonasal function, cosmesis, and quality of life.

A variety of nonvascularized and vascularized tissues can be used to reconstruct the anterior skull base. The radiologist should be familiar with the types of reconstructions used and their typical postoperative

appearances so as not to confuse these with persistent tumor or other complications such as infection. Skull base defects can be described anatomically based on location (ethmoid/cribriform area, sphenoid planum, clivus, petrous apex, pterygopalatine fossa, and infratemporal fossa) and size.

Small dural defects (<1 cm) may be repaired with nonvascularized free grafts. The options include autologous homografts, such as free adipose tissue using the bath-plug technique[21] (Fig. 4.8), tensor fascia lata (Fig. 4.9), or mucoperiosteal free grafts, which have the highest potential to heal well. Bone or cartilage grafts may also be used, as can alloplastic grafts such as a collagen matrix.

Pedicled vascularized flaps may be used for both small and large dural defects and are the workhorse of endonasal skull base reconstruction. In pedicled flaps, the flap remains attached by a vascular pedicle to its donor site after being transposed. The most common pedicled flap used in endoscopic endonasal skull base reconstruction is the nasoseptal flap, popularized by Hadad and Bassagaisteguy,[22] which is based on the posterior septal artery, a branch of the sphenopalatine artery. It is a mucoperichondrial-periosteal flap and owing to its vascularity promotes faster healing, contributing to successful defect closure. Other intranasal pedicled flaps include the inferior turbinate flap, which is based posteriorly on the inferior turbinate artery; the terminal branch of the posterior lateral nasal artery, which arises from the sphenopalatine artery; and the middle turbinate flap based on the middle turbinate and posterolateral nasal arteries. On MRI, nasoseptal flaps have a characteristic C-shaped configuration covering the surgical defect and typically show avid enhancement because of their vascular

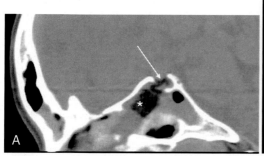 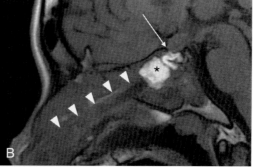

FIG. 4.8 Bath plug technique. Sagittal CT **(A)** and MRI **(B)** images show fat plugging the sphenoidotomy defect (*thin arrows*), supported by a second cube of fat (*asterisk*), bolstered by a Foley catheter (*arrowheads* in **B**).

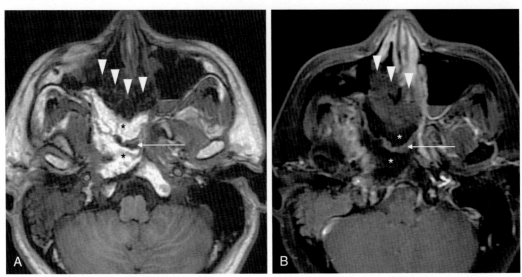

FIG. 4.9 Fascia lata graft. Axial T1-weighted (T1W) **(A)** and fat-suppressed postgadolinium T1W **(B)** images show typical appearances of a fascia lata graft with alternating layers of fat (*asterisk*) and fascia (*thin arrows*), bolstered by removable nasal tampons (*arrowheads*).

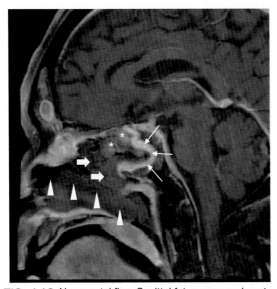

FIG. 4.10 Nasoseptal flap. Sagittal fat-suppressed post-gadolinium T1-weighted image, day 1 post operation. An enhancing "C-shaped" nasoseptal flap (*thin arrows*) is seen bolstered by blood-soaked gelatin sponge (*asterisks*), ribbon gauze (*thick arrows*), and a nasal tampon (*arrowheads*).

pedicle (Fig. 4.10), as opposed to free mucoperiosteal grafts, which do not enhance in the early postoperative period. Nasoseptal flaps vary in thickness and typically contract over time. Although the pattern of enhancement has not been shown to predict CSF leaks,[23] the

absence of enhancement may be used as an indicator of potential vascular compromise (Fig. 4.11). A nonenhancing nasoseptal flap may behave similar to a nonvascularized free mucosal graft in terms of healing and survival of the flap. The position of the flap relative to the surgical defect is another important factor to note, as flap migration or displacement is another potential cause for flap failure. In the long term, both free mucoperiosteal and nasoseptal grafts may develop a covering of enhancing granulation tissue. Understanding the typical patterns of enhancement of the nasoseptal flaps will help distinguish these from residual or recurrent tumor.

Large dural defects (>3 cm in size) are encountered more frequently in the expanded endoscopic endonasal approach, particularly as a result of major oncologic surgery. The complexity of the repair depends on the location of the defect and the ability to define the margins of the defect through the chosen surgical corridor. A multilayered approach is often preferred over a single-layered one, and a combination of nonvascularized and vascularized grafts is common.

The initial layer is the underlay or inlay layer, the purpose of which is to act as a direct subdural or epidural repair and create a water-tight seal. Multiple materials can be used, including autologous homografts, such as bone, cartilage, fat, or fascia, or nonautologous grafts, such as biosynthetic collagen matrix. The options for nonvascularized graft material are the same as those used for small defects, although tensor fascia

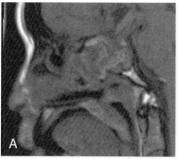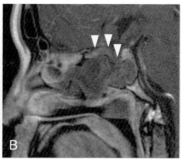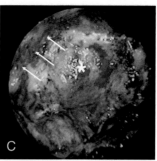

FIG. 4.11 Nonenhancing nasoseptal flap. Postoperative day 1 MRI images, sagittal T1-weighted (T1W) **(A)**, postgadolinium T1W **(B)**, and postoperative day 4 endoscopic **(C)** images showing a nonenhancing nasoseptal flap (*arrowheads* in **B**). On endoscopy, the nasoseptal flap (*asterisk* in **C**) appeared viable, with some areas of bruising and necrosis at the edges (*thin arrows* in **C**). The patient developed a cerebrospinal fluid leak 5 days after surgery.

lata may be preferred over temporalis as a fascia graft because of size, and abdominal fat rather than earlobe fat for the same reason. Bone graft is generally thought to require a longer healing time and can be associated with osteoradionecrosis secondary to radiotherapy.[24] Therefore if bone is used, it is recommended that it be used in combination with a vascularized onlay graft. Rigid mesh repairs have also fallen out of favor, owing to higher rates of extrusion and infection.[25]

The overlay layer aims to cover the entire bony perimeter of the defect with a margin on the extracranial side and can be made of either free or vascularized grafts, although vascularized grafts are preferred for the larger defects. The options for pedicled grafts can be divided into intranasal and extranasal flaps. Intranasal flaps have been discussed earlier for usage in both small and large defects. The nasoseptal flap is preferred for its reliable blood supply and size, as well as its reach to the posterior table of the frontal sinus, whereas the inferior turbinate flap is more useful in posterior sella or clival defects, as it does not tend to reach the anterior cranial fossa. Extranasal or regional flaps include the pericranial flap based on the supraorbital and supratrochlear vessels and the temporoparietal fascial flap based on the superficial temporal artery. Both of these can be harvested endoscopically. For midline defects, the pericranial flap is ideal and can cover most defects. When used in an endoscopic approach, the pericranial flap can be tunneled through the frontal sinus and laid over the defect. Combinations of the frontal pericranial and temporoparietal fascial flaps are also used in very large defects. Free flaps are an option but usually reserved for open approaches.

Multilayered skull base reconstructions can vary considerably in thickness, depending on the surgeon and the size and location of the defect. In typical multilayered reconstructions using pericranial flaps, the different layers can be appreciated on MRI. The inlay graft (often a synthetic collagen matrix) can be seen as a thin, hypointense layer on coronal T2W images, followed by the outer layers of the pericranial flap, comprising a variably thick layer of loose areolar tissue (hyperintense on T2W image, hypointense on T1W image, and variable postgadolinium enhancement), a thin layer of pericranium (hypointense on T2W image, isointense on T1W image), and a variable outermost layer of granulation tissue that develops over time. As with nasoseptal flaps, predicting flap failure based on the imaging characteristics of the pericranial flap is difficult. In our experience, the imaging features associated with flap failure were a very thin or poorly enhancing flap (Fig. 4.12).

## POSTOPERATIVE IMAGING

Imaging in the early postoperative period can be challenging. To understand the postoperative findings, it is essential to have available the complete preoperative imaging workup for comparison, as well as knowledge of the surgical approach, the extent of the surgical excision, and the nature of any reconstruction performed. The radiologist should be familiar with the types of packing materials and bolsters used in the early postoperative period, the different reconstruction options and their imaging appearances, the expected appearance and evolution of early and late postoperative changes over time, and the findings associated with potential early and late complications.

### Early Postoperative Imaging

Early postoperative imaging is typically performed within 48 h of surgery. This provides the best

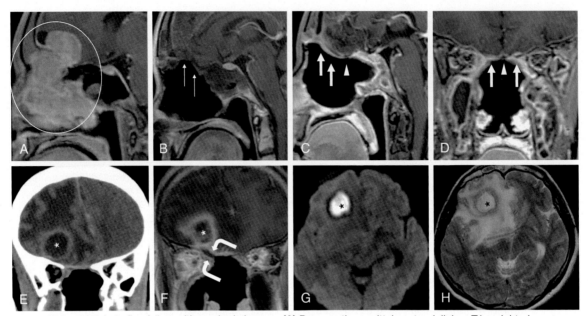

FIG. 4.12 Late flap failure with cerebral abscess. **(A)** Preoperative sagittal postgadolinium T1-weighted imaging (T1WI) shows a large, enhancing esthesioneuroblastoma (*circled*). **(B)** Five days post operation, the tumor has been excised and the skull base reconstructed with a pericranial flap. Note that the flap appears relatively thin and is nonenhancing (*thin arrows*). **(C and D)** Sagittal and coronal postgadolinium T1WI performed 5 months post operation and 3 months post radiotherapy. There is now some enhancement along the flap (*thick arrows*), owing to granulation tissue. Some portions remain poorly enhancing (*arrowheads*), corresponding to necrotic patches endoscopically. **(E–H)** Contrast-enhanced coronal CT **(E)** and T1WI **(F)**, axial DWI **(G)**, and T2WI **(H)** performed 11 months after surgery show typical findings of a cerebral abscess (*asterisk*), with ring enhancement **(E and F)**, central diffusion restriction **(G)** (ADC not shown), and a T2-weighted hypointense capsule with extensive vasogenic edema **(H)**. An enhancing sinus tract is seen leading from the point of flap failure to the abscess **(F)** (*curved arrows*).

opportunity to assess the surgical margins, as any persistent enhancing tumor can easily be distinguished from nonenhancing blood products, temporary surgical bolsters and packing materials, and the reconstructed skull base without needing to worry about potential confounding enhancement from inflammatory or granulation tissues.[26]

Both CT and MR show the expected postoperative changes, including mucoperiosteal thickening; soft tissue density representing debris, fluid, and blood within sinus cavities; bony defects in the septum, the anterior cranial floor, or sinuses (depending on the surgical approach and location of pathology); and, if the dura is breached, pneumocephalus. Depending on the extent of tumor, the endonasal exposure may involve a combination of middle turbinectomy, middle meatal antrostomy, medial maxillectomy, ethmoidectomy, frontal sinusotomy, septectomy, and sphenoidotomy.[20]

Care should be taken to compare the non-contrast-enhanced T1W and postgadolinium T1W sequences, as any postoperative blood products typically show T1W hyperintensity by the time imaging is performed, because of accumulation of the blood breakdown product, methemoglobin. When present, persistent tumor typically retains its preoperative signal and enhancement characteristics and therefore comparison with the preoperative imaging is essential. Particular attention should be paid to the bony margins of the surgery and potential bony recesses, as these may be surgical blind spots for persistent tumor (Fig. 4.13). In some cases in which vascular encasement is involved, a small amount of tumor may be deliberately left behind if deemed unresectable by the surgeon. Careful assessment of these areas on postoperative imaging is essential to guide further management, whether operative or nonoperative (such as with stereotactic radiosurgery).

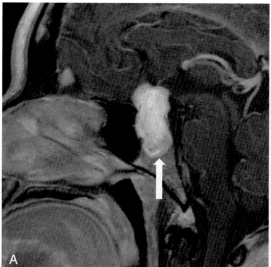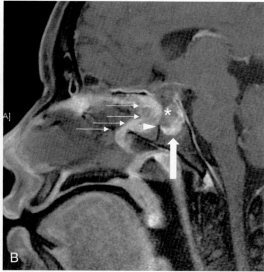

FIG. 4.13 Surgical blind spots: **(A)** Preoperative sagittal postgadolinium T1-weighted image (T1WI) shows an enhancing sellar/suprasellar pituitary macroadenoma. Note that there is remodeling and inferior expansion of the sella, with an intraosseous component that has invaded the clivus, appearing as a slightly darker shade of gray (*thick white arrow*). **(B)** Postoperative sagittal postgadolinium T1WI shows postoperative changes with excision of the tumor and an enhancing "C-shaped" nasoseptal flap (*thin white arrows*). Unfortunately, the invasive component in the clivus (*thick white arrow*) persists, hidden behind a ridge of bone, which indicates the margin of the surgical defect in the sellar floor (*white arrowhead*). Nonenhancing blood clot (*asterisk*) is seen in the clival recess above the enhancing tumor.

Surgical bolsters; dissolvable dressings such as regenerated cellulose (e.g., Surgicel), gelatin sponge (e.g., Gelfoam) or bioresorbables (e.g., Nasopore); and removable packing such as Merocel or Rapid Rhino nasal tampons covered in antibiotic ointment may remain in situ postoperatively. Ribbon gauze impregnated with bismuth iodoform paraffin paste and Foley catheters may also remain in the nasal cavity postoperatively to support flap repairs or for hemostasis. Often a combination of dissolvable and solid removable dressings is used to reinforce flap repairs, and these may be seen for a short time postoperatively on imaging. In contrast, fat or muscle with fascia can be seen for years post procedure.

The appearance of the reconstruction depends on whether a vascularized or nonvascularized flap was used, with vascularized flaps generally showing enhancement even in immediate postoperative scans.

### Late Postoperative Imaging

Many changes can be observed over the course of long-term follow-up for endoscopic endonasal skull base surgery. After the initial surgical packing has been removed and hemorrhage has resolved, enhancing granulation tissue can often be seen in the surgical bed. Exposed and irradiated paranasal sinuses may develop mucoperiosteal thickening and edema. Nonvascularized fat packing generally involutes over time. Most vascularized flaps, such as nasoseptal and pericranial flaps, show mild contraction over time. Granulation tissue often forms over the exposed surfaces of both nonvascularized and vascularized repairs, sometimes resulting in an increased enhancement of the reconstruction over time. This should not be confused with tumor recurrence. Most tumor recurrences occur at the margins of the tumor resection and generally retain the same signal characteristics of the original tumor.

### COMPLICATIONS

Complications of endonasal skull base surgery can be divided into intraoperative, early, and late complications. They can be further subdivided into location of complication and classified as major or minor.

### Intraoperative Complications

Intraoperative complications are frequently identified and managed at the time of surgery. In these cases,

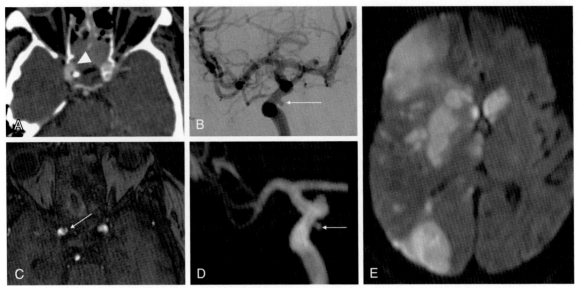

**FIG. 4.14** Internal carotid artery injury. Axial CT angiogram **(A)** shows focal bony defect at the right carotid impression (*arrowhead*) following endoscopic transsphenoidal surgery, with a resultant pseudoaneurysm of the internal carotid artery. Digital subtraction angiogram **(B)** and 3D time-of-flight MR angiography axial and coronal reformatted images **(C and D)** demonstrate the small pseudoaneurysm (*thin arrows*). Axial diffusion-weighted image **(E)** shows the ensuing areas of cerebral infarction.

imaging is not typically required for diagnosis. The most common complication is minor bleeding from the mucosa, obstructing surgical view. Major bleeding may also occur from injury to major vessels such as the anterior and posterior ethmoid arteries, sphenopalatine artery, and ICA. In rare cases, uncontrolled bleeding may require emergent endovascular intervention. Some form of vascular imaging, either digital subtraction angiography or noninvasive CT or MR angiography, may be required to localize the injury and plan any potential interventional therapy. Plain CT or MRI is also helpful to document any hemorrhagic or ischemic complications resulting from vascular injury (Fig. 4.14). Optic nerve and orbital content injury can also occur intraoperatively, as can CSF leaks. These may be recognized intraoperatively and managed immediately. Imaging is useful to document the extent of injury or to diagnose any unrecognized injury.

## Early Postoperative Complications

Early complications (days to weeks) are a common indication for performing imaging postoperatively. Intranasal complications are usually minor and identified on physical examination with endoscopy. These include epistaxis, nasal crusting, or synechiae. Sinusitis may be difficult to differentiate on imaging from postoperative mucosal edema or blood and debris within the sinuses. Early intracranial complications include CSF leak with or without flap failure, infections including meningitis (Fig. 4.15) and brain abscess, encephalocele, pneumocephalus, cavernous sinus thrombosis, and intracranial bleeding, all of which may be identified on imaging.

Early CSF leaks are often suspected clinically when associated with flap failure. CSF leaks are more common when the intracranial pressure is high, and in some cases, a lumbar drain may be deployed to reduce this risk. Patient factors associated with an increased risk of CSF leak include obesity (caused by increased intracranial pressure), Cushing disease (poor tissue healing), and a history of prior surgery or radiation (limited options for vascularized tissue reconstruction and impaired tissue healing).[27] The source of a leak may be identified endoscopically and confirmed clinically by testing for β-2 transferrin, if available. Plain bone algorithm CT scans are generally unhelpful in localizing a CSF leak after skull base surgery and are more useful in identifying the source of spontaneous CSF leaks where a small, isolated bony defect is detected. CT cisternography with intrathecal contrast can be helpful to identify brisk leaks, when there is a relatively constant stream of CSF present. When the source of CSF leak is not obvious endoscopically, MRI

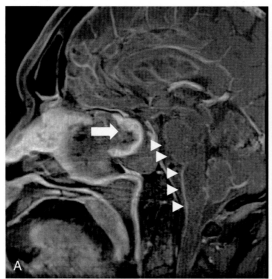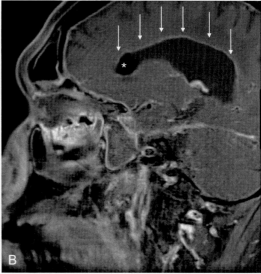

FIG. 4.15 Early postoperative infection **(A** and **B)**. Sagittal fat-suppressed postgadolinium T1-weighted images show an avidly enhancing, "C-shaped" nasoseptal flap (*thick arrow* in **A**). Unfortunately, this has failed to prevent the patient from developing meningitis, as evidenced by the enhancement along the surface of the brainstem (*arrowheads* in **A**), as well as ventriculitis and pneumocephalus, as evidenced by the subependymal enhancement (*thin arrows* in **B**) and gas locule (*asterisk* in **B**) in the frontal horn of the lateral ventricle.

is the imaging modality of choice, particularly with the use of isotropic 3D T2W sequences. Contained CSF leaks may result in a pseudomeningocele (Fig. 4.16). Intracranial hypotension may result in MRI findings of diffuse, smooth pachymeningeal thickening and enhancement, engorgement of the venous sinuses, and sagging of the brainstem and cerebellar tonsils. Subdural effusions and eventual subdural hematomas can also occur. Persistent pneumocephalus can also be a sign of CSF leak or infection. When there is complication by infection, leptomeningeal and ependymal enhancement may be seen (Fig. 4.15), corresponding to meningitis and ventriculitis. Ventriculitis may result in the development of hydrocephalus with periventricular edema and intraventricular debris (Fig. 4.16D). In pyogenic ventriculitis, the intraventricular debris shows restricted diffusion on diffusion weighted imaging. Intracranial abscesses can be epidural, subdural, or intracerebral. When present, intracranial abscesses show rim enhancement on both CT and MRI and are typically associated with vasogenic edema and central restricted diffusion (Fig. 4.12).

Endocrinologic disturbances are relatively common after transsphenoidal surgery. Diabetes insipidus is often transient and may be associated with the absence of the posterior pituitary bright spot on imaging. Panhypopituitarism may result from sacrifice of the pituitary gland or transection of the pituitary stalk.

## Late Postoperative Complications
Late complications (months to years) are much less common than early complications. The intracranial complications include CSF leak and late flap failure, infection (Fig. 4.12), encephalocele (Fig. 4.17), ptosis of the optic chiasm (Fig. 4.18), tumor recurrence, osteoradionecrosis, and secondary tumors induced by radiation. Although some of these may present clinically, these complications can usually be diagnosed on imaging if the radiologist is attentive to the signs.

Intranasal complications include septal necrosis, perforation, saddle nose, and recurrent sinusitis or mucocele caused by obstructed sinus ostia.

## CONCLUSION
Surgical techniques and approaches are constantly evolving. The endoscopic endonasal approach has become one of the preferred approaches to both benign and malignant processes involving the ventral skull base. Radiologists should be familiar with the common endoscopic endonasal surgical approaches and their limitations to provide useful information preoperatively. In addition, radiologists should also be familiar with the expected postoperative appearances of the surgical bed and sinonasal cavity, the commonly used reconstructive techniques, and the imaging features of the common early and late complications.

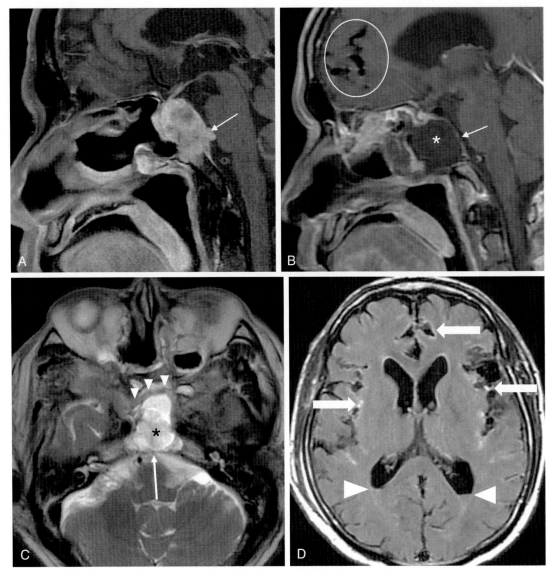

FIG. 4.16 Recurrent chordoma with postoperative pseudomeningocele. **(A)** Preoperative postgadolinium sagittal T1-weighted image (T1WI) shows an enhancing clival mass due to recurrent chordoma. Note the focal nodular area of dural invasion with a nodular intracranial, intradural component (*thin arrow*). There is no invasion of the adjacent brain. **(B)** Postoperative postgadolinium sagittal T1WI shows a focal nonenhancing dural defect (*thin arrow*). A large pseudomeningocele (*asterisk*) has developed, and there is evidence of pneumocephalus (*circled*). **(C)** Postoperative axial T2-weighted (T2W) image shows a contained cerebrospinal fluid (CSF) leak. A large pseudomeningocele has developed between the dural defect (*thin arrow*) and temporoparietal fascia onlay graft (*arrowheads*). Turbulent CSF flow from the cerebellopontine angle cistern can be seen gushing through the dural defect, resulting in loss of T2W signal within the pseudomeningocele (*asterisk*). **(D)** Postoperative postgadolinium T2W fluid-attenuated inversion recovery axial image at the level of the lateral ventricles. Patchy leptomeningeal enhancement is seen as linear hyperintense signal along the surface of the brain (*thick arrows*). Fluid-fluid levels in the occipital horns (*white arrowheads*) may represent postoperative hemorrhage or debris related to ventriculitis.

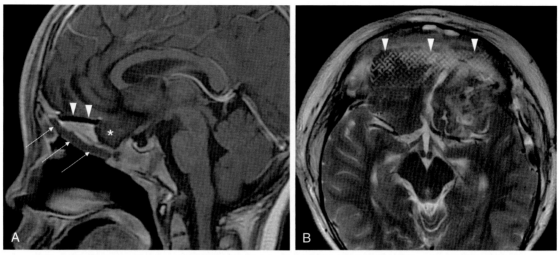

FIG. 4.17 Postoperative encephalocele. Sagittal postgadolinium T1-weighted **(A)** and axial T2-weighted **(B)** images. The skull base has been repaired with titanium mesh (*arrowheads* in **A** and **B**) and a pericranial flap (*thin arrows* in **A**). The posterior edge of the titanium mesh is elevated and fails to cover the posterior skull base defect. A postsurgical encephalocele has developed (*asterisk* in **A**).

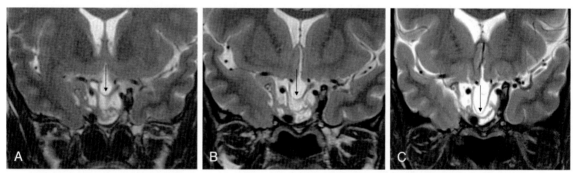

FIG. 4.18 Ptosis of the optic chiasm. Coronal T2-weighted image at 1 year **(A)**, 3 years **(B)**, and 5 years **(C)** after surgery show progressive thinning, elongation, and inferior drooping of the optic chiasm (*thin arrows*) over the course of long-term follow-up post transsphenoidal hypophysectomy. The patient suffered progressive worsening of visual field defects.

## REFERENCES

1. Lindholm J. A century of pituitary surgery: schloffer's legacy. *Neurosurgery.* 2007;61:865–867. Discussion 867–868.
2. Francesco D, Daniel MP, John Jr AJ, Joseph H, Edward Jr RL. A brief history of endoscopic transsphenoidal surgery—from Philipp Bozzini to the First World Congress of Endoscopic Skull Base Surgery. *Neurosurg Focus.* 2005;19:6:E3
3. Liu JK, Das K, Weiss MH, Laws Jr ER, Couldwell WT. The history and evolution of transsphenoidal surgery. *J Neurosurg.* 2002;95:1083–1096.
4. Husain Q, Patel SK, Soni RS, Patel AA, Liu JK, Eloy JA. Celebrating the golden anniversary of anterior skull base surgery: reflections on the past 50 years and its historical evolution. *Laryngoscope.* 2013;123:64–72.
5. Ketcham AS, Wilkins RH, Vanburen JM, Smith RR. A combined intracranial facial approach to the paranasal sinuses. *Am J Surg.* 1963;106:698–703.
6. Govindaraj S, Adappa ND, Kennedy DW. Endoscopic sinus surgery: evolution and technical innovations. *J Laryngol Otol.* 2009;124:242–250.
7. Stammberger H, Posawetz W. Functional endoscopic sinus surgery. Concept, indications and results of the Messerklinger technique. *Eur Arch Otorhinolaryngol.* 1990;247:63–76.
8. McCutcheon IE, Blacklock JB, Weber RS, et al. Anterior transcranial (craniofacial) resection of tumors of the paranasal sinuses: surgical technique and results. *Neurosurgery.* 1996;38:471–479. Discussion 479–480.

9. Thaler ER, Kotapka M, Lanza DC, Kennedy DW. Endoscopically assisted anterior cranial skull base resection of sinonasal tumors. *Am J Rhinol.* 1999;13:303–310.

10. Casiano RR, Numa WA, Falquez AM. Endoscopic resection of esthesioneuroblastoma. *Am J Rhinol.* 2001;15:271–279.

11. Curtin HD, Rabinov JD. Extension to the orbit from paraorbital disease. The sinuses. *Radiol Clin N Am.* 1999; 36:1201–1213. xi.

12. Maroldi R, Ravanelli M, Borghesi A, Farina D. Paranasal sinus imaging. *Eur J Radiol.* 2008;66:372–386.

13. Lund VJ, Stammberger H, Nicolai P, et al. European position paper on endoscopic management of tumors of the nose, paranasal sinuses and skull base. *Rhinol Suppl.* 2010:1–143.

14. Eisen MD, Yousem DM, Montone KT, et al. Use of preoperative MR to predict dural, perineural, and venous sinus invasion of skull base tumors. *AJNR Am J Neuroradiol.* 1996;17:1937–1945.

15. Ong C, Chong VH. Imaging of perineural spread in head and neck tumors. *Cancer Imaging.* 2010;10:S92–S98.

16. Curtin HD. Detection of perineural spread: fat suppression versus no fat suppression. *AJNR Am J Neuroradiol.* 2004;25:1–3.

17. Maroldi R, Farina D, Borghesi A, Marconi A, Gatti E. Perineural tumor spread. *Neuroimaging Clin N Am.* 2008;18: 413–429. xi.

18. Liu CY, Wang MY, Apuzzo ML. The evolution and future of minimalism in neurological surgery. *Childs Nerv Syst.* 2004;20:783–789.

19. Kassam AB, Prevedello DM, Carrau RL, et al. Endoscopic endonasal skull base surgery: analysis of complications in the authors' initial 800 patients. *J Neurosurg.* 2010;114:1544–1568.

20. Learned KO, Lee JYK, Adappa ND, et al. Radiologic evaluation for endoscopic endonasal skull base surgery candidates. *Neurographics.* 2015;5:41–55.

21. Wormald PJ, McDonogh M. 'Bath-plug' technique for the endoscopic management of cerebrospinal fluid leaks. *J Laryngol Otol.* 1998;111:1042–1046.

22. Hadad G, Bassagasteguy L, Carrau RL, et al. A novel reconstructive technique after endoscopic expanded endonasal approaches: vascular pedicle nasoseptal flap. *Laryngoscope.* 2006;116:1882–1886.

23. Adappa ND, Learned KO, Palmer JN, Newman JG, Lee JY. Radiographic enhancement of the nasoseptal flap does not predict postoperative cerebrospinal fluid leaks in endoscopic skull base reconstruction. *Laryngoscope.* 2012;122:1226–1234.

24. Garcia-Garrigos E, Arenas-Jimenez JJ, Monjas-Canovas I, et al. Transsphenoidal approach in endoscopic endonasal surgery for skull base lesions: what radiologists and surgeons need to know. *Radiographics.* 2015;35:1170–1185.

25. Schmalbach CE, Webb DE, Weitzel EK. Anterior skull base reconstruction: a review of current techniques. *Curr Opin Otolaryngol Head Neck Surg.* 2010;18:238–243.

26. Yoon PH, Kim DI, Jeon P, Lee SI, Lee SK, Kim SH. Pituitary adenomas: early postoperative MR imaging after transsphenoidal resection. *AJNR Am J Neuroradiol.* 2001;22: 1097–1104.

27. Kim GG, Hang AX, Mitchell C, Zanation AM. Pedicled extranasal flaps in skull base reconstruction. *Adv Otorhinolaryngol.* 2013;74:71–80.

# CHAPTER 5

# Temporal Bone Inflammatory and Infectious Diseases

DR. MARC LEMMERLING, MD, PHD

## INTRODUCTION

In a wide variety of inflammatory and infectious diseases of the temporal bone, imaging studies are used to determine the extent of the disease and to visualize eventual complications. Imaging protocols for the evaluation of infections in the external ear, the middle ear (and mastoid), and the inner ear are somewhat different, and the interpretation of the images must be done from different viewpoints. In some situations, CT or MRI is the best choice; in others, both techniques are used for different reasons.

## EXTERNAL EAR: EXTERNAL OTITIS

### External Otitis

External otitis is common and can be caused by exposure to polluted water, after trauma (e.g., after the use of cotton swabs), and in a variety of dermatologic diseases. The ear is painful and itches. Diagnosis is in most cases easy, just by inspection or rarely by using an otoscope. Only occasionally imaging is required. On CT, external otitis is seen as a narrowing of the external ear canal that contains a soft tissue opacification (Fig. 5.1). Purely on the basis of imaging the finding is aspecific and cannot be distinguished from any soft tissue obliteration of another origin.

### Necrotizing External Otitis

Necrotizing external otitis, also referred to as malignant external otitis, is a severe infection almost exclusively caused by *Pseudomonas aeruginosa*. The term "malignant" has also been used because of the aggressive behavior of the disease, rapidly spreading from the external ear canal to the ipsilateral deeper soft tissues and bony structures, such as the mastoid, temporomandibular joint, and parotid gland, but the disease can even proceed as far as in the parapharyngeal space or end up as an extensive zone of osteomyelitis of the skull base, rarely with intracranial extension.

Necrotizing external otitis is almost exclusively seen in the diabetic or immunocompromised patient, sometimes in the elderly. Besides local signs of external ear inflammation with otorrhea, ototalgia is the most common symptom.[1]

CT and MRI are both able to visualize the disease, but MRI is superior to provide a detailed view on the exact extent of the disease. On CT, opacification of the external ear canal is seen, as well as bony erosion and destruction of the canal walls and mastoid, and eventually the temporomandibular joint or deeper parts of the skull base, such as the clivus. Pathologic enhancement of the soft tissues surrounding the temporal bone is present, and in more pronounced stages of the disease abscess formation occurs. On MRI the same disease pattern is recognized, but a better contrast resolution leads to a better delineation of the soft tissue changes (Fig. 5.2). Bone marrow changes are also well appreciated on MRI.[2,3] The most common finding on MRI is infiltration of the fat behind the mandibular condyle.[4] Treatment consists of a combination of surgery with intravenous antibiotics.

## MIDDLE EAR AND MASTOID: OTOMASTOIDITIS

### Acute Otomastoiditis and Coalescent Mastoiditis

The middle ear and mastoid are an extension of the upper respiratory tract. Bacteria can infect the middle ear via the Eustachian tube, and can subsequently infect the mastoid antrum and the adjacent pneumatized portions of the petrous bone via the aditus ad antrum. In the case of a mild infection, pain is present and the tympanic membrane is hyperemic. In moderate cases of otomastoiditis, imaging is of no additional value to the clinical findings of the otologist, and a conservative therapy will help. If such an acute infection, however, persists too long, resorption of the ossicles and the

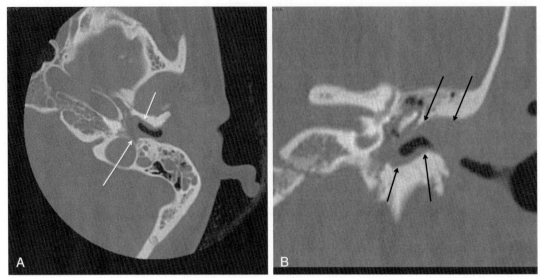

FIG. 5.1 On the axial **(A)** and coronal **(B)** multislice CT images obtained through the left temporal bone in a patient with otomastoiditis obliteration of the external ear canal (*arrows*) is also seen: external otitis.

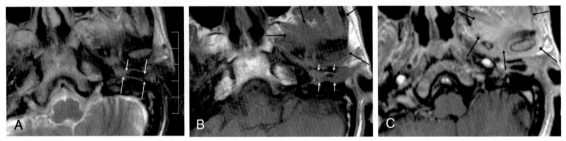

FIG. 5.2 On the axial T2- **(A)** and T1-weighted (T2WI) **(B)** images of the left temporal bone in a diabetic patient opacification is seen in the external ear (*white arrows* in **A** and **B**), as well as infiltration of the left temporomandibular joint and masticator space (*black arrows* in **B**), with loss of the normal fat planes between the muscles of mastication. The T1WI after intravenous injection of gadolinium **(C)** shows strong enhancement of the infiltration in the masticator space (*black arrows* in **C**). The diagnosis of necrotizing external otitis can be made.

mastoid occurs and mastoid cells coalesce, and the term "coalescent mastoiditis" is used. This condition is almost always seen in children. Four clinical signs are indicative of advancing acute mastoiditis: pain and erythema in the mastoid region, tenderness, swelling in the postauricular region with auricle protrusion, and edema of the posterosuperior wall of the external auditory canal.[5] In almost all of these patients the ipsilateral eardrum is inflamed and immobile and bulges.[6]

When this process of coalescence becomes more pronounced, the wall of the tympanic cavity and/or mastoid can be destructed, leading to several severe complications, such as the formation of a subperiostal abscess, thrombosis of the sigmoid sinus, brain abscess,

meningitis, or acute bacterial labyrinthitis. The last one is also referred to as otogenic labyrinthitis and is unilateral (contrary to meningogenic labyrinthitis, which is by rule bilateral). The manifestation of labyrinthitis is discussed later. *Streptococcus pneumoniae* is the most common pathogen causing severe intracranial complications,[7] followed by *Streptococcus pyogenes*.[6]

Temporal bone CT is an excellent technique for the diagnosis of acute coalescent mastoiditis, by demonstrating the air cell septa breakdown, the breakthrough of the sigmoid bony plate, and the lateral cortical wall of the mastoid.[8] Subperiostal abscess is present in half of the patients with coalescent mastoiditis. It is at this point important to make CT images in a soft tissue

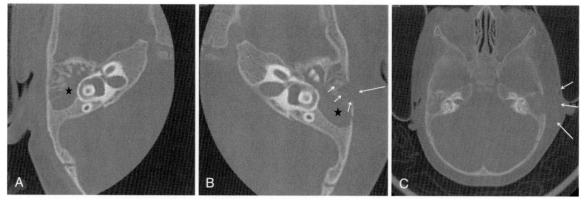

**FIG. 5.3** On the axial multislice CT images from the right **(A)** and left **(B)** temporal bone bilateral otomastoid opacification (*star*) is noted. On the left side, however, coalescence of mastoid cells is seen (*short arrows* in **B**), as well as breakthrough of the lateral bony wall of the mastoid (*long arrow* in **B**). On the overview image **(C)**, asymmetric thickening of the left-sided soft tissues indicates subperiostal abscess formation (*white arrows*).

setting to demonstrate the abscess (Fig. 5.3). MRI can also very well demonstrate such an abscess. In the past, mastoid subperiostal abscess required mastoidectomy, but owing to the use of improved antibiotics the actual treatment consists of tympanostomy with tube insertion, intravenous antibiotics, and postauricular incision with abscess drainage, avoiding morbidity and complications of mastoid surgery in children.[9] Thrombosis of the sigmoid sinus, brain abscess, and meningitis have become increasingly uncommon. MR is the modality of choice to image these conditions. The sigmoid sinus thrombus is spontaneously T1 hyperintense before intravenous (iv) injection of gadolinium and does not enhance after iv injection of gadolinium (Fig. 5.4). An otogenic abscess is not different from a nonotogenic brain abscess and often shows diffusion restriction on MR. Meningitis leads to thickening and increased enhancement of the meninges. Occasionally, late complications are noted, such as ankylosis of the temporomandibular joint (Fig. 5.5).

### Petrous Apicitis

The petrous apex is the most anterior and medial portion of the temporal bone. It articulates with the clivus and is pneumatized to a variable degree, depending on the amount of other pneumatized air cells in the temporal bone. Pneumatization of the petrous apex is present in 33% of all temporal bones.[10] In such a pneumatized petrous apex infection can occur. On CT images the petrous apex becomes opacified, and on MR images classic signs of infection are seen: heterogeneous high signal on T2-weighted image (T2WI), heterogeneous low signal on T1-weighted image (T1WI), and

heterogenous enhancement after intravenous injection of gadolinium (Fig. 5.6). MR enables the differentiation of petrous apicitis from other entities encountered in the petrous apex, such as cholesterol granuloma and cholesterol cyst. How this differentiation can be done is discussed in another dedicated chapter in this book. The frequency of petrous apicitis has decreased with the appropriate use of antibiotics in the treatment of middle ear infections. Nowadays it is extremely rare to see petrous apicitis become aggressive, leading to nasopharyngeal or neck abscess formation or facial nerve paralysis.[11,12]

### Chronic Otomastoiditis Without Cholesteatoma

The natural history of chronic otomastoiditis differs almost completely from acute otomastoiditis. Acute otomastoid disease traditionally develops in well-pneumatized mastoids of children, whereas chronic otomastoiditis usually occurs in a temporal bone with a sclerotic mastoid. Imaging is not mandatory in all patients with chronic otomastoiditis but is well indicated in a preoperative setting in the case of difficult otoscopy or doubtful diagnosis, suspicion for a present malformation, single functional ear, temporal bones after mastoidectomy, and suspicion for the presence of intracranial complications.[13,14]

A wide variety of CT changes is observed in the case of chronic inflammatory/infectious disease of the middle ear and mastoid. These changes occur at the level of the tympanic membrane or in the middle ear cavity. CT can give some information on the tympanic membrane, but the otoscopy is of course able to appreciate such

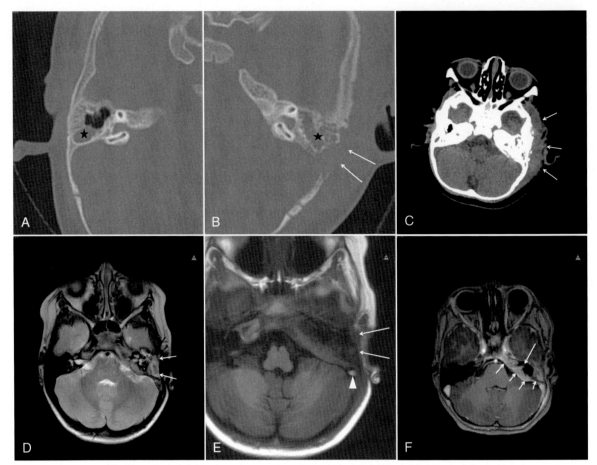

FIG. 5.4 On the axial multislice CT images from the right **(A)** and left **(B)** temporal bone bilateral oto-mastoid opacification is noted (*star*) and is more pronounced on the left side. On the left side, moreover, coalescence of mastoid cells is seen, with breakthrough of the lateral bony wall of the mastoid (*white arrows* in **B**) and with the presence of a subperiostal flegmone **(C)** (*white arrows*). On the corresponding T2-weighted image **(D)** and T1-weighted image (T1WI) **(E)**, respectively, a high and an intermediate signal are present in the opacified left otomastoid (*white arrows*). The high signal on the T1WI indicates the presence of thrombus in the sigmoid sinus (*arrowhead* in **E**). On the postgadolinium T1WI **(F)** important meningeal infiltration is also seen, with strong enhancement and thickening of the meninges along the posterior wall of the temporal bone (*short white arrows*), even extending in the internal auditory meatus (*long white arrow*).

tympanic membrane changes much better, so the CT examination is more dedicated to the evaluation of the various middle ear changes, such as the opacification of the cavity, ossicular chain erosions, and phenomena causing fixation of the ossicular chain, such as formation of fibrous tissue, calcification, or even ossification.

The tympanic membrane is often thickened in the case of chronic otomastoiditis or is perforated. These changes are often seen clearly on CT, but the otologist will for sure be more interested in what is seen behind the membrane. Retraction of the tympanic membrane is another phenomenon often seen in the chronically inflamed middle ear, and this can sometimes lead to confusing CT findings whereby the membrane is positioned on the stapes, whereas the malleus and incus are excluded from the process of sound conduction. In more extreme circumstances, mostly in the case of a coexisting cholesteatoma, the ossicular chain can be absent as a result of autoevacuation and the retracted membrane is positioned on the oval window. The cholesteatoma is also evacuated, but its matrix is not (Fig. 5.7).

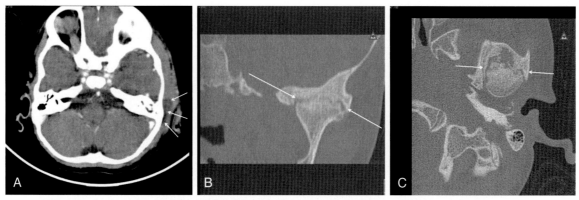

FIG. 5.5 On the axial multislice CT (MSCT) image **(A)** at the temporal bone level and with soft tissue set-ting, obtained in a severely ill child with fever and ear pain, formation of a hypodense subperiostal abscess is shown (*white arrows*). Several months later and after resolution of the acute infectious ear problem, MSCT images of the temporomandibular joint region **(B** and **C)** displayed in bone window setting show a rare complication: temporomandibular joint ankylosis (*white arrows*).

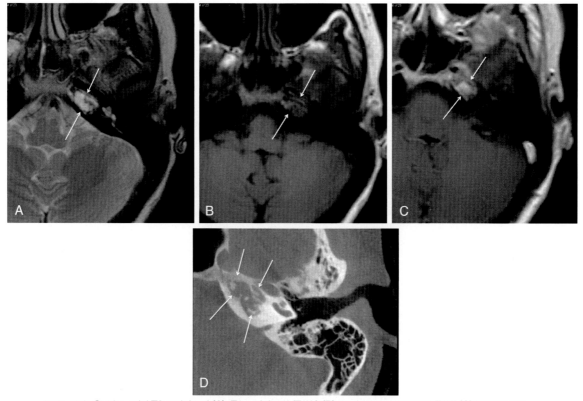

FIG. 5.6 On the axial T2-weighted **(A)**, T1-weighted (T1W) **(B)**, and postgadolinium T1W **(C)** images the opacified left petrous apex, respectively, shows hyperintense and isointense signals and enhances: limited petrous apicitis (*white arrows*). The corresponding axial cone beam CT image is also shown **(D)** (*white arrows*).

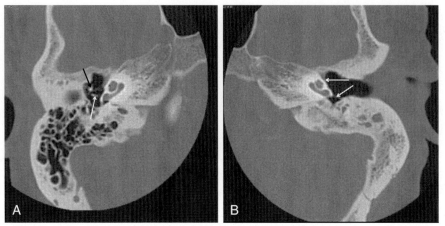

FIG. 5.7 On the axial multislice CT images of the right **(A)** and left **(B)** temporal bones of a patient with chronic left-sided ear discharge and without previous surgical history, the normal malleus neck (*black arrow* in **A**) and incudostapedial joint (*white arrow* in **A**) are seen on the right, whereas on the left side no ossicles are present, and the tympanic membrane is in a retracted position on the window (*white arrows* in **B**): status after autoevacuation.

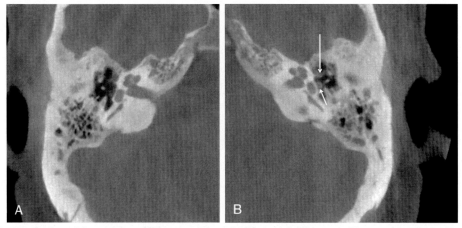

FIG. 5.8 On the axial cone beam CT images of the right **(A)** and left **(B)** temporal bones of a patient with chronic left-sided otomastoiditis normal middle ear findings are seen on the right, but on the left side the stapes is seen too well (*short white arrow* in **B**) and thickening is noted of the tensor tympani muscle tendon (*long white arrow* in **B**) as a result of a nonbony noncalcific soft tissue debris encasing it: fibrous tissue fixation.

In the chronically inflamed middle ear, opacification of the cavity is present and is seen as an effusion with intermediate density. The progressing inflammation can lead to the formation of fibrous tissue, seen on CT as a nonbony noncalcific soft tissue debris encasing some or all of the ossicular chain and its suspensory apparatus, causing fixation of the chain (Fig. 5.8). Ligaments and tendons appear thickened on CT, and it looks as if the stapes is too well seen. A second phenomenon causing ossicular fixation is tympanosclerosis, with deposition of calcifications on the tympanic membrane and in the middle ear cavity, as well on the ossicles itself as on the suspensory apparatus (Fig. 5.9). A third and much rarer phenomenon that causes postinflammatory ossicular fixation is new bone formation. It appears on CT as thick bony webs or general bony encasement (Fig. 5.10).[15,16]

It is known that chronic otitis media can lead to the development of erosions of the ossicular chain, but it is rather rare if no cholesteatoma is present. The observation of ossicular erosions must consequently alert the radiologist that the presence of a cholesteatoma is very probable.

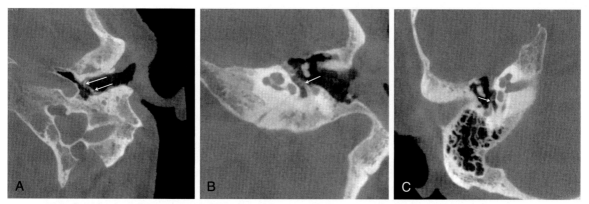

FIG. 5.9 On the axial cone beam CT image obtained at the level of the left eardrum **(A)** thickening and calcification of the tympanic membrane (also called myringosclerosis) (*white arrows*) is present. The stapedius muscle tendon is also thickened and hyperdense because of the presence of calcifications **(B)** (*white arrow*): tympanosclerosis. The contralateral normal stapedius muscle tendon is shown for comparison **(C)** (*white arrow*).

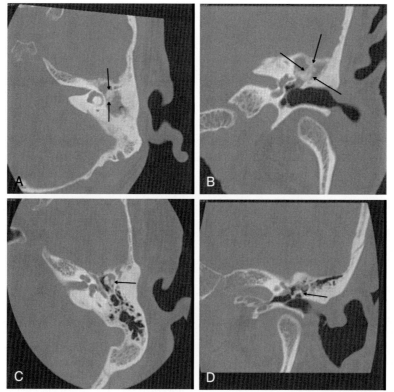

FIG. 5.10 On the axial **(A** and **C)** and coronal **(B** and **D)** multislice CT images obtained through the left temporal bone in two patients with a long history of chronic otomastoiditis large bony webs are present with encasement of the chain: new bone formation (*black arrows*).

### Chronic Otomastoiditis With Cholesteatoma

The vast majority of cholesteatomas are acquired in origin (98%) and result from an ingrowth of keratinizing stratified squamous epithelium through the tympanic membrane into the middle ear cavity. This epithelialized pocket grows faster in an infected middle ear cavity and can cause a mass effect, which can lead to erosion of the ossicles and bony walls of the tympanic cavity and mastoid.[17] Two types of acquired cholesteatoma have been described: pars flaccida cholesteatoma (80%) and pars tensa cholesteatoma (20%). A so-called pars flaccida cholesteatoma originates in the Prussak space (space between the tympanic membrane, the lateral malleal ligament, and the neck of the malleus), grows in the direction of the posterolateral attic, can extend to the mastoid via a route lateral to the incus, and displaces the ossicular chain medially. A pars tensa cholesteatoma originates on the posterosuperior portion of the eardrum, grows in the direction of the facial recess and tympanic sinus, can extend to the mastoid via a route medial to the incus, and displaces the ossicular chain laterally. Patients with cholesteatoma have complaints of ear discharge and hearing loss.

On CT an acquired cholesteatoma appears as a soft tissue mass with a homogeneous density of about 50 HU. Cholesteatoma consequently is undistinguishable from inflammatory tissue, granulation tissue, or scar tissue. As a consequence the beginning of cholesteatoma formation can be missed on CT. Once the cholesteatoma has become larger, and, besides the middle ear opacification, erosion of the ossicles and other bony structures in the tympanic cavity becomes clear, the diagnosis of cholesteatoma can be made with more confidence. The combined finding of opacification on the one hand and erosions on the other indicates the presence of a cholesteatoma in 90% of the cases.

The incus long process and incus lenticular process are the most vulnerable structures in the ossicular chain, followed by the stapes head. The malleus and incus body are more resistant.[18] Pars flaccida cholesteatoma most frequently erodes the incus long process. Pars tensa cholesteatoma primarily erodes the incus long process and stapes superstructure. CT has proved to be very reliable in the evaluation of ossicular chain erosions, and this is also true for the more minute components of the chain, such as the incudostapedial joint and stapes superstructure.[19]

In addition to causing ossicular erosions, cholesteatomas also erode other bony structures in the tympanic cavity. Seen with any frequency are erosions of the scutum and more rarely of the tegmen tympani and of the lateral wall of the lateral semicircular canal. Fistula formation to the membranous labyrinth occurs with an incidence of 0.3 per 100,000 and causes complaints of dizziness.[20] In a large number of patients with fistula to the lateral semicircular canal the facial nerve canal is also eroded.[21] Intracranial complications of cholesteatoma are extremely rare and do not differ from those seen in the case of acute otomastoiditis: sigmoid sinus thrombosis, meningitis, and abscess formation in the brain.

MRI has played an important role in the diagnosis of cholesteatoma for many years. Initially, two completely different MRI techniques were used, one based on the absence of enhancement noted in a cholesteatoma on the T1WI performed 45 min after iv injection of gadolinium and the other based on the high signal seen in cholesteatomas on diffusion-weighted images (DWI). Later the use of a better DWI sequence, so-called non-echo-planar image (EPI) DWI, has become the first choice and gadolinium is no longer used. Non-EPI DWI is widely used, especially in a postoperative setting, before second-look procedures (Figs. 5.11–5.13).[22–24]

## INNER EAR: LABYRINTHITIS

Labyrinthitis is an inflammation of the inner ear. Symptoms of labyrinthitis include loss of balance and dizziness, nausea with vomiting, tinnitus, and vertigo. Of the wide variety of diseases causing labyrinthitis, infection is the most frequent one, and the agent is most frequently of viral (cytomegalovirus, varicella zoster virus) or bacterial origin (*S. pneumoniae*, *Haemophilus influenzae*, *Neisseria meningitides*). Rarely noninfective labyrinthitis is seen in some autoimmune diseases, such as Wegener granulomatosis, polyarteritis nodosa, and Sjögren syndrome.

From an imaging point of view it is most convenient to categorize labyrinthitis by origin/etiology. Four categories are seen: tympanogenic, meningogenic, hematogenous, and traumatic labyrinthitis. The first two are more frequent and are almost always, respectively, unilateral and bilateral. In the case of tympanogenic labyrinthitis, infection spreads from the middle ear into the inner ear through the round or oval window. In the case of meningogenic labyrinthitis, infection is supposed to spread from the meninges to the inner ear through the cochlear aqueduct or via the lamina cribrosa in the vestibule.[25]

Three radiologic stages of labyrinthitis are described based on the histology that also describes three stages of evolution: acute stage, fibrous stage, and ossifying stage.

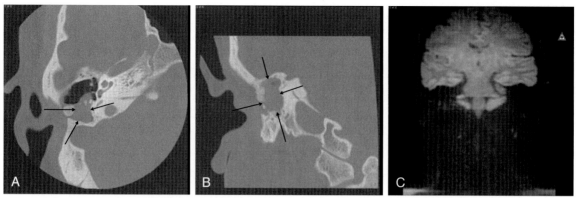

FIG. 5.11 On the axial **(A)** and coronal **(B)** multislice CT images obtained through the right temporal bone in a patient who previously underwent mastoidectomy for cholesteatoma, opacification of the mastoid cavity is seen (*black arrows*). The origin of this opacification is unclear because CT is unable to differentiate cholesteatoma from any other opacification, such as inflammatory tissue, granulation tissue, or scar tissue. The non-echo-planar diffusion-weighted image **(C)** shows no high signal, indicating the absence of a cholesteatoma.

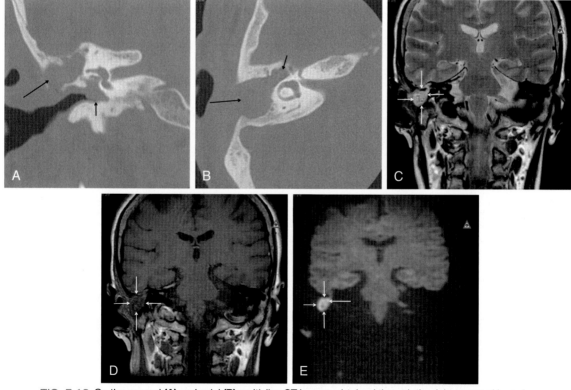

FIG. 5.12 On the coronal **(A)** and axial **(B)** multislice CT images obtained through the right temporal bone in a patient who previously underwent mastoidectomy for cholesteatoma, complete opacification of the middle ear cavity (*short black arrow*) and mastoidectomy cavity (*long black arrow*) is seen. No decision can be made concerning the origin of this opacification, so the eventual underlying recurrent/residual cholesteatoma can neither be confirmed nor excluded. On the corresponding coronal T2-weighted **(C)** and T1-weighted **(D)** images the opacification (*white arrows*), respectively, has a high and intermediate signal. The non-echo-planar diffusion-weighted image **(E)** shows a high signal, indicating the presence of a cholesteatoma (*white arrow*).

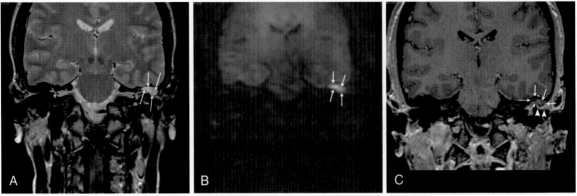

FIG. 5.13 On the coronal T2-weighted (T2WI) **(A)**, non-echo-planar diffusion-weighted (non-EPI DWI) **(B)**, and postgadolinium T1-weighted (T1WI) **(C)** images of a patient with left-sided recurrent cholesteatoma after mastoidectomy the MRI behavior of such a cholesteatoma is clearly shown: high signal on T2WI (*white arrows* in **A**), high signal on non-EPI DWI (*white arrows* in **B**), no enhancement on the postgadolinium T1WI (*white arrows* in **C**), but with an enhancing matrix (*white arrowheads* in **C**).

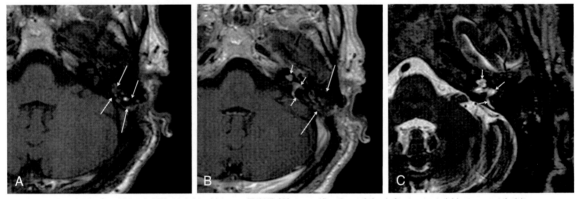

FIG. 5.14 On this axial T1-weighted image (T1WI) **(A)**, opacification of the left otomastoid is present (*white arrows*). The axial postgadolinium T1WI **(B)** shows the enhancing inner ear (*short white arrows*), as well as enhancement of the infected otomastoid (*long white arrows*). The diagnosis of acute stage labyrinthitis can be made because the signal in the fluid-filled spaces of the membranous labyrinth is normal **(C)** (*white arrows*). Because the disease presents unilaterally and with an opacified otomastoid the origin is tympanogenic.

## Acute Stage Labyrinthitis

In the acute stage, edema is present in the membranous labyrinth, and this edema is not visible on CT. On the heavily T2WI on the MRI scan this edema is not distinguishable from the endolymph and perilymph, so this imaging set also shows no anomalies. On the T1WI the signal intensity mostly remains normal or is sometimes slightly increased as a result of hemorrhage. The diagnosis, however, becomes clear on the postgadolinium T1WI showing strong enhancement of the membranous labyrinth. In the case of tympanogenic labyrinthitis the ipsilateral opacification of the otomastoid helps to make the diagnosis (Fig. 5.14).

## Fibrous Stage Labyrinthitis

As labyrinthitis progresses, fibrous tissue invades the membranous labyrinth, causing signal loss on the heavily T2WIs. The enhancement on the postgadolinium T1WI is still present but decreases in intensity. CT mostly remains unremarkable in this stage of the disease (Fig. 5.15).

## Ossifying Stage Labyrinthitis

Frequently after fibrous tissue formation in the inner ear a stage follows in which new bone formation takes place. This ossification obliterates the endolymph and perilymph in the inner ear, causing signal loss on the heavily T2WIs. Contrast enhancement is no longer seen

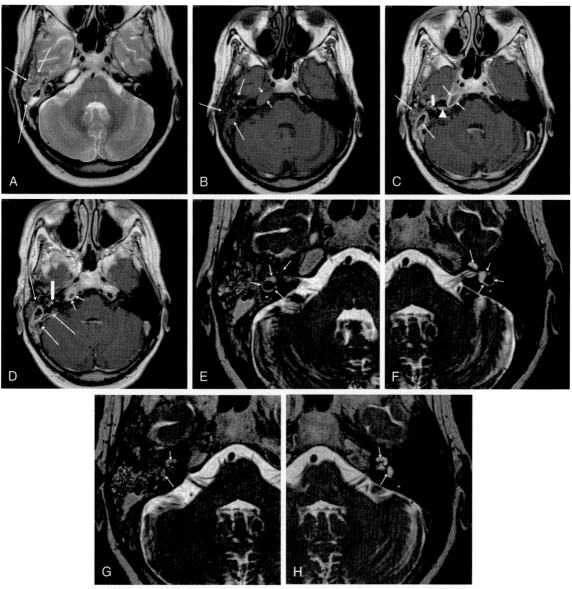

FIG. 5.15 On the axial T2-weighted image (T2WI) **(A)**, infectious opacification of the right otomastoid is seen (*white arrows*). On the axial T1-weighted image (T1WI) **(B)** the otomastoid opacification has an inter-mediate signal (*long white arrows*), as well as the opacification of the petrous apex (*short white arrows*). On the postgadolinium T1WI **(C and D)**, enhancement of the otomastoid is noted (*long white arrows*), including the petrous apex (*short white arrows*). All inner ear structures also enhance (*blocked arrow*), as well as the meninges in the internal auditory meatus (*arrowhead in* **C**). On the high-resolution heavily T2WI from the right **(E and G)** and left **(F and H)** temporal bones the signal in the fluid-filled spaces of the membranous labyrinth, respectively, is decreased and normal (*white arrows*). The diagnosis of fibrous stage labyrinthitis of tympanogenic origin, complicated with petrous apicitis and meningitis, can be made.

on the T1WI. CT finally becomes diagnostically and therapeutically decisive in demonstrating the localization and extent of the ossification process (Fig. 5.16). This information is especially crucial before cochlear implantation.[26,27]

## FACIAL NERVE

Bell palsy is the most common cause of acute facial nerve paralysis (60%).[28] It is a benign, unilateral, usually self-limiting disease, first described by Sir Charles Bell in 1821, most frequently induced by herpes simplex virus. Viral neuronitis of the facial nerve causes nerve swelling, with compression at the nerve's narrowest segments, which are at its foramen in the depth of the internal auditory meatus and along its labyrinthine (second) segment. This nerve compression leads to acute facial weakness.

Ramsay-Hunt syndrome is the combination of acute facial nerve paralysis with herpes zoster infection of the face, with vesicular eruptions over the face, eardrum, and neck. The condition is also referred to as herpes zoster. Often sensorineural hearing loss, dizziness, and facial pain are present. The infection affects most commonly the trigeminal, abducens, and facial nerves.[29]

Facial neuritis cannot be diagnosed with CT. On MRI, facial neuritis presents as a linear contrast enhancement after iv injection of gadolinium because of disruption of the blood-nerve barrier. Such enhancement can be diagnosed with confidence only along segments of the nerve that normally do not enhance, which means in the depth of the internal auditory meatus (Fig. 5.17) and along the first (labyrinthine) segment of the nerve along its course before the geniculate ganglion. A more pronounced perineural vascular plexus is usually present along the second (tympanic) and third (mastoid) segments of the nerve. For that reason, enhancement along these segments is often present in the normal population, so the diagnosis of facial neuritis is not reliable if enhancement is seen there. Purely on the basis of MRI it is also not possible to differentiate the virus causing the enhancement.

Routine imaging of patients with acute facial nerve paralysis is still controversial, as patients with Bell palsy show spontaneous functional recovery in 80% of the cases. Imaging is recommended if the palsy presents in an unusual way or when an etiology other than infection is suspected (e.g., palpable parotid mass).

Lyme disease or Lyme borreliosis is an infection caused by tick bite whereby spirochetes of the *Borrelia* species get transmitted, often *Borrelia burgdorferi*. Approximately a week after the bite, patients can develop erythema migrans. Other symptoms include fever, headache, and fatigue. Involvement of the central nervous system is, together with cardiac and joint involvement, part of the late symptoms when the disease is left untreated. In the case of neuroborreliosis, facial nerve invasion can occur (10%), leading to enhancement of the nerve on MR after iv injection of gadolinium. This is sometimes bilateral, and often other cranial nerves are also affected. It is mandatory to suggest neuroborreliosis if a child presents with an MRI scan on which enhancement is present along the cisternal course of multiple cranial nerves. Treatment is with antibiotics.[30]

## CONCLUSION

In necrotizing external otitis, a rare and severe infection almost exclusively affecting the diabetic and immunocompromised patient, MRI is the best choice to image the extent of the disease. In the case of acute otomastoiditis, a rather rare infection mostly seen in children, CT is helpful to demonstrate coalescence of mastoid cells and the eventual breakthrough of the bony mastoid walls, with risk for formation of a subperiosteal abscess or sigmoid sinus thrombosis. Chronic otomastoiditis is frequently seen and can present without or with cholesteatoma. In patients with chronic otomastoiditis, CT is used to evaluate the ossicular chain and the bony walls of the middle ear and mastoid, and MRI with non-EPI DWI is used to differentiate cholesteatoma from other soft tissue masses. Inner ear inflammation or labyrinthitis is most frequently of tympanogenic or meningogenic origin. In the acute and fibrous stages CT is of no use, but MRI can easily provide the diagnosis. In the ossifying stage of labyrinthitis, both CT and MRI can be used. Facial neuritis cannot be diagnosed with CT, but MRI can show linear contrast enhancement.

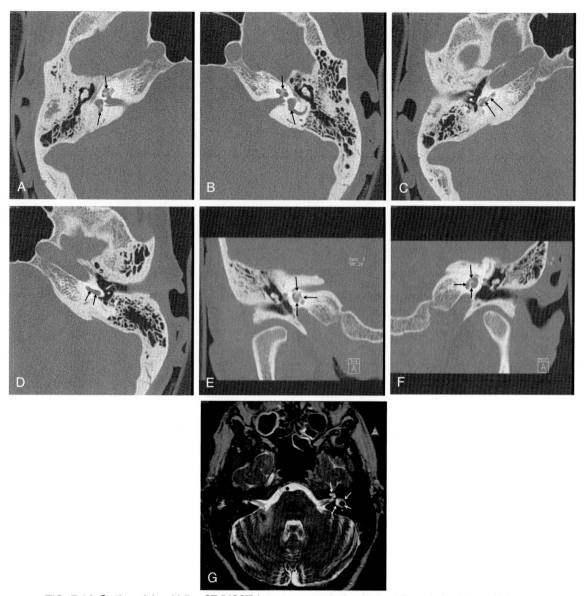

**FIG. 5.16** On the axial multislice CT (MSCT) images, respectively, obtained through the right and left temporal bones at the level of the middle and apical cochlear turns **(A** and **B)** and at the level of the basal cochlear turn **(C** and **D)** ossification is seen in the membranous labyrinth on the right side (*black arrows*). The membranous labyrinth on the left side is normal (*black arrows*). The cochlear ossifying labyrinthitis is also well appreciated on the coronal MSCT image **(E)**, and on the left a normal cochlear density is present **(F)** (*black arrows*). On the high-resolution heavily T2WI **(G)**, complete signal loss is seen in the fluid-filled spaces of the membranous labyrinth on the right side. On the left side the normal high signal is preserved (*white arrows*).

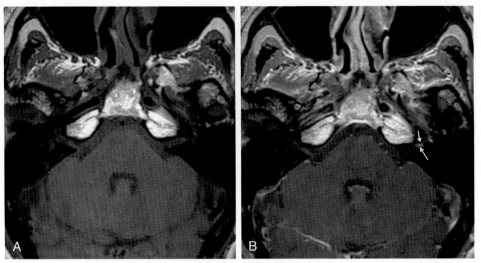

FIG. 5.17 On the axial T1-weighted image (T1WI) before intravenous injection of gadolinium **(A)** no enhancement is seen in the internal auditory meatus bilaterally. On the axial T1WI after intravenous injection of gadolinium **(B)** no enhancement is seen in the internal auditory meatus on the right side, but on the left obvious enhancement (*arrows*) is noted in the depth of the meatus.

## ACKNOWLEDGMENTS

I thank Nancy Verpoort who spent a considerable amount of time editing the figures and texts.

## REFERENCES

1. Rubin J, Yu VL. Malignant external otitis: insights into pathogenesis, clinical manifestations, diagnosis and therapy. *Am J Med.* 1988;85:391–398.
2. Rubin J, Curtin HD, Yu VL, et al. Malignant external otitis: utility of CT in diagnosis and follow-up. *Radiology.* 1990;174:391–394.
3. Grandis JR, Curtin HD, Yu VL. Necrotizing (malignant) external otitis: prospective comparison of CT and MR imaging in diagnosis and follow-up. *Radiology.* 1995;196:499–504.
4. Kwon BJ, Han MH, Oh SH, et al. MRI findings and spreading patterns of necrotizing external otitis: is a poor outcome predictable? *Clin Radiol.* 2006;61:495–504.
5. Cohen-Kerem R, Uri N, Rennert H, et al. Acute mastoiditis in children: is surgical treatment necessary? *J Laryngol Otol.* 1999;113:1081–1085.
6. Bahadori RS, Schwartz RH, Ziai M. Acute mastoiditis in children: an increase in frequency in Northern Virginia. *Pediatr Infect Dis J.* 2000;19:212–215.
7. Kattan H, Drat W. Intracranial otogenic complications: inspite of therapeutic progress still a serious problem. *Laryngorhinootologie.* 2000;79:609–615.
8. Antonelli PJ, Garside JA, Mancuso AA, et al. Computed tomography and the diagnosis of coalescent mastoiditis. *Otolaryngol Head Neck Surg.* 1999;120:350–354.
9. Bauer PW, Brown KR, Jones DT. Mastoid subperiosteal abscess management in children. *Int J Pediatr Otorhinolaryngol.* 2002;63:185–188.
10. Hentona H, Ohkudbo J, Tsutsumi T, et al. Pneumatization of the petrous apex. *Nippon Jibiinkoka Gakkai Kaiho.* 1994;97:450–456.
11. Moore KR, Harnsberger HR, Shelton C, et al. 'Leave me alone' lesions of the petrous apex. *Am J Neuroradiol.* 1998;19:733–738.
12. Muckle RP, De la Cruz A, Lo WM. Petrous apex lesions. *Am J Otol.* 1998;19:219–225.
13. Falcioni M, Taibah A, De Donato G, et al. Preoperative imaging in chronic otitis surgery. *Acta Otorhinolaryngol Ital.* 2002;22:19–27.
14. Rocher P, Carlier R, Attal P, et al. Contribution and role of the scanner in the preoperative evaluation of chronic otitis. Radiosurgical correlation apropos of 85 cases. *Ann Otolaryngol Chir Cervicofac.* 1995;112:317–323.
15. Swartz JD, Wolfson RJ, Marlowe FI, et al. Postinflammatory ossicular fixation: CT analysis with surgical correlation. *Radiology.* 1985;154:697–700.
16. Lemmerling MM, De Foer B, Vandevyver V, et al. Imaging of the opacified middle ear. *Eur J Radiol.* 2008;66:363–371.
17. Schuknecht HF. Infections. In: *Pathology of the Ear.* 2nd ed. Philadelphia: Lea and Febiger; 1993:191–253.
18. Swartz JD. Cholesteatomas of the middle ear: diagnosis, etiology and complications. *Radiol Clin N Am.* 1984;22:15–35.
19. Lemmerling MM, Stambuk HE, Mancuso AA, et al. Normal and opacified middle ears: CT appearance of the stapes and incudostapedial joint. *Radiology.* 1997;203:251–260.

20. Kvestad E, Kvaerner KJ, Mair IW. Labyrinthine fistula detection: the predictive value of vestibular symptoms and computerized tomography. *Acta Otolaryngol.* 2001;121:622–626.

21. Romanet P, Duvillard C, Delouane M, et al. Labyrinthine fistulae and cholesteatoma. *Ann Otolaryngol Chir Cervico-fac.* 2001;118:181–186.

22. Williams MT, Ayache D, Alberti C, et al. Detection of postoperative residual cholesteatoma with delayed contrast-enhanced MR-imaging: initial findings. *Eur Radiol.* 2003;13:169–174.

23. De Foer B, Vercruysse JP, Pilet B, et al. Single-shot, turbo spin-echo, diffusion-weighted imaging versus spin-echo-planar, diffusion-weighted imaging in the detection of acquired middle ear cholesteatoma. *Am J Neuroradiol.* 2006;27:1480–1482.

24. De Foer B, Vercruysse JP, Bernaerts A, et al. Middle ear cholesteatoma: non-echo-planar diffusion-weighted MRI imaging versus delayed gadolinium-enhanced T1-weighted MR imaging: value in detection. *Radiology.* 2010;255:866–872.

25. Lemmerling MM, De Foer B, Verbist BM, et al. Imaging of inflammatory and infectious diseases in the temporal bone. *Neuroimaging Clin N Am.* 2009;19:321–337.

26. Mafee MF. MR imaging of intralabyrinthine schwannoma, labyrinthitis and other labyrinthine pathology. *Otolaryngol Clin N Am.* 1995;28:407–430.

27. Xu HX, Joglekar SS, Paparella MM. Labyrinthitis ossificans. *Otol Neurotol.* 2009;30:579–580.

28. Peitersen E. Bell's palsy: the spontaneous course of 2,500 peripheral facial nerve palsies of different etiologies. *Acta Otolaryngol Suppl.* 2002;549:4–30.

29. Gilchrist JM. Seventh cranial neuropathy. *Semin Neurol.* 2009;29:5–13.

30. Eyselbergs M, Tillemans B, Pals P, et al. Lyme neuroborreliosis. *JBR-BTR.* 2013;96:226–227.

# CHAPTER 6

# Temporal Bone Tumors

BERT DE FOER, MD, PHD • LAURA WUYTS, MD •
ANJA BERNAERTS, MD • JOOST VAN DINTHER, MD •
ERWIN OFFECIERS, MD, PHD • JAN W. CASSELMAN, MD, PHD

## INTRODUCTION

This chapter presents an overview of tumoral lesions of the temporal bone. These lesions can be considered to be rather rare. Imaging plays a crucial role in describing the exact extent of these tumors and can be helpful in specifying some of these lesions.

Classification of temporal bone tumors can be done in various ways. It can be based on the location and origin, age of the patient, histologic findings, and benign or malignant aspect of the lesion. Specific attention should be attributed to the young age group, because several tumoral entities are specific for this age group. Special attention should also be paid to various types of pseudolesions and benign lesions mimicking tumoral pathology. These lesions should definitely not be "touched," as any treatment might be very harmful to the patient. Recognition of these lesions by the radiologist is of utmost importance.

In this chapter, classification of tumoral lesions is made based on the location of the lesion: external ear, middle ear, or petrous bone/membranous labyrinth. The most common tumoral lesions are discussed. Several rare entities are also highlighted. Petrous bone apex lesions are not discussed because they are the subject of a separate chapter in this book.

## IMAGING

### Introduction

For the evaluation of a suspected tumor of the temporal bone, Computed Tomography (CT) and Magnetic Resonance Imaging (MRI) are used.

CT is used to evaluate the osseous invasion by the tumor. The aspect of bone invasion can provide additional information regarding the type of tumor.

MRI is considered to have a superior contrast resolution. Various pulse sequences can be used. The use of intravenously administered gadolinium is highly recommended to see the enhancement of the tumor, soft tissues, meninges, and surrounding vascular structures.

The best way to evaluate a tumoral lesion of the temporal bone is MRI—using various pulse sequences—to detect, delineate, and differentiate the tumor in combination with a high-resolution CT (HRCT) in bone algorithm or cone beam CT (CBCT) to see the osseous delineation and eventual osseous lysis and/or sclerosis of the lesion.

### High-Resolution CT/Cone Beam CT

Multidetector CT (MDCT) uses a combination of a fan beam X-ray configuration and multiple detector rows to acquire slices and to subsequently reconstruct a volume dataset. From this dataset, multiple reconstructions can be made in different planes with various thicknesses.

CBCT uses a combination of a cone beam X-ray configuration and a flat panel detector to directly acquire a volume dataset from which slices can be reconstructed in different planes and with different fields of view. CBCT delivers high-resolution bone images (usually in slice thickness of 0.1 mm) at a dose that is mostly substantially lower than that of MDCT.

CT is best acquired without intravenously administered iodinated contrast by means of a high-resolution bone algorithm to see the exact bony delineation of the tumor.

If access to MRI is not available, CT can be performed using intravenously administered iodinated contrast medium. The dataset should in those cases be acquired in soft tissue as well as high-resolution bone algorithm to allow the evaluation of the soft tissues as well as the bony details of the temporal bone.

Multiplanar reconstructions can give additional information regarding the exact extension of the tumor and the invasion of vascular structures, nerve channels, and the membranous labyrinth.

### Magnetic Resonance Imaging

MRI of the temporal bone should be performed using a dedicated multichannel head coil and a high-field-strength MRI system. The authors use a combination of a multichannel head coil with small surface coils placed inside. Depending on the region to be evaluated, the head coil or the small surface coils can be switched on. Both temporal bones should be imaged to compare both sides. The entire skull base should be included. Evaluation of intracranial extension can also be done similarly.

An MRI of the temporal bone should start with an entire brain examination using a T2-weighted fast spin echo (FSE), a turbo spin echo (TSE), or a fluid-attenuated inversion recovery (FLAIR) sequence to exclude associated brain pathologic processes. A heavily T2-weighted sequence, usually a submillimetric three-dimensional (3D) TSE/FSE T2-weighted sequence, is performed to evaluate the fluid content and the signal intensity characteristics in the membranous labyrinth. Thin-slice (2 mm maximum) spin echo T1-weighted sequences are obtained before and after intravenous administration of gadolinium. A complementary axial submillimetric 3D T1-weighted gradient echo sequence is also scanned, to generate the maximum number of slices through the temporal bone. Fat saturation techniques should be applied in one direction after contrast administration.

The acquisition matrix should be at least 512 × 512 with a field of view of 20 cm or less.

Magnetic resonance angiography (MRA) sequences are obligatory in case of a suspected glomus tumor or in the evaluation of a patient with pulsatile tinnitus. A 3D time-of-flight (TOF) MRA sequence before and after gadolinium administration is mandatory to see the small vessels in various vascular malformations and to evaluate the high- and/or low-velocity status of these vessels.

Diffusion-weighted imaging (DWI) sequences, preferably a non-echo planar DWI sequence (non-EP DWI), should definitely be added in case of a suspected tumoral or pseudotumoral lesion of the temporal bone. Using DWI, differentiation between cholesteatomatous (congenital or acquired) lesions or epidermoid cysts can be easily made. In case of lesions with a high cellularity (e.g., lymphoma), DWI can give a clue to the diagnosis by showing a strong diffusion restriction reflected by a very low apparent diffusion coefficient (ADC) value.

## Tumor Extension

In the temporal bone, specific attention should be paid to tumoral invasion along the facial nerve. Spinocellular and basocellular carcinomas of the external auditory canal (EAC) as well as adenoid cystic carcinomas of the parotid gland have the propensity to spread along the course of the facial nerve (Fig. 6.1). The stylomastoid foramen should always be included in the scanning

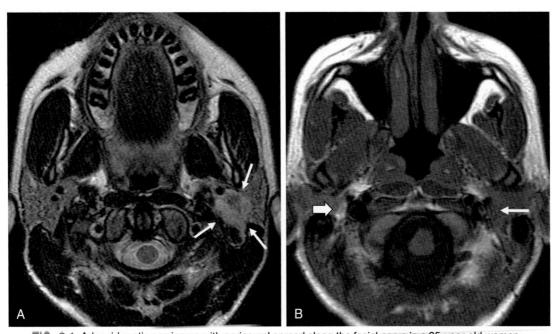

FIG. 6.1 Adenoid cystic carcinoma with perineural spread along the facial nerve in a 35-year-old woman with persistent and painful facial nerve palsy lasting for at least 6 months. **(A)** Axial T2-weighted MR image at the level of the parotid gland shows a slightly hyperintense, heterogeneous, unsharp mass lesion in the left parotid gland (*arrows*): adenoid cystic carcinoma of the left parotid gland. **(B)** Axial unenhanced T1-weighted MR image at the level of the stylomastoid foramen. The right stylomastoid foramen demonstrates normal hyperintense signal because of the fat around the facial nerve (*bold arrow*). This fatty signal on the left side has disappeared because of tumoral infiltration along the facial nerve (*small arrow*).

volume to evaluate its fatty content with the centrally located hypointense facial nerve. Adenoid cystic carcinomas even have the propensity for skip metastases, so careful evaluation of the entire course of the facial nerve is mandatory.

## EXTERNAL EAR AND EXTERNAL AUDITORY CANAL

### Cholesteatoma and Keratosis Obturans

Cholesteatoma and keratosis obturans have been regarded in the past as the same disease process or variations of the same underlying condition. The terms have been used interchangeably in patients presenting with an accumulation of exfoliated keratin within the bony EAC. However, these are two distinct disorders with their own clinical presentations, physical and pathologic findings, and treatment.[1]

Cholesteatomas are most frequently found in the middle ear and mastoid cavity. In rare cases, they originate in the EAC. Typically, this lesion presents in the older age group, is usually unilateral, and is accompanied by a history of chronic ear discharge and otalgia. Several possible causes, such as prior surgery and trauma, have been mentioned.[2] Congenital and acquired cholesteatomas have been reported in cases of congenital stenosis or atresia (Fig. 6.2). Usually external ear canal cholesteatoma requires surgical intervention to remove the cholesteatoma sac and adjacent necrotic bone.[2] Imaging findings are nonspecific, showing a soft tissue mass in the EAC with associated bony erosion on CT.[2,3] Usually the margins of the bony erosion are sharp and regular. In case of associated periostitis, the margins can become irregular. In these cases, differential diagnosis from a malignant tumor is difficult. It is known that accumulated keratin in a cholesteatoma sac causes clear hyperintensity on a $b$1000 DWI MR image[4]; thus non-EP DWI sequences are mandatory to make the diagnosis.

Keratosis obturans commonly occurs in a younger patient group, often in patients with a history of sinusitis or bronchiectasis. Chronic ear discharge is rare. Symptoms are acute severe otalgia and conductive hearing loss. Contrary to cholesteatoma, keratosis obturans is often bilateral. Keratosis obturans more often causes diffuse widening of the EAC and less bone erosion.[1,2]

### Exostoses and Osteomata

Benign bony tumors of the EAC are exostoses and osteomas. Exostoses are by far more common than osteomas.[2]

Exostoses are broad-based lesions in the medial half of the EAC near the tympanic annulus. There is a clear relationship with a history of repetitive exposure to cold water, as in surfing, swimming, and diving. This entity is hence often referred to as "surfer's" or "swimmer's" ear (Fig. 6.3). These lesions are often bilateral and asymptomatic. Occasionally they become large enough to cause obstruction of the EAC with retention of debris. CT demonstrates the broad-based bony lesion nicely and shows the extent of the disease and the eventual retroobstructive pathologic findings in the middle ear. MRI makes little contribution apart from differentiating retroobstructive pathologic findings, such as cholesteatoma and/or inflammation.[2]

Osteomas are much rarer and are situated in the lateral part of the EAC. They occur unilaterally and involve all the layers of normal bone, including bone marrow. Osteomas may also arise in the middle ear and mastoid (Fig. 6.4) and even from the petrous bone pyramid near the porus of the internal auditory canal (IAC). In the middle ear, they can give rise to conductive hearing loss caused by impingement on the ossicles.

### Malignant Tumors of the External Ear and External Auditory Canal

Malignant tumors of the external ear or the external auditory canal (EAC) are considered rared. There are a number of malignant neoplasms originating in the EAC or affecting it secondarily. The most frequently encountered primary malignant neoplasms of the external ear are spinocellular carcinomas (SCCs) (Fig. 6.5) and basal cell carcinomas. The most frequently encountered primary malignant tumors of the EAC are SCCs (Fig. 6.6), basal cell carcinoma, adenoid cystic carcinoma, and ceruminous gland carcinoma.[2,5–7] Malignant melanoma has been reported to arise on the external ear, secondarily invading the EAC. SCC of the EAC and external ear is usually seen in patients with a prior history of therapy-resistant chronic external and middle ear infection.

It is a tumor of the older generation (50–70 years).

Often, these tumors have a locally very aggressive course,[2,5–7] with extensive bone destruction on CT. MRI is superior in demonstrating the exact soft tissue extension.

The most frequently encountered secondary neoplasms are metastatic lesions in the EAC or parotid adenoid cystic carcinoma directly invading the EAC.[2] Breast carcinoma is the most common hematogenous metastatic lesion to occur within the temporal bone.[2]

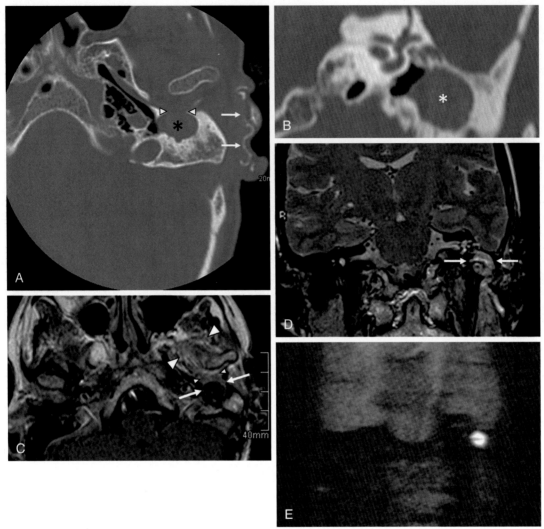

FIG. 6.2 Congenital cholesteatoma of the external auditory canal (EAC) breaking through into the left temporomandibular joint. A 56-year-old female with prior surgery for an external ear atresia now presents with pain at mastication. **(A)** Axial CT image at the level of the left temporomandibular joint and the hypo-tympanum. Note the reconstructed external ear (*arrows*). Instead of an EAC, a sharply delineated punched-out nodular lesion (*asterisk*) is seen at the expected location of the EAC. Note the communication between the lesion and the left temporomandibular joint (*arrowheads*). On this image, further characterization of this lesion cannot be done. **(B)** Coronal CT reformation at the level of the left protympanum. On the expected location of the EAC, a large and sharply delineated punched-out soft tissue lesion (*asterisk*) is found. **(C)** Axial delayed gadolinium-enhanced T1-weighted MR image (same level as in **A**). Note the mixed hypo- to isointensity of the lesion (*arrows*), with some peripheral enhancement. There is a communication with the left temporomandibular joint (*small arrowheads*), with enhancement of the left temporomandibular joint and masticator muscles (*large arrowheads*). **(D)** Coronal T2-weighted MR image (same level as in **B**) shows the moderate to high intensity of the lesion (*arrows*). **(E)** *b*1000 non-EP diffusion-weighted MR image clearly shows the hyperintensity of the lesion in the signal void of the left temporal bone. This hyperintensity is pathognomonic for a cholesteatoma. Final diagnosis based on imaging was a probable congenital chole-steatoma with secondary infection and breakthrough in the left temporomandibular joint. Surgery confirmed these findings.

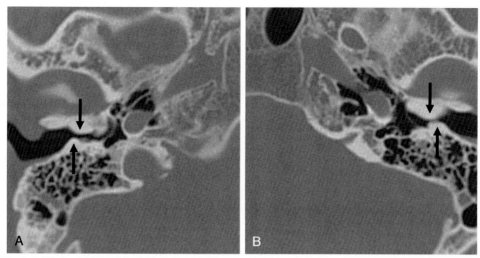

FIG. 6.3 Bilateral external auditory canal (EAC) exostosis. A 57-year-old man was evaluated for conductive hearing loss. Axial high-resolution CT image at the level of the EAC and hypotympanum on the right side **(A)** and on the left side **(B)**. Note the narrowing of the EAC on both sides in its medial part by bony excrescences at the anterior and posterior walls (*arrows*). The patient had a history of diving.

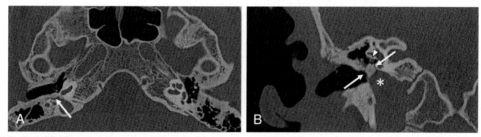

FIG. 6.4 Middle ear osteoma. A 56-year-old man was evaluated for conductive hearing loss. **(A)** Axial CT image at the level of the basal turn of the cochlea. Note the homogeneous round osseous lesion in the posterior part of the mesotympanum (*arrow*). **(B)** Coronal CT reformation at the level of the oval window and vestibule. There is a large protruding jugular bulb (*asterisk*). Note the homogeneous osseous lesion sitting on top of the bony plate on this jugular bulb (*arrows*). The osteoma protrudes in the middle ear. There is an associated dehiscent tympanic segment of the facial nerve (*arrowhead*). The impingement of the osteoma on the ossicles causes the conductive hearing loss.

The prognosis of primary malignant tumors of the EAC depends on the local invasion and the extent of the disease, which can be demonstrated by CT and MRI.[5-7]

Extension of the tumor depends on its site of origin. Tumors originating in the cartilaginous lateral third of the EAC have little or no barriers to extend.

The extension may be anteriorly to the parotid gland.

Currently, there is no staging system for EAC tumors accepted by the American Joint Committee on Cancer or the International Union Against Cancer. Most frequently, the Pittsburgh staging system is used.[6]

When tumors become large, the exact origin of the lesion may be difficult to determine. When extending into the temporomandibular joint and deep spaces of the neck, differentiation from a necrotizing external otitis on imaging can be difficult (Fig. 6.7). Clinical findings, however, differ completely.[2,8] Necrotizing external otitis usually occurs in a younger age group than SCCs of the EAC. The extension pattern toward the temporomandibular joint can also be regarded as rather typical for necrotizing external otitis[8] (Fig. 6.7).

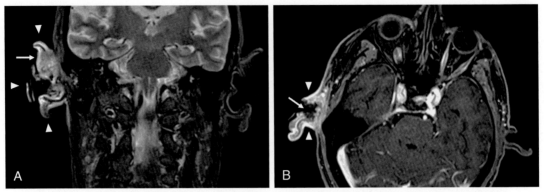

FIG. 6.5 Spinocellular carcinoma of the external ear in a 70-year-old male with swelling and pain of the external ear and central ulceration in the external auditory canal (EAC) opening. Coronal short tau inversion recovery image **(A)** and axial 3D gradient echo T1-weighted image **(B)** after intravenous gadolinium administration. **(A)** There is a diffuse hyperintense signal of the right external ear (*arrowheads*) because of edema with a nodular moderately intense swelling of the superior part of the concha (*arrow*) above the EAC opening. **(B)** Note the enhancement of the concha of the right external ear (*arrowheads*) with the central ulceration toward the EAC opening with some debris in its dependent position (*arrow*).

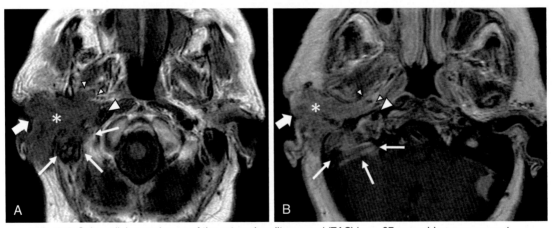

FIG. 6.6 Spinocellular carcinoma of the external auditory canal (EAC) in an 87-year-old woman presenting with right-sided ear pain, itching, and an obliterated EAC. Axial T1-weighted MR image was obtained before **(A)** and after **(B)** intravenous administration of gadolinium. A large hypointense mass lesion is completely obliterating the EAC (*asterisk*) and is secondarily invading the masticator compartment (*small arrowheads*), the external ear (*bold arrow*), and the skull base (*small arrows*). The bulk of the mass lesion is centered on the EAC. The mass lesion is partially encasing the carotid artery (*large arrowhead*). Compare with Fig. 6.7.

In case of skull base osteomyelitis, extension of the pathologic signal intensities on MRI most often spreads toward the skull base rather than to the temporomandibular joint with a low signal on T1-weighted images in the clivus and lateral skull base. Diffusion MRI can in such cases be helpful as ADC values of skull base osteomyelitis are significantly higher than those of tumoral lesions.[9]

## MIDDLE EAR AND MASTOID
### Introduction
The most frequent benign tumor in the middle ear and mastoid is the paraganglioma or glomus tympanicum tumor, followed by facial nerve schwannomas and congenital cholesteatomas. Less frequently adenomatous tumors or adenomas are found. In the entire temporal bone region, the paraganglioma are second in frequency to only vestibulocochlear schwannomas.[10,11]

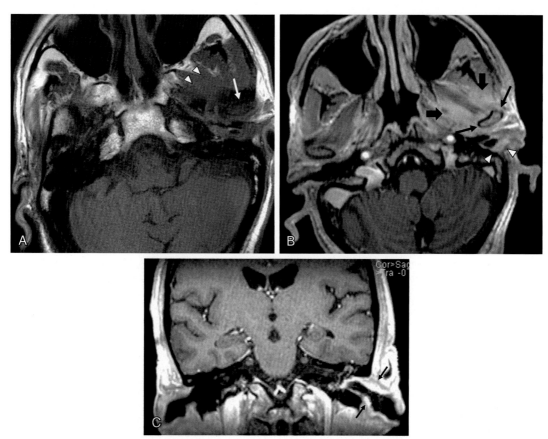

**FIG. 6.7** Necrotizing external otitis in a 57-year-old man with a poorly managed diabetic status. **(A)** Axial unenhanced T1-weighted image: the signal of the left mandibular head is clearly hypointense (*arrow*). The fat planes between the muscles of mastication have disappeared (*arrowheads*). **(B)** Axial enhanced T1-weighted image: there is enhancement in the external auditory canal (EAC) (*arrowheads*), and there is diffuse enhancement of the left mandibular head and temporomandibular joint (*small arrows*). There is diffuse enhancement of the soft tissues around the left temporomandibular joint (*large arrows*). The bulk of this lesion is mainly situated anterior to the EAC. The pattern of spread toward the temporomandibular joint and the space of mastication can be regarded as rather typical for a necrotizing external otitis. **(C)** Coronal reformation of a 3D gradient echo T1-weighted image: there is intense enhancement and slight thickening of the walls of the EAC on the left side (*arrows*).

Malignant tumoral lesions of the middle ear are rare. The most frequent subtypes are the middle ear adenocarcinoma and squamous cell carcinoma.

Specific attention should be paid to tumoral lesions in children and more specifically to rhabdomyosarcoma, Ewing sarcoma, and Langerhans cell histiocytosis.

## Paragangliomas

Paragangliomas arise from the extraadrenal, neural crest-derived paraganglia, the so-called glomus bodies. These glomus bodies lie along the nerves in the inferior temporal bone along the cochlear promontory in the middle ear, giving rise to the glomus tympanicum (Fig. 6.8). They are also situated in the jugular foramen (glomus jugulare), in the common carotid artery bifurcation (glomus caroticum), and along the vagus nerve (glomus vagale). When they involve both the jugular foramen and the middle ear, they are called glomus jugulotympanicum (Fig. 6.9). Most of these jugulotympanic tumors arise in association with the glomus formations of the inferior tympanic branch of the glossopharyngeal nerve (Jacobson nerve) or the mastoid branch of the vagus nerve (Arnold nerve).[11,12]

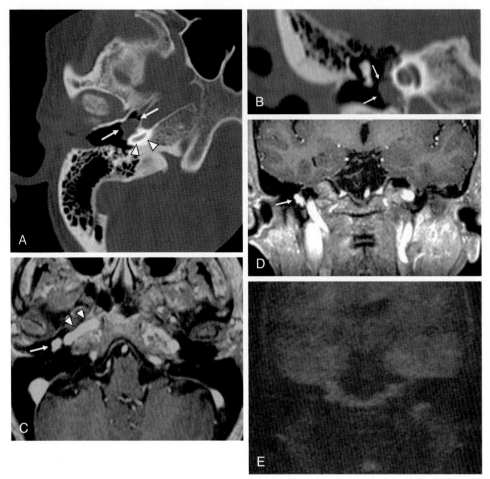

FIG. 6.8 Glomus tympanicum in a 56-year-old woman presenting with pulsatile tinnitus. **(A)** Axial CT image at the level of the basal turn of the cochlea: a nodular soft tissue mass lesion (*arrows*) is found in the anterior inferior part of the middle ear cavity. The lesion is situated against the cochlear promontory. The promontory is caused by the basal turn of the cochlea (*arrowheads*). **(B)** Coronal CT reformation: the nodular soft tissue mass lesion (*arrows*) is seen against the promontory. **(C)** Axial reformation of a gadolinium-enhanced, 3D, T1-weighted gradient echo sequence (magnetization prepared rapid gradient echo [MPRAGE] sequence). A small, strong enhancing mass lesion is found anterior in the signal void of the middle ear and temporal bone pyramid (*arrow*). Compare the strong enhancement of the lesion to the enhancement of the horizontal segment of the internal carotid artery in the skull base (*arrowheads*). **(D)** Coronal reformation of a gadolinium-enhanced MPRAGE sequence. There is a nodular strongly enhancing mass lesion medially in the signal void of the temporal bone (*arrow*). **(E)** Coronal b1000 non-EP diffusion-weighted sequence: no clear hyperintensity can be seen on the location of the lesion. A diagnosis of a cholesteatoma can be excluded.

Paragangliomas account for 0.6% of all neoplasms in the head and neck region. The majority (80%) are situated in the carotid bodies in the common carotid artery bifurcation and in the jugular foramen.[11,12]

The peak age of incidence is in the fifth and sixth decades of life, and there is a clear female predisposition (three to one).

Pulsatile tinnitus is the most important and most common clinical symptom. In case of a large bulky tumor in the middle ear, conductive hearing loss can also be found. Sensorineural hearing loss and vertigo can be caused by inner ear involvement. Numerous cranial nerves may be compromised because of the involvement of the jugular foramen (9th, 10th, and

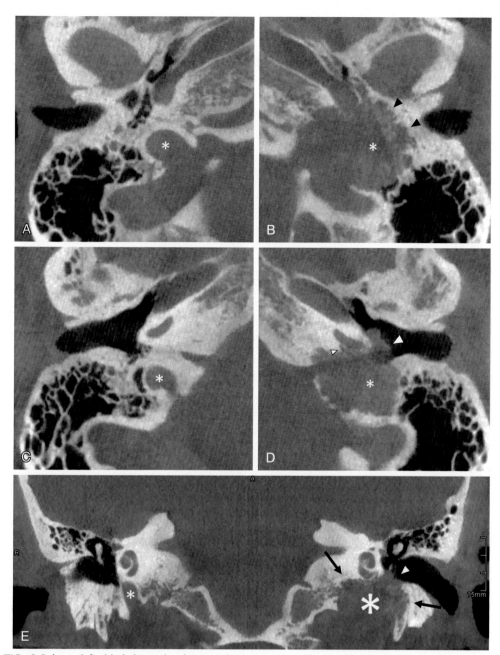

FIG. 6.9 Large left-sided glomus jugulotympanicum tumor in a 26-year-old woman with conductive hearing loss and pulsatile tinnitus. **(A)** Axial cone beam CT (CBCT) image on the right side at the level of the jugular bulb and horizontal carotid canal. Normal right-sided jugular bulb (*asterisk*) with a sharp delineation. **(B)** Axial CBCT image on the left side (same level as in **A**). Note the enlarged jugular foramen (*asterisk*) with its irregular delineation and bone lysis with moth-eaten appearance, most pronounced at its lateral side (*arrowheads*). Compare with the normal side in **(A)**. **(C)** Axial CBCT image on the right side at the level of the basal turn of the cochlea. Normal right-sided jugular bulb (*asterisk*) with a sharp delineation. **(D)** Axial CBCT image on the right side (same level as in **C**). Note the enlarged jugular foramen (*asterisk*) with its irregular delineation already eroding the basal turn of the cochlea (*small arrowhead*). The component of the glomus tumor protruding in the middle ear can be well delineated (*large arrowhead*). **(E)** Coronal CBCT image through the skull base at the level of the cochlea. On the right side, the normal jugular foramen and jugular bulb can be seen (*small asterisk*). Note the enlargement of the jugular foramen on the left side (*large asterisk*) with its clearly irregular delineation and bone lysis with moth-eaten appearance (*arrows*). The component invading the middle ear can easily be evaluated (*arrowhead*).

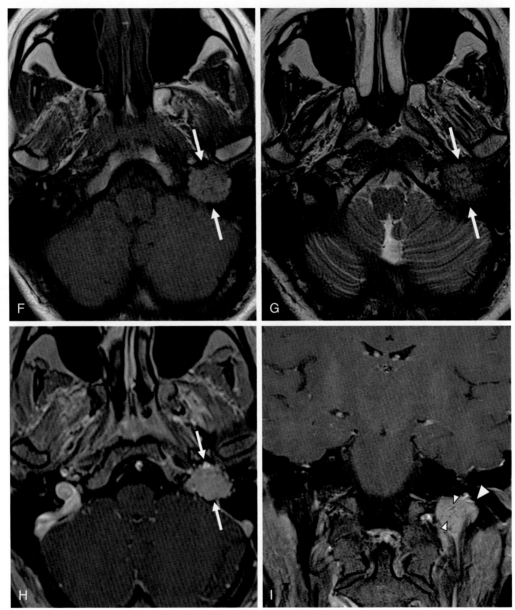

FIG. 6.9, cont'd **(F)** Axial unenhanced spin echo T1-weighted image through the skull base. The glomus tumor can be seen as moderately intense, slightly irregular mass lesions in the enlarged left jugular foramen (*arrows*). **(G)** Axial turbo spin echo T2-weighted image through the skull base (same level as in **F**). The glomus tumor displays intermediate to low signal intensity (*arrows*). **(H)** Axial gadolinium-enhanced 3D gradient echo T1-weighted image (same level as in **F**). Enhancing mass lesion (*arrows*) in the left jugular bulb. The lesion is already touching and compressing the internal carotid artery. **(I)** Coronal gadolinium-enhanced spin echo T1-weighted image: large mass lesion in the left jugular foramen. The small nodular signal voids seen in the tumor represent flow voids in intratumorous arteries (*small arrowheads*). The tumorous component growing in the middle ear can nicely be demonstrated (*large arrowhead*).

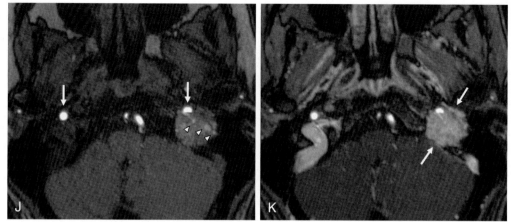

**FIG. 6.9, cont'd (J)** Unenhanced 3D time-of-flight (TOF) MRA demonstrates the high-velocity signal in the right and left internal carotid arteries (*arrows*). Note that the left internal carotid artery is already compressed by the glomus tumor. The small bright dots in the glomus tumor (*arrowheads*) represent the high-velocity vessels in the tumor. **(K)** Gadolinium-enhanced 3D TOF MRA: the jugular bulb is enhancing on both sides with a tumoral enlargement of the left jugular bulb by the glomus tumor (*arrows*).

11th cranial nerves) and the hypoglossal canal (12th cranial nerve). Involvement of the seventh cranial nerve is mostly likely caused by the involvement of the mastoid segment of the facial nerve rather than the tympanic, labyrinthine, and IAC segments.[11,12]

Clinically, the ear, nose and throat (ENT) surgeon will find a blue mass lesion behind the tympanic membrane.

The glomus tympanicum tumor (Fig. 6.8) presents on HRCT/CBCT as a nodular mass lesion situated anteriorly in the hypotympanum against the so-called promontory. The promontory is a bony bulge caused by the cochlea on the medial and anterior hypotympanic wall. The mass lesion can extend into the middle ear cavity, abutting the tympanic membrane. The ossicles are generally spared. If the mass is sufficiently large to fill the epitympanum, attic, and antrum, retention fluid in the mastoid can be found. Bone erosion is usually not present on CT images. Although pulsatile tinnitus is a frequent clinical sign, glomus tympanicum tumors very often cause conductive hearing loss. T1-weighted images show a strongly enhancing mass lesion situated anteriorly in the signal void of the temporal bone pyramid (Fig. 6.8). An appropriate window and level setting makes it possible to situate the lesion against the promotory, even on T1-weighted images. Signal intensities on T2-weighted images may vary but are predominantly intermediate.[10,11]

In case of a glomus jugulotympanicum tumor, HRCT/CBCT clearly demonstrates the moth-eaten erosive appearance of the jugular foramen with extension of the soft tissue mass to the middle ear (Fig. 6.9). Unenhanced T1-weighted images show the mass lesion in the jugular fossa with its characteristic "salt and pepper" appearance. The "pepper" represents the hypointense dots caused by the signal voids of large feeding arteries, whereas the "salt" is secondary to subacute hemorrhage in the tumor.[10–12] On an unenhanced 3D TOF MRA sequence, serpiginous high signal intensities can be found in the tumor, representing the high-velocity flow of the large feeding arteries. In the assessment of paragangliomas, the combination of conventional MRI and contrast-enhanced MRA is significantly superior to conventional MR sequences alone.[13,14] On postgadolinium T1-weighted images, the enhancing mass lesion with its extension to the middle ear can be evaluated (Fig. 6.9).

Care should be taken not to misinterpret normal flow-related signal and enhancement in a large jugular bulb as a meningioma or as a glomus jugulare or jugulotympanicum tumor (Fig. 6.10).[12]

On a clinical basis, it is impossible to make the differentiation between a glomus tympanicum, a glomus jugulotympanicum, and other vascular variants or anomalies, as most of these lesions can present with tinnitus and a retrotympanic bluish or reddish discoloration.

Because a surgical intervention or biopsy can potentially be very harmful in these patients, it is essential that the radiologist is able to recognize these anatomic vascular variants and anomalies.

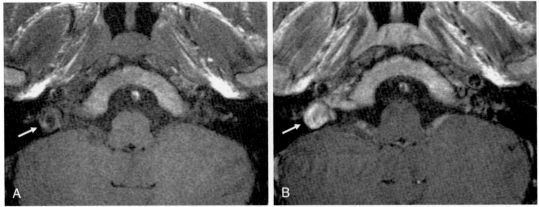

FIG. 6.10 Normal jugular bulb with flow artifacts misinterpreted as a meningioma by a radiologist and several neurosurgeons in a 31-year-old male investigated for vertigo. **(A)** Axial unenhanced T1-weighted image shows a nodular isointense pseudolesion (*arrow*) in the right skull base representing a normal jugular bulb with flow artifacts. **(B)** Axial gadolinium-enhanced T1-weighted image demonstrates enhancement of this nodular pseudolesion. There is indeed a somewhat inhomogeneous signal in the right jugular bulb (*arrow*). This can, however, be regarded as being normal.

A mega jugular bulb can, in the case of deficiency of the bony plate, protrude into the middle ear, giving rise to a blue discoloration of the tympanic membrane.

In those cases, tinnitus has been reported as the most frequent symptom.[15] In case of contact with the ossicular chain, this large protruding dehiscent jugular bulb can even cause conductive hearing loss (Fig. 6.11).[15]

There is also an entity in which an aberrant internal carotid artery can run through the middle ear, presenting as a retrotympanic reddish mass. In this variant, there is an embryologic agenesis of the cervical segment of the internal carotid artery. The embryonic inferior tympanic artery is recruited to bypass the absent carotid segment and runs partially through the middle ear (Fig. 6.12). This hypertrophied vessel may be seen otoscopically and wrongfully considered to be a vascular middle ear tumor.[16]

The persistent stapedial artery is another rare vascular anomaly. Normally, the stapedial artery disappears in the third fetal month; however, it can persist in postnatal life, with the middle meningeal artery arising from it. A persistent stapedial artery originates from the petrous internal carotid artery, enters the hypotympanum in an osseous canal, runs upward between the crurae of the stapes, and then enters the facial canal, running together with the facial nerve (Fig. 6.13) Clinically, it can appear as a reddish retrotympanic pulsatile mass. Its typical course in the middle ear between the crurae of the stapes, together with the absence of the foramen spinosum on imaging, confirms the diagnosis.[17]

Finally, there is another entity in the differential diagnosis of a blue discoloration that also needs to be mentioned.

Middle ear cholesterol granuloma can be regarded as a specific form of chronic middle ear inflammation characterized by the accumulation of blood products and cholesterol with reactive granulation tissue formation. The possible cause is a combination of inflammation, pressure differences, and repetitive microhemorrhage. Findings on CT scan are reported to be nonspecific, with middle ear and mastoid opacification. Expansile scalloping of the surrounding bone and/or ossicular displacement with erosion can occur.[18-20] Clinically, the patient can present with conductive hearing loss, and at otoscopy, the ENT surgeon finds a retrotympanic blue discoloration. On MRI, findings are characteristic, with a spontaneous high signal on T2-weighted and unenhanced T1-weighted images (Fig. 6.14).[18-20] On diffusion-weighted sequences, no high signal on *b*1000 images is found.

### Facial Nerve Schwannoma

The facial nerve schwannoma is the second most common primary middle ear tumor just after glomus tympanicum. It has a predilection for the region of the geniculate ganglion (Fig. 6.15) but can also originate in the tympanic or mastoid segment (Fig. 6.16) of the facial nerve and the internal auditory canal (IAC).

Patients can be asymptomatic or have facial nerve palsy. It should be known, however, that 30% of patients

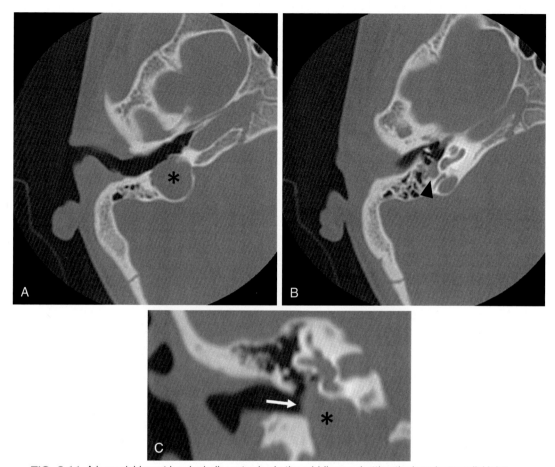

FIG. 6.11 A large dehiscent jugular bulb protrudes in the middle ear abutting the incudostapedial joint and causes conductive hearing loss in a 13-year-old boy. **(A)** Axial CT image on the right side through the hypotympanum and jugular bulb. There is a very large jugular bulb (*asterisk*) protruding in the middle ear cavity. **(B)** Axial CT image on the right side at the level of the round window. A soft tissue density is protruding in the middle ear cavity, abutting the incudostapedial joint (*arrowhead*). **(C)** Coronal CT reformation at the level of the oval window. The large jugular bulb (*asterisk*) is indeed dehiscent and protrudes in the hypotympanum and middle ear (*arrow*).

present without facial nerve palsy. Conductive hearing loss can also be found because, when enlarging, the facial nerve schwannoma can interfere with ossicular function.[21]

Facial schwannomas located in the IAC more likely cause sensorineural hearing loss rather than facial nerve palsy. It should be noted, however, that a tumoral nodular lesion in the fundus of the IAC is more likely to be a vestibulocochlear schwannoma rather than a facial nerve schwannoma. Parasagittal reformations of a high-resolution, 3D, T2-weighted sequence are of help in localizing the lesion in the anterior upper quadrant of the IAC in the case of facial nerve schwannoma

or in the posterior inferior quadrant in the case of the more frequent inferior vestibular nerve schwannoma.

On CT scans, there is an enlargement of the bony delineation of the involved segment of the facial nerve. When situated near the geniculate ganglion, CT usually shows a sharply delineated lytic lesion in the region of the geniculate ganglion. The absence of calcifications makes the differential diagnosis of a facial nerve hemangioma (Fig. 6.17).[19,21] The bony delineation of the enlarged facial nerve canal is usually sharp.[19,21]

To differentiate facial schwannomas from a congenital cholesteatoma, a diffusion-weighted sequence, preferably a non-EP imaging sequence, can be

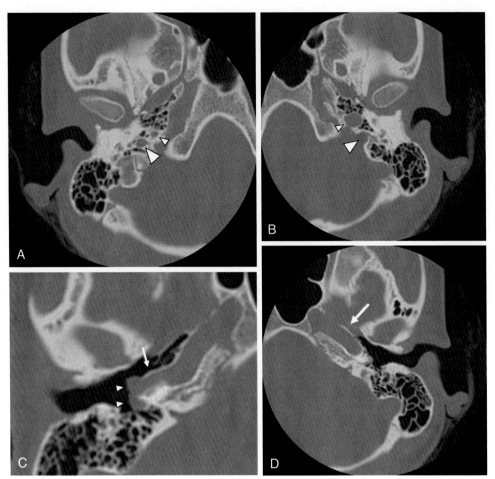

FIG. 6.12 A 21-year-old woman with a subjective feeling of right-sided hearing loss and a normal audiogram. Otoscopy revealed a retrotympanic reddish mass. **(A** and **B)** Axial unenhanced CT scan at the level of the condylar process of the mandible. There is a reduced caliber of the vertical segment of the petrous portion of the right internal carotid artery (ICA) (*small arrowhead*) in comparison with the normal left side. Note the normal jugular bulb (*large arrowheads*). **(C** and **D)** Bilobar mass against the lower medial hypotympanic wall on the right side (*arrowheads* in **C**), representing the hypertrophied inferior tympanic artery as bypass of the agenetic vertical internal carotid artery. Note the lateralized aspect of the bypass on the right side, reaching the horizontal aspect of the ICA (*arrow* in **C**). Compare with the normal horizontal ICA on the left side (*arrow* in **D**).

performed. In case of a facial nerve schwannoma or hemangioma, no clear hyperintensity on a *b*1000 image will be found, contrary to the congenital cholesteatoma (Fig. 6.18).[4,22]

On MRI, diagnosis is mainly made on T1-weighted images, after administration of gadolinium, on which a strongly enhancing mass lesion along the course of the facial nerve can be found.[21]

It should be kept in mind that a focal nodular swelling of the facial nerve can be found in the fundus of the IAC, giving rise to a pseudotumoral swelling in the fundus of the IAC on high-resolution 3D heavily T2-weighted sequences as well as on gadolinium-enhanced T1-weighted sequences in cases of idiopathic facial nerve palsy or Bell paralysis. This is caused by retrograde swelling of the nerve before the narrowest part of its entire course: the bony canal of the labyrinthine segment of the facial nerve. Typically, this nodular swelling is limited to the fundus of the IAC without enlargement of the labyrinthine segment of the facial nerve.[23]

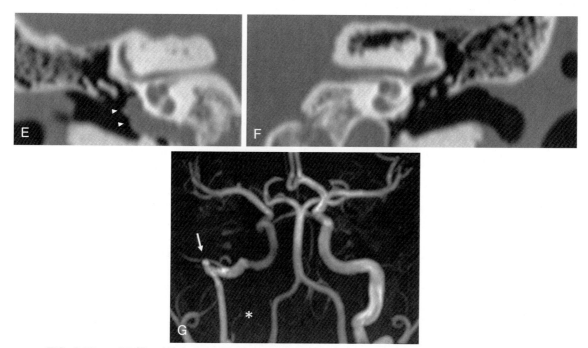

FIG. 6.12, cont'd **(E** and **F)** Coronal CT reformation at the level of the protympanum. Note the bypass running in the right caudal middle ear (*arrowheads* in **E**). Compare with the normal middle ear on the left side. **(G)** Unenhanced 3D time-of-flight MRA of the intracranial arteries shows the hypoplastic vertical segment of the internal carotid artery running clearly more laterally (*asterisk*) than the normal-sized left ICA. Note also the more lateral aspect of the bypass in the middle ear (*arrow*).

The facial nerve can be secondarily involved in tumoral pathology of the petrous bone. It can be involved by direct invasion of contiguous lesions, such as naso- or oropharyngeal carcinomas, or by invasion via retrograde perineural spread, such as in adenoid cystic carcinoma of the parotid gland (Fig. 6.1). Hematogeneous spread from a breast, bronchus, or prostate carcinoma can manifest on imaging as a facial nerve schwannoma (Fig. 6.19).

Another entity that requires mentioning is the epineurial pseudocyst of the mastoid segment of the facial nerve. These lesions are benign and attached to the epineurium of the facial nerve. On imaging, the location posterior to the mastoid segment of the facial nerve is characteristic (Fig. 6.20). On MRI, their cystic nature is confirmed by their high signal intensity on T2-weighted sequences (Fig. 6.20). The majority of epineurial pseudocysts are asymptomatic. Knowledge of their location and aspect are, however, important, as they are located on the access path of mastoidectomy.[24] Although epineurial pseudocysts are reported to be rare, they seem to be much more frequent than reported.

## Congenital Cholesteatoma

Acquired cholesteatoma often originates from a posterosuperior retraction pocket of the tympanic membrane (pars flaccida cholesteatoma) (Fig. 6.21). A less frequent variant originates at the lower part of the tympanic membrane (pars tensa cholesteatoma). Acquired pars flaccida cholesteatoma originates out of retractions of the tympanic membrane, progressively evolving into the Prussak space. Because of its expansion, the cholesteatoma starts eroding the surrounding structures, such as the bony spur of the scutum, lateral epitympanic wall, and ossicular chain (mainly the head of the malleus and the long process and body of the incus). By definition, acquired cholesteatoma is always associated with tympanic membrane abnormalities and associated infection.[4,22]

Congenital cholesteatoma is a congenital anomaly originating at the time of neural tube closure when a part of the ectoderm gets entrapped in the temporal bone. By definition, congenital cholesteatomas are found behind an intact tympanic membrane. They can be found anywhere in the middle ear cavity but are preferably found anteroinferiorly in the

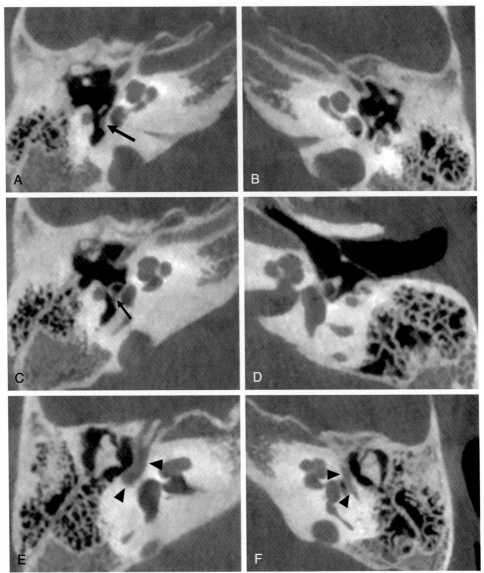

FIG. 6.13 A 9-year-old boy investigated for conductive hearing loss on the right side. Imaging demonstrated a persistent stapedial artery. **(A and B)** Axial cone beam CT (CBCT) image at the level of the sinus tympani, slightly below the oval window, **(A)** right side, **(B)** left side. The persistent stapedial artery can be seen as a tiny soft tissue density against the posterior medial wall of the middle ear (*arrow* in **A**). Note the absence of this structure on the normal left side in **(B)**. **(C and D)** Axial CBCT image at the level of the oval window, **(C)** right side, **(D)** left side. The persistent stapedial artery can be seen as a tiny soft tissue density running through the crurae of the stapes on the right side (*arrow* in **C**). Compare with the normal left side in **(D)**. **(E and F)** Axial CBCT image at the level of the tympanic segment of the facial nerve, **(E)** right side, **(F)** left side. The anterior half of the tympanic segment of the facial nerve on the right side is thickened, reflecting the course of the persistent stapedial artery together with the tympanic segment of the facial nerve (*arrowheads*). Note the normal caliber of the tympanic segment of the facial nerve on the left side in **(F)** (*arrowheads*).

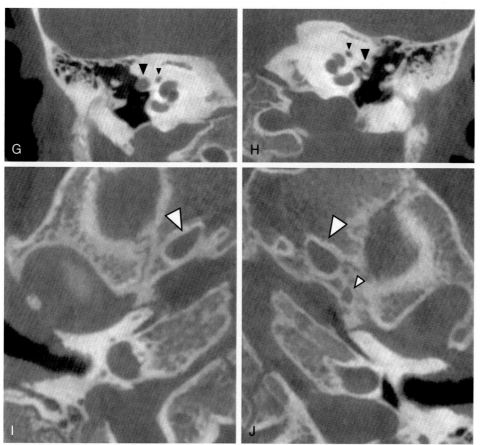

FIG. 6.13, cont'd **(G and H)** Coronal CBCT image at the level of the cochlea, **(G)** right side, **(H)** left side. There is a clear thickening of the anterior portion of the tympanic segment of the facial nerve on the right side (*large arrowhead*) when compared with the labyrinthine segment (*small arrowhead*). Note the normal findings on the left side in **H. (I and J)** Axial CBCT image through the skull base at the level of the foramen ovale, **(I)** right side, **(J)** left side. On the normal left side **(J)**, a normal foramen ovale (*large arrowhead*) and foramen spinosum (*small arrowhead*) can be seen. On the right side **(I)**, only a foramen ovale (*large arrowhead*) can be found.

middle ear (Fig. 6.22) or posterosuperiorly toward the antrum.[3,4,22] Another preferential location is around the region of the geniculate ganglion, very often with a component invading the middle ear associated to a component invading the petrous bone pyramid (Fig. 6.18). However, lesions can be found in any part of the temporal bone pyramid, even invading the membranous labyrinth (Fig. 6.23). Congenital cholesteatoma should always be included in the differential diagnosis of a sharply delineated lytic lesion in the petrous bone or a middle ear soft tissue lesion behind an intact tympanic membrane.

Congenital cholesteatoma is the third most common primary middle ear tumor.

On CT, middle ear congenital cholesteatoma usually presents as a small nodular soft tissue mass very often without any associated ossicular erosion (Fig. 6.22). The Prussack's space is not involved, and the scutum is sharply delineated with a normal pars flaccida of the tympanic membrane.[3,4,22]

MRI can be used to differentiate these middle ear lesions because cholesteatomas appear hyperintense on *b*1000 diffusion-weighted images (Figs. 6.18, 6.22, and 6.23). A non-echo planar diffusion-weighted sequence should be preferred over an echo planar diffusion-weighted sequence, as the former has no susceptibility artifacts at the interface of the temporal lobe and temporal bone and it is able to demonstrate cholesteatomas as small as 2 mm.[3,4,22]

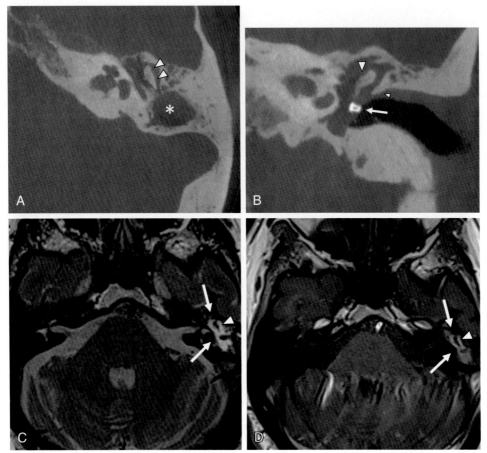

FIG. 6.14 A 42-year-old male with a history of chronic middle ear infection on the left side and a conductive hearing loss on audiogram. Otoscopy revealed a retrotympanic bluish discoloration. **(A)** Axial cone beam CT (CBCT) image at the level of the oval window. There is a complete and homogeneous opacification of the left middle ear and mastoid (*asterisk*). The ossicular chain (*arrowheads*) is not eroded nor is the lateral epitympanic wall. **(B)** Coronal CBCT image at the level of the basal turn of the cochlea. There is complete and homogeneous opacification of the middle ear with an intact scutum (*small arrowhead*) and ossicular chain (*large arrowhead*). Note the metallic intratympanic ventilation tube (*arrow*). **(C)** Axial turbo spin echo (SE) T2-weighted MR image at the level of the internal auditory canal (IAC). There is a complete and homogeneous hyperintensity of the left middle ear (*arrows*). Note the central signal void caused by the ossicles (*arrowhead*). **(D)** Axial SE T1-weighted MR image at the level of the IAC (same level as in **C**). There is a complete and homogeneous hyperintensity of the left middle ear (*arrows*). Note the central signal void caused by the ossicles (*arrowheads*).

On T2-weighted MR images, a congenital cholesteatoma (as well as an acquired cholesteatoma) displays a moderate intensity, clearly lower than that of inflammatory middle ear changes. On T1-weighted images, a congenital cholesteatoma (as well as an acquired cholesteatoma) is hypointense without any contrast enhancement apart from some peripheral enhancement.[3,4,22]

To summarize, the most frequent primary middle ear tumors are (in descending order of frequency) (1) glomus tympanicum, (2) facial nerve schwannoma, and (3) congenital cholesteatoma.

There is, however, another entity that needs to be mentioned in the differential diagnosis of primary middle ear tumors because it has similar (but also slightly different) imaging features and that is the middle

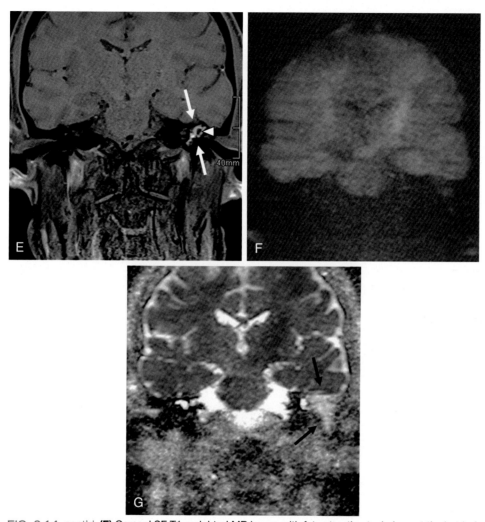

FIG. 6.14, cont'd **(E)** Coronal SE T1-weighted MR image with fat saturation technique at the level of the external auditory canal. The signal intensity of the left middle ear remains high on this fat-saturated T1-weighted image, reflecting the presence of blood (*arrows*). Note again the signal void of the ossicles (*arrowhead*). **(F)** Coronal *b*1000 diffusion-weighted image (same level as in **E**) demonstrates the lack of clear hyperintensity. **(G)** Coronal ADC map. High signal intensity on ADC map (*arrows*), there are no signs of diffusion restriction. The spontaneous high signal intensity on T1- and T2-weighted MR image together with the lack of diffusion restriction is pathognomonic for a cholesterol granuloma.

ear adenoma. It is a very rare, benign, slow-growing lesion arising from the mucosa of the middle ear lining. Rarely, this tumor may progress to a malignant adenocarcinoma. Clinically, the patient presents with conductive hearing loss and a middle ear mass lesion that may have a reddish discoloration. Imaging findings are nonspecific, with a middle ear soft tissue lesion on CT. On MRI, findings are also nonspecific with a

T1-hypointense, T2-hyperintense mass lesion, with enhancement after gadolinium administration[19,25,26] (Fig. 6.24). DWI displays no hyperintensity on *b*1000 images.

## Meningioma

Temporal bone meningiomas are common tumors in an uncommon location.

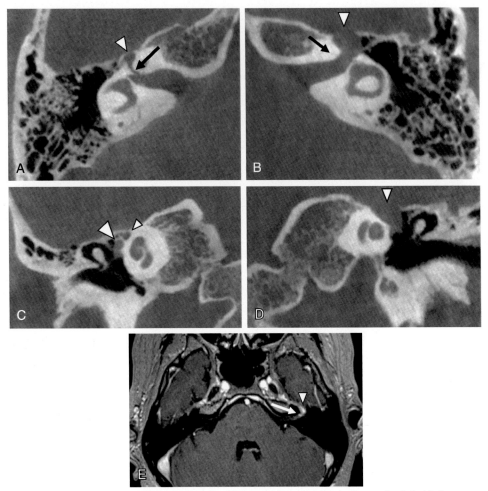

FIG. 6.15 Facial nerve schwannoma centered on the geniculate ganglion region on the left side in a 32-year-old female investigated for relapsing facial nerve palsy. **(A)** Axial CT image on the right side (same level as in **B**). Note the normal aspect of the labyrinthine segment (*arrow*) and geniculate ganglion (*arrowhead*). Compare with **(B)**. **(B)** Axial cone beam CT (CBCT) image at the level of the geniculate ganglion (same level as in **A**). There is an enlargement of the tympanic segment of the facial nerve (*arrow*) and a sharply delineated lytic lesion centered on the geniculate ganglion (*arrowhead*). The lesion has no internal calcifications. Compare with the normal side in **(A)**. **(C)** Coronal CBCT image on the right side through the geniculate ganglion (same level as in **D**). The labyrinthine segment (*small arrowhead*) and the proximal tympanic segment (*large arrowhead*) adjacent to the geniculate ganglion have a normal size (compare with **D**). **(D)** Coronal CBCT image on the left side through the geniculate ganglion (same level as in **C**). Note the enlargement of the geniculate ganglion (*arrowhead*). The labyrinthine segment and the proximal tympanic segment can no longer be distinguished (compare with the normal findings in **C**). **(E)** Axial multiplanar reconstruction of a 3D gradient echo T1-weighted sequence at the level of the geniculate ganglion (same level as in **A** and **B**). There is a fusiform enlargement of the geniculate ganglion (*arrowhead*) as well as the labyrinthine segment (*arrow*).

Meningiomas gain access to the temporal bone by means of three potential sites of origin: the tegmen tympani (or other temporal bone walls), the jugular fossa, and the IAC. Only meningiomas that originate from tegmen tympani/temporal bone walls and jugular fossa meningiomas will be discussed and illustrated in this chapter. The tegmen tympanic meningioma originates from the middle cranial fossa dura and inferomedially spreads through the tegmen tympani. As such, bone infiltration in meningioma most commonly occurs by secondary spread, although primary intradiploic tumors are reported. Bony changes are characterized by a lack of

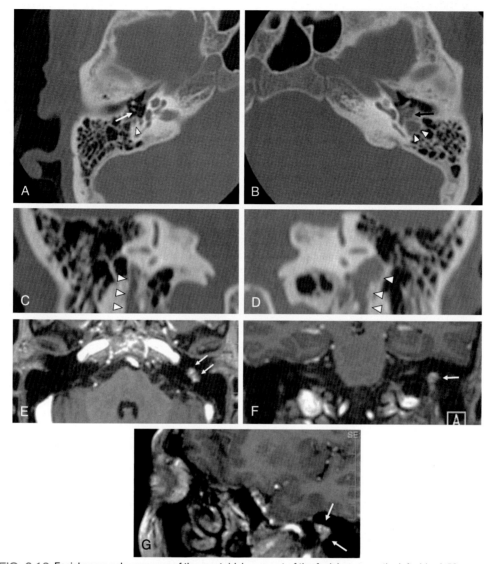

FIG. 6.16 Facial nerve schwannoma of the mastoidal segment of the facial nerve on the left side. A 52-year-old male investigated for conductive hearing loss on the left side. The patient had no facial nerve palsy. **(A)** Axial CT image at the level of the incudostapedial joint on the right side (same level as in **B**). Normal aspect of the mastoidal or third segment of the facial nerve in the pyramidal eminence (*arrowhead*). Note the normal aeration of the middle ear and the normal incudostapedial joint (*arrow*). Compare with **(B)**. **(B)** Axial CT image at the level of the incudostapedial joint on the left side (same level as in **A**). There is a clear enlargement of the bony deline-ation of the third or mastoidal segment of the facial nerve (*arrowheads*). The mass lesion is extending into the middle ear and surrounds the incudostapedial joint (*arrow*). This extension explains the conductive hearing loss on the left side. Compare with the normal side in **(A)**. **(C)** Coronal CT reformation on the right side at the level of the mastoidal segment of the facial nerve (same level as in **D**). Note the normal size and delineation of the mastoid segment of the facial nerve (*arrowheads*) (compare with **D**). **(D)** Coronal CT reformation on the left side (same level as in **C**). There is a clear enlargement of the second genu and mastoid segment of the facial nerve, located under the lateral semicircular canal (*arrowheads*). Compare with the normal findings in **(C)**. **(E)** Axial mulitplanar reformation (MPR) of a 3D gradient echo T1-weighted sequence demonstrating the enhancing mass lesion in the signal void of the left temporal bone (*arrows*). **(F)** Coronal MPR of a 3D gradient echo T1-weighted sequence at the level of the vestibule. A nodular enhancing mass lesion in the signal void of the left temporal bone can be seen (*arrow*). **(G)** Sagittal MPR of a 3D Gradient echo T1-weighted sequence at the level of the second genu of the facial nerve showing the enhancement and thickening of the second genu (*arrows*). Findings on CT and MRI are compatible with a facial nerve schwannoma located on the second genu of the facial nerve.

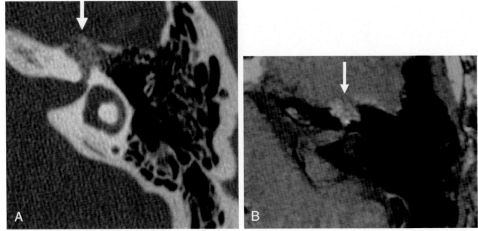

FIG. 6.17 Facial nerve hemangioma at the level of the geniculate ganglion in a patient investigated for conductive hearing loss. **(A)** Axial CT image at the level of the geniculate ganglion. A lytic lesion centered on the geniculate ganglion region (*arrow*) can be found. Note that the lesion has internal dot-like calcifications. **(B)** Axial gadolinium-enhanced T1-weighted image (same level as in **A**). The lesion shows a homogeneous contrast enhancement (*arrow*). There are some small internal nodular hypointensities reflecting the internal dot-like calcifications in the hemangioma. Characteristic appearance of a facial nerve hemangioma on CT and on MRI.

frank bone destruction and sclerosis. The irregular bone deposition occurring along the inner and outer table with speculated margins is regarded highly typical (Figs. 6.25 and 6.26).[27-29] This irregular bone deposition is not seen in fibrous dysplasia of the temporal bone (Fig. 6.27). Clinically, tegmen tympanic meningiomas cause conductive hearing loss because of encasement of the ossicular chain (Figs. 6.25 and 6.26). Complaints of chronic otitis media are also frequently found and may be the main reason for consulting the ENT surgeon.[28,29]

In the differential diagnosis, apart from fibrous dysplasia, cholesteatoma should also be considered. However, on CT, meningiomas lack the destructive bone and ossicular changes as seen in cholesteatoma.

On MRI, an intracranial enhancing dural-based lesion can be found with slight hyperintensity on T2-weighted images, isointensity on T1-weighted images, and strong enhancement after intravenous administration of gadolinium (Figs. 6.25 and 6.26).[27-29]

Another way of gaining access to the temporal bone for a meningioma is extension from the jugular foramen intra- and extracranially (Fig. 6.28). Jugular foramen meningiomas are rare lesions and are the third most frequent jugular foramen tumor after glomus jugulare tumors and schwannomas of the lower cranial nerves.[30,31]

Although these lesions are histologically benign, they are considered locally aggressive, very often with infiltration of the temporal bone (Fig. 6.28). Imaging features are comparable with those of the classic temporal bone meningioma, with a sclerotic aspect of the lesion and its characteristic irregular bony delineation as one of the most characteristic features. MRI characteristics are dominated by the mainly hypointense aspect of the lesion both on T1- and T2-weighted images because of the very often heavily calcified aspect of the lesion (Fig. 6.28). Sometimes, differential diagnosis with other skull base tumors is difficult because of the overlapping imaging features (Fig. 6.29).[32]

## Rhabdomyosarcoma

Rhabdomyosarcomas are the second most common malignant head and neck tumor in children, after malignant lymphoma. In the temporal bone, they originate from intrinsic middle ear and/or Eustachian tube musculature or from primitive pluripotent mesenchymal remnants. Other locations in the head and neck region, such as the orbit, paranasal sinuses, or the nasopharynx, are far more common.[33,34] They usually present clinically as a chronic otitis media, often with a sudden onset of facial palsy or symptoms of involvement of other cranial nerves during the course of the disease. These neurologic "alarm" symptoms, which develop in about 30% of patients, should draw the attention of the clinician (Fig. 6.30).[33,34] Because these tumors have had time to develop, indiscriminate bony destruction is often extensive. The extent of the soft tissue mass is best seen on MRI. MRI characteristics are nonspecific,

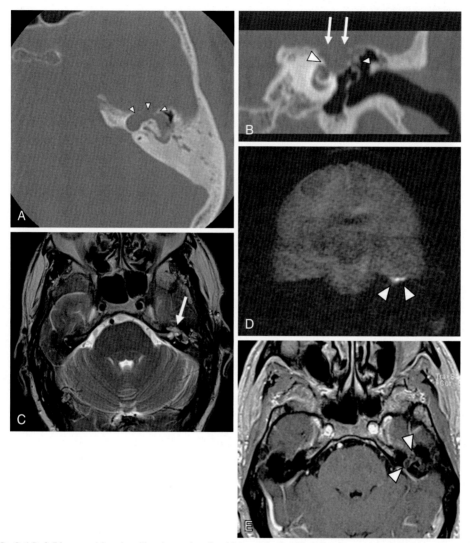

FIG. 6.18 A 51-year-old male with a long-standing history of mixed hearing loss on the left side and a sudden onset of a facial nerve paralysis on the left side (House-Brackmann grade III). **(A)** Axial CT image at the level of the superior semicircular canal on the left side. A sharply delineated semilunar punched-out soft tissue lesion (*arrowheads*) is located anteriorly in the petrous bone apex around the anterior limb of the superior semicircular canal. **(B)** Coronal CT image at the level of the geniculate ganglion and cochlea. Note the large sharply delineated punched-out soft tissue lesion in the region of the geniculate ganglion (*arrows*). The lesion is abutting the cochlea (*large arrowhead*). There is a small component of soft tissue extending in the middle ear attic (*small arrowhead*). The delineation of the ossicles is lost because of the partial evacuation of the middle ear component of the congenital cholesteatoma. **(C)** Axial turbo spin echo T2-weighted image at the level of the membranous labyrinth on the left side. There is a small moderately intense nodular lesion anterior in the petrous bone apex (*arrow*). **(D)** Coronal *b*1000 non-echo planar diffusion-weighted image (same level as in **B**). Bilobular hyperintense lesion, under the tegmen (*arrowheads*), pathognomonic for a congenital cholesteatoma. **(E)** Axial T1-weighted image 45 min after intravenous administration of gadolinium. Anterior and medial in the petrous bone apex, a bilobular peripherally enhancing low-intensity lesion is noted (*arrowheads*). The lesion displays the signal characteristics and the enhancement pattern of a cholesteatoma. The sharply delineated punched-out lesion on CT in the left petrous bone apex, near the region of the geniculate ganglion with invasion in the membranous labyrinth anterior to the superior semicircular canal is highly suspicious of a congenital cholesteatoma. The lesion probably had a large middle ear component, which was partially evacuated through the tympanic membrane into the external auditory canal. MR findings confirm the presence of a congenital cholesteatoma as the lesion displays a clear hyperintense signal on *b*1000 diffusion-weighted images.

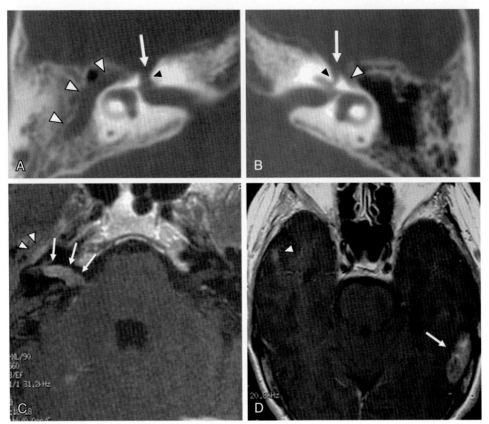

FIG. 6.19 Metastases of a bronchus carcinoma along the course of the facial nerve. A 64-year-old male presenting with a right-sided facial nerve palsy. **(A)** Axial CT image at the level of the tympanic segment of the facial nerve and lateral semicircular canal on the right side. There is a clear enlargement of the labyrinthine segment of the facial nerve (*small arrowhead*), the geniculate ganglion (*arrow*), and the tympanic segment (*large arrowheads*). Compare with the normal side in **(B)**. **(B)** Axial CT image (same level as in **A**). Note the normal size and aspect of the labyrinthine segment (*small arrowhead*), the geniculate ganglion (*arrow*), and the tympanic segment (*large arrowhead*). Compare with **(A)**. **(C)** Axial gadolinium-enhanced T1-weighted MR image at the level of the internal auditory canal. The entire internal auditory canal is filled up with enhancing tissue (*arrows*) The proximal part of the tympanic segment (*arrowheads*) is also enhancing. **(D)** Axial gadolinium-enhanced T1-weighted MR image through the temporal lobe. Large enhancing mass lesion in the left temporal lobe (*arrow*) and second small enhancing mass lesion in the right temporal lobe (*arrowhead*). Brain metastasis of a bronchus carcinoma.

however, with a hyperintensity on T2-weighted images and a moderate intensity on T1-weighted images, with strong enhancement after intravenous administration of gadolinium.[33,34] On imaging, differential diagnosis with Langerhans cell histiocytosis is sometimes impossible, although it is said that the occurrence of neurologic "alarm" symptoms of cranial nerve palsy are far less frequent in Langerhans cell histiocytosis.[35,36] Langerhans cell histiocytosis is often found bilaterally on CT scan, often with sparing of the ossicles as a striking

imaging feature. In the case of an aggressive looking middle ear mass lesion in a child, however, diagnosis of a rhabdomyosarcoma definitely should be considered. There are other rare primary malignant temporal bone tumors such as Ewing sarcoma (Fig. 6.31)[37,38] and hemangioendothelioma, often presented in the literature as case reports. These lesions present with nonspecific complaints of therapy-resistant chronic middle ear infection with often a sudden onset of cranial nerve palsy (Fig. 6.31). Again, the sudden onset of

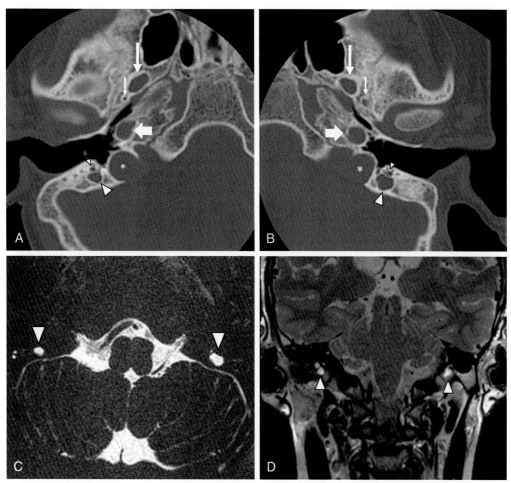

FIG. 6.20 A 14-year-old girl investigated for the presence of residual cholesteatoma, before second-look surgery. **(A)** Axial CT image at the level of the hypotympanum and the skull base on the right side. There is a clear aerated external ear and middle ear cavity. Note the normal structures in the skull base—from anterior to posterior—the foramen ovale (*large arrow*), the foramen spinosum (*small arrow*), the vertical portion of the internal carotid artery (*thick arrow*), the prominent but nondehiscent jugular bulb (*asterisk*) and the mastoidal segment of the facial nerve (*small arrowhead*). Posterior to the mastoidal segment, a nodular and sharply delineated hypodensity can be noted (*large arrowhead*). **(B)** Axial CT image at the level of the hypotympanum and the skull base on the left side (same level as in **A**). There is a clear aerated external ear and middle ear cavity. Again, from anterior to posterior, one recognizes the foramen ovale (*large arrow*), the foramen spinosum (*small arrow*), the vertical portion of the internal carotid artery (*thick arrow*), the prominent but nondehiscent jugular bulb (*asterisk*), and the mastoidal segment of the facial nerve (*small arrowhead*). Posterior to the mastoidal segment of the facial nerve, a nodular and sharply delineated hypodensity can be noted, partially surrounding the mastoidal segment of the facial nerve (*large arrowhead*). **(C)** Axial 3D turbo spin echo (TSE) T2-weighted MR image (same level as in **A** and **B**). Bilateral nodular hyperintensity posterior in the signal void of the temporal bone pyramid (*arrowheads*). The hyperintensity reflects the cystic nature of the lesion. **(D)** Coronal TSE T2-weighted MR image. Bilateral clear nodular hyperintensity posterior and inferior in the temporal bone (*arrowheads*). The aspect and location on CT and MRI with the fluid signal intensity on T2-weighted images is compatible with bilateral epineurial pseudocysts of the facial nerve. Final diagnosis: bilateral epineurial pseudocyst of the intratemporal facial nerve on both sides.

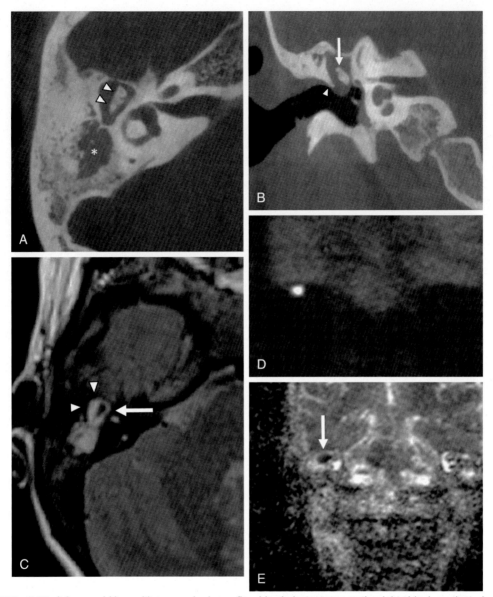

FIG. 6.21 A 9-year-old boy with an acquired pars flaccida cholesteatoma on the right side, investigated for a deep pars flaccida retraction pocket and conductive hearing loss on the right side. **(A)** Axial cone beam CT (CBCT) image on the right side, at the level of the lateral semicircular canal, the maleus head, and the incus body and short process. There is a complete opacification of the middle ear and mastoid (*asterisk*). There is flattening of the maleus head, the incus body, and short process along its lateral side (*arrowheads*) as a subtle sign of ossicular erosion. The lateral epitympanic space is also slightly enlarged. **(B)** Coronal CBCT image on the right side at the level of the cochlea. There is a nodular soft tissue lesion in the Prussak space. The scutum is blunted (*arrowhead*), and there is a small erosion of the maleus head (*arrow*). **(C)** Axial turbo spin echo T2-weighted image at the level of the superior semicircular canal (same level as in **A**). There is a small nodular lesion with moderate intensity in the anterior epitympanic space (*arrowheads*) with a central signal void of the ossicles (*arrow*). **(D)** Coronal *b*1000 non-echo planar diffusion weighted (non-EP DW) image (same level as in **B**): nodular and strongly hyperintense lesion under the tegmen, compatible with a cholesteatoma. **(E)** Coronal ADC map (same level as in **B** and **D**): nodular hypointense lesion (*arrow*) on the same location as the hyperintensity in **(D)**, compatible with diffusion restriction in the middle ear cholesteatoma. The finding of subtle erosions on CBCT together with the characteristic hyperintensity on *b*1000 non-EP DW image and the diffusion restriction on the ADC map are pathognomonic for an acquired pars flaccida cholesteatoma.

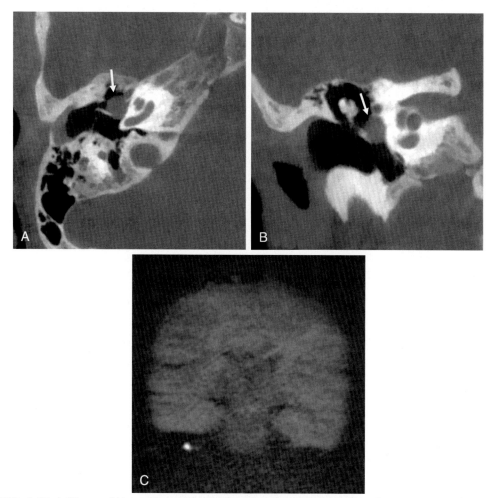

FIG. 6.22 A 12-year-old boy with a conductive hearing loss on the right side and at otoscopy a whitish nodular lesion in the protympanum behind an intact tympanic membrane. **(A)** Axial cone beam CT (CBCT) at the level of the basal turn of the cochlea demonstrates a small nodular lesion against the promontory, anterior to the malleus handle (*arrow*). **(B)** Coronal CBCT at the level of the cochlea showing a small nodular lesion lying against the cranial aspect of the promontory, medial to the malleus handle (*arrow*). **(C)** Coronal *b*1000 non-echo planar diffusion-weighted image (same level as in **B**): small hyperintense nodular lesion in the signal void of the temporal bone pyramid. The aspect, location, delineation, and signal intensity of this lesion is pathognomonic for a congenital middle ear cholesteatoma.

cranial nerve palsy should raise suspicion of an underlying lesion and prompt imaging. Imaging aspects of these rare lesions are variable, but an aggressive looking lesion is usually found (Fig. 6.31).

## Langerhans Cell Histiocytosis

Langerhans cell histiocytosis is another disease entity encountered in children, with an often aggressive-looking appearance on cross-sectional imaging, making the differential diagnosis with rhabdomyosarcoma difficult.[35,36]

Although the etiology and pathogenesis is still not well established, it is supposed to be caused by an abnormal immune regulation. The disease is not considered to be truly neoplastic. It includes disorders formerly known as histiocytosis X in its three subforms: eosinophilic granuloma, Hand-Schüller-Christian disease, and Letterer-Siwe disease.

Temporal bone involvement can be solitary (in 5%–25% of patients), but it can be a part of systemic disease. Patients with disease limited to the temporal bone should always have a complete

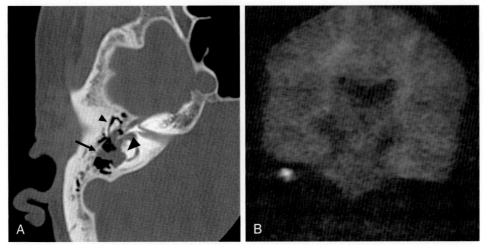

FIG. 6.23 Congenital middle ear cholesteatoma invading the membranous labyrinth. A 52-year-old male with conductive hearing loss and a sudden onset of vertigo. **(A)** Axial CT image at the level of the lateral semicircular canal showing soft tissues in the mastoid antrum (*arrow*). Note that there is no soft tissue in the Prussak space and that there is no erosion of the lateral epitympanic wall (*small arrowhead*), a finding characteristic of an acquired cholesteatoma. The lesion invades the lateral semicircular canal (*large arrowhead*). These soft tissues are highly nonspecific but suspicious of a congenital cholesteatoma. **(B)** Coronal *b*1000 non-echo planar diffusion-weighted imaging (non-EP DWI). The diagnosis of a congenital cholesteatoma is confirmed by non-EP DWI showing a clear hyperintense lesion. The final diagnosis of a congenital cholesteatoma suggested on CT and MRI was confirmed at surgery. Vertigo could be explained by the invasion of the membranous labyrinth.

examination to exclude systemic involvement.[35,36] Clinically it presents as chronic otitis media, with massive osseous destruction and associated soft tissue mass on imaging. Findings on cross-sectional imaging very often seem to be disproportionate to the clinical findings. As mentioned, cranial nerve deficit is uncommon. Another major imaging feature compared with rhabdomyosarcoma is the fact that the lesions are often bilateral. On CT, extensive osseous destruction with associated soft tissue mass lesion is seen (Fig. 6.32). However, involvement of the auditory ossicles and the inner ear is not as frequent as might be expected from the extensive bony damage. MR signal intensities are nonspecific: variable signal intensity on T1-weighted imaging and high signal intensity on T2-weighted imaging, with strong enhancement after intravenous gadolinium administration (Fig. 6.32).[35,36]

### Other Tumors

Several other tumoral lesions can be found in the temporal bone region, such as non-Hodgkin lymphoma (Fig. 6.33). Signs on CT and MRI are highly nonspecific, showing a relatively homogeneous soft tissue mass destroying all bony structures.[39,40]

Various types of osseous and soft tissue tumors can be found in the temporal bone: Ewing sarcoma, fibrosarcoma, osteosarcoma, and chondrosarcoma. Benign lesions include osteoblastoma, giant cell tumor, and hemangiomas. Several tumors may show intratumoral calcifications, such as Ewing sarcoma, chondrosarcoma, and osteosarcoma.

Secondary tumors of the temporal bone are not uncommon. Breast carcinomas, as well as lung, kidney, and prostate carcinoma and melanoma, may invade the temporal bone (Fig. 6.34). Lesions can be lytic, blastic, or mixed depending upon the type of primary tumor. The temporal bone invasion can be the primary manifestation of the tumor.[40]

The temporal bone can be directly invaded by surrounding tumors. Nasopharyngeal carcinoma may invade the temporal bone, growing through foramina and fissures and following the course of vessels and nerves (Fig. 6.35).[40]

## INNER EAR
### Congenital Cholesteatoma

In the petrous bone and inner ear, congenital cholesteatoma usually presents as a sharply delineated

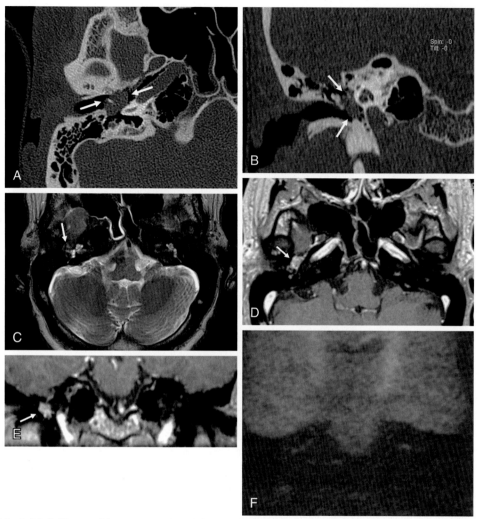

**FIG. 6.24** A 42-year-old man presenting with ear pain and chronic ear discharge. At otoscopy, a soft tissue lesion protruding through the tympanic membrane was noted. The lesion displayed no whitish pearly aspect, nor did it display a bluish aspect. There was no tinnitus or facial nerve palsy. **(A)** Axial CT image at the level of the basal turn of the cochlea. There is a small nodular lesion in the anterior hypotympanum (*arrows*). The lesion, however, does not seem to be lying against the promontory. **(B)** Coronal CT image at the level of the cochlea. On this image, the lesion seems to be lying against the promontory (*arrows*) but is not completely attached to it in its lower portion. **(C)** Axial turbo spin echo T2-weighted MR image at the level of the basal turn of the cochlea (same level as in **A**). Moderate-intensity nodular lesion anterior in the hypotympanum on the right side (*arrow*). **(D)** Axial gadolinium-enhanced 3D gradient echo T1-weighted image (same level as in **A**). Nodular strongly enhancing mass lesion in the middle ear (*arrow*). **(E)** Coronal gadolinium-enhanced 3D gradient echo T1-weighted image demonstrating the nodular strongly enhancing mass lesion in the middle ear (*arrow*). **(F)** Coronal *b*1000 non-echo planar diffusion-weighted (DW) image (same level as in **E**) shows no evident hyperintense signal, excluding a cholesteatoma. The lesion has clinically no signs of a cholesteatoma or a glomus tumor. The lack of a hyperintense signal on a *b*1000 DW image excludes the presence of a cholesteatoma. Although the lesion strongly enhances, CT shows that the lesion is not entirely abutting the promontory. CT also demonstrates that the lesion does not have a relationship with the facial nerve canal. Surgery demonstrated a middle ear adenomatous tumor.

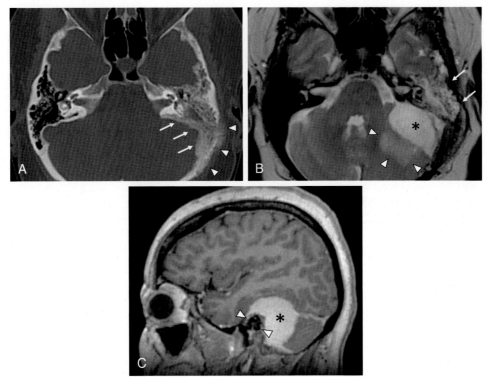

FIG. 6.25 Temporal bone meningioma. A 42-year-old female presenting with chronic and therapy-resistant otitis media. **(A)** Axial CT image through both temporal bones at the level of the internal auditory canal (IAC). There is a subtotal opacification of the left middle ear, antrum, and mastoid. Sclerotic changes and thickening of the bone can be found along the posterior side of the left temporal bone (*arrows*). Note the irregularities of the bone along the outer cortex (*arrowheads*). These irregularities are considered characteristic of temporal bone meningioma. **(B)** Axial T2-weighted MR at the level of the IAC (same level as in **A**). A large extraaxial mass lesion is found in the posterior fossa along the posterior side of the temporal bone (*asterisk*). There is limited edema in the adjacent cerebellar hemisphere (*small arrowheads*). Note the hyperintense signal intensity in the left middle ear and mastoid (*arrows*). **(C)** Sagittal gadolinium-enhanced T1-weighted MR image through the left temporal bone. Large enhancing mass lesion posterosuperior (*asterisk*) of the left temporal bone. Central in the temporal bone signal void, the hypointense signal of the membranous labyrinth, vestibule, can be found (*arrowheads*).

punched-out lesion. It can be found anywhere in the petrous bone pyramid, but there is a predilection for the region around the facial nerve geniculate ganglion (Fig. 6.18).[4,22] Its sharp delineation enables the differentiation from metastatic lesions in the petrous bone pyramid. The lesion can invade the membranous labyrinth (Fig. 6.23) and the segments of the facial nerve (Fig. 6.18). Contrary to the hemangioma of the facial nerve, it does not have calcification in it on CT scan.

In the case of a petrous bone congenital cholesteatoma, MRI is superior in characterizing the lesion and in describing its exact extension and invasion on the surrounding structures of the membranous labyrinth (Figs. 6.18 and 6.23). Signal intensities of cholesteatoma on standard MR sequences are rather nonspecific, whereas signal intensities on DWI, and more specifically *b*1000 images, are highly sensitive and specific.[4,22]

## Endolymphatic Sac Tumor

An endolymphatic sac tumor (ELST) is a rare tumor arising from the epithelium of the endolymphatic sac. It is an adenomatous neoplasm with papillary histologic findings. Its typical location is the posteromedial part of the temporal bone.

The endolymphatic sac is derived from the ectoderm and is the terminal enlargement of the endolymphatic duct. It consists of proximal and distal segments. The proximal or rugose segment is continuous with the

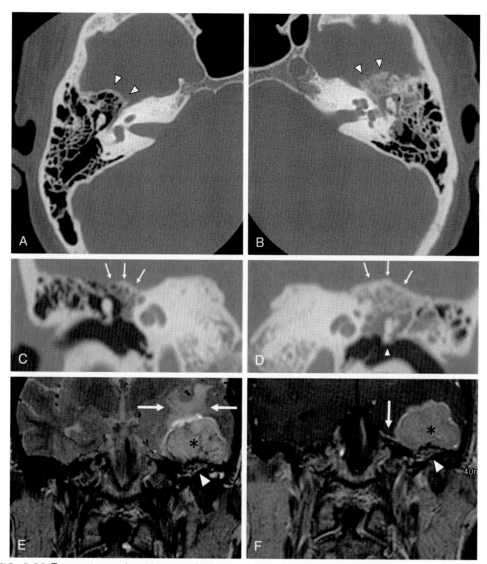

FIG. 6.26 Tegmen tympani meningioma. A 55-year-old female presenting with mixed hearing loss on the left side, investigated by CT and MRI. **(A)** Axial CT image at the level of the malleus and incus. Normal ossicular chain with normal aspect of the bone of the anterior epitympanic wall (*arrowheads*). **(B)** Axial CT image (same level as in **A**) demonstrating a partially opacified middle ear without any ossicular erosion. Note the thickened and sclerotic aspect of the anterior epitympanic wall (*arrowheads*). Compare with the normal side in **(A)**. **(C)** Coronal CT reformation at the level of the cochlea. There is complete aeration of the middle ear and epitympanic space with a normal aspect of the bone of the tegmen tympani (*arrows*). **(D)** Coronal CT reformation (same level as in **C**). There is partial opacification of the middle ear around the ossicular chain (*arrowhead*). Note the sclerotic and thickened aspect of the bone of the tegmen tympani (*arrows*). Compare with the normal side in **(C)**. **(E)** Coronal T2-weighted MR image through the middle ear. There is a large hyperintense mass lesion (*asterisk*) in the middle cranial fossa on top of the tegmen tympani with surrounding edema in the left temporal lobe (*arrows*). Note the hyperintense signal alterations in the middle ear (*arrowhead*). **(F)** Coronal T1-weighted MR image (same level as in **E**). The mass lesion is strongly enhancing (*asterisk*). There is a component of the mass lesion in the middle ear (*arrowhead*). Note the small dural tail at the medial side of the mass lesion (*arrow*). Findings on CT and MRI are characteristic of a tegmen tympanic meningioma. Clinical signs are caused by the meningioma invading the middle ear.

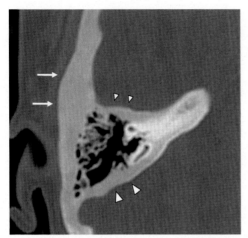

FIG. 6.27 Fibrous dysplasia. A 17-year-old female investigated for a conductive hearing loss. Thickening of the right squama temporalis (*arrows*) and anterior (*small arrowheads*) and posterior wall (*large arrowheads*) of the right temporal bone pyramid. Note the absence of any irregularities of the bone (compare with the meningioma in Fig. 6.25A). Findings are typical of fibrous dysplasia.

distal endolymphatic duct. This particular location is important, as it explains the propensity of the tumor to involve the petrous bone as well as the cerebellopontine angle structures.[41]

The ELST is found in almost any age group, in patients between 20 and 80 years. There is an equal distribution between males and females.

Clinically, patients usually present with unilateral hearing loss and tinnitus. Large tumors may also cause symptoms attributable to cerebellopontine angle extension. The clinical course can be indolent with a long-standing symptom history attributable to slow progression of the tumors. There is a known higher incidence in von Hippel-Lindau disease, but this is not a prerequisite, as these tumors also occur sporadically. Patients with von Hippel-Lindau disease are more likely to have bilateral ELSTs.[41]

The imaging hallmark of these lesions is that they are, by definition, centered on the endolymphatic duct location with a retrolabyrinthine mass with osseous erosion. On CT, bony spicules within the lesion can be found, representing residual bone fragments rather than new bone formation. Part of the tumor can be surrounded by a thin rim of expanded bone, caused by the slow progression of the tumor. This thin rim of bone differentiates these lesions of more aggressive lesions involving the temporal bone, such as high-grade chondrosarcoma or metastatic lesions.[41]

On MRI, smaller lesions show a heterogeneous signal intensity on unenhanced T1-weighted images with a peripheral rim of increased signal intensity and strong enhancement after intravenous administration of gadolinium (Fig. 6.36). Despite the high vascular status of these lesions, signal voids are absent, making this a clue in the differential diagnosis with glomus tumors. Another clue in the differential diagnosis with glomus jugulare tumors is the fact that smaller ELSTs usually spare the jugular foramen. Larger tumors have more variable imaging features. Often, the center of larger tumors is difficult to localize. Bone destruction can be extensive with a less clear bony rim, making the differential diagnosis with more aggressive lesions much more difficult. In larger tumors, vascular flow voids can be found, making the differential diagnosis with a large glomus jugulotympanicum difficult. Smaller ELSTs have peripheral zones of high intensity on unenhanced T1-weighted images, whereas the high-intensity zones on unenhanced T1-weighted images in larger lesions are more scattered. The high intensity on T1-weighted images is caused by the presence of breakdown products of subacute hemorrhage throughout the hypervascular tumor (Fig. 6.36).[41]

The treatment of choice is extensive surgical resection, preferably after preoperative embolization. In the case of large tumors, the recurrence rate is high.

ELST can be easily confused at histopathologic examination with other papillary lesions; thus, the imaging features of these lesions are of great help to make the diagnosis.[41]

### Intralabyrinthine Schwannomas

Intralabyrinthine schwannomas (ILSs) develop from the Schwann cells of the intralabyrinthine branches of the vestibulocochlear nerve and initially do not have a component in the IAC. Primary ILSs are extremely rare. It is estimated that they account for about 10% of all vestibulocochlear schwannomas.[42] Sensorineural hearing loss is the most frequent presenting symptom. Tinnitus and vertigo are reported less frequently.

ILSs meet the imaging criteria of vestibulocochlear schwannomas. They have a slightly higher signal intensity than normal intralabyrinthine fluid on unenhanced T1-weighted images, with a strong enhancement after intravenous gadolinium administration. On very thin, high-resolution, 3D, heavily T2-weighted sequences, ILSs appear as hypointense lesions with sharp borders replacing the high signal intensity of the fluid (Figs. 6.37 and 6.38). These sequences also make it possible to distinguish in which scala ILSs are located (Fig. 6.37).

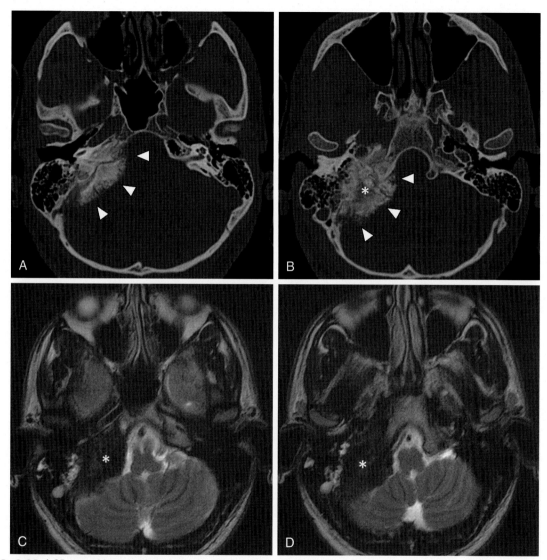

FIG. 6.28 A 25-year-old man with complaints of increasing sensorineural hearing loss and episodes of rotatory vertigo. **(A)** Axial unenhanced CT image through the temporal bone at the level of the basal turn of the cochlea. There is a large lesion located against the posterior side of the temporal bone. The lesion demonstrates a sun-ray appearance (arrowheads) (see also Fig. 6.25A). **(B)** Axial unenhanced CT image through the skull base. The lesion has an aggressive-looking appearance, with invasion in the base of the skull and the posterolateral aspect of the clivus (asterisk). Again a sun-ray appearance toward the posterior fossa can be noted (arrowheads) (see also Fig. 6.25A). This aggressive sun-ray appearance can be regarded as being typical for a temporal bone meningioma. **(C)** Axial turbo spin echo (TSE) T2-weighted image (same level as in **A**). The lesion is predominantly hypointense (asterisk) because of the calcification in the mass. **(D)** Axial TSE T2-weighted image (same level as in **B**). Hypointense aspect of the lesion (asterisk) caused by the heavily calcified aspect of the tumor.

*Continued*

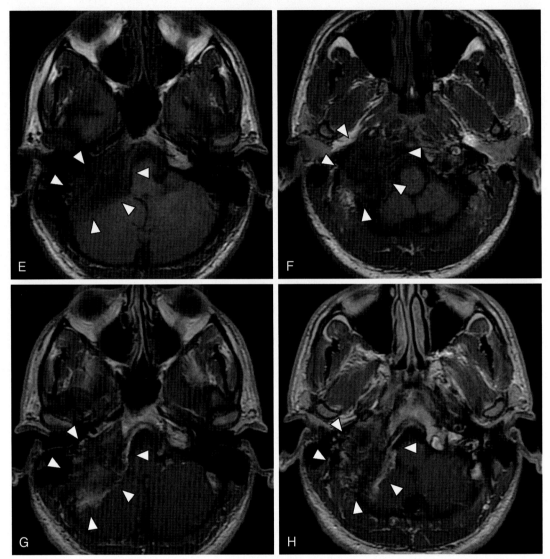

FIG. 6.28, cont'd **(E)** Axial unenhanced spin echo (SE) T1-weighted image (same level as in **A** and **C**). Note the mixed isointense, mainly peripheral, and hypointense, mainly central, aspect of the lesion (*arrowheads*). **(F)** Axial unenhanced SE T1-weighted image (same level as in **B** and **D**). Mixed isointense, mainly peripheral, and hypointense, mainly central, aspect of the lesion (*arrowheads*). **(G)** Axial gadolinium-enhanced T1-weighted image through the temporal bone at the level of the basal turn of the cochlea (*arrowheads*) (same level as in **A**, **C**, and **E**). The lesion shows a faint to moderate enhancement, mainly in the periphery of the mass. **(H)** Axial gadolinium-enhanced T1-weighted image through the skull base (*arrowheads*) (same level as in **B**, **D**, and **F**) demonstrating a faint enhancement of the lesion. The aspect of the lesion on CT with the predominant low signal intensities on MR is highly typical for a meningioma. In this case, it proved to be a calcified jugular foramen meningioma, with extension outside the skull into the poststyloidal parapharyngeal space. Surgical intervention resulted in only partial resection of the tumor.

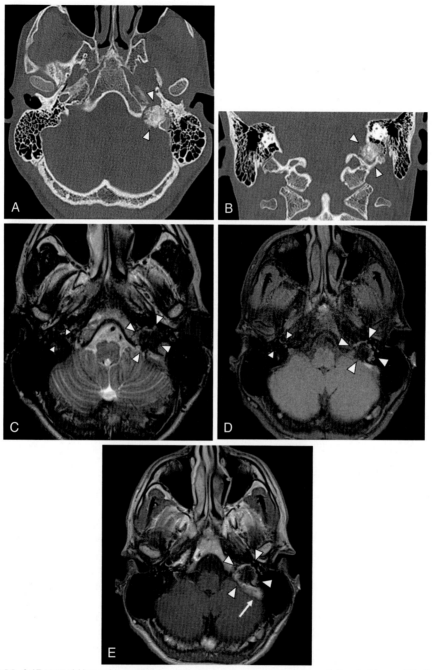

FIG. 6.29 A 17-year-old boy with swallowing difficulties. **(A)** Axial CT scan through the skull base at the level of the jugular foramen. On the left side, the jugular foramen is filled with a calcified nodular mass lesion with a slightly irregular delineation toward its medial and posterior border (*arrowheads*). **(B)** Coronal CT scan through the skull base at the level of the jugular foramen. The left-sided jugular foramen is filled with a calcified mass lesion (*arrowheads*). **(C)** Axial turbo spin echo (SE) T2-weighted MR image through the skull base (same level as in **A**). The left jugular foramen is filled with a slightly inhomogeneous hypointense lesion (*large arrowheads*). Its intensity is slightly higher than the flow void in the normal jugular bulb on the right side (*small arrowheads*). **(D)** Unenhanced SE T1-weighted MR image with fat-saturation technique through the skull base (same level as in **A** and **C**). The left jugular foramen is filled with a slightly inhomogeneous hypointense lesion (*large arrowheads*). Its intensity is again slightly higher than the normal jugular bulb on the right side (*small arrowheads*). **(E)** Gadolinium-enhanced SE T1-weighted MR image. Enhancement is noted only around or in the periphery of the lesion (*arrowheads*) as well as in the adjacent sigmoid sinus (*arrow*). Although this lesion may look like a jugular foramen meningioma, the young age of the patient makes this diagnosis rather unlikely. Transmastoid biopsy revealed an osteosarcoma.

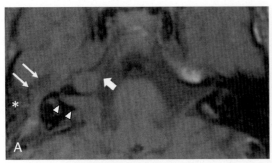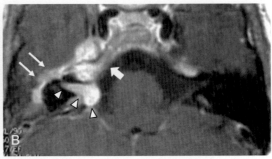

**FIG. 6.30** Rhabdomyosarcoma. A 6-year-old girl presenting with deafness on the right side and a sudden onset of facial paralysis. **(A)** Unenhanced spin echo (SE) T1-weighted image. The hypointense fluid signal in the internal auditory canal on the right side is replaced by soft tissue with an isointensity to brain tissue (*arrowheads*). The fat signal in the petrous apex on the right side is replaced by soft tissue (*thick arrow*). Compare with the normal fatty marrow signal in the left petrous apex. There seems to be an extension in the anterior side of the petrous bone, probably along the course of the facial nerve (*small arrows*). The middle ear signal void is replaced by an isointense signal (*asterisk*). **(B)** Gadolinium-enhanced SE T1-weighted image. Strong enhancement of the mass lesion in the internal auditory canal and cerebellopontine angle (*arrowheads*). There is also enhancement of the mass lesion in the petrous apex (*thick arrow*) and in the anterior part of the petrous bone, probably along the course of the facial nerve (*small arrows*). Although the lesion mimics a facial nerve schwannoma, these lesions are considered extremely rare in young children. The differential diagnosis of a middle and inner ear mass lesion in a child should always include rhabdomyosarcoma.

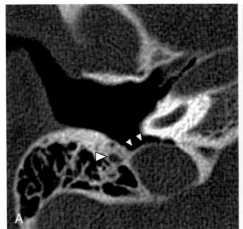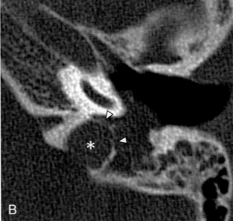

**FIG. 6.31** A 9-year-old child with left-sided ear pain lasting for a week with a sudden onset of facial paralysis. **(A)** Axial CT image at the level of the basal turn of the cochlea on the right side. Normal bony delineation of the jugular bulb (*small arrowheads*) and the third segment of the facial nerve in the mastoid (*large arrowhead*). **(B)** Axial CT image at the level of the basal turn of the cochlea on the left side. Irregular soft tissue mass lesion (*asterisk*) posterior in the hypotympanum. The mass clearly erodes the posterior part of the mastoid. By doing so, it also erodes the third segment of the facial nerve, which no longer can be delineated. Compared with the normal right side in **(A)**, the bony plate covering the jugular bulb seems to be eroded (*small arrowheads*). Biopsy revealed Ewing sarcoma. This mass lesion has aggressive features, which, together with the alarm symptom of a sudden onset of facial paralysis, should alert the radiologist toward a malignant lesion. Differential diagnosis should also include rhabdomyosarcoma. (Courtesy of R. Hermans, Leuven, Belgium.)

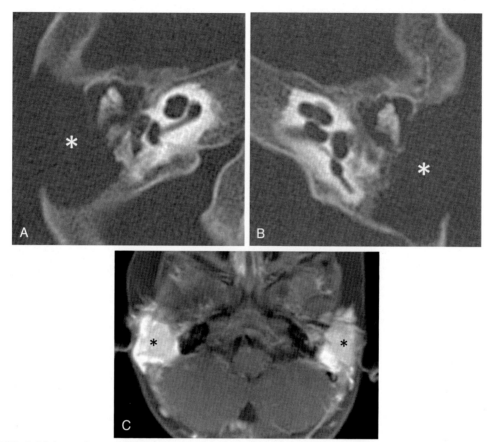

FIG. 6.32 Langerhans cell histiocytosis. A 3-year-old child with chronic ear discharge and a skin rash. **(A)** Axial CT image on the right side at the level of the basal and middle turn of the cochlea. Large soft tissue lesion (*asterisk*) centered on the mastoid with erosion of the mastoid cells and the lateral mastoid wall. There is extension of the soft tissue toward the external ear. Note that there is no clear evidence of ossicular chain erosion. **(B)** Axial CT image on the left side at the level of the basal and middle turn of the cochlea (same level as in **A**). Large soft tissue lesion (*asterisk*) centered on the mastoid with erosion of the mastoid cells and the lateral mastoid wall. There is extension of the soft tissues toward the external ear. There is no clear evidence of ossicular chain erosion. **(C)** Axial gadolinium-enhanced T1-weighted images with fat saturation. Bilateral strongly enhancing large soft tissue masses in the temporal bone (*asterisks*). The lack of cranial nerve palsy and the bilateral large enhancing mass lesions in the temporal bone area are highly suggestive of Langerhans cell histiocytosis. (Courtesy of R. Hermans, Leuven, Belgium.)

About 80% of ILSs are located in the cochlea, with a predilection for the transition area between the basal and second turns of the cochlea (Fig. 6.37). All of these intracochlear schwannomas are located in the scala tympani or in both the scala tympani and scala vestibuli. Involvement of the vestibular labyrinth, vestibule, and/or semicircular canals is far less frequent (about 15%) (Fig. 6.38).[42]

Based on the study of MR follow-up examinations, it is estimated that about 50% of the ILSs grow and start to fill up the cochlea gradually before invading the vestibular labyrinth.[42] The other 50% of ILSs remain stable.

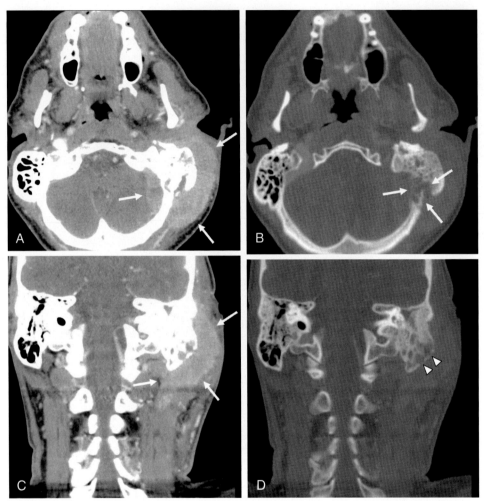

FIG. 6.33 Temporal bone non-Hodgkin lymphoma. A 49-year-old male with hemophilia A and HIV presenting with facial paralysis on the left side. At clinical examination, a swelling behind the left ear was found. **(A)** Axial CT image after intravenous administration of iodinated contrast. A large mass lesion is found centered on the mastoid process with a large surrounding soft tissue component (*arrows*). **(B)** Axial CT image after intravenous administration of iodinated contrast, bone window settings (same level as in **A**). There is a clear lysis of the bone between the mastoid process and the occipital bone (*arrows*). **(C)** Coronal CT reformation after intravenous administration of iodinated contrast. Mass lesion centered on the left mastoid process with associated bone defects. Note the large associated soft tissue mass (*arrows*). **(D)** Coronal CT reformation after intravenous administration of iodinated contrast: bone window settings. A complete opacification of the left mastoid is found. Bone defects at the level of the mastoid tip are found (*arrowheads*).

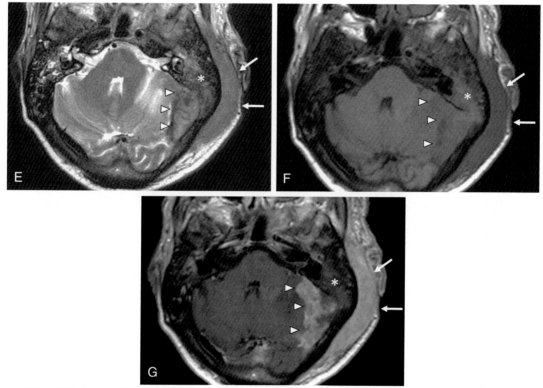

**FIG. 6.33, cont'd  (E)** Axial T2-weighted MR image at the level of the membranous labyrinth. The entire mastoid on the left side is filled with a hypointense lesion *(asterisk)*: compare with the hyperintense inflammatory material on the right side. There is a soft tissue component with a hypointense aspect on the exterior side *(arrows)* as well as on the interior side in the posterior fossa *(arrowheads)*. **(F)** Axial T1-weighted MR image (same level as in **E**). The entire mastoid is filled up with a hypointense lesion *(asterisk)* with an external *(arrows)* and internal *(arrowheads)* component. **(G)** Axial gadolinium-enhanced T1-weighted MR image (same level as in **E** and **F**). There is a strong enhancement of the external *(arrows)* and internal *(arrowheads)* components. The mastoid component of the mass lesion demonstrates no enhancement *(asterisk)*. At biopsy, this aggressive-looking lesion was proved to be a non-Hodgkin lymphoma.

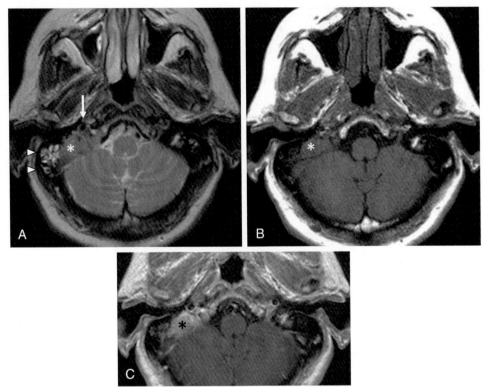

FIG. 6.34 Temporal bone metastases. A 68-year-old female with headache and tinnitus. **(A)** Axial T2-weighted MR image through the skull base at the level of the mastoid tip. There is a large isointense to slightly hyperintense mass lesion in the skull base on the right side (*asterisk*), partly surrounding the internal carotid artery (*arrow*). Note the retroobstructive fluid in the mastoid tip (*arrowheads*). **(B)** Axial unenhanced T1-weighted MR image (same level as in **A**). The mass lesion is isointense to brain tissue (*asterisk*). **(C)** Axial gadolinium-enhanced T1-weighted MR image (same level as in **A**). Strong enhancement of the mass lesion in the right skull base (*asterisk*). This metastatic lesion was the first manifestation of a bronchus carcinoma. This lesion was detected during an investigation for tinnitus. Probably, the tinnitus was caused by the high degree of vascularity of the lesion.

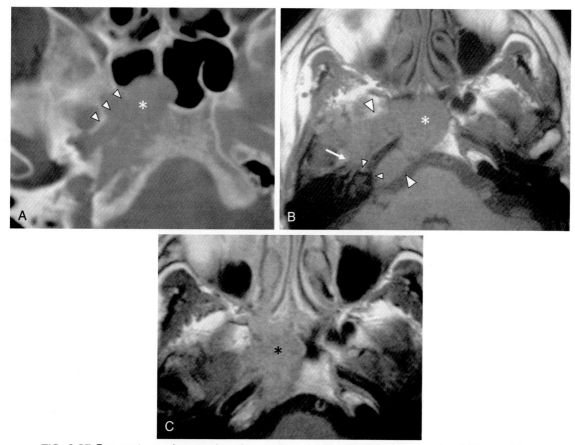

FIG. 6.35 Recurrent nasopharyngeal carcinoma with secondary temporal bone invasion. A 56-year-old male with sudden onset of facial nerve palsy with a prior history of nasopharyngeal carcinoma treated with radiotherapy. **(A)** Axial CT image at the level of the skull base. Large mass lesion invading the clivus and adjacent lower temporal bone apex. The mass (*asterisk*) follows the course of the horizontal segment of the internal carotid artery (*arrowheads*). **(B)** Axial unenhanced T1-weighted image. Large isointense mass lesion (*asterisk*) extending (*large arrowheads*) anterior and posterior into the skull base and temporal bone, along the course of the horizontal segment of the internal carotid artery. The mass abuts the otic capsule without invading it (*small arrowheads*). It invades the region of the geniculate ganglion (*arrow*), causing the facial nerve palsy. **(C)** Axial gadolinium-enhanced T1-weighted image (same level as in **B**). The mass lesion strongly enhances (*asterisk*), invades the right side of the skull base, and follows the course of the horizontal segment of the internal carotid artery.

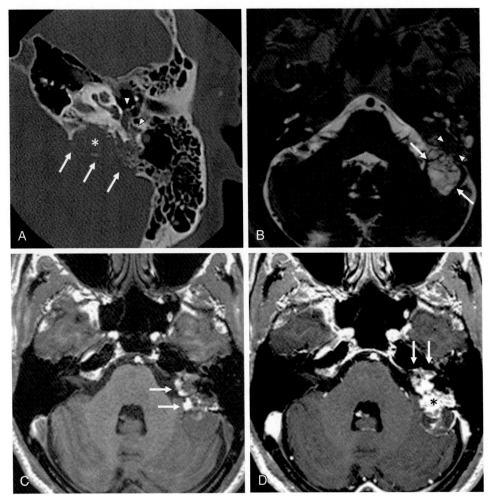

FIG. 6.36 Endolymphatic sac tumor. A 27-year-old female with left-sided facial nerve paralysis. **(A)** Axial CT image at the level of the basal turn of the cochlea and round window. There is a large mass lesion (*asterisk*) situated in the posterior part of the temporal bone. Note the associated irregular lysis of the temporal bone (*arrows*). There is invasion in the pyramidal eminence and the middle ear (*arrowheads*), causing the facial paralysis. **(B)** Axial 3D turbo spin echo (SE) T2-weighted MR image through the membranous labyrinth. There is a large mass lesion partially situated in the posterior side of the temporal bone with a hypointense aspect (*arrowheads*). There is a second hyperintense component of the mass lesion in the left posterior cerebellopontine angle with a clear hyperintensity (*arrows*). **(C)** Axial SE T1-weighted MR image through the left temporal bone at the level of the internal auditory canal. The lesion shows a characteristic peripheral hyperintensity of the mass lesion in the left cerebellopontine angle (*arrows*). **(D)** Axial gadolinium-enhanced SE T1-weighted MR image (same level as in **C**). There is strong enhancement of the mass lesion (*asterisk*) on the posterior side of the left temporal bone. Note the extension of the mass lesion into the left internal auditory canal (*arrows*). Patient was known with Von Hippel Lindau's disease.

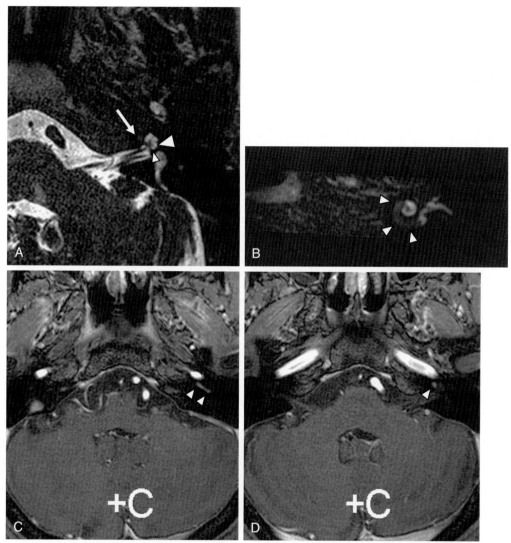

**FIG. 6.37** Intralabyrinthine schwannoma located in the basal and middle turns of the cochlea. A 42-year-old male with sensorineural hearing loss on the left side. **(A)** Axial 0.6-mm 3D turbo spin echo (TSE) T2-weighted MR image at the level of the middle turn of the cochlea demonstrates a small zone of signal loss in the anterior part of the middle turn of the cochlea (*arrow*). Discrimination between the scala vestibuli (*large arrowhead*) and scala tympani (*small arrowhead*) cannot be made. **(B)** Curvilinear MPR along the 2½ turns of the cochlea demonstrates the zone of signal loss caused by the intralabyrinthine schwannoma in the basal and middle turns of the cochlea (*arrowheads*). **(C)** Axial gadolinium-enhanced 3D gradient echo T1-weighted image through the skull base demonstrating the enhancing tumor in the basal turn of the cochlea on the left side (*arrowheads*). **(D)** Axial gadolinium-enhanced 3D gradient echo T1-weighted image through the internal auditory canal (same level as in **A**) shows the enhancing tumor in the middle turn of the cochlea (*arrowhead*) corresponding to the area of signal loss in the 3D TSE T2-weighted MR image.

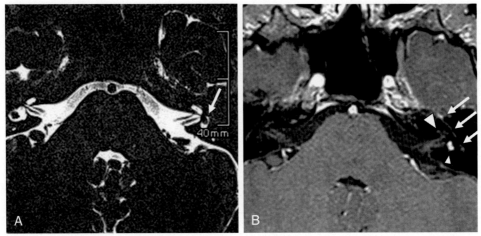

FIG. 6.38 Intralabyrinthine schwannoma located in the vestibule on the left side. A 32-year-old airline pilot investigated for profound sensorineural hearing loss on the left side. **(A)** Axial 0.4-mm 3D turbo spin echo T2-weighted MR image at the level of the vestibule. There is a nodular hypointense lesion in the anterior part of the left vestibule (*arrow*). Compare with the normal right side with normal signal intensities of the right vestibule. **(B)** Axial 1-mm-thick MPR of a gadolinium enhanced 3D gradient echo T1-weighted sequence through the vestibule (same level as in **A**). There is a small nodular mass lesion in the left vestibule (*small arrowhead*). Note the normal aspect of the middle and apical turns of the cochlea (*large arrowhead*). There is a normal aspect of the left facial nerve (*arrows*). Based on this MR examination, the airline pilot was grounded. He was later operated on for removal of the schwannoma. He also received a cochlear implant on the operated side and was allowed to fly again.

## SUMMARY

Although temporal bone tumors often have a non-specific imaging appearance, cross-sectional imaging plays an important role in describing the exact extent of these lesions. In several lesions, the location, aspect, and imaging features of those lesions, on MRI as well as on CT, may add a clue to diagnosis.

## REFERENCES

1. Persaud RA, Hajioff D, Thevasagayam MS, et al. Keratosis obturans and external ear cholesteatoma: how and why we should distinguish between these conditions. *Clin Otolaryngol Allied Sci.* 2004;29:577–581.
2. Hermans R. External ear imaging. In: Lemmerling M, De Foer B, eds. *Temporal Bone Imaging.* New York: Springer Verlag, Berlin, Heidelberg; 2015:35–51.
3. Baráth K, Huber AM, Stämpfli P, et al. Neuroradiology of cholesteatomas. *Am J Neuroradiol.* 2011;32:221–229.
4. De Foer B, Vercruysse JP, Spaepen M. Diffusion-weighted magnetic resonance imaging of the temporal bone. *Neuroradiology.* 2010;52:785–807.
5. Nyrop M, Grontved A. Cancer of the external auditory canal. *Arch Otolaryngol Head Neck Surg.* 2002;128:834–837.
6. Lobo D, Llorente JL, Suárez C. Squamous cell carcinoma of the external auditory canal. *Skull Base.* 2008;18:167–172.
7. Chang CH, Shu MT, Lee JC, et al. Treatments and outcome of malignant tumors of external auditory canal. *Am J Otolaryngol.* 2009;30:44–48. Epub 2008 Jul 22.
8. Franco-Vidal V, Blanchet H, Bebear C, et al. Necrotizing external otitis: a report of 46 cases. *Otol Neurotol.* 2007;28:771–773.
9. Ozgen B, Oguz KK, Cila A. Diffusion MR imaging features of skull base osteomyelitis compared with skull base malignancy. *Am J Neuroradiol.* 2011;32:179–184.
10. Tuan AS, Chen JY, Mafee MF. Glomus tympanica and other intratympanic masses: role of imaging. *Oper Tech Otolaryngol.* 2014;25:49–57.
11. Rao AB, Koeller KK, Adair CF. From the archives of the AFIP. Paragangliomas of the head and neck: radiologic-pathologic correlation. *Radiographics.* 1999;19:1605–1632.
12. Caldemeyer KS, Mathews VP, Azzarelli B, et al. The jugular foramen: a review of anatomy, masses, and imaging characteristics. *Radiographics.* 1997;17:1123–1139.
13. Neves F, Huwart L, Jourdan G, et al. Head and neck paragangliomas: value of contrast-enhanced 3D MR angiography. *Am J Neuroradiol.* 2008;29:883–889.
14. Aschenbach R, Basche S, Esser D, et al. Usefullness of ultrafast dynamic 3D-T1w data acquisition in detection of hypervascular lesions of the middle ear: first experience. *Eur J Radiol.* 2012;81:257–261.
15. Sayit AT, Gunbey HP, Fethallah B, et al. Radiological and audiometric evaluation of high jugular bulb and dehiscent jugular bulb. *J Laryngol Otol.* 2016;130:1059–1063.

16. Nicolay S, De Foer B, Bernaerts A, et al. Aberrant carotid artery presenting as a retrotympanic vascular mass. *Acta Radiol Short Rep.* 2014;3(10). http://dx.doi.org/10.1177/2047981614553695. pii: 2047981614553695.

17. Yilmaz T, Bilgen C, Savas R, et al. Persistent stapedial artery: MR angiographic and CT findings. *Am J Neuroradiol.* 2003;24:1133–1135.

18. Lemmerling MM, De Foer B, Verbist BM, VandeVyver V. Imaging of inflammatory and infectious diseases in the temporal bone. *Neuroimaging Clin N Am.* 2009;19:321–337.

19. Lo AC, Nemec SF. Opacification of the middle ear and mastoid: imaging findings and clues to differential diagnosis. *Clin Radiol.* 2015;70:e1–e13.

20. Lemmerling MM, De Foer B, VandeVyver V, et al. Imaging of the opacified middle ear. *Eur J Radiol.* 2008;66:363–371.

21. Wiggins 3rd RH, Harnsberger HR, Salzman KL, et al. The many faces of facial nerve schwannoma. *Am J Neuroradiol.* 2006;27:694–699.

22. De Foer B, Nicolay S, Vercruysse JP, et al. Imaging of cholesteatoma. In: Lemmerling M, De Foer B, eds. *Temporal Bone Imaging.* New York: Springer Verlag, Berlin, Heidelberg; 2015:69–87.

23. Sartoretti-Schefer S, Kollias S, Wichmann W, et al. T2-weighted three-dimensional fast spin echo MR in inflammatory facial nerve palsy. *Am J Neuroradiol.* 1998;19:491–495.

24. Pertzborn SL, Reith JD, Mancuso AA, et al. Epineurial pseudocysts of the intratemporal facial nerve. *Otol Neurotol.* 2003;24:490–493.

25. Bierry G, Riehm S, Marcellin L, et al. Middle ear adenomatous tumour: a not so rare glomus tympanicum-mimicking lesion. *J Neuroradiol.* 2010;37:116–121.

26. Maintz D, Stupp C, Krueger K, et al. MRI and CT of adenomatous tumours of the middle ear. *Neuroradiology.* 2001;43:58–61.

27. Hamilton BE, Salzman KL, Patel N, et al. Imaging and clinical characteristics of temporal bone meningeoma. *Am J Neuroradiol.* 2006;24:490–493.

28. Ayache D, Trablazini F, Bordure P, et al. Serous otitis media revealing temporal en plaque meningioma. *Otol Neurotol.* 2006;27:992–998.

29. Nicolay S, De Foer B, Bernaerts A, et al. A case of a temporal bone meningioma presenting as a serous otitis media. *Acta Radiol Short Rep.* 2014;3(10). http://dx.doi.org/10.1177/2047981614555048. pii: 204798161455048.

30. Fayad JN, Keles B, Brackmann DE. Jugular foramen tumors: clinical characteristics and treatment outcomes. *Otol Neurotol.* 2010;31:299–305.

31. Sanna M, Bacciu A, Falcioni M, et al. Surgical management of jugular foramen meningiomas: a series of 13 cases and review of the literature. *Laryngoscope.* 2007;117:1710–1719.

32. Chennupati SK, Norris R, Dunham B, et al. Osteosarcoma of the skull base: case report and review of literature. *Int J Pediatr Otorhinolaryngol.* 2008;72:115–119.

33. Sbeity S, Abella A, Arcand P, et al. Temporal bone rhabdomyosarcoma in children. *Int J Pediatr Otorhinolaryngol.* 2007;71:807–814.

34. Freling JM, Merks JHM, Saeed P, et al. Imaging findings in craniofacial childhood rhabdomyosarcoma. *Pediatr Radiol.* 2010;40:1723–1738.

35. Hermans R, De Foer B, Smet MH, et al. Eosinophilic granuloma of the head and neck: CT and MRI features in three cases. *Pediatr Radiol.* 1994;24:33–36.

36. Fernandez-Latorre F, Menor-Serrano F, Alonso-Charterina S, et al. Langerhans' cell histiocytosis of the temporal bone in pediatric patients: imaging and follow-up. *Am J Roentgenol.* 2000;174:217–221.

37. Pfeiffer J, Boedeker CC, Ridder GJ. Primary Ewing sarcoma of the petrous temporal bone: an exceptional cause of facial palsy and deafness in and nursing. *Head Neck.* 2006;28:955–959.

38. Kadar AA, Hearst MJ, Collins MH, et al. Ewing's sarcoma of the petrous bone: case report and literature review. *Skull Base.* 2010;20:213–217.

39. Sritharan N, Moghadam A, Choroomi S, et al. Primary non-Hodgkin lymphoma of the petrous temporal bone. *Otol Neurotol.* 2012;33(2):e11–e12. http://dx.doi.org/10.1097/MAO.0b013e31821d9fbc.

40. Imhof H, Czerny C, Dirisamer A, et al. Tumorous lesions of the temporal bone. In: Lemmerling M, Kolias S, eds. *Radiology of the Petrous Bone.* New York: Springer Verlag, Berling, Heidelberg; 2004:69–81.

41. Van Rensburg PJ, Van Der Meer G. Magnetic resonance and computed tomography imaging of a grade IV papillary endolymphatic sac tumour. *J Neurooncol.* 2008;89:199–203.

42. Tieleman A, Casselman JW, Somers T, et al. Imaging of intralabyrinthine schwannomas: a retrospective study of 52 cases with emphasis on lesion growth. *Am J Neuroradiol.* 2008;29:898–905.

# CHAPTER 7

# Temporal Bone Trauma

BERT DE FOER, MD, PHD • ABDELLATIF BALI, MD •
ANJA BERNAERTS, MD • JOOST VAN DINTHER, MD •
ERWIN OFFECIERS, MD, PHD • JAN W. CASSELMAN, MD, PHD

## TEMPORAL BONE PSEUDOFRACTURES— FRACTURE MIMICS

An important challenge in detecting and classifying temporal bone fractures is the inherent complexity of the temporal bone anatomy. Although the evaluation of symmetry is helpful to distinguish normal anatomy from acute injury, temporal bone sutures or fissures and canals can still be wrongly interpreted as fractures.

The temporal bone has a complex structure. It is a part of the lateral wall of the skull and forms an important part of the skull base.

The temporal bone consists of five parts: squamous, mastoid, petrous, tympanic, and styloid parts.[1-3]

There are so-called external fissures or sutures that separate the temporal bone from its neighboring skull bones.[1-3]

These include the sphenosquamosal suture, formed by the greater wing of the sphenoid and the squamous temporal bone, located lateral to the foramen spinosum (Fig. 7.1A).

The occipitomastoid suture separates the mastoid process from the occipital bone (Fig. 7.1A).

The sphenopetrosal suture, which courses anteromedially along the anterior margin of the petrous bone, between the foramen ovale and the carotid canal, contains the deeper petrosal nerve (Fig. 7.1B).

The petrooccipital suture also runs anteromedially, coursing superior to the sphenopetrosal suture and along the posterior aspect of the temporal bone, posterior to the carotid canal (Fig. 7.1B).

The five portions of the temporal bone are separated by several internal sutures and fissures.[1-3]

The tympanosquamous and tympanomastoid fissures run parallel to the anterior and posterior walls of the external auditory canal, respectively. Of these two, the tympanosquamous fissure, being the most anterior one, is more consistently seen and more likely to be mistaken for an external auditory canal fracture (Fig. 7.2). It follows the tympanosquamous fissure

medially and divides to form the petrosquamosal and petrotympanic fissures.

The tympanomastoid fissure runs posterior and parallel to the external auditory canal (Fig. 7.2).

The petrosquamosal fissure is occasionally seen on axial images extending anteromedially from the mandibular fossa toward the greater wing of the sphenoid (Fig. 7.2).

The petrotympanic fissure is best seen on sagittal images as a short-segment channel connecting the upper tympanic cavity with the mandibular fossa.

There are also intrinsic channels or canals that might be mistaken for a fracture.[1-3]

These include the cochlear aqueduct, the glossopharyngeal sulcus, the vestibular aqueduct, the singular nerve canal, the subarcuate canal, the mastoid canaliculus, the inferior tympanic canaliculus, the canal for the chorda tympani, and the groove for the superior petrosal sinus.

The cochlear aqueduct contains perilymph and is obliquely oriented. It extends from the subarachnoid space to the region close to the round window membrane. The medial aspect of the cochlear aqueduct is funnel shaped and almost invariably visible. Its lateral part is usually very thin (Fig. 7.3A).

It runs in the same direction as the internal auditory canal, but in a lower position in the temporal bone and is usually much thinner. Its size and delineability can be variable.

The glossopharyngeal sulcus represents the point of entry of the glossopharyngeal nerve into the pars nervosa of the jugular foramen. It is consistently seen on axial images a few millimeters below the cochlear aqueduct (Fig. 7.3B).

The vestibular aqueduct contains the endolymphatic duct and sac, which allows passage of endolymph. It runs from the vestibule to the posterior surface of the temporal bone, parallel and posterior to the posterior semicircular canal. Again, its size and delineability can be variable (Fig. 7.4).

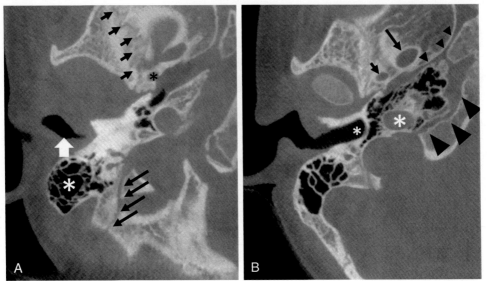

FIG. 7.1 **(A)** Axial cone beam CT (CBCT) image through the lower skull base at the level of the mastoid tip (*large asterisk*) and the lower external auditory canal (*bold arrow*). Two of the external fissures, separating the temporal bone from its neighboring skull bones, can clearly be seen. The sphenosquamosal suture (*small arrows*), formed by the greater wing of the sphenoid and the squamous temporal bone, is located lateral to the foramen spinosum (*small asterisk*). The occipitomastoid suture (*large arrows*) separates the mastoid from the occipital bone. **(B)** Axial CBCT image through the hypotympanum (*small asterisk*), the foramen ovale (*large arrow*), and the foramen spinosum (*small arrow*) in a different patient. The sphenopetrosal suture (*small arrowheads*) courses anteromedially, along the anterior margin of the petrous bone, between the foramen ovale (*large arrow*) and the carotid canal (*large asterisk*). The petrooccipital suture (*large arrowheads*) is running along the posterior aspect of the temporal bone, separating the os petrosum from the occipital bone.

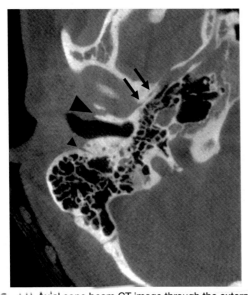

FIG. 7.2 Axial cone beam CT image through the external auditory canal and the temporomandibular joint. The lateral part (*large arrowhead*) of the tympanosquamous fissure as well as its medial extension, the petrosquamous fissure, is seen (*arrows*). The tympanomastoid fissure is also seen in its lateral part (*small arrowhead*).

The singular canal carries the singular or posterior ampullary nerve. It extends from the posterior inferior wall of the fundus of the internal auditory canal to the junction of the vestibule with the ampulla of the posterior semicircular canal (Fig. 7.5A).

The subarcuate canal is a dura-lined canal for the subarcuate artery, which has an anterior convex course between the two limbs of the superior semicircular canal (Fig. 7.5B). It is prominent in children, in contrast to adults, where it is significantly reduced in size.

The mastoid canaliculus contains the nerve of Arnold, a branch of the 10th cranial nerve, and can be seen as a linear canal connecting the jugular foramen with the mastoid segment of the facial nerve canal (Fig. 7.6A).

The inferior tympanic canaliculus contains the inferior tympanic branch, also called Jacobson nerve. It runs from the spina in the jugular foramen between the pars vascularis and pars nervosa upward to the middle ear and can be evaluated on coronal (Fig. 7.6B–E) as well as on axial images.

A glomus jugulare tumor extends along this pathway from the jugular foramen toward the middle ear cavity. It also forms the point of entry of the aberrant internal carotid artery, when present.

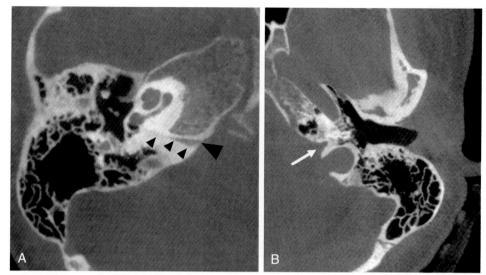

FIG. 7.3 **(A)** Axial cone beam CT (CBCT) image on the right side through the basal turn of the cochlea and the oval window. The cochlear aqueduct can be seen almost along its entire course (*small arrowheads*). Note the funnel-shaped appearance of its medial opening (*large arrowhead*). **(B)** Axial CBCT image on the left side through the jugular foramen (slightly lower than in **A**) showing the funnel-shaped appearance of the glossopharyngeal sulcus (*arrow*). It runs parallel to, but lower than, the cochlear aqueduct.

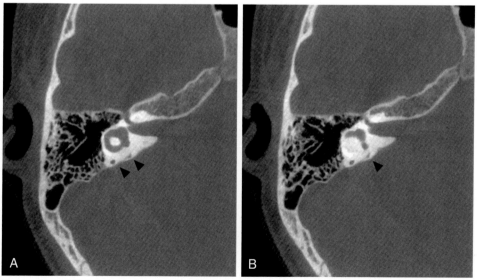

FIG. 7.4 **(A and B)** Axial cone beam CT image at the level of the vestibule and lateral semicircular canal. Note the narrow vestibular aqueduct (*arrowheads*) running parallel to the posterior semicircular canal.

The canal for the chorda tympani runs from the third or mastoid segment of the facial nerve upward, laterally and anteriorly to the middle ear cavity where it runs through the middle ear just medial to the tympanic membrane. It can be evaluated in the axial (Fig. 7.7A–D) as well as in the coronal planes (Fig. 7.7E–G).

The groove for the superior petrosal sinus is a deep groove that runs on the upper edge of the petrosal pyramid in which the superior petrosal vein runs (Fig. 7.8). The depth of the groove may be variable, and the superior semicircular canal may be dehiscent into the sinus.

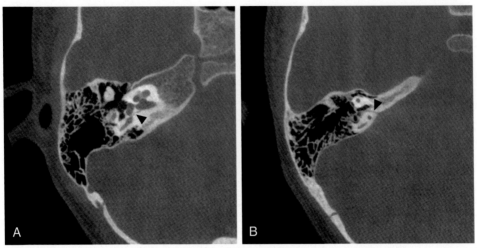

FIG. 7.5 **(A)** Axial cone beam CT (CBCT) image at the level of the oval window. The singular nerve canal (*arrowhead*), containing the posterior ampullary nerve, runs from the posterior part of the internal auditory canal to the ampulla of the posterior semicircular canal. **(B)** Axial CBCT image at the level of the superior semicircular canal. The subarcuate canal is running through both limbs of the superior semicircular canal as an anterior curvilinear hypodense line (*arrowhead*).

## TEMPORAL BONE FRACTURES

Temporal bone fractures have been traditionally classified as longitudinal or transverse, reflecting the relationship of the fracture line with regard to the long axis of the petrous bone.

Longitudinal fractures form the majority of the fractures. They are caused by a temporoparietal blow on the head, and the forces are diverted along the long axis of the temporal bone. Longitudinal fractures comprise 70%–90% of the temporal bone fractures and extend anteromedially, often involving the external auditory canal and the middle ear cavity (Fig. 7.9).[1-6]

The ossicles are frequently involved with subsequent conductive hearing loss. Evaluation of ossicular damage is best done using CT or cone beam CT (CBCT) after resorption of the hemotympanum, as the opacification caused by the blood in the middle ear might obscure subtle ossicular dislocations (Fig. 7.10).

The inner ear is spared in most cases of longitudinal fractures, and facial paralysis is rather rare (10%–20%) and, if present, often delayed and incomplete.

Longitudinal fractures have been further classified as anterior and posterior subtypes. The anterior subtype arises anterior to the external auditory canal, coursing medially, along the tegmen tympani and toward the petrous apex. The posterior subtype arises posterior to the external auditory canal, coursing through the middle ear and terminating in the foramen lacerum of the foramen ovale.[1-6]

Transverse fractures are less frequent; they comprise 10%–30% of the temporal bone fractures. Transverse fractures typically result from a trauma to the frontal or occipital region. The forces run perpendicular to the long axis of the temporal bone.

Very often, there is involvement of the otic capsule and labyrinth, with subsequent severe sensorineural hearing loss or even deafness (Fig. 7.9). Vertigo is also a frequent complaint. Facial paralysis is frequent (40%–50%) and often immediate and complete with a high House-Brackmann grade. The ossicles are often spared, without any conductive hearing loss. Air in the membranous labyrinth can be frequently found in cases of transverse fractures (Fig. 7.11).[1-4]

Transverse fractures have further been subdivided into a medial and a lateral subtype, where the medial subtype passes medial to the arcuate eminence, traversing the internal auditory canal and often injuring cranial nerves VII and VIII, whereas the lateral subtype passes lateral to the arcuate eminence, traversing the bony labyrinth.

Often, fractures are neither purely longitudinal nor purely transverse and some are very complicated to describe.

The most important feature of a classification system lies in its ability to predict clinical outcome.[1,4-6]

Subdivision of fractures into those that violate the otic capsule and those that do not is described to have a more accurate prediction of the likelihood of serious or long-term complications.[1,4-6]

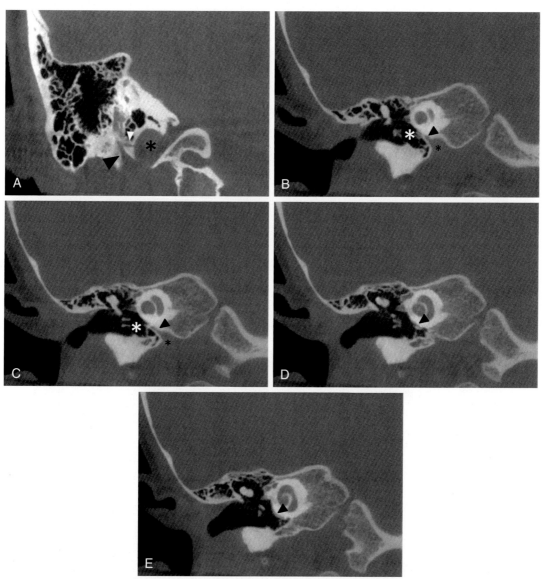

FIG. 7.6  **(A)** Coronal cone beam CT (CBCT) image through the jugular foramen (*asterisk*). The mastoid canaliculus (*small arrowhead*), containing the Arnold nerve, is seen as a linear lucency between the mastoid segment of the facial nerve (*large arrowhead*) and the jugular foramen. **(B–E)** Coronal CBCT image through the anterior hypotympanum and the cochlea. The inferior tympanic canaliculus is seen as a small linear canal (*arrowhead*) running upward and laterally from the jugular foramen (*small asterisk*) and the hypotympanum (*large asterisk*).

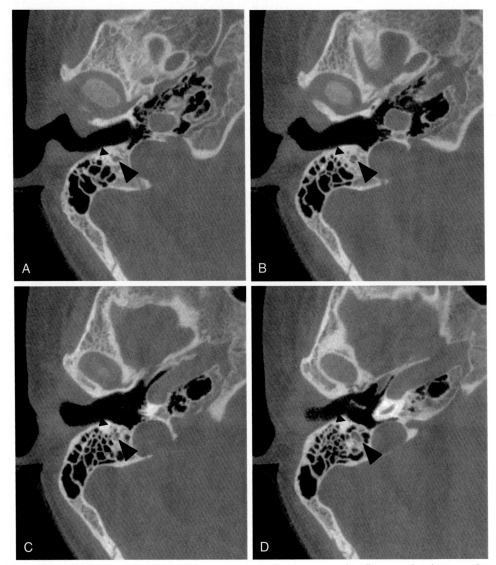

FIG. 7.7 **(A–D)** Axial cone beam CT (CBCT) image through the lower external auditory canal and consecutive slices upward until the level of the manubrium of the malleus. The canal for the chorda tympani can be seen from its origin at the facial nerve canal (*large arrowhead*) running upward toward the middle ear (*small arrowhead*).

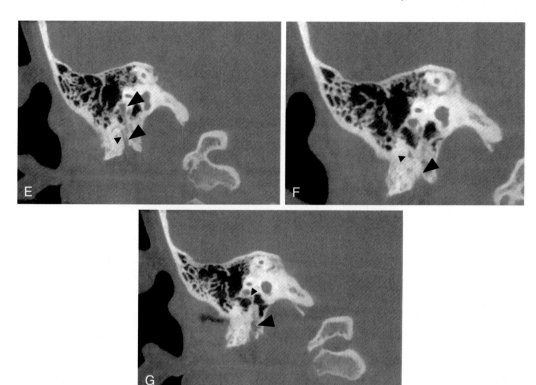

FIG. 7.7, cont'd **(E–G)** Coronal CBCT image through the mastoid segment of the facial nerve canal (*large arrowheads*). The canal for the chorda tympani (*small arrowhead*) can be seen running upward and laterally from the stylomastoid foramen.

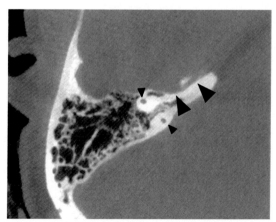

FIG. 7.8 Axial cone beam CT image through the limbs of the superior semicircular canal (*small arrowheads*). The sulcus for the superior petrosal sinus can be seen running anteriorly, on the superior edge of the petrosal bone pyramid (*large arrowheads*).

Sometimes, the hearing loss is detected only long after the original trauma, in some cases even after years (Fig. 7.12).

It should be noted that temporal bone fractures have little ability to form a callus. So, a temporal bone fracture can still be detected years after the initial trauma (Fig. 7.13).[2]

There is also a tendency for squamous epithelial cell invasion of the fracture site so that acquired cholesteatoma is a potential delayed complication. Such cholesteatomas are extremely rare but have the tendency to become large and extensive, as most of these patients lack a history of chronic otitis media and have hence well pneumatized middle ears.[2]

## COMPLICATIONS OF TEMPORAL BONE FRACTURES
### Fistulous Communications

Two types of fistulous communications after a trauma exist: cerebrospinal fluid (CSF) leak and perilymphatic fistula.[1–3,5,7,8]

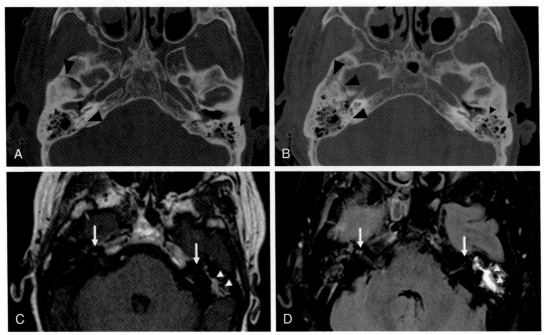

FIG. 7.9 A 54-year-old female who fell down the stairs. Clinically, the patient had a facial and abducens nerve paralysis on the right side, which gradually recovered. She also had a transmeatal liquor leakage, which stopped spontaneously after a few days, and a total hearing loss on the right side. **(A)** Axial CT image through the skull base at the level of the horizontal carotid canal. On the right side, a transverse fracture running anteroposteriorly can be seen (*large arrowheads*). On the left side, a longitudinal fracture can be seen in the lateral wall of the mastoid (*small arrowhead*). **(B)** Axial CT image through the skull base at the level of the basal turn of the cochlea (slightly higher than on the left side). The transverse fracture on the right side can clearly be seen (*large arrowheads*). The longitudinal fracture can be seen in the mastoid cells (*small arrowheads*). Note that both middle ears and mastoid cells are opacified, representing a bilateral hemotympanum. **(C)** Axial unenhanced T1-weighted image at the level of the internal auditory canal and the middle turn of the cochlea. On the right side, the apical and middle turns of the cochlea (*arrow*) display a higher signal intensity than on the left side (*arrow*) owing to blood deposition in the membranous labyrinth as a consequence of the transverse fracture. Note that the entire middle ear and mastoid on the left side (*arrowheads*) is displaying a spontaneous higher intensity, representing the hemotympanum. **(D)** Axial fluid-attenuated inversion recovery (FLAIR) image at the level of the internal auditory canal and the middle turn of the cochlea (same level as in **C**). The apical and middle turns of the cochlea display a higher signal intensity on the right side (*arrow*) than on the left side (*arrow*) owing to blood deposition in the membranous labyrinth. The entire middle ear and mastoid on the left side (*arrowheads*) is displaying a spontaneous higher signal intensity representing the hemotympanum. It should be noted that the signal intensity is higher on the FLAIR image than on the T1-weighted image. FLAIR sequences are known to have a higher sensitivity for blood in the acute phase.

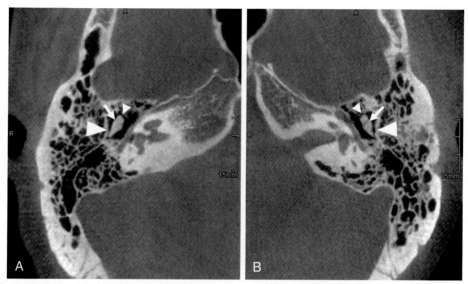

FIG. 7.10 A 28-year-old male with persistent conductive hearing loss after a longitudinal temporal bone fracture on the left side. **(A)** Axial cone beam CT (CBCT) image at the level of the incudomalleolar joint on the right side. Normal-appearing incudomalleolar joint with close apposition of the malleus head (*small arrowhead*) to the incus body and short process (*large arrowhead*). There is no dissociation of the joint between the malleus and incus (*arrow*). **(B)** Axial CBCT image at the level of the incudomalleolar joint on the left side (same level as in **A**). There is a minimal separation (*arrow*) between the malleus head (*small arrowhead*) and the incus body and short process (*large arrowhead*). Compare with the normal situation in **(A)**. Conclusion: subtle incudomalleolar dissociation on the left side.

CSF leak is usually secondary to disruption of the roof of the middle ear, the tegmen tympani. A tegmen tympani disruption can be asymptomatic. Most frequently, however, it causes CSF leakage. In the case of an associated tear of the tympanic membrane, there will also be CSF otorrhea. However, when the tympanic membrane is intact, fluid may egress anteriorly via the Eustachian tube and may cause CSF rhinorrhea. If the defect in the tegmen tympani is large, a meningoencephalocele may herniate in the middle ear (Fig. 7.14). This can also be asymptomatic, but it may be the cause of a subsequent meningitis. If the meningoencephalocele impinges on the ossicles, it may also cause conductive hearing loss.[1-3,5,7]

The second type of fistulous communication is a perilymphatic fistula. It is caused by a leakage of perilymph from the inner ear to the middle ear. Clinically, it may be associated with fluctuating sensorineural hearing loss and vertigo. The oval and round windows are the most common sites of origin for a perilymphatic fistula. Diagnosis can be very difficult. If there is clinical suspicion, imaging may show on CT or CBCT an opacification in the oval or round window

niche, which is a highly aspecific finding. Heavily T2-weighted sequences may demonstrate fluid accumulation in the oval or round window niche. Again, this can be regarded as aspecific, but in the appropriate clinical setting, these findings can give the clue to diagnosis.[1-3,5,7,8]

## Conductive Hearing Loss

Posttraumatic conductive hearing loss is very common after traumatic injury. It can be caused by hemotympanum, tympanic membrane damage, and ossicular discontinuity.[1-7]

In the acute phase of a longitudinal temporal bone fracture, conductive hearing loss is usually caused by the hemotympanum.

Clinical evaluation and audiogram should always be repeated after the resorption of the hemotympanum, as the conductive hearing loss may persist because of ossicular dissociation.

The malleus has a ligamentous apparatus consisting of the anterior, lateral, and superior malleal ligaments. Furthermore, the manubrium is also partially embedded in the tympanic membrane. The stapes is well fixed

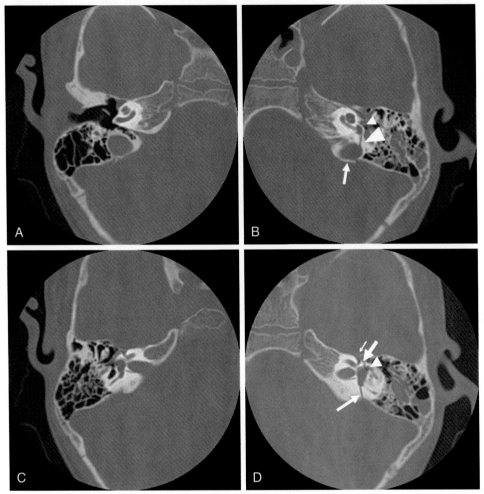

FIG. 7.11 An 8-year-old boy who fell down from the upper bed of a bunk bed with immediate headache, vertigo, and vomiting. Left-sided deafness was noted only afterward. **(A)** Axial CT image at the level of the basal turn of the cochlea on the right side demonstrating the normal otic capsule, the well-aerated hypo-tympanum, and the normal malleus handle. **(B)** Axial CT image at the level of the basal turn of the cochlea on the left side (same level as in **A**). Note the transverse fracture line running anteroposterior from the round window niche (*small arrowhead*) through the otic capsule (*large arrowhead*) in the fossa of the jugular bulb (*arrow*). There are some opacified mastoid air cells representing some blood deposition in some mastoid air cells. **(C)** Axial CT image at the level of the vestibule on the right side. Note the normal vestibule and posterior semicircular canal. The mastoid air cells display no opacification. **(D)** Axial CT image at the level of the vestibule on the left side (same level as in **C**). The transverse fracture is running from the region of the geniculate ganglion (*small arrow*) through the vestibule (*bold arrow*) and the posterior part of the tempo-ral bone pyramid (*large arrow*). Note the small air bubble anterior in the vestibule, at the junction with the lateral semicircular canal (*arrowhead*).

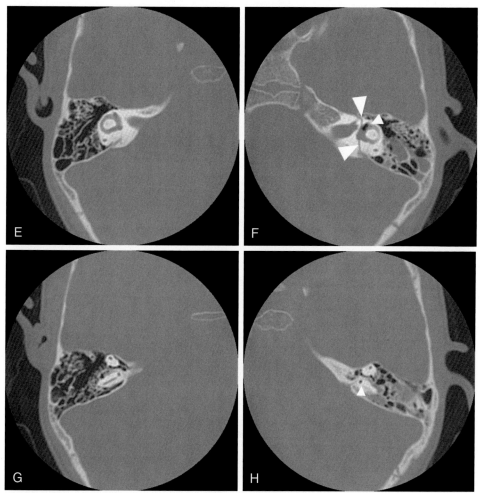

FIG. 7.11, cont'd **(E)** Axial CT image at the level of the lateral semicircular canal on the right side. Normal aspect of the lateral semicircular canal. **(F)** Axial CT image at the level of the lateral semicircular canal on the left side (same level as in **E**). The transverse fracture line is clearly visible (*large arrowheads*) and is running through the vestibule. Note the air in the anterior part of the vestibule (*small arrowhead*). **(G)** Axial CT image at the level of the superior semicircular canal on the right side. There is a well-aerated petrous bone pyramid with aerated cells extending between the superior semicircular canal. **(H)** Axial CT image at the level of the superior semicircular canal on the left side (same level as in **G**). The posterior limb of the superior semicircular canal displays a hypodense aspect, reflecting the presence of air in the superior semi-circular canal (*small arrowhead*). Compare with the normal isodense aspect of the anterior limb. Conclusion: transverse fracture of the temporal bone on the left side, with air in the vestibule and the anterior limb of the superior semicircular canal.

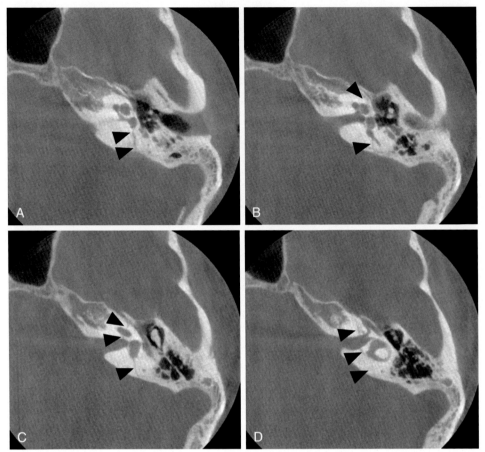

FIG. 7.12 A 40-year-old female with severe sensorineural hearing loss after a car crash. The hearing loss was not detected until 3 years after the trauma. **(A–D)** Axial cone beam CT images from caudal to cranial. The transverse fracture (*arrowheads*) is running through the basal turn of the cochlea, the vestibule and posterior semicircular canal, the apical turn of the cochlea, and the internal auditory canal. Conclusion: transverse fracture of the temporal bone.

between the footplate and the incudostapedial articulation; it is also supported by the stapedius muscle. The incus, however, is relatively heavy and has only minor ligamentous support.

Types of ossicular discontinuity include incudostapedial subluxation, malleoincudal subluxation, incus dislocation, stapes fracture and dislocation, and the rare malleus fracture.[1–4,7]

One of the most frequent types of ossicular dissociation is the dissociation between the incus and malleus. This is because in most cases the forces of the trauma run through the incudomalleolar joint (Fig. 7.15). This dissociation can be clear with the classical image of the ice cream falling off its cone

(Fig. 7.16). It can, however, also be very discrete and often can be diagnosed only by carefully comparison of the fractured with the normal site. A subtle separation on axial high-resolution CT/CBCT image of the malleus head from the incus body can be the only sign (Fig. 7.10).[1–4,7,8]

Another frequent type of dissociation is the separation between the long apophysis of the incus and the capitulum of the stapes. The presumed cause is a simultaneous tetanic contraction of the tensor tympani and stapedius tendon. Again, this can be very clear and also very subtle (Fig. 7.17). Double-oblique reconstructions through the joint of the incus and stapes have been proved to be superior in the evaluation of

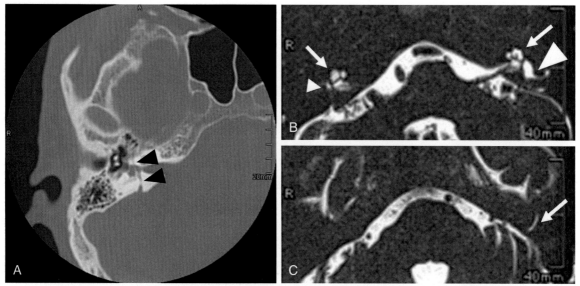

FIG. 7.13 A 49-year-old male with a prior history of a craniofacial trauma at the age of 6 years with complete deafness on the right side. Investigation was planned to evaluate the membranous labyrinth before a possible cochlear implant. **(A)** Axial CT image at the level of the vestibule. The transverse fracture line (*arrowheads*) is still visible, even more than 40 years later. Temporal bone fractures do not have the tendency to form callus. **(B)** Axial 3D turbo spin echo (TSE) T2-weighted image at the level of the vestibule. The vestibule on the left side can clearly be seen (*large arrowhead*). Note that the vestibule on the right side has nearly completely lost its fluid signal apart from a small area anteriorly (*small arrowhead*), owing to fibrosis. The signal in the cochlea remains high on both sides. **(C)** Axial 3D TSE T2-weighted image at the level of the superior semicircular canal. There is a normal-intensity signal in both limbs of the superior semicircular canal on the left side (*arrow*). The right superior semicircular canal can no longer be delineated. Conclusion: extensive fibrosis in the vestibule and semicircular canals on the right side owing to fibrosis caused by a right-sided transverse temporal bone fracture, 40 years prior. A cochlear implant still can be performed on the right side because the cochlea is fluid filled and the nerve can be delineated (not shown).

the separation of this joint. These can show the long apophysis of the incus, the stapes capitullum, and both crura of the stapes, as well as the foot plate in one plane without any partial volume effect of the tympanic segment of the facial nerve (Fig. 7.17).[9]

Complete incus dislocation requires a separation of the incudostapedial and the malleoincudal attachments. If the incus dislocation is complete, the incus can be found in the attic, the middle ear, or the external auditory canal (Fig. 7.18). In rare cases it can be completely absent, presumably resorbed over time.[1,2]

Stapes fractures are rare and often difficult to diagnose. Double-oblique reconstructions are highly valuable in demonstrating the normal stapes configuration, eventual fractures, and displaced fragments. The integrity of the foot plate can also be evaluated on these images.

## Sensorineural Hearing Loss

Sensorineural hearing loss can be caused by a fracture through the internal auditory canal, a fracture through the membranous labyrinth, or a cochlear concussion. The last entity occurs often without any imaging manifestations.[1,2]

Sensorineural hearing loss can be caused by a labyrinthine hemorrhage in the case of a transverse temporal bone fracture. Unenhanced T1-weighted MR images display in those cases a higher signal intensity in the membranous labyrinth. It is, however, known that fluid-attenuated inversion recovery sequences have a higher sensitivity for membranous labyrinth bleeding (Fig. 7.9).[8] Membranous labyrinth bleeding can, however, also spontaneously be caused in patients administered anticoagulant medication and in patients with coagulopathy or

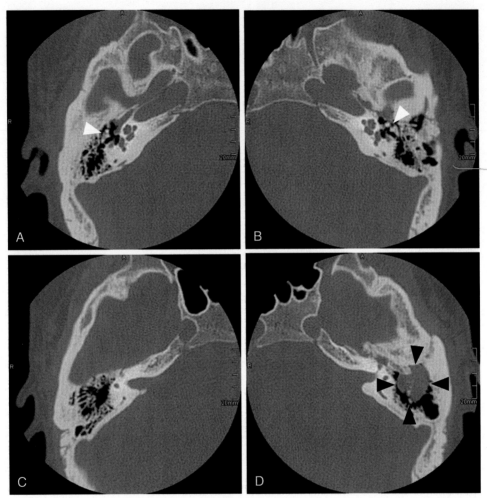

FIG. 7.14 A 29-year-old male with persistent conductive hearing loss after a severe craniofacial trauma.
**(A)** Axial CT image at the level of the incudomalleolar joint on the left side. There is a well-aerated middle
ear with a normal aspect of the incudomalleolar articulation (*arrowhead*). **(B)** Axial CT image at the level of
the incudomalleolar joint on the left side (same level as in **A**). There is a dissociation of the incudomalleolar
articulation, with medial displacement of the malleus head (*arrowhead*). Compare with the normal situation
in **(A)**. **(C)** Axial CT image at the level of the superior semicircular canal on the right side. There is a well-
aerated antrum and mastoid. **(D)** Axial CT image at the level of the superior semicircular canal on the left
side (same level as in **C**). There is a large, nodular, soft tissue mass lesion in the antrum (*arrowheads*)

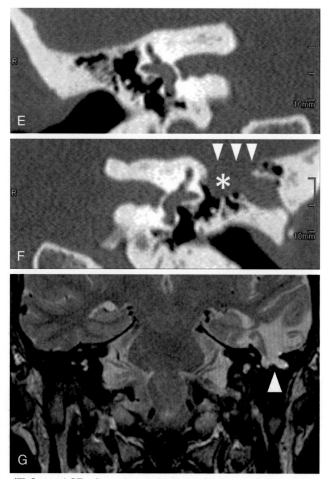

FIG. 7.14, cont'd **(E)** Coronal CT reformation at the level of the oval window on the right side. There is an intact delineation of the tegmen tympani with a well-aerated antrum and mastoid. **(F)** Coronal CT reformation at the level of the oval window on the left side. There is loss of delineation of the tegmen tympani (*arrowheads*) with a large soft tissue mass in the antrum (*asterisk*). **(G)** Coronal T2-weighted image through the brain stem. There is a region of tissue loss in the left temporal lobe, with herniation of brain and meninges through the large defect (*arrowhead*). Conclusion: left-side posttraumatic incudomalleolar dissociation with a posttraumatic tissue loss in the left temporal lobe. There is a large tegmen tympani defect with a meningoencephalocele herniating through the defect.

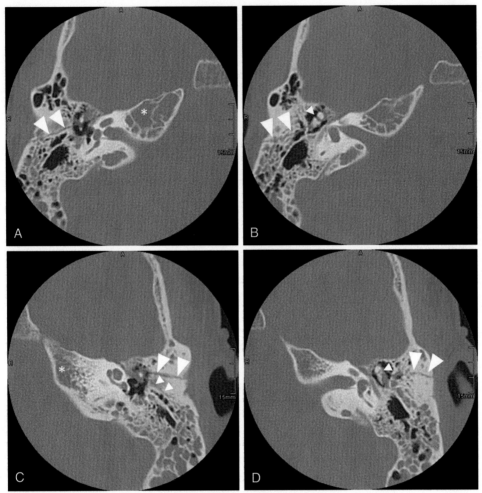

FIG. 7.15 A 40-year-old male with bilateral severe conductive hearing loss after crashing with his scooter on the trunk of a car. **(A)** Axial cone beam CT (CBCT) image at the level of the oval window on the right side. A longitudinal fracture (*arrowheads*) can be seen in the roof of the external auditory canal. The extension of the fracture runs exactly between the malleus and incus. Note also the aerated but opacified petrous bone apex (*asterisk*). **(B)** Axial CBCT image at the level of the incudomalleolar joint on the right side (slightly higher than in **A**). The fracture line can be seen in the lateral epitympanic wall (*large arrowheads*). Note the dissociation of the incudomalleolar joint (*small arrowhead*). **(C)** Axial CBCT image at the level of the round window on the left side (slightly lower than in **A**). A V-shaped longitudinal fracture with one broad anterior component (*large arrowheads*) and one thinner posterior component (*small arrowheads*) can be seen running through the roof of the external auditory canal. The medial extension of both fracture lines runs directly between the malleus and incus. Note the nonaerated petrous apex (*asterisk*). **(D)** Axial CBCT image at the level of the incudomalleolar joint on the left side (slightly higher than in **C**). The fracture line can be seen in the lateral epitympanic wall (*large arrowheads*). Note the subtle dissociation of the incudomalleolar joint (*small arrowhead*). Conclusion: bilateral longitudinal temporal bone fracture. The fracture line and fracture's force runs on both sides almost immediately through the incudomalleolar joint causing the incudomalleolar dislocation on both sides.

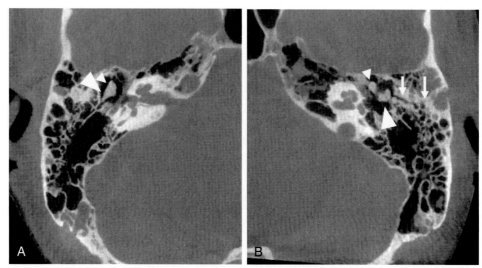

FIG. 7.16 A 31-year-old male with a prior history of a severe craniofacial trauma after falling off a rooftop. He presents with persistent left-sided conductive hearing loss and tinnitus. **(A)** Axial cone beam CT (CBCT) image at the level of the oval window on the right side showing the normal ice cream cone appearance composed of the incus corpus and short process (*large arrowhead*) and the malleus head (*small arrowhead*). **(B)** Axial CBCT image at the level of the oval window on the left side (same level as in **A**). The longitudinal fracture line can easily be seen (*arrows*). Note the displaced ice cream, malleus head (*small arrowhead*), separated from the cone, incus corpus and short process (*large arrowhead*). Conclusion: clear posttraumatic separation of the incudomalleolar joint on the left side.

sickle cell disease. The clinical history of the patient, however, will add to the differential diagnosis.[1,2,5,8]

CT or CBCT may demonstrate, in addition to bleeding, air in the membranous labyrinth (Fig. 7.11).

Other, albeit rare, causes of posttraumatic sensorineural hearing loss are brain stem injuries specifically to the cochlear nuclei of the inferior colliculi. The entity of a hemorrhage in the inferior colliculi of the brain stem caused by sudden deceleration with the inferior colliculi hitting the tentorium and a subsequent bleeding is a rare but devastating cause of acute deafness.

## Ossicular Fractures

Ossicular fractures without an associated temporal bone fracture may also occur.

Most of these ossicular fractures and/or displacements are caused by accidental perforation of the tympanic membrane. Most frequently, perforation of the tympanic membrane is caused by a cotton wool tip accidently perforating the tympanic membrane. Other causes of perforation have also been described and can been variable (Fig. 7.19).[2,8]

There is another entity that needs to be mentioned, and that is the fracture of the malleus handle. It can

be part of a longitudinal temporal bone fracture, but it can also be isolated.[2] In the latter case, it is most often caused by the pressure difference that results from a sudden retraction of the index finger out of the external auditory canal.[8] The clinical and otoscopical diagnosis can be confirmed by CBCT or CT showing the discontinuity of the malleus handle (Fig. 7.20).

## Facial Nerve Injury

The facial nerve has a very long trajectory in the temporal bone and can be injured at any point, from the root entry zone at the level of the pons, over the cisternal/canalicular segment, throughout the temporal bone and extracranially in the parotid gland.

Because the facial nerve gives off branches at various points with different functions (lacrimation, taste, stapedius muscle function), careful clinical evaluation may sometimes localize the site of damage.

The nature of damage is variable, ranging from complete transection to stretching, compression by hematoma or fracture fragments, and neuronal edema.[1–5]

The timing of the facial nerve palsy to the trauma is highly predictive of long-term prognosis. In transverse fractures, the onset of facial nerve palsy is usually immediate. Immediate onset usually suggests nerve

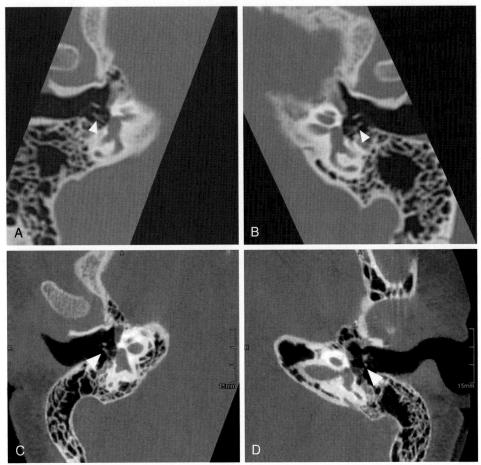

**FIG. 7.17** Two patients (aged 56 years, in **A** and **B**; aged 13 years in **C** and **D**) with persistent left-sided conductive hearing loss after a head trauma with a longitudinal fracture. The patient in **A** and **B** was scanned using CT scan. The patient in **C** and **D** was scanned using cone beam CT (CBCT). **(A)** Axial double-oblique CT reformation at the level of the incudostapedial joint on the right side. Note the normal alignment from lateral to medial (*arrowhead*) of the long apophysis of the incus, the stapes capitulum, and both crura of the stapes. **(B)** Axial double-oblique CT reformation at the level of the incudostapedial joint on the left side. On this side, there is a small gap between the long apophysis of the incus and stapes capitulum, compatible with an incudostapedial dissociation (*arrowhead*). **(C)** Axial double-oblique CBCT reformation at the level of the incudostapedial joint on the right side. Note the normal alignment from lateral to medial (*arrowhead*) of the long apophysis of the incus, the stapes capitulum, and both crura of the stapes. **(D)** Axial double-oblique CBCT reformation at the level of the incudostapedial joint on the left side. On this side, there is a small gap between the long apophysis of the incus and stapes capitulum compatible with an incudostapedial dissociation (*arrowhead*). Conclusion: Both patients have an incudostapedial dissociation explaining the conductive hearing loss. Double-oblique reformations are regarded as highly sensitive for (subtle) ossicular chain and footplate abnormalities.

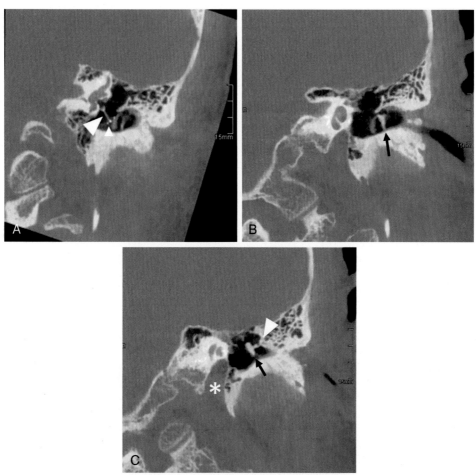

FIG. 7.18 A 56-year-old male with a history of prior surgery for cholesteatoma and ossicular reconstruction using a partial ossicular replacement prosthesis (PORP). The patient was evaluated after a head trauma with a longitudinal temporal bone fracture (not shown) because of severe persistent conductive hearing loss after the trauma. **(A)** Coronal cone beam CT (CBCT) image at the level of the round window. The PORP (*large arrowhead*) is clearly seen. It is no longer in contact with the stapes or (*small arrowhead*) with the reconstructed tympanic membrane. **(B)** Coronal CBCT image at the level of the cochlea (slightly anterior to the level in **A**). The incus (*arrow*) can be seen as a Y-shaped bony structure in the external auditory canal. **(C)** Coronal CBCT image at the level of the anterior hypotympanic space. Note the jugular bulb (*asterisk*). The malleus (*arrow*) is sitting on the edge of the anterior delineation of the scutum (*arrowhead*) and is hence partially located in the middle ear and in the external ear. Conclusion: displacement of the malleus, between the middle and external ear, and the incus, in the external auditory canal, is due to the trauma. The PORP is also displaced.

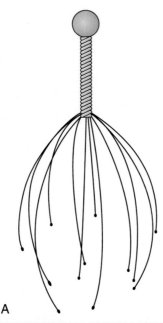

A

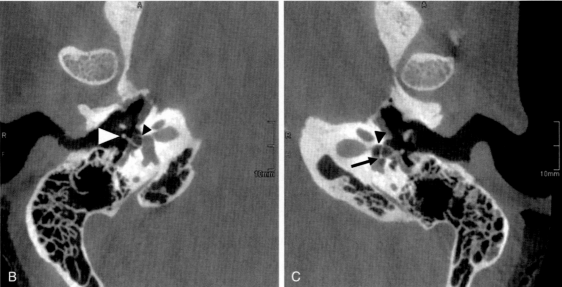

FIG. 7.19 A 32-year-old female presenting after a penetrating trauma to her left ear canal. Her child had accidentally perforated her ear drum with the pin of a head massage device. The patient reported immediate otalgia, hearing loss, tinnitus, and vertigo. **(A)** Head massage device. **(B)** Axial double-oblique reformation of a cone beam CT at the level of the incudostapedial joint (*large arrowhead*) demonstrating the normal situation on the right side. Note the intact footplate (*small arrowhead*). **(C)** Axial double-oblique reformation of a cone beam CT on the left side at the level of the incudostapedial joint. Note the depression of the footplate into the vestibule (*arrow*) and the air in the vestibule (*arrowhead*). The posterior crus of the stapes seems depressed into the vestibule. Conclusion: protrusion of the footplate and posterior crus of the vestibule after tympanic membrane perforation by a pin of a scalp massage tool. At surgery, reconstruction of the footplate and retraction of the stapes could be performed, with hearing restoration up to 80%. Vertigo and tinnitus disappeared in the weeks after surgery.

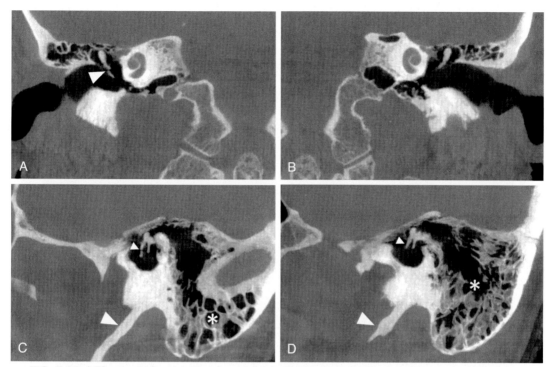

FIG. 7.20 A 52-year-old female with pain and conductive hearing loss after forceful retraction of the index finger out of the external auditory canal on the right side. At otoscopy, a malleus fracture was suspected. **(A)** Coronal cone beam CT (CBCT) image at the level of the malleus handle and the cochlea on the right side. There is a fracture running through the malleus handle (*arrowhead*) with slight distraction of the fragments. **(B)** Coronal CBCT image at the level of the malleus handle and the cochlea on the left side (same level as in **A**). Normal aspect of the malleus handle (compare with **A**). **(C)** Sagittal maximum intensity projection (MIP) reformation of the temporal bone on the right side. The ossicular chain can easily be detected in the middle ear. The fracture of the malleus handle is clearly seen (*small arrowhead*). Note the mastoid cells (*asterisk*) as well as the styloid process (*large arrowhead*). **(D)** Sagittal MIP reformation of the temporal bone on the left side (same level as in **C**). The normal ossicular chain can easily be detected in the middle ear. The normal malleus handle (*small arrowhead*), the mastoid cells (*asterisk*), and the styloid process (*large arrowhead*) can be seen (compare with **C**). Conclusion: fracture of the malleus handle.

transection, whereas delayed onset (more than 24h later) suggests nerve edema or compression by a hematoma. A high-grade facial nerve palsy may benefit from early facial nerve decompressive surgery (Fig. 7.21).[1-5]

The majority of injuries occur in the region of the geniculate ganglion, followed by the second genu, the tympanic segment, and the mastoid segment.

Radiologically, facial nerve involvement can be suspected when a fracture line approaches or traverses a segment of its course (Fig. 7.21).

Unenhanced T1-weighted images theoretically may be able to demonstrate a spontaneous hyperintense lesion in or around the facial nerve segments representing a hematoma.[1-5]

Gadolinium-enhanced T1-weighted images may demonstrate a thickened and strongly enhancing facial nerve caused by the edema (Fig. 7.21). It must be kept in mind that the region of the geniculate ganglion and tympanic facial nerve normally enhances, because of the presence of a venous plexus. A comparison of the traumatic side with the normal side is hence mandatory.

## CONCLUSION

Temporal bone anatomy is complex, with multiple fissures and canals that can be confused with fractures. Knowledge of normal temporal bone anatomy

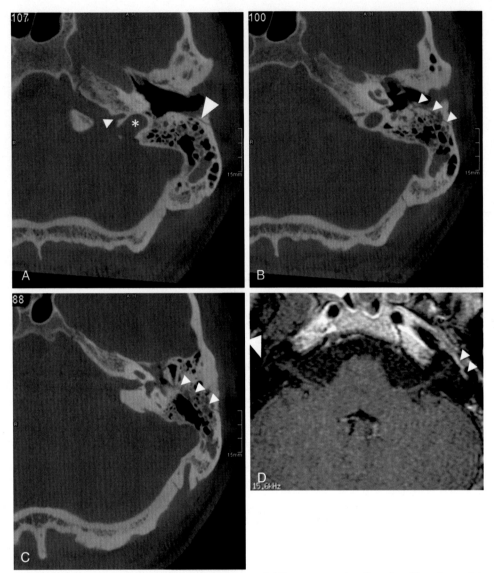

FIG. 7.21 A 54-year-old male who fell down from a scaffolding on a construction site with an immediate severe facial nerve palsy (House-Brackmann grade V). **(A)** Axial cone beam CT (CBCT) image at the level of the jugular bulb (*asterisk*). The longitudinal fracture line can be seen running anterior in the mastoid tip (*large arrowhead*). Note again the glossopharyngeal sulcus (*small arrowhead*). See also Fig. 7.3B. **(B)** Axial CBCT image at the level of the basal turn of the cochlea. The longitudinal fracture line is seen running through the posterosuperior wall of the external auditory canal (*arrowheads*). Its expected course is running through the region of the geniculate ganglion. **(C)** Axial CBCT image at the level of the incudomalleolar joint. The fracture line has a characteristic course along the long axis of the temporal bone (*arrowheads*) and is running through the region of the geniculate ganglion. **(D)** Axial gadolinium-enhanced 3D gradient echo T1-weighted image through the internal auditory canal at the level of the tympanic segment of the facial nerve. The tympanic segment of the facial nerve on the left side displays an intense enhancement (*small arrowheads*). Compare with the tympanic segment of the facial nerve on the right side (*large arrowhead*).

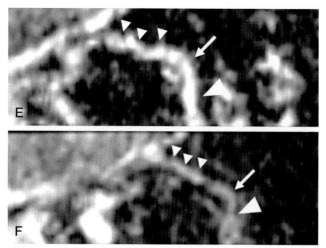

FIG. 7.21, cont'd **(E)** Sagittal reformation of the tympanic (*small arrowheads*) segment, second genu (*arrow*), and mastoid segment (*large arrowhead*) of the facial nerve on the right side. The facial nerve is thickened over its entire course and is strongly enhancing. **(F)** Sagittal reformation of the tympanic (*small arrowheads*) segment, second genu (*arrow*), and mastoid segment (*large arrowhead*) of the facial nerve on the normal right side. The tympanic and mastoid segments display a subtle enhancement because of the presence of a venous plexus. Compare with the thickened and enhancing facial nerve on the right side in **(E)**. Conclusion: longitudinal fracture of the temporal bone with a course running through the tympanic segment of the facial nerve and the geniculate ganglion with an almost immediate high-grade facial nerve palsy (House-Brackmann grade V). MRI demonstrates thickening and enhancement of the facial nerve in its tympanic and mastoid segment. After decompressing surgery, the facial nerve palsy gradually disappeared. Immediate high-grade facial nerve palsies are usually seen in transverse fractures and are less common in longitudinal fractures.

and comparison of both temporal bones is of utmost importance. Careful and systematic evaluation of the external ear, ossicles and other middle ear structures, and the inner ear structures and facial nerve segments is mandatory. CT or CBCT and MRI are complementary in the complete radiologic evaluation of a patient with a temporal bone trauma.

## REFERENCES

1. Collins JM, Krishnamoorthy AK, Kubal WS, et al. Multidetector CT of temporal bone fractures. *Semin Ultrasound Ct MR*. 2012;33:418–431.
2. Swartz JD. Temporal bone trauma. *Semin Ultrasound CT MR*. 2001;22:219–228.
3. Zimmer A, Reith W. Trauma of the temporal bone. *Radiology*. 2010;54:340–345.
4. Zayas JO, Feliciano YZ, Hadley CR, et al. Temporal bone trauma and the role of multidetector CT in the emergency department. *Radiographics*. 2011;31:1741–1755.
5. Juliano AF, Ginat DT, Moonis G. Imaging review of the temporal bone: Part II. Traumatic, postoperative and noninflammatory nonneoplastic conditions. *Radiology*. 2015;276:655–672.
6. Sung EK, Nadgir RN, Sakai O. Computed tomographic imaging in head and neck trauma: what the radiologist needs to know. *Semin Roentgenol*. 2012;47:320–329.
7. Jeevan S, Ormond R, Kim AH, et al. Cerebrospinal fluid leaks and encephalocele of temporal bone origin: nuances to diagnosis and management. *World Neurosurg*. 2015;83:560–566.
8. Maillot O, Attyé A, Boyer E, et al. Post traumatic deafness: a pictorial review of CT and MRI findings. *Insights Imaging*. 2016;7:341–350.
9. Henrot PH, Iochum S, Batch T, et al. Current multiplanar imaging of the stapes. *Am J Neuroradiol*. 2005;26:2128–2133.

# CHAPTER 8

# Update on Imaging of Hearing Loss

LUBDHA M. SHAH, MD • RICHARD H. WIGGINS III, MD, CIIP, FSIIM

## INTRODUCTION

In the imaging evaluation of hearing loss, the radiologic examination is complementary to the physical examination. The clinical evaluation includes not only an accurate history of the hearing loss itself (unilateral or bilateral, slow onset or fast onset, etc.) but also the patient's medical history (possible trauma, ototoxic drugs, associated facial nerve palsies, etc.). Hearing loss can be described as sensorineural, conductive, or mixed, and this will guide the choice of imaging modality to correlate with the clinical history and symptoms. In this chapter, we will review the more common hearing loss entities, and divide these pathologies into those presenting with sensorineural hearing loss (SNHL), conductive hearing loss (CHL), and mixed hearing loss (MHL). The pathologies for SNHL and CHL will be further grouped and discussed as either congenital or acquired entities. In very simplistic terms, CHL is frequently initially evaluated with CT, whereas SNHL is most frequently initially evaluated with MRI. When reviewing the imaging studies, a systematic "outside-in" approach along the hearing pathway is helpful, from the external anatomic structures to the internal structures.

## IMAGING MODALITIES

Thin-section CT and MRI provide complementary information in evaluating skull base and temporal bone (TB) pathologies. On evaluation of a patient with hearing loss, CT of the TB is particularly helpful to evaluate the osseous structures (external auditory canal [EAC], middle ear, and otic capsule), whereas MRI is useful to evaluate the inner ear structures, internal auditory canal (IAC), cerebellopontine angle (CPA), and brainstem.

CT of the TBs can be performed with the patient lying supine, in the anatomic axial plane. Multidetector CT scanners acquire submillimeter slices with low radiation dose and reduced scan time. It is important for the imager to be wary of low-dose techniques, as these will limit the accurate evaluation of the normally dense TB osseous structures. Submillimeter multiplanar reconstructions can be performed with minimal overlap. Although parameters vary by institution, suggested TB CT parameters are described in Box 8.1. This technique is capable of revealing a broad spectrum of EAC and middle ear lesions that may not be apparent on the basis of clinical findings alone. Radiation dose in TB CT imaging can be high because of the requirement of high spatial resolution. Leng et al. demonstrated an ultrahigh-resolution scan mode with an iterative reconstruction algorithm to improve the quality of the TB CT image with decreased radiation dose.[1] Axial acquisitions with multiple plane reconstructions can effectively evaluate the osseous TB anatomy and pathology (Fig. 8.1).

MRI is a fundamental method of evaluating the inner ear structures as well as the cerebrospinal fluid (CSF) spaces, IAC, CPA, and adjacent brain parenchyma. Dedicated head and temporomandibular joint coils are important for achieving an optimal signal to noise ratio. Screening MRI (noncontrasted thin-section CSF bright sequences) of the CPA/IAC can be performed in the initial evaluation of SNHL in the appropriately screened patient (i.e., older patient with progressive asymmetric hearing loss). When there is a suspected or known retrocochlear lesion, MRI of the CPA/IAC

> **BOX 8.1**
> **CT Parameters**
>
> Submillimeter (0.6 mm) slices
> Multiplanar reconstructions with minimal overlap (0.5 mm)
> >    Axial
> >    Coronal
> >    Long-axis (Stenver) projection
> >    Short-axis (Pöschl) projection
> >    Scout image
> >    Standard algorithm large field of view thicker
> >       sections (2–3 mm)

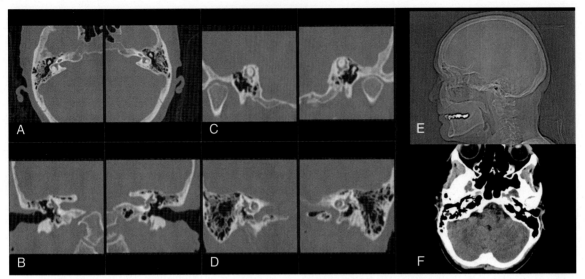

FIG. 8.1 Routine Picture archiving and communication system (PACS) temporal bone hanging protocol: **(A)** Axial right and left thin-section (submillimeter) bone algorithm acquisition images, **(B)** right and left coronal thin-section bone algorithm reconstructions, **(C)** right and left thin-section short-axis (similar to Pöschl projection) reconstructions, **(D)** right and left thin-section long axis (similar to Stenver projection), **(E)** scout image, and **(F)** axial standard algorithm large field of view thicker section (2–3 mm).

without and with contrast can be performed. In addition, in cases of complicated SNHL, or when there are other symptoms such as cranial neuropathy, long tract signs, and/or headache, imaging should include whole brain and posterior fossa sequences (axial T2 and/or fluid-attenuated inversion recovery [FLAIR]). Although parameters vary by institution, suggested screening MRI IAC parameters are described in Box 8.2. Imaging is critical in the assessment of hearing loss, and when a pathology is identified, the most commonly encountered tumor is vestibular schwannoma (VS).[2] One diagnostic review and meta-analysis concluded that nonimaging screening protocols, including pure-tone audiometry, auditory brainstem response, clinical symptoms, electronystagmography, caloric irrigation, and hyperventilation tests, were not accurate in detecting VSs.[3]

MRI is widely used for the evaluation of asymmetric SNHL. There are, however, drawbacks of risks, cost, and time associated with MRI. Non-contrast-enhanced MRI studies have been shown to be adequate in the detection of CPA/IAC masses using thin CSF bright sequences.[4,5] A prospective, blinded study using fast spin echo (FSE) T2-weighted (T2W) MRI demonstrated a threefold decreased cost while maintaining 98% sensitivity for schwannomas.[5] A screening high-resolution FSE T2W MRI was also shown to be adequate to detect other pathologies, including other CPA/IAC

lesions, inner ear lesions, and intraaxial lesions (such as infarctions, multiple sclerosis, mesial temporal sclerosis, and colloid cysts).[6] Daniels et al. concluded that this high-resolution FSE screening technique, used in conjunction with appropriate clinical prescreening and referral, can provide an equally sensitive method of evaluating unilateral SNHL compared with contrast-enhanced T1-weighted (T1W) MRI while reducing costs and providing distinct advantages in evaluating non-VS causes of SNHL.[6] They also showed that false positives on contrast-enhanced T1W MRI (true negatives on FSE T2W MRI) can lead to unnecessary diagnostic tests, intervention, and increased costs of care. Similarly, in a study comparing T2W MRI with contrast-enhanced MRI in 146 patients with asymmetric SHNL, Verret et al. demonstrated that only T2W MRI instead of contrast-enhanced MRI would have decreased costs over $100,000.[7] With the addition of multiple planes (i.e., axial and coronal) and advances in MRI techniques (e.g., constructive interference in steady state [CISS], fast imaging employing steady-state acquisition [FIESTA], and sampling perfection with application optimized contrast using different flip angle evolutions [SPACE]), 100% sensitivity and excellent interrater agreement can be achieved with high-resolution MRI protocols.[8]

Contrast-enhanced MRI has been shown by other studies to provide useful information for nonneoplastic lesions. Annesley-Williams et al. found that 2- to 5-mm lesions may be missed on two-dimensional (2D) FSE T2W MRI and that contrast-enhanced MRI may be needed to further investigate findings on three-dimensional (3D) and 2D MRI (9% and 15%, respectively).[9] However, in considering patient care related to non-neoplastic CPA/IAC pathologies, such as inflammatory pathologies that are typically acute in onset and of viral etiology, these cases are treated regardless of the MRI findings.

Imaging pitfalls should also be considered when evaluating MRI. For example, the petrous apex marrow adjacent to the IAC can enhance on postcontrast T1W MRI (especially bright on cases without fat saturation) and be erroneously interpreted as a CPA/IAC tumor. Similarly, asymmetric aeration of the petrous apices with unilateral benign trapped fluid can also be mistaken for pathology. The enhancement of a prominent anterior inferior cerebellar artery (AICA) loop may be mistaken for a small VS.[10] Other pseudomasses include the choroid plexus protruding through the lateral recesses of the fourth ventricle and the cerebellar flocculus normally projecting into the posterolateral aspect of the CPA cistern. The vestibular nerve ganglion (Scarpa ganglion) in the IAC should also not be mistaken as a small VS. If there is a punctate (<2 mm) enhancing lesion in the CPA/IAC, it can safely be followed over time. Pathologies arising from the jugular foramen may also extend superiorly into the CPA/IAC region.

## SENSORINEURAL HEARING LOSS

SNHL indicates dysfunction of the cochlea, cochlear nerve, and/or brain and can be measured with a tuning fork touched to the top of the head, by conduction through bone, so that the sound will localize to the normal side in these patients. The structures of note include the cochlea and the cochlear nerve from the origin nucleus through the CPA/IAC cistern into the modiolus. In addition to CT of the TBs, thin-section MRI with T1W pre- and postcontrast with fat-saturation sequences, T2W sequences, and 3D CISS/3D T2 FSE/3D fourier transformation CISS/SPACE sequences are essential for the thorough evaluation of SNHL.

### Congenital SNHL Pathologies

Congenital hearing loss is defined as hearing loss present at birth and is generally divided into genetic and nongenetic forms. Congenital SNHL etiologies include membranous labyrinth dysplasias, cochlear/vestibular aplasia/dysplasia, enlarged vestibular aqueduct, IAC atresia/stenosis, and perilymphatic fistula. Genetic anomalies cause approximately half of the cases of congenital SNHL[11]; of these approximately 75%–80% demonstrate an autosomal recessive inheritance, 15%–20% demonstrate an autosomal dominant inheritance, and 1%–2% demonstrate an X-linked inheritance.[12] Approximately 30% of inherited forms of hearing loss are syndromic, and the remaining 70% are considered nonsyndromic.[13]

Although the cause is unknown in 25%–40% of cases,[14] intrauterine toxin exposure, infections, and perinatal insults account for many cases of pediatric SNHL.[11] Cytomegalovirus (CMV) infection is the most common environmental cause of prelingual hearing loss in the United States, implicated in approximately 10% of infants with congenital hearing loss and 34% of children with moderate to severe late-onset idiopathic hearing loss.[15] Among children with clinically apparent congenital CMV infection, the prevalence of SNHL is ~30%.[16]

Cross-sectional imaging is an integral tool in the clinical evaluation of congenital SNHL. Otolaryngologists utilize CT and/or MRI to identify potential etiologies and abnormalities that may predict hearing loss progression or prognosis, to define TB anatomy and the central auditory pathway and to identify additional intracranial abnormalities that may require further workup and/or intervention. Abnormalities on CT and/or MRI are found in 20%–50% of children with SNHL and correlate with the degree of hearing loss.[17] Although traditionally bone algorithm CT is the modality of choice in demonstrating inner ear dysplasias in children with SNHL, dual-technique imaging with high-resolution TB CT and MRI has been show to identify a substantially larger number of abnormalities in children being evaluated for cochlear implantation than either technique alone.[18]

The spectrum of inner ear anomalies ranges from complete aplasia to subtle dysplasia. Sennaroglu and Saatci[19] proposed a classification for cochleovestibular malformations that included, in order of decreasing severity: labyrinthine aplasia, cochlear aplasia, common cavity deformities, cystic cochleovestibular malformations (incomplete partition type-1), cochleovestibular hypoplasia, and incomplete partition type-2 (IP-II), each of which is thought to result from an insult occurring at a progressively later stage of development.

Labyrinthine aplasia (Michel deformity) is the complete absence of the cochlea, vestibule, and semicircular canals (SCCs). In cases of labyrinthine aplasia, there is SNHL from birth without the option of cochlear implantation in the affected ear. The bony labyrinth is

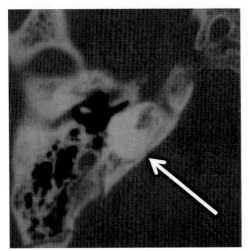

FIG. 8.2 Labyrinthine aplasia. Axial bone algorithm thin-section CT of the right temporal bone through the petrous apex demonstrates dense bone without inner ear formation (*arrow*), consistent with labyrinthine aplasia.

featureless, and the petrous apex may be hypoplastic or absent, and the IAC is small. The middle ear may be normal in the mild form to abnormal with fused ossicles in the more severe form. In these cases, the lateral wall of the inner ear is flat and the facial nerve geniculate ganglion is displaced posterior to its normal expected location.[20] There is no normal high-signal-intensity fluid in the membranous labyrinth on high-resolution T2W MR. Labyrinthine aplasia occurs when there is arrest of the otic placode development at the third gestational week. It may be associated with Klippel-Feil syndrome and/or thalidomide exposure (Fig. 8.2).

Cochlear aplasia occurs in late third week arrest, with absent cochlea, dysmorphic vestibule, and SCCs.[21,22] The vestibule and IAC may be dilated. In these cases, the cochlear promontory is flat and the facial nerve labyrinthine segment, geniculate ganglion, and anterior tympanic portions are located at the expected location of the cochlea. The EAC, middle ear, ossicular chain, bony vestibular aqueduct, and endolymphatic duct are normal in size (Fig. 8.3).

If there is an arrest in the fourth week after differentiation of the otic placode into the otocyst, a common cavity deformity occurs and an ovoid single inner ear cavity is formed. The SCCs are usually absent but may be present and dysplastic. The IAC size is concordant with the size of the common cavity and enters the cavity at the center portion; however, the modiolus is absent (Fig. 8.4).[23] Oblique sagittal T2W images perpendicular to the IAC are important to assess the presence or absence of the cochlear nerve if cochlear implantation is planned (Fig. 8.5).[12]

A cystic cochleovestibular anomaly results if there is arrest in the fifth gestational week. A "figure 8"-shaped

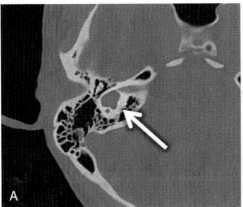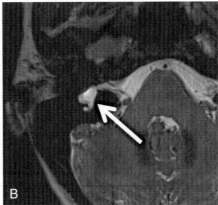

FIG. 8.3 Cochlear aplasia. Axial thin-section bone algorithm CT **(A)** and correlating axial cerebrospinal fluid bright constructive interference in steady state MRI **(B)** through the inner ear structures demonstrates a dysplastic dilated vestibule (*arrow*) without anterior and medial cochlear formation, consistent with cochlear aplasia.

dysplastic and cystic cochlea and vestibule with SCC dysplasia is seen.[19] There are no internal features, and no modiolus is identified in these cases. The vestibule is cystic and dilated, and the SCCs are variable in shape and degree of dilatation. The IAC is normal or small in size with a normal facial nerve; however, the cochleovestibular nerves are deficient or absent. The EAC,

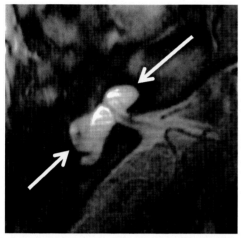

FIG. 8.4 Common cavity deformity. Axial thin-section cerebrospinal fluid bright CISS image through the right temporal bone demonstrates a common cavity deformity with an ovoid single inner ear cystic structure (*arrows*) of a combined dysplastic cochlea and vestibule.

middle ear, ossicular chain, bony vestibular aqueduct, and endolymphatic duct are normal in size.

SCC dysplasia is a spectrum of congenital deformities. The embryologic insult occurs at 6–8 weeks of gestation. The SCCs begin as disk-shaped evaginations arising from the vestibular appendage in the sixth gestational week. The central portion of each disk is resorbed and replaced by the mesenchyme, which results in the formation of the characteristic SCC. Failure of formation of one of these disks results in the absence of the involved SCC, whereas incomplete absorption of the central portion of the disk results in a dysplastic or pocket-shaped SCC. The superior SCC is the first to form, followed by the posterior SCC and then the lateral SCC. The most common and least severe dysplasia in this spectrum is a common cavity formed by the lateral SCC and the vestibule (Fig. 8.6). On axial CT images, subtle SCC abnormalities may be indicated by an absent or small bony island between the vestibule and the lateral SCC (Fig. 8.7). Normally, the transverse diameter of this bony island measures between 2.6 and 4.8 mm.[24] As an internal standard for comparison, the osseous bony island between the vestibule and inside the loop of the lateral SCC should be wider from right to left than the vestibule width from right to left. In these cases, there may be associated oval window atresia (OWA) and the cochlea may be affected with incomplete partition of the apical and middle turns. There may also be ossicular anomalies. In addition to SNHL, there may be CHL due

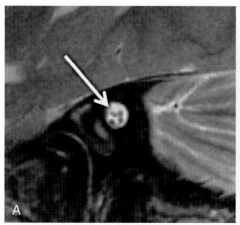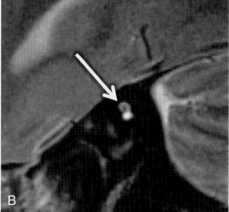

FIG. 8.5 Cochlear nerve aplasia. Oblique thin-section cerebrospinal fluid bright MRI sections through the midportion of the bilateral internal auditory canals (IACs) demonstrates a normal IAC on the right **(A)** with four nerves seen in cross-section, with the facial nerve identified (*arrow*) superiorly and anteriorly. The cochlear nerve is seen anteriorly and inferiorly, inferior to the facial nerve, and the superior and inferior vestibular nerves are seen posteriorly within the IAC. The correlating small IAC on the left **(B)** shows a single nerve in cross-section (*arrow*), consistent with the facial nerve in this pediatric patient with normal bilateral facial motion but left congenital SNHL.

to this OWA and ossicular chain anomalies.[19] It can be sporadic or associated with congenital syndromes (e.g., CHARGE, Alagille, Waardenburg, Crouzon, Apert). In CHARGE syndrome (coloboma, heart defects, choanal atresia, retardation of growth and development, and ear abnormalities), for instance, there is absence of the SCC bilaterally, dysmorphic vestibule, and cochlear anomalies with absence of the cochlear nerve canal.[25]

Large endolymphatic sac anomaly (often used when found on MRI), or large vestibular aqueduct syndrome (often used when found on CT), is seen when there is arrest in the seventh gestational week (Fig. 8.8). This is the most common inner ear malformation seen in children with nonsyndromic hearing loss and is bilateral in 90% of cases. The prevalence of enlarged vestibular aqueducts

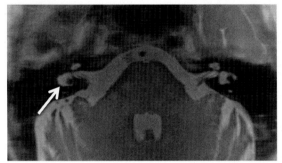

FIG. 8.6 Lateral semicircular canal (SCC) dysplasia. Axial cerebrospinal fluid bright thin-section MRI through the IACs and vestibules demonstrates a cystic vestibule, consistent with a right lateral SCC dysplasia with no osseous island or lateral SCC formation (*arrow*).

in children with SNHL is estimated to be 10%–15%.[26] There are often associated other inner ear anomalies, such as IP-II, vestibular enlargement, and SCC dysplasias.[12] It is a familial lesion with autosomal recessive inheritance. Patients are able to hear at birth, but their hearing deteriorates over the early years of life. The typical clinical presentation is a child or teenager with progressive SNHL. There may be posttraumatic potentiation of SNHL. It is the most commonly missed cause of congenital deafness. Rarely, patients have distal renal tubular acidosis resulting in varying degrees of metabolic acidosis. There is also an association with Pendred syndrome, which is severe SNHL with thyroid pathology.

The criteria to determine an enlarged vestibular aqueduct (in which the endolymphatic sac lies) are variable. On CT, a bony vestibular aqueduct diameter measuring greater than 1.5 mm in the transverse dimension at the midpoint or an opercular measurement greater than 2 mm is generally considered to be the defining characteristics.[27,28] The vestibular aqueduct is usually found at the level of the vestibule and lateral SCC, so it is easy to simply compare the diameter of the duct/sac with the lateral and posterior SCC width, which should be larger than the aqueduct (Fig. 8.8A and B).[28] There is no relationship between the size of the endolymphatic sac and the severity of the SNHL. The aqueduct itself is best evaluated with CT, whereas the sac is best seen as bright signal intensity on thin-section T2W MRI. In greater than 75% of cases, there is an associated cochlear dysplasia.[29] The apical turn of the cochlea in these cases is dysmorphic with modiolar deficiency (Fig. 8.9).[30] High-resolution T2W MRI may be able to distinguish more

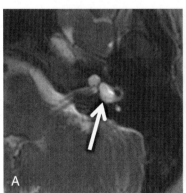
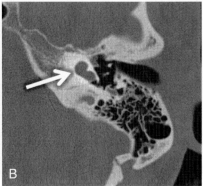
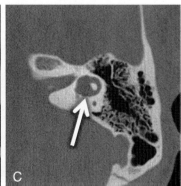

FIG. 8.7 Mild lateral semicircular canal (SCC) dysplasia. Axial thin-section cerebrospinal fluid bright MRI (**A**) through the left cochlea and vestibule (*arrow*), correlating axial thin-section bone algorithm CT through the dysplastic cochlea (**B**, *arrow*), and thin-section CT through the mildly dysplastic vestibule (**C**, *arrow*) demonstrate abnormal dysplasia of the cochlea and vestibule, with cystic changes, and abnormal architecture of the inner ear structures, in this case of mild lateral SCC dysplasia. The osseous island inside the inner ring of the lateral SCC in (**C**) should be wider from right to left than the vestibule width from right to left. In this case, the vestibule (*arrow*) is wider than the osseous island, consistent with mild lateral SCC dysplasia.

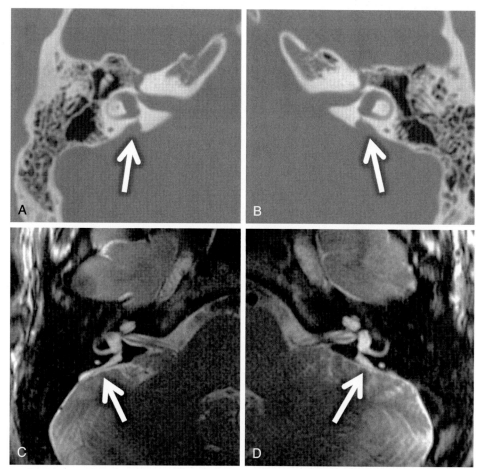

FIG. 8.8 Large endolymphatic sac anomaly (LESA) or large vestibular aqueduct syndrome (LVAS). Axial thin-section bone algorithm CT of the right **(A)** and left **(B)** temporal bones demonstrates bilateral LVAS (*arrows*) extending posterior from the vestibules (LVAS is wider than the internal standard of the lateral semicircular canal). The correlating axial thin-section cerebrospinal fluid (CSF) bright MRI of the right **(C)** and left **(D)** temporal bones demonstrates the corresponding CSF-like bright LESA bilaterally (*arrows*).

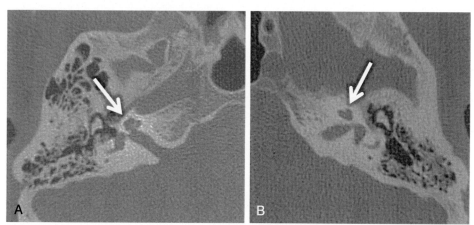

FIG. 8.9 Cochlear dysplasia. Axial thin-section bone algorithm CT images of the right **(A)** and left **(B)** temporal bones at the level of the cochleas and vestibules demonstrate a normal right cochlea (**A**, *arrow*) and a dysplastic left cochlea (**B**, *arrow*), with less than two turns to the cochlea itself.

subtle abnormalities of scalar chamber asymmetry with the more anterior scala vestibuli larger than the more posterior scala tympani.[31] Approximately 50% of cases have associated vestibular and/or SCC anomalies. In patients with sudden hearing loss, studies have shown wider vestibular aqueducts in the affected ear as compared with controls.[32] The endolymphatic sac can show enhancement,[32,33] which may be due to inflammation of the endolymphatic tissue or venous engorgement. It is hypothesized that a wide vestibular aqueduct may be associated with insufficient maturation of the inner ear.[34] The congenital "fragile" inner ear may receive abnormal pressure transmission through the vestibular aqueduct.[35]

Cochlear nerve deficiency (CND) is noted in 12%–18% of pediatric patient ears with SNHL.[36,37] It is usually congenital and refers to the absence or reduction in caliber of the cochlear nerve. Because cochlear implants are generally contraindicated in CND, it is important to identify this condition in children being considered for implantation.[38,39] There will be an associated narrowing of the IAC on CT (IAC diameter of <4 mm), which is theorized to occur because the IAC width depends on the presence of the vestibulocochlear nerve cells to form normally.[40,41] In general, pediatric patients with narrow IACs on CT perform worse after implantation than those with normal-caliber IACs, presumably because the cochlear nerve is likely to be absent or small when the IAC is narrow.[42] With CND, CT may also show a stenotic or absent bony cochlear canal (normally between 1.4 and 3.0 mm).[43] The osseous anatomy must be assessed with caution, as cochlear nerve-deficient ears may demonstrate normal caliber of the bony cochlear canal in ≤23% of cases[44] and normal-sized IACs in ≤73% of cases.[45] Heavily T2W or CSF bright MRI sequences, such as SPACE, CISS, and FIESTA, can be used to identify the cochlear nerve, which should be located in the anterior inferior quadrant of the IAC, as well as the intracanalicular segment of the facial nerve (anterior and superior) and the superior and inferior divisions of the vestibular nerve posteriorly within the IAC (Fig. 8.5A). Although CND can be seen in isolation, it can occur in conjunction with aplasia of the vestibular nerve (complete absence of the eighth cranial nerve) (Fig. 8.5B).

Rarely, it has been reported that an intrameatal AICA loop can cause asymmetric SNHL because of neurovascular compression of the cochlear nerve.[46] The study by Gorrie et al. found a statistically significant association between AICA loops that ran between the facial and vestibulocochlear nerves and hearing loss but found no statistically significant association between AICA loops that made no contact with the nerve, ran adjacent to the nerve, or displaced the nerve.[47]

## Acquired SNHL Pathologies

Acquired SNHL etiologies include tumors, infectious/inflammatory processes, trauma, autoimmune/immune disorders, and degenerative/idiopathic processes. Tumors can cause SNHL, including vestibular (acoustic) schwannomas (60%–90%), meningiomas (3%–6%), epidermoids (3%–6%), schwannomas of cranial nerves 5, 7, 9, 10, 11, and 12, lymphoma, leukemia, metastases, and meningeal carcinomatosis.[48]

VS is the most common tumor of the IAC/CPA, accounting for 60%–90% of tumors in this region.[49–51] In sporadic cases, the incidence is highest in patients in the fifth through the seventh decades.[52] However, in patients with neurofibromatosis type II, patients commonly present in the first 2 decades with bilateral VSs (Fig. 8.10) along with other cranial nerve schwannomas, meningiomas, and ependymomas of the central nervous system.[53] In addition to SNHL, patients can have symptoms of tinnitus, dysequilibrium, and/or decreased speech discrimination, because of the mass effect of the tumor on the cochlear and vestibular divisions of cranial nerve 7.[54]

On CT, VSs are isoattenuating compared with the brain parenchyma and can be difficult to delineate without contrast material enhancement.[50] Lateral extension of the VS from the CPA into the IAC results in

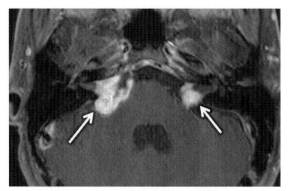

FIG. 8.10 Bilateral vestibular schwannomas. Axial postcontrasted fat-saturated T1W MRI through the level of the bilateral internal auditory canals (IACs) shows bilateral enhancing lesions of the cerebellopontine angle/IACs consistent with bilateral schwannomas in this patient with known neurofibromatosis type-II (better referred to as the MISME syndrome, or multiple inherited schwannomas, meningiomas, and ependymomas; because patients with neurofibromatosis type-II do not get neurofibromas, it is another poorly named thing in medicine).

widening of the porus acusticus (Fig. 8.11). The spherical cisternal component forms an acute angle with the petrous bone.[55] Hemorrhage and calcification are rare in untreated tumors.[56] Enhancement is typically avid and homogenous and better seen on MRI. On T1W MRI, VSs are usually isointense or mildly hypointense compared with brain parenchyma and hyperintense compared with CSF. On T2W MRI, they are mildly hyperintense compared with brain parenchyma and isointense to hypointense compared with CSF. If large, the tumors may have a heterogeneous internal architecture with cystic components (Fig. 8.11).[50] Deformity and mass effect on the adjacent structures can result in facial numbness if the trigeminal nerve is compressed, cerebellar signs if the lower cranial nerves are affected, or hydrocephalus if there is compression of the fourth ventricle. Heavily T2W or CSF bright MRI sequences can outline the tumor relative to adjacent structures (Fig. 8.12). There may be decreased labyrinthine signal intensity, which may be due to increased protein content.[57]

The VSs are slow-growing lesions, with growth rates ranging from 0.2 mm to a few millimeters per year. Surgical resection for complete cure is performed, if feasible.[58] Of the three main surgical approaches (retrosigmoid, middle cranial fossa, and translabyrinthine),[59–61] the translabyrinthine approach is reserved for patients with poor hearing or complete hearing loss, because it leads it to hearing sacrifice. When the VS is "impacted," extending laterally into the cochlear aperture, there is a decreased chance of hearing preservation after surgery.[62] Stereotactic radiosurgery is an option in high-risk patients, those with bilateral tumors, and those with residual tumors after initial treatment.[63]

The VSs can also arise from Schwann cells within the membranous labyrinth, described as an intralabyrinthine schwannoma (you may have noticed on the right if you were looking closely at Fig. 8.6).[64] This benign tumor appears on MRI as a soft tissue density lesion within the high-signal inner ear fluid and shows focal enhancement. It appears as a focal enhancing mass within the membranous labyrinth on contrast-enhanced T1WI MRI and as a filling defect on high-resolution T2W MRI. These can be subdivided according to location within the inner ear structures: intracochlear, vestibulocochlear, transmodiolar, transmacular, and transotic.[65] Intralabyrinthine schwannomas result in progressive hearing loss.

Meningiomas are also found in the CPA but are most commonly found eccentric to the medial opening of the IAC, the porus acusticus (Fig. 8.13). Possible

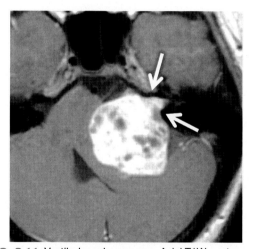

FIG. 8.11 Vestibular schwannoma. Axial T1W postcontrasted MRI through the cerebellopontine angle/internal auditory canal (IAC) demonstrates a large enhancing lesion with internal cystic foci extending into the IAC with widening of the porus acusticus (the opening of the IAC) (*arrows*), consistent with a vestibular schwannoma. Although these are often referred to as vestibular schwannomas, the schwannoma may be arising from any of the four nerves within the IAC; therefore it is important to check for possible enhancing extension along the labyrinthine segment of the facial nerve to distinguish a facial nerve schwannoma from a vestibulocochlear nerve schwannoma. Facial nerve schwannomas within the IAC may present clinically with sensorineural hearing loss, as the facial nerve interestingly is less sensitive to internal derangement than the cochlear nerve is to external compression.

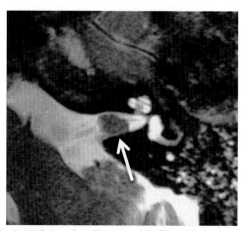

FIG. 8.12 Internal auditory canal (IAC) vestibular schwannoma. Axial thin-section cerebrospinal fluid (CSF) bright (T2 FSE, SPACE, CISS, or FIESTA) MRI through the left IAC shows a well-defined filling defect within the normally bright CSF of the IAC (*arrow*), consistent with a vestibular schwannoma.

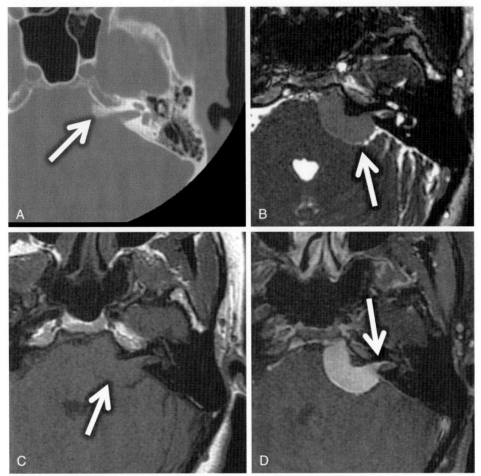

FIG. 8.13 Cerebellopontine angle (CPA) meningioma. Axial thin-section bone algorithm CT image **(A)** through the left CPA/internal auditory canal (IAC) demonstrates a focal region of hyperostotic change (*arrow*) anterior to the IAC porus acusticus. Axial thin-section cerebrospinal fluid (CSF) bright SPACE MRI **(B)** demonstrates a CSF/vascular cleft (*arrow*) between the extraaxial lesion and the brain parenchyma. The axial T1W precontrast MRI **(C)** shows the lesion to be isointense compared with brain parenchyma (*arrow*), and the corresponding axial thin-section postcontrasted T1W MRI **(D)** with fat saturation shows avid homogeneous enhancement with an enhancing dural tail (*arrow*) extending along the anterior wall of the left IAC, consistent with a CPA meningioma.

IAC extension of a meningioma usually does not result in widening of the porus acusticus as it does with VSs. These meningiomas are characteristically broad based along the petrous wall with a hemispheric morphology and form an obtuse angle at the bone-tumor interface.[66] Meningiomas are hyperattenuating or isoattenuating compared with brain parenchyma[66] and may be calcified on CT. A helpful imaging feature is the adjacent bone, which may be sclerotic or hyperostotic (Fig. 8.13A). On MRI, meningiomas are isointense or slightly hypointense compared with

gray matter on T1W MRI and isointense or hypointense compared with gray matter on T2W MRI. Typically, meningiomas show homogeneous enhancement unless there is internal calcification or microcystic change. A "dural tail" of dural enhancement extending from the margins of the lesion is often seen and may extend into the IAC itself (Fig. 8.13D). Surface CSF cleft and flow voids from marginal pial vessels may be seen, often described as a CSF/vascular cleft between the extraaxial meningioma and the adjacent normal brain parenchyma (Fig. 8.13B).[67–69]

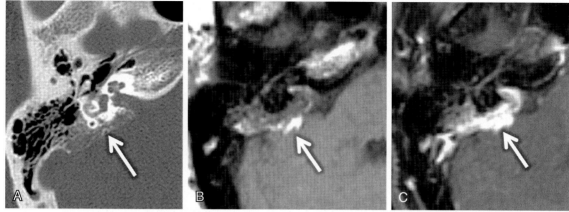

FIG. 8.14 Endolymphatic sac tumor (ELST). Axial thin-section bone algorithm CT image **(A)** through the right cerebellopontine angle/internal auditory canal demonstrates abnormal permeative changes (*arrow*) to the posterior wall of the petrous apex. Correlating axial thin-section T1W precontrasted MRI **(B)** shows peripheral abnormal bright T1W signal intensity (*arrow*) consistent with blood products, whereas the corresponding axial thin-section T1W postcontrasted MRI **(C)** with fat saturation shows avid heterogeneous enhancement (*arrow*), consistent with an ELST.

An endolymphatic sac tumor (ELST) is a locally invasive papillary cystadenomatous tumor of the endolymphatic sac in a retrolabyrinthine location.[70,71] These lesions are centered in the fovea of the endolymphatic sac along the posterior surface of the petrous TB. Larger lesions (greater than 3 cm) can spread to involve the middle ear, CPA cistern, and/or jugular foramen. On CT, this lesion shows intratumoral bone spicules with a moth-eaten, lytic appearance of the invaded bone.[48] A thin rim of calcification along the posterior margin of the tumor is common (Fig. 8.14A). A vascular catheter or CT angiogram may exhibit enlarged distal vessels from the ascending pharyngeal and occipital arteries feeding the vascular tumor.[72] Flow voids can be seen when the tumor is greater than 2 cm in size. On T1W MRI, lesions greater than 3 cm and along the margin when the lesion is less than 3 cm may show high-signal foci, reflecting blood products (Fig. 8.14B). The majority of ELSTs (80%) have these foci of increased signal intensity. Low-intensity foci in the tumor matrix may represent hemosiderin staining. These lesions show heterogeneous enhancement (Fig. 8.14C).[73]

Virtually all patients with ELSTs will have SNHL. Other symptoms include facial nerve palsy, pulsatile tinnitus, and vertigo. Hearing loss and ELST are frequently associated with von Hippel-Lindau syndrome (VHL) and should be considered when screening individuals at risk for VHL and when monitoring patients with an established diagnosis of VHL. Although most cases are sporadic, ~7% ELSTs may be seen in the setting of VHL. Bilateral ELSTs are seen in VHL. Audiologic evaluation and MRI should allow early detection and enhance management of hearing loss in these patients. Many patients with VHL have hearing loss without radiographic evidence of an ELST. Whether it is caused by an ELST that is too small to be detected by MRI or is produced by some other etiology is still unknown.[74]

Labyrinthine ossificans (LO) is also a potential cause of acquired SNHL (Fig. 8.15). There are three stages to labyrinthitis (vestibulocochlear neuritis). In the acute stage, MRI may show inner ear enhancement. In the intermediate stage, fibrous tissue results in loss of the fluid signal on heavily T2W MRI (e.g., SPACE, CISS, or FIESTA) (Fig. 8.15C and D). However, there is higher T2 signal than as seen with an intralabyrinthine schwannoma.[75,76] CT may appear normal in these early stages. In the late stage, the inner ear structures show bone attenuation on CT (Fig. 8.15A and B). The most extensive cases are seen as a complication of meningitis. TB trauma (e.g., a unilateral fracture with a perilymphatic fistula or postoperatively after stapedectomy or other inner ear surgery) and autoimmune inner ear disease have also been attributed to the development of LO. The scala tympani of the basal turn is the most common region of cochlear ossification.[48] Patients present acutely with profound SNHL, vertigo, and tinnitus. LO can complicate or may preclude cochlear implantation.

Labyrinthitis ossificans is fibrous and eventual bony proliferation in the endolymphatic structures. It may arise from purulent material reaching the endolymph via CSF and from adjacent inflammatory disease. It begins with fibrosis and progresses to ossification in

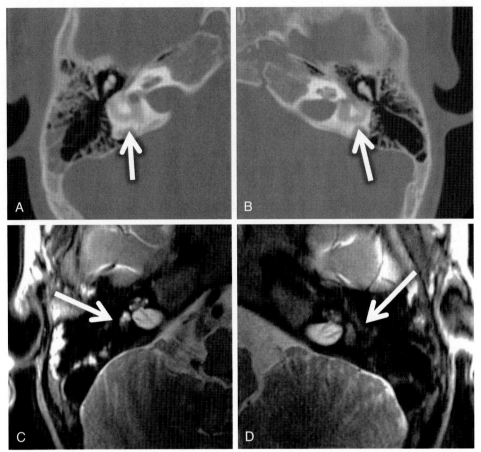

FIG. 8.15 Labyrinthine ossificans (LO). Axial thin-section bone algorithm right **(A)** and left **(B)** CT images show bilateral increased density within the vestibules and lateral semicircular canals (SCCs) (*arrows*). The correlating axial thin-section cerebrospinal fluid (CSF) bright MRI sections on the right **(C)** and left **(D)** show correlating loss of the expected CSF-like bright signal intensity within the bilateral vestibules and lateral SCCs, consistent with LO.

as early as 2 months.[77,78] In cochlear labyrinthitis ossificans, the fluid spaces of the cochlea are affected. In noncochlear labyrinthitis ossificans, the fluid spaces of the SCC or vestibule are affected (Fig. 8.15). Labyrinthitis ossificans can contraindicate or complicate cochlear implantation; therefore, pre-cochlear implant evaluation of the TB with CT is essential.[79] A hazy increased density within the normally fluid-filled spaces of the membranous labyrinth is seen in mild cases, whereas severe cases show complete obliteration with bone replacement. On CSF bright thin sequences, there is loss of normal fluid signal intensity within the cochlea because of fibrous proliferation within the labyrinth (Fig. 8.15C and D). The modiolus can appear "enlarged."[80] The enhancement of the membranous

labyrinthitis can persist in the ossifying stages of labyrinthitis ossificans.

Otosyphilis caused by the bacterium spirochete *Treponema pallidum* can cause acute and fluctuating hearing loss and vertigo. CT shows permeative demineralization of the otic capsule.[81] Contrast-enhanced MRI demonstrates enhancement of cranial nerves 7 and 8. There may be syphilitic labyrinthitis with enhancement of the membranous labyrinth.[82]

Posttraumatic SNHL can be the result of injury to the inner ear structures. Transverse fractures through the TBs often involve the inner ear with SNHL, and facial nerve canal involvement is also common.[83] In the medial subtype, the fracture extends along the posterior or petrous surface through the fundus of the IAC to the first genu of the facial nerve, with permanent

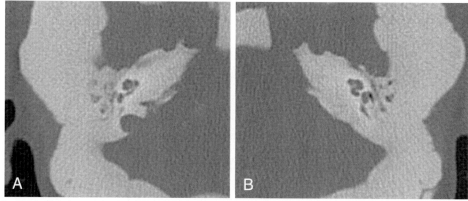

FIG. 8.16 Osteopetrosis. Axial thin-section bone algorithm CT images through the right **(A)** and left **(B)** temporal bones at the level of the cochleas demonstrate diffuse osseous thickening and increased density, consistent with a rare case of skull base and temporal bone osteopetrosis.

hearing loss commonly found.[84] In the lateral subtype, the fracture extends along the posterior petrous surface through the labyrinth with a perilymphatic fistula more commonly found.[84]

CT can sometimes detect the TB fracture extending through the oval window or round window and pneumolabyrinth. SNHL may occur in the absence of a TB fracture,[85,86] possibly due to injury to the membranous labyrinth.[87] A perilymph fistula, which is an abnormal communication between the middle and inner ear either with leakage of perilymph into the middle ear or pneumolabyrinth in the inner ear, could also cause SNHL. MRI may be needed to detect perilymph inside the middle ear.[88,89]

In posttraumatic cases, MRI is helpful to detect subtle lesions within the inner ear, such as labyrinthine hemorrhage or localized brain axonal damage along central auditory pathways. MRI with 3D FLAIR acquisition can aid in the detection of inner ear hemorrhage and posttraumatic lesions of the brain parenchyma (axonal damage and brain hematoma) that may lead to auditory agnosia.[90] Unenhanced T1W MRI will detect hyperintensity, representing hemorrhage, in the cochlea or vestibule. Damage to the central auditory pathways involving the cochlear nerve, brainstem, and thalamus could result in SNHL and, depending on the location of the damage, may cause hearing loss on the contralateral side.[91] Intralabyrinthine hemorrhage can also occur in patients with a history of anticoagulation, sickle cell disease, trauma, leukemia, or other hyperviscosity syndromes. Patients experience an acute onset of unilateral SNHL. There is high signal within normally fluid-filled spaces of the labyrinth on T1 MRI.

Demyelinating processes such as multiple sclerosis or a suboptimally located cavernous malformation can cause SNHL if the lesion involves the cochlear nucleus. MRI of the brain will reveal additional white matter plaques in a characteristic periventricular and pericallosal distribution. A cavernous malformation will demonstrate the characteristic speckled appearance caused by varying ages of blood products and a hemosiderin rim.

Autoimmune SNHL has been described in studies in which the clinical pattern did not fit with known entities.[92–94] These patients responded to treatment for an autoimmune disease, namely, chronic cortisone and cyclophosphamide therapy. Clinical results in the study by Kataoka et al. suggested that endolymphatic hydrops may have a role in autoimmune SNHL.[92] Immune-mediated audiovestibular dysfunction may be either a separate disease entity or a part of a more generalized (auto-) immune process.[93]

Osteopetrosis is also associated with SNHL.[95] Bones may be uniformly sclerotic, but alternating sclerotic and lucent bands may be noted in iliac wings and near the ends of long bones. The bones might be club-like or appear like a bone within bone (endobone). In type 1 autosomal recessive osteopetrosis, the entire skull is thickened and dense, especially at the base (Fig. 8.16).[95] In type 2, the calvarium is spared. Contrast-enhanced MR may show extramedullary hematopoiesis with enhancing extracerebral spaces.[96] Flared IACs and large subarcuate fossae are classically seen.[95] Sinuses are small and underpneumatized. Vertebrae are extremely radiodense and may show alternating bands, known as the rugger-jersey sign. In autosomal recessive osteopetrosis, MR angiogram can demonstrate compromise

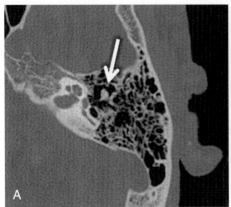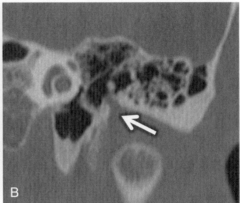

FIG. 8.17 External auditory canal (EAC) dysplasia. Axial thin-section bone algorithm CT image **(A)** and coronal reconstruction **(B)** through the left temporal bone shows a case of EAC dysplasia with a small middle ear cavity and malformed ossicles (**A**, *arrow*) and complete EAC atresia (**B**, *arrow*).

of the petrous segment of the internal carotid artery.[97] MR venogram may show stenosis of the dural venous sinuses.

Presbycusis can occur as a sequela of aging, infectious processes, inflammatory processes, trauma, toxicity of certain medications, and long-term exposure to loud noise. Often high-frequency hearing loss in older adults reveals nothing on MRI of the CPA/IAC. However, cortical MRI reveals a significant hearing loss–related increase in functional connectivity between the auditory cortex and the right motion-sensitive visual area MT+ (the probable human homologue of visual motion-responsive macaque motion-responsive visual areas: the middle temporal area [MT] and the medial superior temporal area) when processing matching audiovisual input. The work by Puschmann and Thiel suggests there are permanent, task-independent changes in coupling between visual and auditory sensory areas with an increasing degree of hearing loss.[98] Growing evidence suggests that hearing loss is associated with reduced cognitive functioning and incident dementia. There appear to be functional alterations in the engagement of the auditory cortex in age-associated hearing impairment, especially during processing of sounds. Cognitive decline and age-related hearing loss may be expressions of widespread neural degeneration that occurs during aging, an idea referred to as the common cause hypothesis.[99,100] Emerging evidence suggests that functional alterations are also seen in other brain regions including frontal cortices and the limbic system, lending support to information degradation and sensory deprivation theories. These ideas suggest that hearing loss results in compromised cognitive performance and functional decline because cognitive resources are increasingly dedicated to auditory processing to the detriment of other processes (e.g., executive function).[99,101–104]

## CONDUCTIVE HEARING LOSS

Conductive hearing loss may be due to transmission fixation or transmission discontinuity. Key anatomic structures to be assessed include the EAC, tympanic membrane, ossicular chain, and oval window. In CHL, there is likely to be a CT abnormality. If upon initial review there is no abnormality, *look again*. MRI findings depend on the pathology, such as inflammatory disorders or tumors.

### Congenital Conductive Hearing Loss

Congenital CHL pathologies include EAC dysplasia, OWA, ossicular anomalies (e.g., malleoincudal fixation, stapes fixation, and incudostapedial dislocation),[105] congenital cholesteatoma, and fenestral otosclerosis (rare in childhood).

EAC dysplasia can be mild or complete EAC atresia with associated auricle deformity (Fig. 8.17). The severity of the auricular dysplasia parallels the degree of deformity of the middle ear and ossicles.[106] The spectrum of this congenital malformation ranges from the mildest form with a narrowed EAC to no identifiable EAC owing to bone, soft tissue, or mixed components. There may be hypoplasia of the middle ear and mastoid complex. The ossicular chain may be dysmorphic; for example, the malleus and incus may be fused and/or rotated. Congenital cholesteatoma can be seen in up to 10% of these cases.[106] The facial nerve has an aberrant course and may exit the skull base into

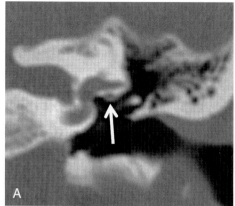 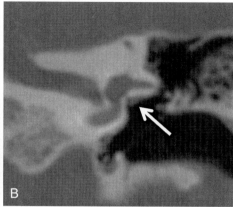

FIG. 8.18 Normal comparison and oval window atresia (OWA). Coronal reconstruction CT of a normal temporal bone **(A)** and an OWA case **(B)**. The normal coronal section through the vestibule shows the normal anatomy with the "duck head" shape of the inner ear structures (**A**, the head of the duck is the vestibule, the beak of the duck is the lateral semicircular canal [SCC], and the neck of the duck is the basal turn of the cochlea), with the tympanic segment of the facial nerve normally positioned below the lateral SCC (*arrow*) and lateral to the oval window at the duck head shape of the vestibule. The comparison OWA case shows an osseous bar covering the oval window niche, but there is also medial displacement of the tympanic segment of the facial nerve drawn into the OWA (*arrow*).

the glenoid fossa or lateral to the styloid process. The tympanic segment may be dehiscent, bowing into the middle ear cavity, or it may overly the oval window, especially in cases of OWA. The descending (or mastoid) segment of the facial nerve is often anteriorly displaced in EAC atresia cases. The inner ear and IAC are usually normal. In unilateral cases, the affected side shows CHL and the other ear has normal hearing. In every EAC atresia case, thorough evaluation needs to address the type and thickness of the atretic plate, the size of the mastoid complex and middle ear cavity, the status of the ossicular chain, the status of the oval and round windows, the course of the facial nerve, the possible presence of a cholesteatoma, and the status of the inner ear.[107]

In OWA, there is an absent cleavage plane between the lateral SCC above and the cochlear promontory below, with an associated anomalous stapes and malpositioned facial nerve.[108] The oval window is covered by a thin bony plate in these cases. The stapes superstructure and distal incus are usually malformed in OWA. There is absence of the normal paired crura of the stapes. The tympanic segment of the facial nerve (CN 7) is inferomedially positioned overlying the expected position of the oval window (Fig. 8.18), which complicates surgical repair. Embryologically, it is hypothesized that the primitive stapes fails to fuse with the primitive vestibule during the seventh week of gestation.[109] Congenital stapes fixation will result if the stapes forms

but the annular ligament does not. In malleoincudal fixation, the malleus head and incus body are fused or fixed to the epitympanic wall.

Congenital cholesteatomas arise from epithelial rests in the middle ear of pediatric patients. There is no history of otorrhea, tympanic membrane perforation, or otologic procedures. The patient may present with CHL, or it can be an incidental finding of a pearly white lesion at otoscopy. Congenital cholesteatoma is suggested by the presence of a homogenous mass of soft tissue attenuation within the middle ear on CT scans with osseous destruction. These lesions are identified in the anterior superior quadrant of the middle ear cavity above the Eustachian tube opening (Fig. 8.19). They occur around the incudostapedial joint, manifesting as unilateral CHL.[110] Small cholesteatomas are encapsulated masses in the anterior tympanic cavity. Larger congenital cholesteatomas may erode the ossicles, the middle ear wall, the lateral SCC, and/or the tegmen tympani. Bone erosion is less common than with acquired cholesteatomas and occurs late in the disease course.[111] The long process of the incus and the stapes superstructure are the most commonly destroyed. The lesion is isointense to hypointense on T1W imaging and intermediate on T2W imaging and may show peripheral enhancement.

A persistent stapedial artery (PSA) can cause CHL and may be found in association with an aberrant internal carotid artery. In the embryo, the stapedial

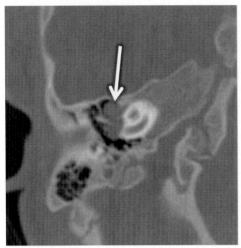

FIG. 8.19 Congenital cholesteatoma. Axial thin-section bone algorithm CT image through the middle ear cavity shows a soft tissue density mass (*arrow*) medial to the ossicles in a child with conductive hearing loss, consistent with a congenital cholesteatoma.

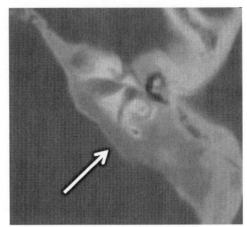

FIG. 8.20 Fibrous dysplasia (FD). Axial thin-section bone algorithm CT image through the left temporal bone at the level of the internal auditory canal shows diffuse expansile and ground-glass changes (*arrow*) to the osseous anatomy surrounding the inner ear structures and otic capsule, consistent with FD. Fibrous dysplasia will interestingly often spare the dense otic capsule itself surrounding the inner ear structures.

artery runs through the stapes and regresses by the third month of gestation.[112] A PSA courses across the floor of the middle ear and cochlear promontory and passes between the crura of the stapes,[113] where it can present with CHL. The lack of regression of this anomalous vessel may replace the normal blood supply of the middle meningeal artery, leading to an ipsilateral absence of the foramen spinosum posterolateral to foramen ovale on CT of the skull base.[113,114]

Fibrous dysplasia is a rare cause of congenital CHL.[115] Bone CT shows increased bone volume with a "ground glass" appearance (Fig. 8.20). There is osseous expansion of the TB with relative sparing of the otic capsule. In this slowly progressing, inherited bony disease, there is fibroosseous replacement of bone. Although there is usually conductive hearing loss and/or EAC bony stenosis, hearing loss may be sensorineural or mixed as well. Cystic, pagetoid, and sclerotic appearances represent the phases of the disease in descending order of activity.[116]

## Acquired Conductive Hearing Loss

Acquired CHL etiologies include EAC pathologies, neoplasm, trauma, tympanosclerosis, effusion, malleus fixation, acquired cholesteatoma, and fenestral otosclerosis.

EAC exostoses are broad-based osseous masses associated with chronic irritation and classically described in cases of repeated cold water exposure, such as in scuba divers and surfers. These lesions cause bony stenosis of

EAC with increased wall thickness and bone density (Fig. 8.21).[117]

External auditory (EAC) cholesteatoma is characterized by local invasion of the squamous epithelium lining the EAC, resulting in canal wall erosions and periostitis. Although most cases are spontaneous or idiopathic, these lesions can occur as a sequela of prior trauma, surgery, or radiation.[118] Most patients, typically older patients, present with chronic dull ear pain and otorrhea, often unilateral.[118] CT will reveal focal soft tissue within the EAC, often along the inferior wall, with adjacent osseous erosion. There are bony flecks in approximately 50% of cases (Fig. 8.22).[119] The cholesteatoma may extend into the mastoid and middle ear or may involve the facial nerve or tegmen tympani.[120] It is important to correlate with clinical symptoms, as imaging mimics include carcinoma and otitis externa.

Keratosis obturans (KO) is an expansile accumulation of keratin debris within the EAC and is associated with sinusitis and bronchiectasis.[121,122] As compared with patients with EAC cholesteatoma, patients with KO are younger and present with severe pain, CHL, and rarely otorrhea. The findings are typically bilateral, with widening of the EAC by a soft tissue epidermal plug and smooth osseous scalloping on CT (Fig. 8.23).[122]

Medial canal fibrosis (MCF) is characterized by fibrous tissue in the medial osseous EAC, which presents in the early stages as a thickened tympanic membrane with

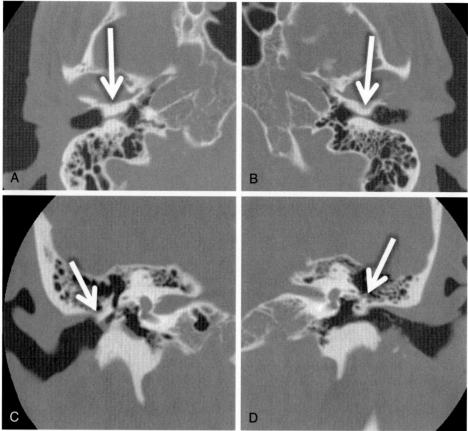

FIG. 8.21 External auditory canal (EAC) exostoses. Axial thin-section bone algorithm CT images through the right **(A)** and left **(B)** temporal bones (TBs) demonstrate osseous overgrowth (*arrows*) of the bony EAC canal. This is also shown on the coronal reconstructions of the right **(C)** and left **(D)** TBs (*arrows*), consistent with EAC exostosis with osseous overgrowth partially protecting the tympanic membranes (TMs) from repetitive exposure to cold water.

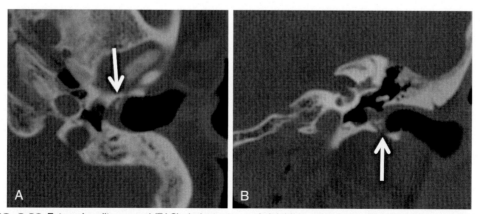

FIG. 8.22 External auditory canal (EAC) cholesteatoma. Axial thin-section bone algorithm CT image **(A)** and coronal reconstruction **(B)** of the left temporal bone (TB) demonstrates osseous erosion of the anterior (**A**, *arrow*) and inferior (**B**, *arrow*) medial osseous EAC with bony flecks within the adjacent soft tissue density mass, consistent with EAC cholesteatoma.

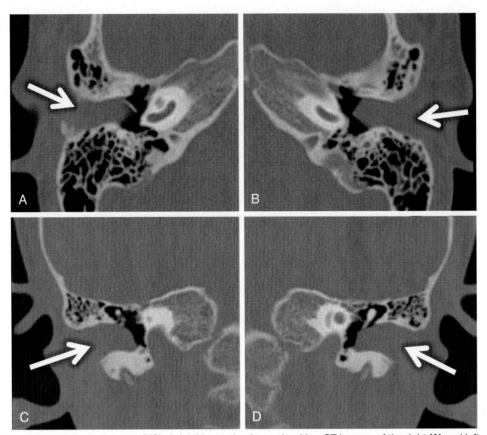

**FIG. 8.23** Keratosis obturans (KO). Axial thin-section bone algorithm CT images of the right **(A)** and left **(B)** temporal bones (TBs) demonstrate nonaggressive soft tissue filling the external auditory canals (EACs) bilaterally (*arrows*). The coronal thin-section reconstructions of the right **(C)** and left **(D)** TBs appear to show slight expansion of the osseous EACs (*arrows*) without underlying osseous changes, consistent with KO.

edematous and mildly thickened medial EAC mucosa. In the later stages, there is a crescent of thickened soft tissue overlying the lateral tympanic membrane surface and extending laterally to fill the EAC (Fig. 8.24). MCF can be seen in patients with CHL and otorrhea. There may be a history of chronic otitis media.[123] Approximately 60% of cases have bilateral involvement.[124] Rarely, squamous cell carcinoma and ceruminous adenomas can involve the EAC, possibly leading to CHL on presentation.

Tympanosclerosis is a healing variant of chronic otitis media characterized by the deposition of hyalinized collagen in the tympanic cavity. The suspensory ligaments and tendons may ossify or calcify. The tympanosclerosis surrounding the ossicles can make it appear as if there are extra ossicles or "hairy ossicles" (Fig. 8.25). This postinflammatory new bone deposition is seen in the tympanic membrane, middle ear, ossicles, mastoids, and oval and round windows.

In contradistinction to fenestral otospongiosis, new bone deposition within the oval window is irregular. A calcified degenerative stapes footplate arthritis may mimic this disorder.[125] Recurrent inflammation and healing lead to calcification of the tympanic membrane (myringosclerosis), which can cause CHL.[126]

Trauma can also result in CHL. Initially after injury, hearing may be difficult to evaluate, especially if there is hemotympanum, which may lead to a transient CHL. TB trauma is frequently associated with brain and cervical spine injuries[127] that sometimes require surgical management. Persistent CHL occurs in 50% of patients 6 months after a TB trauma.[128] The prediction of future hearing loss with TB fractures is better related to whether the fracture is otic capsule involving or otic capsule sparing, but TB fractures are classically described as longitudinal, transverse, and oblique, depending on their relationship to the petrous apex. Longitudinal fractures are along the

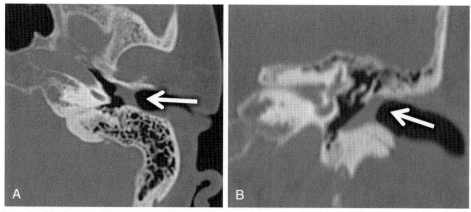

FIG. 8.24 Medial canal fibrosis. Axial thin-section bone algorithm CT image **(A)** and coronal reconstruction **(B)** demonstrate nonaggressive soft tissue within the medial left external auditory canal (*arrows*) adjacent to the TM without underlying osseous changes and a crescent shape lateral to the soft tissue density mass (*arrows*).

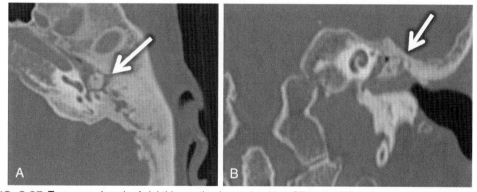

FIG. 8.25 Tympanosclerosis. Axial thin-section bone algorithm CT image **(A)** and coronal reconstruction **(B)** demonstrate abnormal osseous densities (*arrows*) within the left middle ear cavity, with surrounding soft tissue or fluid density, in an appearance described as "hairy ossicles" or extra ossicles, consistent with tympanosclerosis.

long axis of the petrous portion of the TB and comprise approximately 80% of TB fractures (Fig. 8.26A).[115] These are more likely to involve the ossicles and result in CHL. Longitudinal fractures that disrupt the tympanic membrane may allow an ingrowth of the squamous epithelium that can also lead to an acquired cholesteatoma.[129] Transverse fractures are perpendicular to the long axis of the petrous portion and are more likely to involve the bony labyrinth to result in SNHL (Fig. 8.26B). Approximately 20% of longitudinal fractures and 50% of transverse fractures are associated with facial nerve injury.[83]

CHL is caused by the disruption of the ossicular chain. The most common middle ear injuries are incudomalleolar and incudostapedial joint subluxation. The best view of the incudostapedial joint is the oblique plane (perpendicular to the oval window). In this plane, the ossicular chain usually represents a "V" formed by the long process of the incus and the stapes. A "gap" between the incus and stapes may be due to subluxation. On the axial plane, the incudomalleolar joint looks like an ice cream cone: the head of the malleus corresponds to the ice cream and the body and the short process of the incus correspond to the cone. With subluxation, there is a lack of osseous continuity. Incudomalleolar dislocation can be seen with a longitudinal TB fracture. In such cases, the malleus head and the incus body remain fixed together but the entire bloc is displaced, typically inward. On the coronal reconstruction, the separation of the malleus and incus may resemble a "broken heart" (Fig. 8.27).

Pathology of the ossicles can also result in hearing loss. Malleus fixation can be idiopathic, posttraumatic, developmental, or postinfectious secondary to chronic otitis media. Syphilis can cause adhesions between the footplate and oval window, which can be difficult to detect on CT.[130]

Middle ear effusions may impede the movement of ossicles and decrease tympanic membrane compliance.[131] Fluid in the middle ear and mastoid air cells is easily demonstrated on CT and MR examinations; however, infected effusions (mastoiditis) are a clinical distinction (Fig. 8.28) and are only rarely diagnosed on cross-sectional imaging when infectious changes are seen with osseous changes over time. Myringotomy or tympanostomy tubes allow middle fluid to drain into the EAC.

Chronic otitis media can lead to middle ear atelectasis with retraction of the tympanic membrane onto the ossicles and/or cochlear promontory. In cases that are

long-standing, there may be erosion of the incus and stapes with pockets of desquamated keratin and epithelium in which acquired cholesteatomas can develop.[129] Middle ear cholesteatoma (MEC) is characterized by the accumulation of desquamated keratin epithelium in the middle ear cavity or other pneumatized portions of the TB. The majority of MEC are acquired (98%), whereas only 2% are congenital.[48] According to the invasion theory, acquired MEC may develop from chronic Eustachian tube dysfunction, which produces a vacuum phenomenon in the middle ear cavity and leads to a retraction pocket in the pars flaccida. There is squamous metaplasia of the inflamed middle ear epithelium over time.[132] The epithelial invasion theory hypothesizes that keratinizing stratified squamous epithelium grows into the middle ear cavity after perforation of the tympanic membrane.[48] Approximately 80% of acquired MEC are associated with the more loosely attached pars flaccida

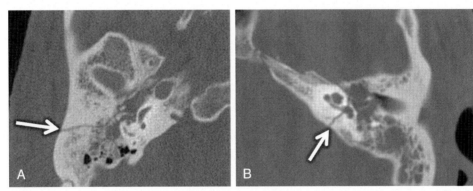

FIG. 8.26 Temporal bone (TB) longitudinal and transverse fractures. Axial thin-section bone algorithm CT images from two patients with conductive hearing loss demonstrate a longitudinal oriented fracture (**A**, *arrow*) on the right TB image and a transverse oriented fracture (**B**, *arrow*) on the left TB separate case image.

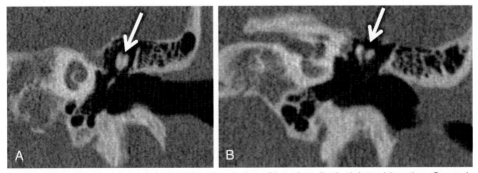

FIG. 8.27 Normal comparison and the broken heart sign of incudomalleolar joint subluxation. Coronal reconstructions from temporal bone (TB) CT studies of a normal comparison left TB (**A**) and an abnormal incudomalleolar joint subluxation (**B**) TB image. The normal comparison (**A**) reconstruction image shows the expected "heart-shaped" (**A**, *arrow*) relationship between the malleus and the incus articulation. The abnormal image (**B**) shows the "broken-heart" shape (**B**, *arrow*) of incudomalleolar joint subluxation in this patient with conductive hearing loss.

of the tympanic membrane, whereas ~20% are associated with the more tightly attached pars tensa. Patients may present with chronic otorrhea, tympanic membrane perforation, a pars flaccida retraction pocket, and a pearly white lesion at otoscopy.

The pars flaccida is the anterior and superior aspect of the tympanic membrane. A perforation in the pars flaccida provides the squamous epithelium access to the lateral epitympanic recess (often mistakenly called Prussak space), which is the recess between the

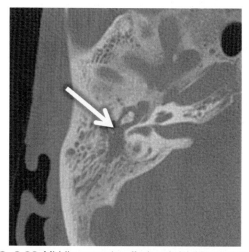

FIG. 8.28 Middle ear cavity effusion. Axial thin-section bone algorithm CT image through the right temporal bone shows fluid density filling the middle ear cavity and mastoid air cells (*arrow*) without osseous destruction, consistent with middle ear effusion.

ossicles and the lateral wall of the epitympanum (or attic). On CT, the acquired MEC of the pars flaccida appears as a lobulated expansile lesion in the lateral epitympanic recess with erosion of the scutum and ossicles (Fig. 8.29).[133] Careful attention should be made to the scutum, as erosion of this bony "spur" is one of the earliest abnormalities of a cholesteatoma to be detected on CT, particularly on the coronal images. It can extend superiorly through the aditus ad antrum into the attic and mastoid air cells. Pars tensa MEC laterally displace and erode the ossicles[133] and can extend into the sinus tympani.

On MRI, MEC is a nonenhancing T1 hypointense and mildly T2 hyperintense lesion. These lesions demonstrate similar MRI characteristics, independent of location within the TB, with reduced diffusivity on diffusion-weighted imaging (DWI).[134] Nonechoplanar turbo spin echo DWI has less susceptibility artifact at the air-bone interface even with thinner slice acquisitions. Although there may be decreased sensitivity in the postoperative setting, DWI can be helpful to evaluate for residual cholesteatoma (Fig. 8.30).[135,136] MRI features are helpful to distinguish between MEC, cholesterol granuloma, and granulation tissue (Table 8.1).

In addition to ossicular destruction, other complications of cholesteatomas include facial nerve paralysis and labyrinthine fistula. Erosion of the tegmen tympani can occur, resulting in intracranial complications such as meningitis, thrombosis, and/or abscess. MRI, particularly coronal thin-section T2W images, is helpful to reveal complications of MEC, such as meningoencephaloceles from tegmen tympani erosion. SNHL

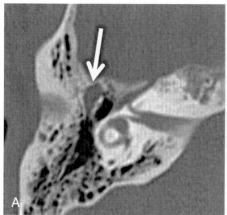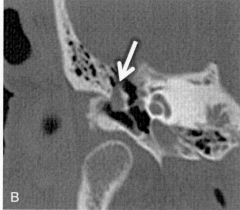

FIG. 8.29 Acquired pars flaccida middle ear cholesteatoma (MEC). Axial thin-section bone algorithm CT image of the right temporal bone **(A)** and coronal reconstruction **(B)** demonstrate a soft tissue density mass (*arrows*), which is non-gravity dependent and filling the lateral epitympanic recess while destroying the scutum (the superior attachment of the TM) and the ossicles from laterally, consistent with an MEC.

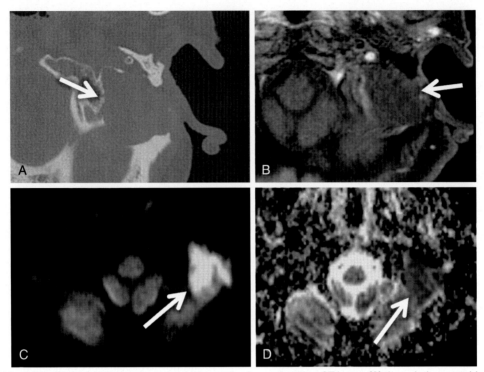

FIG. 8.30 Mastoid cholesteatoma. Axial thin-section bone algorithm CT image **(A)** through the mastoid process demonstrates a marrow-replacing process (**A**, *arrow*), with loss of the expected mastoid trabeculation. The correlating axial T1-weighted postcontrast MRI **(B)** with fat saturation shows the lesion to have no internal enhancement (**B**, *arrow*), with a small amount of linear medial enhancement. The correlating axial diffusion-weighted image (DWI) **(C)** and ADC image **(D)** show bright DWI signal (**C**, *arrow*) and corresponding dark apparent diffusion coefficient (ADC) signal intensity (**D**, *arrow*), consistent with a cholesteatoma.

**TABLE 8.1**
**MRI Features of Middle Ear Cholesteatoma Versus Cholesterol Granuloma Versus Granulation Tissue**

| Pathology | T1W MRI | T2W MRI | Enhancement | DWI |
|---|---|---|---|---|
| Cholesteatoma | Hypointense | Hyperintense | No | Yes |
| Cholesterol Granuloma | Hyperintense | Hyperintense | No | Variable |
| Granulation Tissue | Hypointense | Hyperintense | Yes | No |

*DWI*, diffusion-weighted imaging; *T1W*, T1-weighted; *T2W*, T2-weighted.

may result if there is erosion into the labyrinth causing a labyrinthine fistula. The cholesteatoma may drain spontaneously or may erode into the EAC, possibly leading to an automastoidectomy.

Otospongiosis (or otosclerosis) is an osteodystrophy of the otic capsule/perifenestral bony labyrinth of unknown cause. It is typically bilateral (85%) and predominantly affects Caucasian women (65%–72%).[137] Seventy percent of cases are inherited (autosomal dominant with incomplete penetrance); the remaining are sporadic.[126] Hearing loss in the second to the fourth decades is the presenting symptom. The CHL predominates initially and then progresses to mixed and SNHL.[138] In 70% cases, patients have early tinnitus, and a majority are bilateral (85%). Some patients may have vestibular symptoms, such as vertigo.[139,140]

The normal otic capsule has an outer periosteum layer, a middle endochondral bone layer, and an inner endosteum layer. The middle endochondral bone layer is resorbed and replaced by spongy vascular bone, hence

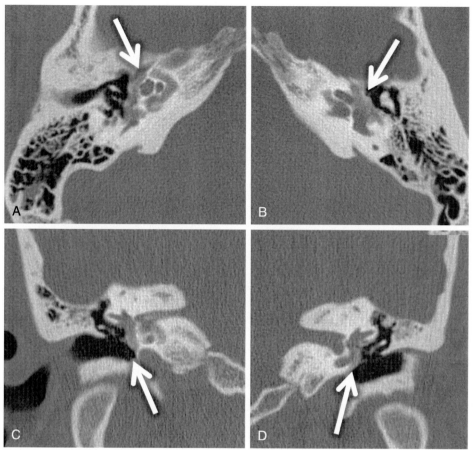

**FIG. 8.31** Otospongiosis. Axial thin-section bone algorithm CT images of the right **(A)** and left **(B)** temporal bones (TBs) demonstrate abnormal low densities surrounding the cochleas (*arrows*) bilaterally within the otic capsules. The coronal thin-section reconstructions of the right **(C)** and left **(D)** TBs show an abnormal low density involving the bilateral cochlear promontories (*arrows*) with extension of abnormal density into the bilateral oval window niches, consistent with otospongiosis in this patient with bilateral conductive hearing loss.

the "otospongiosis." Early in the disease spongy bone foci appear as abnormal bony density at the fissula ante fenestram,[141] a cleft of fibrocartilaginous tissue anterior to the oval window. The oval window may appear too wide (osteoclastic resorption). When the disease is limited to this area under the oval window, it is fenestral otospongiosis. This bone resorption can spread posteriorly along the oval window margins toward the round window; involvement of the otic capsule indicates cochlear otospongiosis (Fig. 8.31A and B). Abnormal bone impinges on the stapes footplate, causing mechanical fixation to the oval window, and results in progressive CHL. Late in the course of the disease, there is heaped up new bone along the oval and round window margins on CT and plugging of oval window

(obliterative otosclerosis) (Fig. 8.31C and D). There is no bony encroachment of the membranous labyrinth, which would indicate labyrinthitis ossificans. On contrast-enhanced MRI, there may be punctate enhancing foci in the medial wall of the middle ear cavity in the active phase. Fenestral otospongiosis (85%) is more common than cochlear otospongiosis (15%).[142] Fenestral otospongiosis is always present in cases of cochlear otosclerosis, but the cochlear type is present in less than 15% of cases of fenestral otospongiosis.[143] Cochlear (retrofenestral) otospongiosis presents clinically with progressive SNHL. The SNHL is postulated to be the result of metabolic substances, toxins, and proteolytic enzymes in the cochlear fluid causing hyalinization of the spiral ligament.[144–146]

## MIXED HEARING LOSS

MHL occurs when there is a combination of conductive and sensorineural hearing loss. There may be damage in the outer ear, middle ear, and/or inner ear (cochlea), as well as the auditory nerve.

### MHL Pathologies

The classic cause of MHL is otospongiosis. As mentioned earlier, otospongiosis progresses to MHL and SNHL.[138]

Age-related SNHL compounded with factors such as overexposure to loud noise, genetic predisposition, and medications can contribute to MHL. Other causes of both CHL and SNHL are birth defects, diseases or infections, tumors, and head injuries. The presentation of MHL depends on the degree of each component of hearing loss. Hearing loss that is more sensorineural will create difficulties in understanding speech, even though the volume often seems loud enough. Conversely, hearing loss that is more conductive may not greatly affect understanding of speech, but it will require sounds to be louder than normal. The CHL is typically addressed first.

Osseous fixation of the malleus can be a cause of a combined conductive and sensorineural hearing loss. Katzke et al. described the characteristic clinical, audiologic, and histologic findings, as well as the etiology of 66 patients with an idiopathic fixation of the head of the malleus.[147] Ninety-four percent of these patients had a sensorineural component to their hearing loss, far greater than the loss that could be attributed to presbycusis.

## CONCLUSION

A myriad of etiologies can cause sensorineural, conductive, and/or mixed hearing loss. The correlation of clinical examination and imaging are important in the complete evaluation of a patient with hearing loss. In addition to knowledge of the important TB anatomic landscape, recognizing the imaging findings on dedicated CT and MRI of the TBs is helpful in making the diagnosis and in understanding the pathophysiology.

## DISCLOSURE

Disclosure of any relationship with a commercial company that has a direct financial interest in subject matter or materials discussed in article or with a company making a competing product.

## REFERENCES

1. Leng S, Diehn FE, Lane JI, et al. Temporal bone CT: improved image quality and potential for decreased radiation dose using an ultra-high-resolution scan mode with an iterative reconstruction algorithm. *AJNR Am J Neuroradiol.* 2015;36(9):1599–1603.
2. Watanabe K, Cobb MIH, Zomorodi AR, Cunningham CD RD, Nonaka Y, Satoh S, Friedman AH, Fukushima T. Rare Lesions of the Internal Auditory Canal. *World Neurosurg.* 2017 Mar;99:200–209. http://dx.doi.org/10.1016/j.wneu.2016.12.003. Epub 2016 Dec 10. PubMed PMID: 27965072.
3. Hentschel M, Scholte M, Steens S, Kunst H, Rovers M. The diagnostic accuracy of non-imaging screening protocols for vestibular schwannoma in patients with asymmetrical hearing loss and/or unilateral audiovestibular dysfunction: a diagnostic review and meta-analysis. *Clin Otolaryngol.* 2016. http://dx.doi.org/10.1111/coa.12788.
4. Fukui MB, Weissman JL, Curtin HD, Kanal E. T2-weighted MR characteristics of internal auditory canal masses. *AJNR Am J Neuroradiol.* 1996;17(7):1211–1218.
5. Shelton C, Harnsberger HR, Allen R, King B. Fast spin echo magnetic resonance imaging: clinical application in screening for acoustic neuroma. *Otolaryngol Head Neck Surg.* 1996;114(1):71–76.
6. Daniels RL, Swallow C, Shelton C, Davidson HC, Krejci CS, Harnsberger HR. Causes of unilateral sensorineural hearing loss screened by high-resolution fast spin echo magnetic resonance imaging: review of 1,070 consecutive cases. *Am J Otol.* 2000;21(2):173–180.
7. Verret DJ, Adelson RT, Defatta RJ. Asymmetric sensorineural hearing loss evaluation with T2 FSE-MRI in a public hospital. *Acta Otolaryngol.* 2006;126(7):705–707.
8. Abele TA, Besachio DA, Quigley EP, et al. Diagnostic accuracy of screening MR imaging using unenhanced axial CISS and coronal T2WI for detection of small internal auditory canal lesions. *AJNR Am J Neuroradiol.* 2014;35(12):2366–2370.
9. Annesley-Williams DJ, Laitt RD, Jenkins JP, Ramsden RT, Gillespie JE. Magnetic resonance imaging in the investigation of sensorineural hearing loss: is contrast enhancement still necessary? *J Laryngol Otol.* 2001;115(1):14–21.
10. Parnes LS, Shimotakahara SG, Pelz D, Lee D, Fox AJ. Vascular relationships of the vestibulocochlear nerve on magnetic resonance imaging. *Am J Otol.* 1990;11(4):278–281.
11. Nadol JB Jr. Hearing loss. *N Engl J Med.* 1993;329(15):1092–1102.
12. Huang BY, Zdanski C, Castillo M. Pediatric sensorineural hearing loss, part 1: practical aspects for neuroradiologists. *AJNR Am J Neuroradiol.* 2012;33(2):211–217.
13. Lalwani AK, Castelein CM. Cracking the auditory genetic code: nonsyndromic hereditary hearing impairment. *Am J Otol.* 1999;20(1):115–132.
14. Brookhouser P. *Sensorineural Hearing Loss in Children.* St Louis, Mo: Mosby Year Book; 1993.

15. Barbi M, Binda S, Caroppo S, Ambrosetti U, Corbetta C, Sergi P. A wider role for congenital cytomegalovirus infection in sensorineural hearing loss. *Pediatr Infect Dis J*. 2003;22(1):39–42.

16. Peckham CS, Stark O, Dudgeon JA, Martin JA, Hawkins G. Congenital cytomegalovirus infection: a cause of sensorineural hearing loss. *Arch Dis Child*. 1987;62(12):1233–1237.

17. DeMarcantonio M, Choo DI. Radiographic evaluation of children with hearing loss. *Otolaryngol Clin N Am*. 2015;48(6):913–932.

18. Trimble K, Blaser S, James AL, Papsin BC. Computed tomography and/or magnetic resonance imaging before pediatric cochlear implantation? Developing an investigative strategy. *Otol Neurotol*. 2007;28(3):317–324.

19. Sennaroglu L, Saatci I. A new classification for cochleovestibular malformations. *Laryngoscope*. 2002;112(12):2230–2241.

20. Hudgins PA. *Labyrinthine Aplasia*. Salt Lake City: Amirsys; 2004.

21. Chan KH. Sensorineural hearing loss in children. Classification and evaluation. *Otolaryngol Clin N Am*. 1994;27(3):473–486.

22. Curtin HD. Congenital malformations of the ear. *Otolaryngol Clin N Am*. 1988;21(2):317–336.

23. Hudgins PA. *Common Cavity, Inner Ear*. Salt Lake City: Amirsys; 2004.

24. Purcell DD, Fischbein NJ, Patel A, Johnson J, Lalwani AK. Two temporal bone computed tomography measurements increase recognition of malformations and predict sensorineural hearing loss. *Laryngoscope*. 2006;116(8):1439–1446.

25. Huang BY, Zdanski C, Castillo M. Pediatric sensorineural hearing loss, part 2: syndromic and acquired causes. *AJNR Am J Neuroradiol*. 2012;33(3):399–406.

26. Arcand P, Desrosiers M, Dube J, Abela A. The large vestibular aqueduct syndrome and sensorineural hearing loss in the pediatric population. *J Otolaryngol*. 1991;20(4):247–250.

27. Valvassori GE, Clemis JD. The large vestibular aqueduct syndrome. *Laryngoscope*. 1978;88(5):723–728.

28. Swartz JD. An overview of congenital/developmental sensorineural hearing loss with emphasis on the vestibular aqueduct syndrome. *Semin Ultrasound CT MR*. 2004;25(4):353–368.

29. Harnsberger HR. *Large Endolymphatic Sac Anomaly*. Salt Lake City: Amirsys; 2004.

30. Naganawa S, Ito T, Iwayama E, et al. MR imaging of the cochlear modiolus: area measurement in healthy subjects and in patients with a large endolymphatic duct and sac. *Radiology*. 1999;213(3):819–823.

31. Davidson HC, Harnsberger HR, Lemmerling MM, et al. MR evaluation of vestibulocochlear anomalies associated with large endolymphatic duct and sac. *AJNR Am J Neuroradiol*. 1999;20(8):1435–1441.

32. Sugiura M, Naganawa S, Ishida IM, et al. Vestibular aqueduct in sudden sensorineural hearing loss. *J Laryngol Otol*. 2008;122(9):887–892.

33. Naganawa S, Koshikawa T, Fukatsu H, Ishigaki T, Nakashima T, Ichinose N. Contrast-enhanced MR imaging of the endolymphatic sac in patients with sudden hearing loss. *Eur Radiol*. 2002;12(5):1121–1126.

34. Ishida IM, Sugiura M, Naganawa S, Teranishi M, Nakashima T. Cochlear modiolus and lateral semicircular canal in sudden deafness. *Acta Otolaryngol*. 2007;127(11):1157–1161.

35. Boston M, Halsted M, Meinzen-Derr J, et al. The large vestibular aqueduct: a new definition based on audiologic and computed tomography correlation. *Otolaryngol Head Neck Surg*. 2007;136(6):972–977.

36. Parry DA, Booth T, Roland PS. Advantages of magnetic resonance imaging over computed tomography in preoperative evaluation of pediatric cochlear implant candidates. *Otol Neurotol*. 2005;26(5):976–982.

37. McClay JE, Booth TN, Parry DA, Johnson R, Roland P. Evaluation of pediatric sensorineural hearing loss with magnetic resonance imaging. *Arch Otolaryngol Head Neck Surg*. 2008;134(9):945–952.

38. Gray RF, Ray J, Baguley DM, Vanat Z, Begg J, Phelps PD. Cochlear implant failure due to unexpected absence of the eighth nerve–a cautionary tale. *J Laryngol Otol*. 1998;112(7):646–649.

39. Maxwell AP, Mason SM, O'Donoghue GM. Cochlear nerve aplasia: its importance in cochlear implantation. *Am J Otol*. 1999;20(3):335–337.

40. Glastonbury CM, Davidson HC, Harnsberger HR, Butler J, Kertesz TR, Shelton C. Imaging findings of cochlear nerve deficiency. *AJNR Am J Neuroradiol*. 2002;23(4):635–643.

41. Walton J, Gibson WP, Sanli H, Prelog K. Predicting cochlear implant outcomes in children with auditory neuropathy. *Otol Neurotol*. 2008;29(3):302–309.

42. Papsin BC. Cochlear implantation in children with anomalous cochleovestibular anatomy. *Laryngoscope*. 2005;115(1 Pt 2 suppl 106):1–26.

43. Stjernholm C, Muren C. Dimensions of the cochlear nerve canal: a radioanatomic investigation. *Acta Otolaryngol*. 2002;122(1):43–48.

44. Adunka OF, Jewells V, Buchman CA. Value of computed tomography in the evaluation of children with cochlear nerve deficiency. *Otol Neurotol*. 2007;28(5):597–604.

45. Huang BY, Roche JP, Buchman CA, Castillo M. Brain stem and inner ear abnormalities in children with auditory neuropathy spectrum disorder and cochlear nerve deficiency. *AJNR Am J Neuroradiol*. 2010;31(10):1972–1979.

46. Esposito G, Messina R, Carai A, et al. Cochleovestibular nerve compression syndrome caused by intrameatal anterior inferior cerebellar artery loop: synthesis of best evidence for clinical decisions. *World Neurosurg*. 2016;96:556–561.

47. Gorrie A, Warren 3rd FM, de la Garza AN, Shelton C, Wiggins 3rd RH. Is there a correlation between vascular loops in the cerebellopontine angle and unexplained unilateral hearing loss? *Otol Neurotol*. 2010;31(1):48–52.

48. Juliano AF, Ginat DT, Moonis G. Imaging review of the temporal bone: part I. Anatomy and inflammatory and neoplastic processes. *Radiology.* 2013;269(1):17–33.

49. Schuknecht HF. *Pathology of the Ear.* Cambridge, Mass: Harvard University Press; 1974.

50. Valavanis ASO, Naidich TP. *Clinical Imaging of the Cerebello-pontine Angle.* Berlin, Germany: Springer-Verlag; 1987.

51. Brackmann DEBL. Rare tumors of the cerebellopontine angle. *Otolaryngol Head Neck Surg.* 1980;88(5):555–559.

52. Propp JM, McCarthy BJ, Davis FG, Preston-Martin S. Descriptive epidemiology of vestibular schwannomas. *Neuro Oncol.* 2006;8(1):1–11.

53. Martuza RL, Ojemann RG. Bilateral acoustic neuromas: clinical aspects, pathogenesis, and treatment. *Neurosurgery.* 1982;10(1):1–12.

54. Selesnick SH, Jackler RK. Clinical manifestations and audiologic diagnosis of acoustic neuromas. *Otolaryngol Clin N Am.* 1992;25(3):521–551.

55. Hatam A, Bergstrom M, Moller A, Olivecrona H. Early contrast enhancement of acoustic neuroma. *Neuroradiology.* 1978;17(1):31–33.

56. Castillo R, Watts C, Pulliam M. Sudden hemorrhage in an acoustic neuroma. Case report. *J Neurosurg.* 1982;56(3):417–419.

57. Somers T, Casselman J, de Ceulaer G, Govaerts P, Offeciers E. Prognostic value of magnetic resonance imaging findings in hearing preservation surgery for vestibular schwannoma. *Otol Neurotol.* 2001;22(1):87–94.

58. National Institutes of Health Consensus Development Conference Statement on Acoustic Neuroma, December 11-13, 1991. The Consensus Development Panel. *Arch Neurol.* 1994;51(2):201–207.

59. Cohen NL, Hammerschlag P, Berg H, Ransohoff J. Acoustic neuroma surgery: an eclectic approach with emphasis on preservation of hearing. The New York University-Bellevue experience. *Ann Otol Rhinol Laryngol.* 1986;95(1 Pt 1):21–27.

60. Harner SG, Ebersold MJ. Management of acoustic neuromas, 1978-1983. *J Neurosurg.* 1985;63(2):175–179.

61. Glasscock 3rd ME, Kveton JF, Jackson CG, Levine SC, McKennan KX. A systematic approach to the surgical management of acoustic neuroma. *Laryngoscope.* 1986;96(10):1088–1094.

62. Dubrulle F, Ernst O, Vincent C, Vaneecloo FM, Lejeune JP, Lemaitre L. Cochlear fossa enhancement at MR evaluation of vestibular schwannoma: correlation with success at hearing-preservation surgery. *Radiology.* 2000;215(2):458–462.

63. Noren G, Arndt J, Hindmarsh T. Stereotactic radiosurgery in cases of acoustic neurinoma: further experiences. *Neurosurgery.* 1983;13(1):12–22.

64. Harnsberger HR. *Intralabrinthine Schwannoma. Diagnostic Imaging: Head and Neck.* Salt Lake City, UT, USA: Amirsys; 2004.

65. Fitzgerald DC, Grundfast KM, Hecht DA, Mark AS. Intralabyrinthine schwannomas. *Am J Otol.* 1999;20(3):381–385.

66. Valavanis A, Schubiger O, Hayek J, Pouliadis G. CT of meningiomas on the posterior surface of the petrous bone. *Neuroradiology.* 1981;22(3):111–121.

67. Zimmerman RD, Fleming CA, Saint-Louis LA, Lee BC, Manning JJ, Deck MD. Magnetic resonance imaging of meningiomas. *AJNR Am J Neuroradiol.* 1985;6(2):149–157.

68. Spagnoli MV, Goldberg HI, Grossman RI, et al. Intracranial meningiomas: high-field MR imaging. *Radiology.* 1986;161(2):369–375.

69. Gentry LR, Jacoby CG, Turski PA, Houston LW, Strother CM, Sackett JF. Cerebellopontine angle-petromastoid mass lesions: comparative study of diagnosis with MR imaging and CT. *Radiology.* 1987;162(2):513–520.

70. Luff DA, Simmons M, Malik T, Ramsden RT, Reid H. Endolymphatic sac tumours. *J Laryngol Otol.* 2002;116(5):398–401.

71. Pelosi S, Koss S. Adenomatous tumors of the middle ear. *Otolaryngol Clin N Am.* 2015;48(2):305–315.

72. Baltacioglu F, Ekinci G, Ture U, Sav A, Pamyr N, Erzen C. MR imaging, CT, and angiography features of endolymphatic sac tumors: report of two cases. *Neuroradiology.* 2002;44(1):91–96.

73. Lo WW, Applegate LJ, Carberry JN, et al. Endolymphatic sac tumors: radiologic appearance. *Radiology.* 1993;189(1):199–204.

74. Manski TJ, Heffner DK, Glenn GM, et al. Endolymphatic sac tumors. A source of morbid hearing loss in von Hippel-Lindau disease. *JAMA.* 1997;277(18):1461–1466.

75. Mafee MF. MR imaging of intralabyrinthine schwannoma, labyrinthitis, and other labyrinthine pathology. *Otolaryngol Clin N Am.* 1995;28(3):407–430.

76. Swartz JD. *Labyrinthitis.* Salt Lake City: Amirsys; 2004.

77. Paparella MM, Sugiura S. The pathology of suppurative labyrinthitis. *Ann Otol Rhinol Laryngol.* 1967;76(3):554–586.

78. deSouza C, Paparella MM, Schachern P, Yoon TH. Pathology of labyrinthine ossification. *J Laryngol Otol.* 1991;105(8):621–624.

79. Harnsberger HR, Dart DJ, Parkin JL, Smoker WR, Osborn AG. Cochlear implant candidates: assessment with CT and MR imaging. *Radiology.* 1987;164(1):53–57.

80. Harnsberger HR. *Labyrinthine Ossificans. Diagnostic Imaging: Head and Neck.* Salt Lake City, UT, USA: Amirsys; 2004.

81. Levenson MJ, Parisier SC, Jacobs M, Edelstein DR. The large vestibular aqueduct syndrome in children. A review of 12 cases and the description of a new clinical entity. *Arch Otolaryngol Head Neck Surg.* 1989;115(1):54–58.

82. Swartz JD. *Otosyphilis. Diagnostic Imaging: Head and Neck.* Salt Lake City, UT, USA. Amirsys; 2004.

83. Darrouzet V, Duclos JY, Liguoro D, Truilhe Y, De Bonfils C, Bebear JP. Management of facial paralysis resulting from temporal bone fractures: our experience in 115 cases. *Otolaryngol Head Neck Surg.* 2001;125(1):77–84.

84. Swartz JD. *Temporal Bone Fractures.* Salt Lake City: Amirsys; 2004.

85. Ulug T, Ulubil SA. Contralateral labyrinthine concussion in temporal bone fractures. *J Otolaryngol.* 2006;35(6):380–383.

86. Mark AS, Seltzer S, Harnsberger HR. Sensorineural hearing loss: more than meets the eye? *AJNR Am J Neuroradiol.* 1993;14(1):37–45.

87. Fitzgerald DC. Head trauma: hearing loss and dizziness. *J Trauma.* 1996;40(3):488–496.

88. Algin O, Bercin S, Akgunduz G, Turkbey B, Cetin H. Evaluation of labyrinthine fistula by MR cisternography. *Emerg Radiol.* 2012;19(6):557–560.

89. Mark AS, Fitzgerald D. Segmental enhancement of the cochlea on contrast-enhanced MR: correlation with the frequency of hearing loss and possible sign of perilymphatic fistula and autoimmune labyrinthitis. *AJNR Am J Neuroradiol.* 1993;14(4):991–996.

90. Maillot O, Attye A, Boyer E, et al. Post traumatic deafness: a pictorial review of CT and MRI findings. *Insights Imaging.* 2016;7(3):341–350.

91. Mil'bert ML. An instrument for cornea transplantation. *Oftalmol Zh.* 1966;21(5):397–398.

92. Kataoka H, Takeda T, Nakatani H, Saito H. Sensorineural hearing loss of suspected autoimmune etiology: a report of three cases. *Auris Nasus Larynx.* 1995;22(1):53–58.

93. Veldman J. Immune-mediated sensorineural hearing loss. *Auris Nasus Larynx.* 1998;25(3):309–317.

94. McCabe BF. Autoimmune sensorineural hearing loss. *Ann Otol Rhinol Laryngol.* 2007;116(12):875–879.

95. Swartz JD. *Osteopetrosis, Temporal Bone. Diagnostic Imaging: Head and Neck.* Salt Lake City, UT, USA: Amirsys; 2004.

96. Cure JK, Key LL, Goltra DD, VanTassel P. Cranial MR imaging of osteopetrosis. *AJNR Am J Neuroradiol.* 2000;21(6):1110–1115.

97. Cure JK, Key LL, Shankar L, Gross AJ. Petrous carotid canal stenosis in malignant osteopetrosis: CT documentation with MR angiographic correlation. *Radiology.* 1996;199(2):415–421.

98. Puschmann S, Thiel CM. Changed crossmodal functional connectivity in older adults with hearing loss. *Cortex.* 2016;86:109–122.

99. Lindenberger U, Baltes PB. Sensory functioning and intelligence in old age: a strong connection. *Psychol Aging.* 1994;9(3):339–355.

100. Anstey KJ, Luszcz MA, Sanchez L. A reevaluation of the common factor theory of shared variance among age, sensory function, and cognitive function in older adults. *J Gerontol B Psychol Sci Soc Sci.* 2001;56(1):P3–P11.

101. Pichora-Fuller MK. Cognitive aging and auditory information processing. *Int J Audiol.* 2003;42(suppl 2). 2S26–32.

102. Tun PA, McCoy S, Wingfield A. Aging, hearing acuity, and the attentional costs of effortful listening. *Psychol Aging.* 2009;24(3):761–766.

103. Humes LE, Busey TA, Craig J, Kewley-Port D. Are age-related changes in cognitive function driven by age-related changes in sensory processing? *Atten Percept Psychophys.* 2013;75(3):508–524.

104. Lin FR, Yaffe K, Xia J, et al. Hearing loss and cognitive decline in older adults. *JAMA Intern Med.* 2013;173(4):293–299.

105. Kurosaki Y, Tanaka YO, Itai Y. Malleus bar as a rare cause of congenital malleus fixation: CT demonstration. *AJNR Am J Neuroradiol.* 1998;19(7):1229–1230.

106. Hudgins PA. *EAC Atresia.* Salt Lake City,UT: Amirsys; 2004.

107. Jahrsdoerfer RA, Yeakley JW, Aguilar EA, Cole RR, Gray LC. Grading system for the selection of patients with congenital aural atresia. *Am J Otol.* 1992;13(1):6–12.

108. Swartz JD. *Oval Window Atresia. Diagnostic Imaging: Head and Neck.* Salt Lake City, UT, USA: Amirsys; 2004.

109. Lambert PR. Congenital absence of the oval window. *Laryngoscope.* 1990;100(1):37–40.

110. Hudgins PA. *Congential Cholesteatoma. Diagnostic Imaging: Head and Neck.* Salt Lake City, UT, USA: Amirsys; 2004.

111. Koltai PJ, Nelson M, Castellon RJ, et al. The natural history of congenital cholesteatoma. *Arch Otolaryngol Head Neck Surg.* 2002;128(7):804–809.

112. Guinto FC Jr, Garrabrant EC, Radcliffe WB. Radiology of the persistent stapedial artery. *Radiology.* 1972;105(2):365–369.

113. Silbergleit R, Quint DJ, Mehta BA, Patel SC, Metes JJ, Noujaim SE. The persistent stapedial artery. *AJNR Am J Neuroradiol.* 2000;21(3):572–577.

114. Thiers FA, Sakai O, Poe DS, Curtin HD. Persistent stapedial artery: CT findings. *AJNR Am J Neuroradiol.* 2000;21(8):1551–1554.

115. Swartz JD. Temporal bone trauma. *Semin Ultrasound CT MR.* 2001;22(3):219–228.

116. Swartz JD. *Fibrous Dysplasia, Temporal Bone.* Salt Lake City: Amirsys; 2004.

117. Wiggins RH. *EAC Exostoses. Diagnostic Imaging: Head and Neck.* Salt Lake City, UT, USA: Amirsys; 2004.

118. Dubach P, Hausler R. External auditory canal cholesteatoma: reassessment of and amendments to its categorization, pathogenesis, and treatment in 34 patients. *Otol Neurotol.* 2008;29(7):941–948.

119. Wiggins RH. *EAC Cholesteatoma. Diagnostic Imaging: Head and Neck.* Salt Lake City, UT, USA: Amirsys; 2004.

120. Heilbrun ME, Salzman KL, Glastonbury CM, Harnsberger HR, Kennedy RJ, Shelton C. External auditory canal cholesteatoma: clinical and imaging spectrum. *AJNR Am J Neuroradiol.* 2003;24(4):751–756.

121. Piepergerdes MC, Kramer BM, Behnke EE. Keratosis obturans and external auditory canal cholesteatoma. *Laryngoscope.* 1980;90(3):383–391.

122. Tran LP, Grundfast KM, Selesnick SH. Benign lesions of the external auditory canal. *Otolaryngol Clin N Am.* 1996;29(5):807–825.

123. Trojanowska A, Drop A, Trojanowski P, Rosinska-Bogusiewicz K, Klatka J, Bobek-Billewicz B. External and middle ear diseases: radiological diagnosis based on clinical signs and symptoms. *Insights Imaging.* 2012;3(1):33–48.

124. Wiggins RH. *EAC Medial Canal Fibrosis.* Salt Lake City: Amirsys; 2004.

125. Goodhill V. *Ear, Diseases, Deafness, and Dizziness*. New York: Harper and Row; 1979.

126. Weissman JL. Hearing loss. *Radiology*. 1996;199(3):593–611.

127. Sun GH, Shoman NM, Samy RN, Cornelius RS, Koch BL, Pensak ML. Do contemporary temporal bone fracture classification systems reflect concurrent intracranial and cervical spine injuries? *Laryngoscope*. 2011;121(5):929–932.

128. Cvorovic L, Jovanovic MB, Markovic M, Milutinovic Z, Strbac M. Management of complication from temporal bone fractures. *Eur Arch Otorhinolaryngol*. 2012;269(2):399–403.

129. Chole RA. *Chronic Otitis Media, Mastoiditis, and Petrositis*. St Louis, Mo: Mosby Year Book; 1993.

130. Nadol J. St Louis, Mo: Mosby-Year Book; 1993.

131. Kerschner JE. Bench and bedside advances in otitis media. *Curr Opin Otolaryngol Head Neck Surg*. 2008;16(6):543–547.

132. Semaan MT, Megerian CA. The pathophysiology of cholesteatoma. *Otolaryngol Clin N Am*. 2006;39(6):1143–1159.

133. Barath K, Huber AM, Stampfli P, Varga Z, Kollias S. Neuroradiology of cholesteatomas. *AJNR Am J Neuroradiol*. 2011;32(2):221–229.

134. De Foer B, Vercruysse JP, Spaepen M, et al. Diffusion-weighted magnetic resonance imaging of the temporal bone. *Neuroradiology*. 2010;52(9):785–807.

135. Alzahrani M, Alhazmi R, Belair M, Saliba I. Postoperative diffusion weighted MRI and preoperative CT scan fusion for residual cholesteatoma localization. *Int J Pediatr Otorhinolaryngol*. 2016;90:259–263.

136. Vercruysse JP, De Foer B, Pouillon M, Somers T, Casselman J, Offeciers E. The value of diffusion-weighted MR imaging in the diagnosis of primary acquired and residual cholesteatoma: a surgical verified study of 100 patients. *Eur Radiol*. 2006;16(7):1461–1467.

137. Juliano AF, Ginat DT, Moonis G. Imaging review of the temporal bone: Part II. Traumatic, postoperative, and noninflammatory nonneoplastic conditions. *Radiology*. 2015;276(3):655–672.

138. Purohit B, Hermans R, Op de Beeck K. Imaging in otosclerosis: a pictorial review. *Insights Imaging*. 2014;5(2):245–252.

139. Goh JP, Chan LL, Tan TY. MRI of cochlear otosclerosis. *Br J Radiol*. 2002;75(894):502–505.

140. Sando I, Hemenway WG, Miller DR, Black FO. Vestibular pathology in otosclerosis temporal bone histopathological report. *Laryngoscope*. 1974;84(4):593–605.

141. Swartz JD, Faerber EN, Wolfson RJ, Marlowe FI. Fenestral otosclerosis: significance of preoperative CT evaluation. *Radiology*. 1984;151(3):703–707.

142. Harnsberger HR. *Fenestral Otosclerosis. Diagnostic Imaging: Head and Neck*. Salt Lake City, UT, USA: Amirsys; 2004.

143. Harnsberger HR. *Cochlear Otosclerosis. Diagnostic Imaging: Head and Neck*. Salt Lake City, UT, USA: Amirsys; 2004.

144. Causse JR, Causse JB, Bretlau P, et al. Etiology of otospongiotic sensorineural losses. *Am J Otol*. 1989;10(2):99–107.

145. Parahy C, Linthicum FH Jr. Otosclerosis: relationship of spiral ligament hyalinization to sensorineural hearing loss. *Laryngoscope*. 1983;93(6):717–720.

146. Abd el-Rahman AG. Cochlear otosclerosis: statistical analysis of relationship of spiral ligament hyalinization to hearing loss. *J Laryngol Otol*. 1990;104(12):952–955.

147. Katzke D, Plester D. Idiopathic malleus head fixation as a cause of a combined conductive and sensorineural hearing loss. *Clin Otolaryngol Allied Sci*. 1981;6(1):39–44.

# CHAPTER 9

# Imaging of the Facial Nerve

THERESA KOUO, MD • ROBERT E. MORALES, MD •
PRASHANT RAGHAVAN, MBBS

## ANATOMY

The facial nerve comprises motor, sensory, and para-sympathetic fibers. The dominant motor component comprises 70% of the total axons. The sensory compo-nent makes up much of the remaining portion of the nerve and includes the nervus intermedius (nerve of Wrisberg). The motor division supplies somatic motor fibers to the muscles of the face, scalp, and auricle; the buccinators; the platysma; the stapedius; the stylohyoi-deus; and the posterior belly of the digastric. The motor division also contains sympathetic motor fibers, which constitute the vasodilator nerves of the submandibular and sublingual glands, conveyed through the chorda tympani nerve. The nerve of Wrisberg contains lacrimal secretomotor parasympathetic fibers and sensory fibers carrying input from the external auditory canal, the nasopharynx, and palate and taste sensation from the anterior two-thirds of the tongue and oral cavity. The facial nerve also has many clinically relevant communi-cations with other cranial and cervical spinal nerves.[1–3]

## Supranuclear Control

The supranuclear contribution from the motor cortex (Fig. 9.1) originates from pyramidal neurons in the lower third of the precentral gyrus. The cortical pro-jection fibers pass within the posterior genu of the internal capsule and descend in the pontine pyramidal tracts. The fibers for the lower facial muscles completely decussate to the contralateral facial nucleus. However, some cortical projection fibers for the upper face proj-ect to the ipsilateral as well as the contralateral facial nuclei. This explains why supranuclear lesions spare the motor functions of the upper face.[1,3,4]

## Motor Component

The motor nucleus of the facial nerve is located within the pontine tegmentum, just superior to the nucleus ambiguus, posterior to the superior olivary nucleus, and medial to the spinal trigeminal nucleus. The fibers course posteromedially and loop (the internal genu) around the medial aspect of the abducens nucleus to form the facial colliculus, a shallow bulge in the floor of the fourth ventricle, easily identified on axial MR images. This close anatomic relationship explains how both the facial and abducens nerves may be simulta-neously affected by disease processes. The motor fibers exit the lateral border of the pons in the cerebellopon-tine angle cistern, where they lie medial to cranial nerve (CN) VIII (Fig. 9.2).

## Sensory, Special Sensory, and Parasympathetic

The nerve of Wrisberg exits the pons between the motor root and CN VIII and courses parallel to the motor root, to the internal auditory canal. It also carries somato-sensory fibers (from the trigeminal nucleus, having received them from the posterior auricular nerve) and special sensory taste fibers, received from the chorda tympani from the anterior tongue and oral cavity, to the nucleus tractus solitarius in the medulla.[1,4]

The parasympathetic secretomotor component comprises fibers to the lacrimal and submandibular glands that originate in the superior salivatory nucleus. At the geniculate ganglion, the fibers to the lacrimal gland do not synapse but leave via the greater super-ficial petrosal nerve. They then join the deep petrosal nerve (comprising sympathetic nerve fibers) to form the vidian nerve (of the pterygoid canal) and synapse in the pterygopalatine ganglion. Postganglionic fibers reach the lacrimal gland via the zygomatic branch of the maxillary nerve (V2), which communicates with the lacrimal nerve (branch of the V1).[1,3,4]

The preganglionic fibers for the submandibular and sublingual glands continue along the facial nerve, passing through the geniculate ganglion, and exit at the mastoid segment within the chorda tympani. The chorda tympani travels medial to the handle of mal-leus in the tympanic cavity and enters the infratempo-ral fossa through the petrotympanic/glaserian fissure, where it joins the lingual nerve (CN V3). The fibers synapse within the submandibular ganglion, innervat-ing the submandibular and sublingual salivary glands.[1]

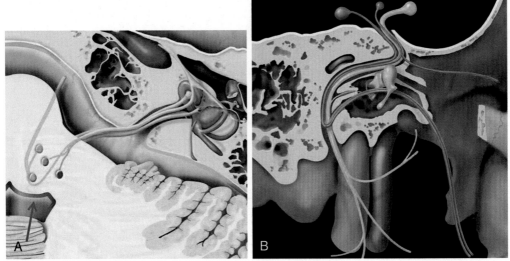

FIG. 9.1 The nuclei of the facial nerve **(A)**. Motor nucleus (orange), nucleus tractus solitarius (blue), superior salivatory nucleus (pink). Note that the facial nerve loops around the abducens nucleus (*red arrow*) to form the facial colliculus. Image **(B)** is a sagittal oblique graphic image demonstrating the components of the facial nerve with the motor component (yellow), the secretomotor fibers in the chorda tympani (blue), and the parasympathetic fibers that exit through the greater superficial petrosal nerve (purple). (From Harnsberger H, Osborn A, Macdonald A, et al. *Diagnostic and Surgical Imaging Anatomy: Brain, Head and Neck, Spine*. Salt Lake City, Utah: Amirsys; 2006:224–231; with permission.)

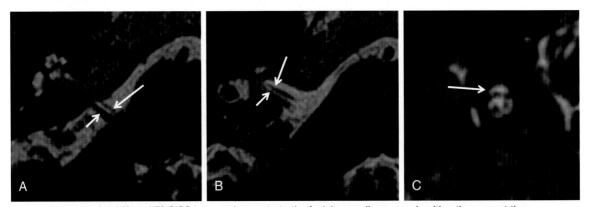

FIG. 9.2 Axial **(A** and **B)** CISS images demonstrate the facial nerve (*long arrow*) exiting the pons at the cerebellopontine angle to enter the internal auditory canal (IAC), anterior to the vestibulocochlear nerve (*short arrow*). **(C)** An oblique sagittal reformatted image derived from axial 3D CISS images depicting the position of the facial nerve in the anterosuperior quadrant of the IAC.

## Peripheral Course

The facial nerve may be conveniently divided into cisternal, intracanalicular, labyrinthine, tympanic, mastoid, and extracranial segments (Fig. 9.3). The facial nerve exits from the pontomedullary sulcus at the root exit point. The nerve remains adherent to the undersurface of the pons for 8–10 mm, through the attached segment. The nerve then detaches from the pons at the root detachment point. The transition zone extends for approximately 2 mm, followed by the cisternal segment, which extends anterolaterally to the porus acusticus.[5] The cisternal segment is typically 24 mm in length.[6]

The nerve of Wrisberg exits between the motor root and the vestibulocochlear nerve. The nerve joins the

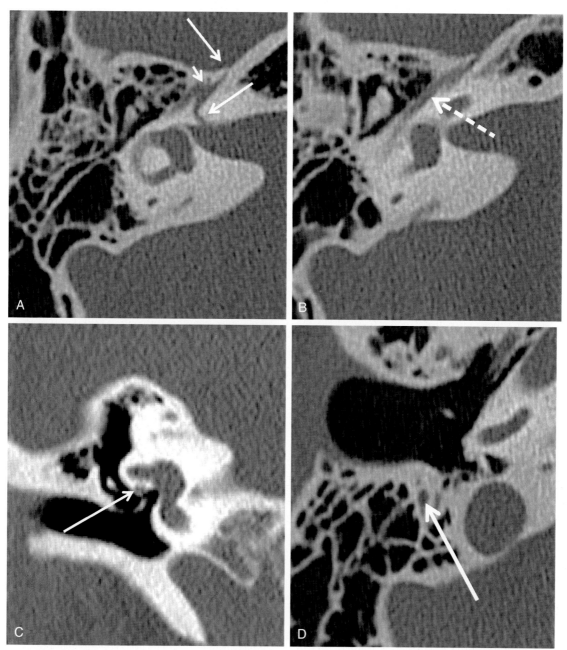

FIG. 9.3 Intratemporal course of the facial nerve. High-resolution CT images demonstrating labyrinthine **(A)**, tympanic **(B** and **C)**, and mastoid **(D)** segments of the facial nerve. The geniculate ganglion (*short arrow*, **A**) resides in the geniculate fossa at the junction of the labyrinthine and tympanic segments. Note the greater superficial petrosal nerve canal arising from the geniculate fossa in **(A)** (*dotted arrow*). In **(C)**, the relationship between the tympanic segment of the nerve, the lateral semicircular canal, and the oval window is demonstrated. The nerve passes under the canal, where it is contained within a bony canal that may sometimes be dehiscent.

motor root as it exits the brainstem or at the porus acusticus and becomes a common trunk, the nervi facialis.[2] The intracanalicular segment travels within the anterior and superior quadrants of the internal auditory canal (IAC) for approximately 8 mm.

Within the lateral IAC, the nerve is separated from the cochlear nerve inferiorly by a horizontal partition of dura and bone, the transverse or falciform crest. A vertical dural and osseous crest known as Bill bar separates the facial nerve from the superior vestibular nerve, which lies posteriorly (Fig. 9.3).

The facial/fallopian canal consists of three segments: labyrinthine, tympanic, and mastoid, extending from Bill bar to the stylomastoid foramen (Fig. 9.3).[7] The labyrinthine segment is the narrowest and shortest segment within the facial canal, 3–5 mm in length.[8] It extends from the anterosuperior fundus to the geniculate ganglion. It passes between the ampulla of the superior semicircular canal and the cochlea to travel forward and downward. Exiting anteriorly from the geniculate ganglion is the first branch of CN VII, the greater superficial petrosal nerve (GSPN). At the geniculate ganglion, the nerve makes a sharp 75 degree turn posteriorly (anterior or first genu). This marks the beginning of the tympanic segment. The tympanic segment (Fig. 9.3) is 10 mm in length. The nerve traverses the medial wall of the tympanic cavity superolateral to the oval window and inferior to the lateral semicircular canal.[8] It then enters the facial recess, medial to the pyramidal eminence, and then turns inferiorly 95–125 degrees (posterior or second genu) to become the mastoid segment. The mastoid segment courses posteromedial to the external auditory canal and lateral to the inferior aspect of the tympanic annulus, extending for 13 mm in adults.[9] The mastoid segment gives rise to the nerve to the stapedius and the chorda tympani.

The extracranial facial nerve exits the temporal bone at the stylomastoid foramen, situated between the styloid process anteriorly and the mastoid process posteriorly. The nerve immediately enters the substance of the parotid gland, after which it divides into two terminal branches: the upper temporofacial branch and the lower cervicofacial branch. In the parotid gland, these nerves further divide into temporal, zygomatic, buccal, marginal mandibular, and cervical branches.[1,4,7]

The peripheral nerve is composed of three layers, the endoneurium, the perineurium, and the epineurium. The intracranial and intracanalicular segments of the nerve lack the perineurium and epineurium, making them more susceptible to injury.[8]

### Vascular Supply of the Facial Nerve

The cortical motor area of the face is supplied by the middle cerebral artery. The facial nucleus within the pons is supplied primarily by the anterior inferior cerebellar artery (AICA), a branch off the basilar artery. The AICA enters the IAC with the facial nerve and gives rise to the labyrinthine (internal auditory) artery and supplies the cisternal, intracanalicular, and labyrinthine segments. The tympanic and mastoid segments are fed from the stylomastoid artery, typically arising from the posterior auricular artery. The extracranial facial nerve is supplied by posterior auricular, occipital, and superficial temporal arteries.

Venous drainage parallels the arterial blood supply. Within the IAC, the veins drain into branches of the internal auditory vein. At and distal to the geniculate ganglion, the nerve is surrounded by a tough connective tissue sheath, which is contiguous with the facial canal periosteum and the epineurium. Within this sheath lies a venous network, which drains into veins accompanying the petrosal and stylomastoid arteries. This accounts for normal enhancement of the geniculate ganglion and distal nerve segments on postcontrast MRI (Fig. 9.4).[1,4,7,10,11]

### CLINICAL AND IMAGING EVALUATION

Facial paralysis may occur in a variety of acute and chronic clinical settings. A variety of infectious, autoimmune, granulomatous, neoplastic, and vascular disease can present with facial palsy. The first step in clinical evaluation is the determination of whether the facial palsy is consequent to an upper or lower motor neuron process. Clinical evaluation of facial weakness centers on the determination of whether the weakness is caused by a central (supranuclear) or a peripheral (nuclear, lower motor neuron) lesion. A useful clinical tenet is that a central lesion will spare the forehead and brow, whereas a peripheral lesion will result in complete facial weakness in addition to loss of emotional or involuntary facial motion. These presentations result from bilateral supranuclear innervation to the upper facial musculature. The clinician may also be able to localize the lesion to a segment of the nerve based on whether lacrimation is impaired (implying a lesion proximal to the GSPN-suprageniculate), hyperacusis is present (suprastapedia), or if taste and salivation are affected (suprachordal). The severity of facial paralysis is typically graded using the House-Brackmann Facial Nerve Grading System (Table 9.1). Central causes are best investigated with MRI, whereas peripheral causes may require a combination of MRI and CT. Often, disease processes may affect long segments of the nerve and such precise localization is not possible. The most commonly encountered cause

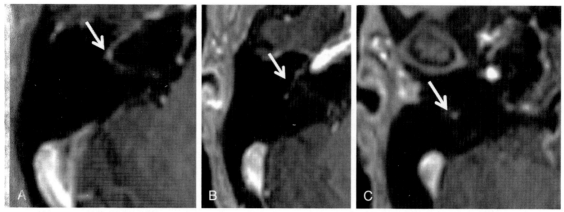

FIG. 9.4 Normal facial nerve enhancement. The presence of a perineural venous plexus around the geniculate ganglion and tympanic and mastoid segments (**A**, **B**, and **C**, respectively, *arrows*) accounts for normal enhancement on postgadolinium T1-weighted images. This may be more pronounced on volumetric T1-weighted images, as shown. Enhancement of the nerve in the cerebellopontine angle, internal auditory canal, or labyrinthine segment is an abnormal finding.

## TABLE 9.1
## House-Brackmann Grading of Facial Nerve Dysfunction

| Grade/Degree of Dysfunction | Clinical Findings |
| --- | --- |
| I. Normal | Normal function |
| II. Mild | Slight weakness noticeable on close inspection<br>Normal symmetry and tone at rest<br>Slight mouth asymmetry with motion |
| III. Moderate | Obvious, but not disfiguring facial asymmetry<br>Moderate synkinesis, hemifacial spasm<br>Normal symmetry and tone at rest<br>Slight forehead and mouth weakness with motion |
| IV. Moderate to severe | Obvious weakness and/or disfiguring asymmetry<br>No forehead motion, incomplete eye closure, asymmetric mouth motion with maximum effort |
| V. Severe | Only barely perceptible motion<br>Asymmetry at rest<br>No forehead movement, only slight mouth movement, incomplete eye closure |
| VI. Complete paralysis | No facial movement |

of lower motor neuron facial paralysis is Bell palsy, discussed in detail later.[12]

A typical MRI protocol for evaluating the facial nerve and temporal bone should comprise diffusion-weighted images (DWIs); axial and coronal pre- and postcontrast thin-section (3-mm) T1-weighted images, the latter with fat suppression; and a heavily T2-weighted volumetric sequence. In the evaluation of hemifacial spasm (HFS), MR angiography is useful in the identification of a compressive vascular loop. The intraparotid segment of the nerve is not usually well demonstrated on routine MRI but may be visualized using a steady state gradient echo sequence, such as three-dimensional (3D)-reversed fast imaging with steady-state precession (PSIF)-DWI (Siemens, Erlangen, Germany) or a 3D FIESTA (fast imaging employing steady state precession; GE, Milwaukee, USA) sequence or its equivalent.[13,14] MR Diffusion Tensor Imaging (DTI) tractography has been used to demonstrate the position of the facial nerve in relation to CerebelloPontine Angle (CPA) tumors.[15]

The normal facial nerve on contrast-enhanced MRI exhibits enhancement in its tympanic segment and beyond because of the presence of a circumneural venous plexus. It is important to note that on both unenhanced and contrast-enhanced 3D inversion recovery-prepared fast spoiled gradient-echo, the normal nerve may appear increased in signal intensity (Fig. 9.4).[16]

CT is best performed with a multidetector CT scanner, with images acquired axially parallel to the hard palate, with an edge-enhancing algorithm. Images are viewed at a wide window level and width and are displayed with a small field of view. The axial images are reconstructed typically in coronal and sagittal planes (although they may be reconstructed in any plane, given that the voxels are isotropic).

## CONGENITAL ANOMALIES

Congenital malformations of the facial nerve may occur in isolation or in association with more complex abnormalities of the brain and temporal bones. They may be asymptomatic or present at birth with profound facial paralysis. Bifurcations and trifurcations of the nerve may occur as isolated phenomena, most commonly distal to the geniculate ganglion, in the tympanic segment, although rare labyrinthine and mastoid segment bifurcations have also been reported.[17,18]

Incomplete closure of the fallopian canal caused by a malformation of Reichert cartilage results in dehiscence of the canal, most commonly at the level of the oval window. A pure dehiscence without prolapse of the nerve cannot be reliably diagnosed using CT because the wall of the normal facial nerve canal is extremely thin.[19–21] The nerve can prolapse into the middle ear cleft and lie directly over the oval window and may be at risk for inadvertent injury at surgery. Although this is typically an incidental finding, the occasional patient may present with conductive hearing loss consequent to the stapedial crura being attached to the nerve. On coronal CT images, the prolapsed nerve is readily identified as a smoothly convex soft tissue structure inferior to the lateral semicircular canal, overlying the oval window and stapes,

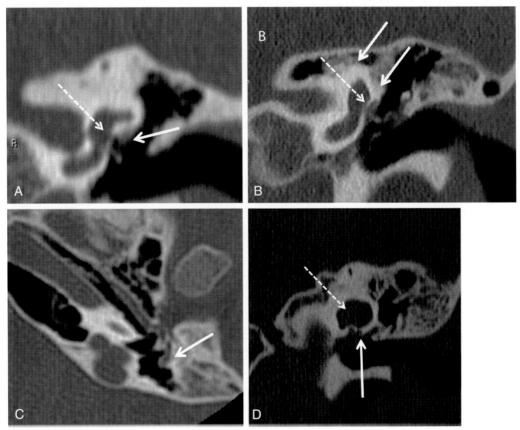

FIG. 9.5 The facial nerve in congenital anomalies of the inner ear. **(A)** Isolated oval window atresia. Note the dehiscence of the facial canal (*arrow*) and the abnormal position of the nerve (*solid arrow*) overlying the stenotic oval window (*dashed arrow*). **(B)** CHARGE association. Note the absence of lateral and superior semicircular canals (*arrows*) with stenosis of the oval window with the facial nerve directly overlying it (*dashed arrow*). **(C)** Aural atresia. Note the relatively anterior location of the mastoid segment of the facial nerve (*arrow*). **(D)** Cystic cochleovestibular dysplasia (*dashed arrow*) with the facial nerve displaced inferiorly to lie lateral to the stenotic oval window.

contiguous with the facial nerve canal (Fig. 9.5). Facial nerve prolapse is also a feature of oval window atresia and the CHARGE syndrome (colobomas, heart defects, choanal atresia, mental retardation, and genitourinary and ear anomalies) (Fig. 9.5).[20-24]

The course of the facial nerve is frequently altered in congenital aural atresia and is an important variable that determines surgical planning.[25] Typically, the angle at the first genu is excessively obtuse, the tympanic segment is displaced inferiorly to lie over the oval window, and the second genu and mastoid segments are displaced anteriorly. The nerve may therefore exit the temporal bone more anteriorly, at the level of the round window, increasing the risk of injury at surgery when the auricle is elevated. The course of the nerve is also altered with malformations of the oval window and inner ear structures (Fig. 9.5).[26,27]

The facial nerve and its nucleus may be congenitally absent, as has been noted in Mobius (where the abducens nerve is also abnormal), DiGeorge, Poland, Goldenhar, and trisomy 13 and 18 syndromes, among others.[28-30] Absence or hypoplasia of the nerve is best demonstrated on high-resolution 3D T2-weighted sequences. On sagittal reformatted images derived from such a sequence, the nerve will be absent from its usual position in the anterosuperior quadrant of the IAC (Fig. 9.6). The facial nerve also may demonstrate an anomalous course when the vestibulocochlear nerve is absent. Aplasia, aberrant origin, and course of the facial nerve may be a feature of pontine tegmental cap dysplasia, a rare hindbrain malformation. In such patients, the facial

and vestibular nerves course in two separate anomalous bony canals (duplicated IAC) (Fig. 9.7).[31,32]

## VASCULAR DISORDERS OF THE FACIAL NERVE

HFS is characterized by severe unilateral involuntary twitching of some or all of the facial musculature. Often this begins insidiously in the orbicularis oculi muscle and spreads to involve the lower muscles of the face. Vascular compression of the facial nerve is the most common cause of HFS. Most commonly, the culprit vessel is the AICA, posterior inferior cerebellar artery, or vertebral artery.

The extent of nerve compression required to produce symptoms is unclear; HFS may occur despite the absence of significant nerve deformation on imaging. Imaging is an important component in patient selection for microvascular decompression. Optimal protocol selection is critical for visualization of the facial nerve and determination of the presence of vascular compression. Thin-section multiplanar Steady-State Free Procession (SSFP) sequences are excellent for depicting both the nerve and the compressing vessel (Fig. 9.8). Reconstruction of source images to generate oblique or curved reformatted images can provide valuable additional characterization for preoperative planning. Historically, microvascular decompression for HFS has targeted the "root exit zone," corresponding to the root detachment point and transition zone of the facial nerve, spanning approximately a 4-mm segment. Distal nerve compression along the cisternal segment has shown relatively lower rates of HFS. However, more recent studies have shown proximal nerve involvement in patients with HFS, including compression at the root exit point within the pontomedullary sulcus or along the subsequent attached segment, which extends 8–10 mm along the undersurface of the pons.[5,33-35]

### Venous Vascular Malformations

These rare lesions, previously referred to as hemangiomas, may present with gradual facial palsy, tinnitus, HFS, or hearing loss. They account for 0.7% of temporal bone masses and usually present between the third and sixth decades of life. Histologic features include irregularly shaped, dilated lesional vessels with flattened endothelial cells, scant smooth muscle, and absence of the internal elastic lamina. Intralesional bone spicules (hence the term "ossifying" hemangioma) may also be present.[36-39] These lesions may infiltrate the facial nerve, in contrast to schwannomas, which compress

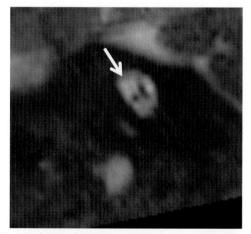

FIG. 9.6 Congenital absence of the facial nerve. Oblique sagittal reformatted 3D CISS image demonstrating absence of the facial nerve in the anterosuperior quadrant of the internal auditory canal (*arrow*).

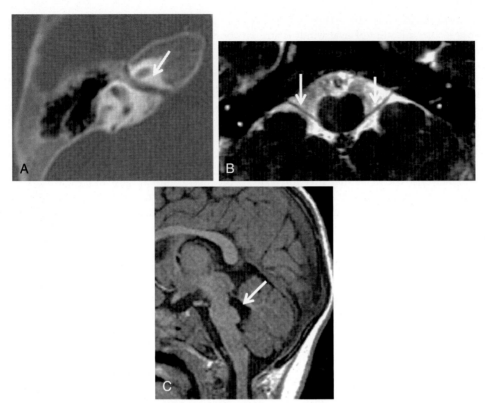

FIG. 9.7 Pontine tegmental cap dysplasia. The internal auditory canal is dimunitive (*arrow*, **A**), transmitting only the facial nerve. On the axial 3D CISS images **(B)**, the facial nerves are present (*arrows*) but the vestibulocochlear nerves are absent. Note the characteristic dorsal pontine hump (*arrow*, **C**). (Modified from Leiva-Salinas C, et al. Abnormalities of the cochlear nerves and internal auditory canals in pontine tegmental cap dysplasia. *Otol Neurotol*. 2012;33(9):e73–e74.)

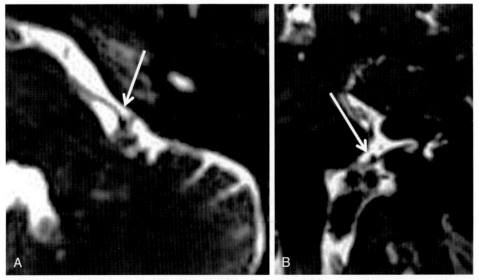

FIG. 9.8 Hemifacial spasm. Axial **(A)** and coronal **(B)** reformatted CISS images demonstrating deformation of the left facial nerve in the cerebellopontine angle cistern by the anterior inferior cerebellar artery (*arrows*).

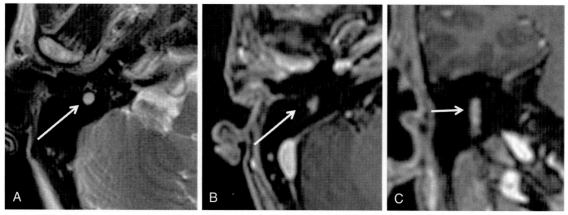

FIG. 9.9 Venous vascular malformation of the mastoid segment of the facial nerve (facial nerve hemangioma). The lesion is hyperintense on the axial T2-weighted image (*arrow*, **A**) and demonstrates intense enhancement on the axial and coronal postcontrast images (*arrows*, **B** and **C**). These lesions may sometimes demonstrate a spiculated bone reaction on CT but may otherwise be indistinguishable from schwannomas.

the nerve. The most common locations are the geniculate ganglion, the fundus of the IAC, and the posterior genu. Intratumoral bone spicules on CT images are pathognomonic of this entity. They are best evaluated with contrast-enhanced MRI whereby they demonstrate marked enhancement. Low-signal-intensity foci may be seen on T1- and T2-weighted images, corresponding to the ossific matrix of the lesion. A "honeycomb" or "spoke-wheel" pattern of ossification on CT is typical of this entity (Fig. 9.9). This finding is present, however, in only about 50% of cases. In its absence, these lesions may be indistinguishable from schwannomas, although more focal lesions as opposed to fusiform expansion may favor a venous vascular malformation. Most surgeons advocate early intervention to preserve facial function.[40] Although the lesion can be successfully separated from the nerve with no loss of function, resection of the nerve and cable grafting may be necessary when nerve infiltration or an intense perineural reaction is present.[41,42]

## FACIAL NERVE TRAUMA

Both blunt and penetrating craniofacial trauma may lead to severe facial nerve injury and paralysis. Facial paralysis may occur in up to 50% of patients with temporal bone fractures. Most cases of posttraumatic facial paralysis are delayed, incomplete, and transient and are due to intraneural hematomas. When paralysis is immediate, the nerve is usually transected. In patients with deteriorating facial function, surgical exploration

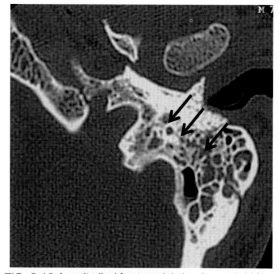

FIG. 9.10 Longitudinal fracture violating the mastoid facial nerve canal in a patient who presented with facial palsy 2 days after a motor vehicle accident (*arrows*).

and neurorrhaphy or decompression, best performed within 2 weeks after injury and by 2 months at the latest, is necessary.[43,44] Facial nerve injury is more likely to occur with transverse (38%–50% of cases) rather than longitudinal (20%) fractures. The most common site of nerve injury with transverse fractures is the labyrinthine segment, whereas longitudinally oriented fractures tend to involve the facial canal in the geniculate fossa (Fig. 9.10). Posttraumatic facial palsy

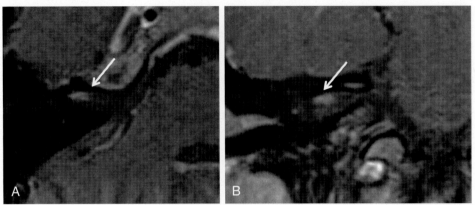

FIG. 9.11 Bell palsy. Note the typical tuft-like enhancement of the facial nerve (*arrows*) in the fundus of the internal auditory canal on axial **(A)** and coronal **(B)** postcontrast images.

is best evaluated with high-resolution CT (HRCT). MRI has been used to visualize intraneural hematoma. It has been suggested that intense enhancement of the nerve may imply nerve fiber degeneration and regeneration.[45–47]

## INFLAMMATORY DISORDERS

Bell palsy, an acute-onset peripheral facial neuropathy, is the most common cause of lower motor neuron facial palsy, characterized by an abrupt onset of facial weakness, which peaks by 48–72 h, as a general rule. It affects approximately 25 people per 100,000. Symptoms reflect the mixed profile of the facial nerve and the complex connections that exist with other CNs. Associated symptoms include postauricular pain, dysgeusia, hyperacusis, decreased lacrimation and salivation, subjective change in facial sensation (CN V), vestibular dysfunction (CN VIIII), and pharyngeal symptoms (CNs IX and X). These are present in 50%–60% of cases and are reassuring as to the diagnosis of Bell palsy. The severity of facial palsy correlates with the duration of the disease and degree of recovery.[48]

Inflammatory edema of the facial nerve, with resultant ischemia of the nerve caused by vascular compression, especially in the tight labyrinthine segment, is believed to be responsible for the disease. The exact pathogenesis of the disease is controversial. Infection (HSV-1 DNA has been found in the endoneural fluid and in the pot auricular musculature), herpes simplex type-1, nerve compression, and autoimmune factors may all play a role.[49]

Although the clinical picture is strongly suggestive in most cases, Bell palsy is a diagnosis of exclusion. Acute lower motor neuron facial palsy is not unique to Bell palsy and may be seen with brainstem infarction and multiple sclerosis.[50] Almost all patients with the condition demonstrate improvement in 6 months. If improvement does not occur or the symptoms are progressive, further investigation is warranted to exclude other diagnoses, the most worrisome of which is tumor. Contrast-enhanced MRI in Bell palsy is of limited value but typically demonstrates enhancement of the nerve in the fundus of the IAC and in the geniculate ganglion, labyrinthine, and tympanic segments (Fig. 9.11). The nerve is not usually thickened, and any enlargement should raise suspicion for tumor. Such enhancement, it must be stressed, is not unique to Bell palsy and may be seen with any inflammatory affliction of the nerve (Fig. 9.12). These include, among others, Lyme disease, Ramsay Hunt syndrome, sarcoidosis, Guillain-Barré syndrome, autoimmune diseases such as Sjögren disease, and infections such as leprosy.[51–54]

Herpes zoster oticus (Ramsay Hunt syndrome) results from reactivation of latent varicella zoster virus in the geniculate ganglion. It may be triggered by stress, aging, or immunosuppression. Typical symptoms include burning external ear pain followed by a vesicular rash in the pinna and external auditory canal, facial palsy, vertigo, tinnitus, sensorineural hearing loss, and nystagmus. MRI demonstrates thickening and enhancement of the facial nerve in any or all of its segments, the vestibulocochlear nerve (especially the superior vestibular nerve),[55] the inner ear structures, and also

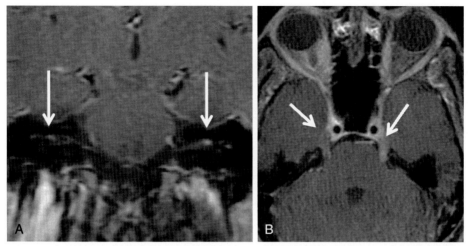

FIG. 9.12 Lyme disease. Enhancement of the facial nerves in the fundus of the internal auditory canal is evident in **(A)** (*arrows*). The cisternal segments of the trigeminal nerves also enhance abnormally (*arrows*, **B**).

the lesions of the external auditory canal (Fig. 9.13). Enhancement has been observed to extend into the pons along the intrapontine course of the facial nerve and its pontine nucleus.[56] Abnormalities of the facial and vestibulocochlear nerves and inner ear structures may also be evident on pre- and post-contrast 3D fluid-attenuated inversion recovery images and may correlate with symptom severity.[57]

The facial nerve may also be secondarily involved in acute and chronic otomastoiditis. The incidence of such involvement in acute mastoiditis has decreased in the antibiotic era. Facial palsy reportedly occurs in only 0.005% of such patients. About 1% of patients who have cholesteatoma may present with facial nerve paralysis. Facial palsy may occur with skull base osteomyelitis with or without malignant external otitis (Fig. 9.14). Subtle osseous erosion of the facial canal, especially in the tympanic segment, where the wall is inherently thin, may be difficult to detect. However, gross invasion of the fallopian canal is usually evident on HRCT. Enhancement of the nerve may be present on contrast-enhanced MRI.[58,59]

## TUMORS OF THE FACIAL NERVE

Tumors of the facial nerve usually present with progressive facial paresis or paralysis. Facial paralysis that does not evolve in a pattern typical of Bell palsy (e.g., insidious onset, progression for more than 3 weeks, persistence for longer than 6 months) must be investigated. However, tumors have been known to precipitate facial paralysis acutely. The facial nerve may be afflicted by primary neoplasms and also be secondarily involved by tumors of the temporal bone or by perineural spread (PNS) of malignancy. Only the more frequent of them will be considered here.

### Schwannomas

Facial nerve schwannomas (FNSs) account for 64% of facial nerve tumors.[60] They can occur along any portion of the nerve and often involve multiple segments, most commonly the geniculate ganglion.[61] The symptoms, imaging appearance, and treatment approach are highly dependent upon the location of the lesion.

MRI protocols should include 2-mm axial and coronal T1 pre- and postcontrast and 3D 0.6-mm heavily T2-weighted imaging Constructive Interference in Steady-State (CISS) through the temporal bone. HRCT, with multiplanar reformations, is useful to evaluate for expansion of the facial canal and aid in ruling out other lesions such as cholesteatoma and hemangioma.

Intradural FNSs involving the cisternal or intracanalicular segments may be indistinguishable from vestibular schwannomas on imaging. However, imaging may demonstrate extension of the mass into the labyrinthine segment, confirming the schwannoma as facial in origin. It is important to recognize this "labyrinthine tail" to distinguish these two entities. FNSs may also present with a "dumbbell" shape, extending from the fundus of the IAC, through the labyrinthine segment, into the geniculate fossa (Fig. 9.15).[62,63]

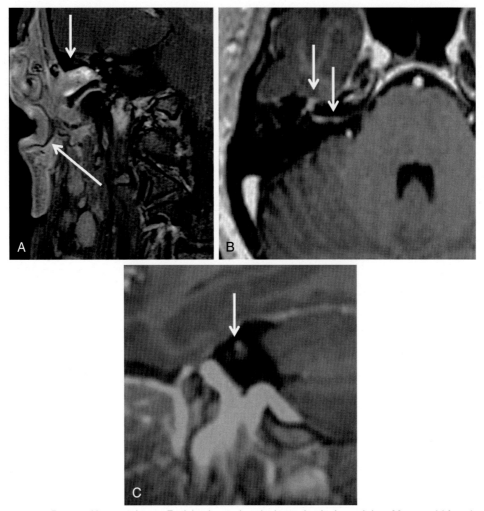

FIG. 9.13 Ramsay Hunt syndrome. Facial palsy and vesicular periauricular rash in a 30-year-old female patient. In **(A)**, extensive thickening and enhancement of the soft tissues of the external auditory canal and pinna are evident (*arrows*). Enhancement of the facial nerve is visible in the geniculate ganglion and internal auditory canal on axial and sagittal postcontrast sequences (*arrows*, **B** and **C**).

FNSs confined to the geniculate ganglion or GSPN are usually clinically silent until late in the disease, presenting as a middle cranial fossa mass on imaging, often mistaken for meningiomas. When evaluating an enhancing extraaxial lesion in the middle cranial fossa, radiologists should evaluate for bony scalloping and enlargement of the geniculate fossa, which may indicate FNS (Fig. 9.15).

Tympanic segment FNSs appear as multilobulated masses, because of the lack of solid bony architecture of the surrounding facial canal. These lesions may extend inferolaterally, resulting in ossicular displacement and conductive hearing loss, or superomedially, resulting in erosion and fistula formation with the lateral semicircular canal.[63] An FNS along the mastoid segment may give the deceptive appearance of a destructive, invasive lesion due to extension through the fragile, thin mastoid septations. FNSs within the parotid gland may present as palpable masses, less commonly facial paralysis (Fig. 9.15).[63,64]

Treatment options include observation, stereotactic radiosurgery, and surgical resection. The surgical approach depends on the size and location of the lesion and hearing status. Tumors proximal to the geniculate ganglion with less than 1 cm CPA component with preserved hearing are resected with a middle

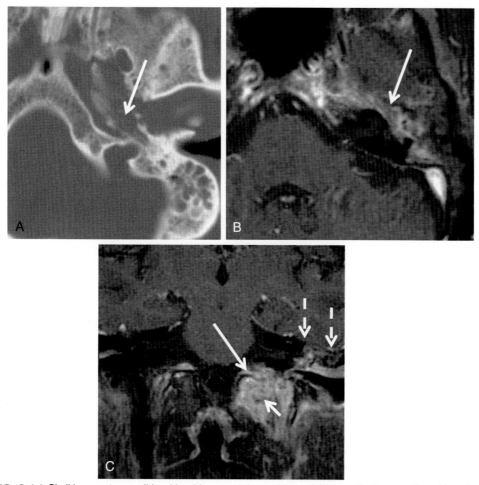

FIG. 9.14 Skull base osteomyelitis with otitis externa in an elderly diabetic patient presenting with multiple lower cranial nerve palsies. The axial CT image (*arrow*, **A**) demonstrates osseous destruction in the petrous apex. Note the abnormally increased enhancement of the geniculate ganglion and tympanic facial nerve in (*arrow*, **B**). Abnormal enhancement is also noted in the jugular foramen (*long arrow*) and hypoglossal canal (*short arrow*) in (**C**). Inflammation is also seen in the external auditory canal and middle ear cavity (*dashed arrows*).

cranial fossa approach. In patients with large CPA components, a retrosigmoid approach is necessary, whereas in patients without salvageable hearing, a translabyrinthine approach is taken. Mastoid FNSs are resected via a transmastoid approach.[65]

Other rare lesions that may present as an enhancing mass involving the facial nerve include glomus tumors, choristomas (usually in the geniculate ganglion), and geniculate meningiomas.[66]

### Perineural Spread of Malignancy

PNS of tumor is a well-recognized pattern of tumor spread of head and neck malignancies, often portending

a poor prognosis and decreased survival rates. The presence of PNS may mandate the use of wider margins of resection, prophylactic lymph node dissection, and adjuvant chemotherapy or radiation therapy. Several malignancies are known for this pattern of tumor spread, including squamous cell carcinoma, adenoid cystic carcinoma, lymphoma, melanoma, and some sarcomas. The facial and trigeminal nerves are most commonly involved. Pain, paresthesia, or weakness in a specific CN distribution in the setting of known head and neck malignancy is strongly suggestive of PNS. However, patients may be initially asymptomatic, emphasizing the importance for radiologists to

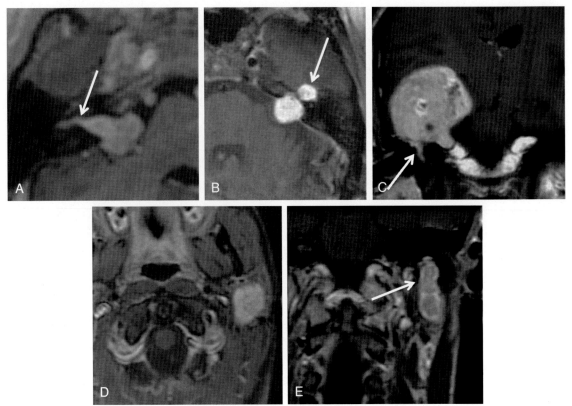

FIG. 9.15 Facial nerve schwannoma. In **(A)**, note the extension of the tumor beyond the fundus of the internal auditory canal into the labyrinthine facial canal (*arrow*), indicating the facial nerve origin of the schwannoma. In **(B)**, the schwannoma involves the canalicular and labyrinthine segments and the geniculate ganglion (*arrow*). In **(C)**, it arises from the geniculate fossa (*arrow*) to present as a large middle cranial fossa mass. The radiologist should always scrutinize the geniculate fossa when evaluating an extraaxial mass in this region. In **(D)**, the schwannoma appears as a nonspecific solidly enhancing parotid space mass. However, the facial nerve origin of the mass is evident from its extension along and smooth expansion of the mastoid facial nerve canal (*arrow*, **E**).

perform surveillance evaluation for potential PNS in patients with head and neck cancer. Occasionally, identification of PNS may precede the detection of the primary tumor.[67,68]

Typically, in PNS, the tumor extends in a centripetal fashion toward the brain; however, the tumor may also extend in a centrifugal manner at branch points. There may be segments of uninvolved or only microscopically involved nerve separating the primary tumor and the metastatic mass. Because these "skip" areas may occur, clear surgical margins do not guarantee that PNS spread has not occurred.

PNS involving the facial nerve classically results from the spread of malignant tumors of the parotid space along the extracranial nerve branches. The tumor spreads in a retrograde fashion from the peripheral rami into the facial canal (Fig. 9.16). Alternatively, the tumor may reach the facial nerve by way of the GSPN. An additional important pathway for PNS along the extracranial nerve is from the auriculotemporal nerve, a branch of the mandibular division of the trigeminal nerve (V3). Branches of the auriculotemporal nerve join the facial nerve within the parotid gland, serving as a direct route for PNS to the facial nerve (Fig. 9.17).[69]

MRI is the imaging modality of choice for PNS. Radiologic findings of perineural tumor include nerve thickening, nerve enhancement, enlargement or destruction of the foramina, obliteration of fat planes, and facial muscle denervation atrophy. Precontrast T1-weighted images should include the parotid region and the pterygopalatine

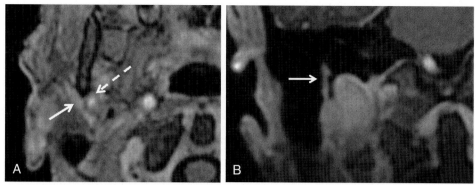

FIG. 9.16 Perineural spread of primary parotid squamous cell carcinoma. On the axial contrast-enhanced image (*arrow*, **A**), a small focus of enhancement representing recurrent tumor is evident lateral to the retromandibular vein (*dashed arrow*). In (**B**), spread along the mastoid segment of the facial nerve is evident (*arrows*).

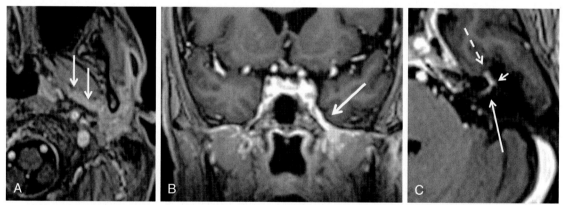

FIG. 9.17 Perineural spread via the auriculotemporal nerve in a patient with adenoid cystic carcinoma. In (**A**), note the extension of enhancing tumor medially from the parotid gland into the masticator space along the course of the auriculotemporal nerve toward the mandibular division of the trigeminal nerve (*arrows*). In (**B**), perineural spread along V3 into Meckel cave is evident (*arrow*). Also noted, in (**C**), is perineural spread along the facial nerve to the geniculate ganglion (*short arrow*), to the greater superficial petrosal nerve (*dashed arrow*), and to the canalicular segment (*long arrow*).

fossa for careful evaluation of facial and trigeminal branches and the pterygopalatine ganglion. Loss of fat signal in the PterygoPalatine Fossa (PPF) or the various neural canals in the skull base is an important clue in the diagnosis of PNS. Postcontrast imaging with fat suppression is of benefit to increase sensitivity for PNS. 3T MRI may be superior to 1.5T in the detection of PNS.[70,71]

## CONCLUSION

The facial nerve is a complex structure, affected by a variety of disease processes. The radiologist must possess a thorough knowledge of its anatomy, the clinical picture, and appropriate imaging protocols to narrow differential diagnoses.

## REFERENCES

1. Curtin H, Sanelli P, Som P. Temporal bone: embryology and anatomy. In: Som PM, Curtin HD, eds. *Head and Neck Imaging.* 4th ed. St Louis, MO: Mosby; 2003:1057–1092.
2. Jager L, Reiser M. CT and MR imaging of the normal and pathologic conditions of the facial nerve. *Eur J Radiol.* 2001;40(2):133–146.
3. May M. Anatomy of the facial nerve for the clinician. In: May M, Schaitlin B, eds. *The Facial Nerve, May's Second Edition.* New York: Thieme Medical Publishers; 2000.

4. Swartz JD, Harnsberger HR. *Imaging of the Temporal Bone.* New York: Thieme Medical Publishers; 1998.

5. Hughes M, Branstetter BF, Frederickson AM, et al. Imaging hemifacial spasm. *Neurographics.* 2015;5(1):2–8.

6. Al-Noury K, Lotfy A. Normal and pathological findings for the facial nerve on magnetic resonance imaging. *Clin Radiol.* 2011;66(8):701–707.

7. Harnsberger H, Osborn A, Macdonald A, et al. *Diagnostic and Surgical Imaging Anatomy: Brain, Head and Neck, Spine.* Salt Lake City, UT: Amirsys; 2006.

8. Gupta S, Mends F, Hagiwara M, Fatterpekar G, Roehm PC. Imaging the facial nerve: a contemporary review. *Radiol Res Pract.* 2013;2013:248039.

9. Nager GT, Proctor B. Anatomic variations and anomalies involving the facial canal. *Otolaryngol Clin N Am.* 1991;24(3):531–553.

10. Hendrix P, Griessenauer CJ, Foreman P, et al. Arterial supply of the lower cranial nerves: a comprehensive review. *Clin Anat.* 2014;27(1):108–117.

11. Blunt MJ. The blood supply of the facial nerve. *J Anat.* 1954;88(4):520–526.

12. Hashisaki GT. Medical management of Bell's palsy. *Compr Ther.* 1997;23(11):715–718.

13. Chu J, Zhou Z, Hong G, et al. High-resolution MRI of the intraparotid facial nerve based on a microsurface coil and a 3D reversed fast imaging with steady-state precession DWI sequence at 3T. *AJNR Am J Neuroradiol.* 2013;34(8):1643–1648.

14. Li C, Li Y, Zhang D, Yang Z, Wu L. 3D-FIESTA MRI at 3 T demonstrating branches of the intraparotid facial nerve, parotid ducts and relation with benign parotid tumours. *Clin Radiol.* 2012;67(11):1078–1082.

15. Hilly O, Chen JM, Birch J, et al. Diffusion tensor imaging tractography of the facial nerve in patients with cerebellopontine angle tumors. *Otol Neurotol.* 2016;37(4):388–393.

16. Dehkharghani S, Lubarsky M, Aiken AH, Kang J, Hudgins PA, Saindane AM. Redefining normal facial nerve enhancement: healthy subject comparison of typical enhancement patterns–unenhanced and contrast-enhanced spin-echo versus 3D inversion recovery-prepared fast spoiled gradient-echo imaging. *AJR Am J Roentgenol.* 2014;202(5):1108–1113.

17. Glastonbury CM, Fischbein NJ, Harnsberger HR, Dillon WP, Kertesz TR. Congenital bifurcation of the intratemporal facial nerve. *AJNR Am J Neuroradiol.* 2003;24(7):1334–1337.

18. Jakkani RK, Ki R, Karnawat A, Vittal R, Kumar AD. Congenital duplication of mastoid segment of facial nerve: a rare case report. *Indian J Radiol Imaging.* 2013;23(1):35–37.

19. Baxter A. Dehiscence of the falloplan canal. An anatomical study. *J Laryngol Otol.* 1971;85(6):587–594.

20. Di Martino E, Sellhaus B, Haensel J, Schlegel J-G, Westhofen M, Prescher A. Fallopian canal dehiscences: a survey of clinical and anatomical findings. *Eur Arch Oto-Rhino-Laryngol.* 2005;262(2):120–126.

21. Swartz JD. The facial nerve canal: CT analysis of the protruding tympanic segment. *Radiology.* 1984;153(2):443–447.

22. Booth TN, Vezina LG, Karcher G, Dubovsky EC. Imaging and clinical evaluation of isolated atresia of the oval window. *AJNR Am J Neuroradiol.* 2000;21(1):171–174.

23. Raghavan P, Mukherjee S, Phillips CD. Imaging of the facial nerve. *Neuroimaging Clin N Am.* 2009;19(3):407–425.

24. Joshi VM, Navlekar SK, Kishore GR, Reddy KJ, Kumar ECV. CT and MR imaging of the inner ear and brain in children with congenital sensorineural hearing loss. *Radiographics.* 2012;32(3):683–698.

25. Shonka DCJ, Livingston 3rd WJ, Kesser BW. The Jahrsdoerfer grading scale in surgery to repair congenital aural atresia. *Arch Otolaryngol Head Neck Surg.* 2008;134(8):873–877.

26. Jahrsdoerfer RA. The facial nerve in congenital middle ear malformations. *Laryngoscope.* 1981;91(8):1217–1225.

27. Romo LV, Curtin HD. Anomalous facial nerve canal with cochlear malformations. *AJNR Am J Neuroradiol.* 2001;22(5):838–844.

28. Verzijl HTFM, Valk J, de Vries R, Padberg GW. Radiologic evidence for absence of the facial nerve in Mobius syndrome. *Neurology.* 2005;64(5):849–855.

29. Ouanounou S, Saigal G, Birchansky S. Mobius syndrome. *AJNR Am J Neuroradiol.* 2005;26(2):430–432.

30. Verzijl HTFM, van der Zwaag B, Cruysberg JRM, Padberg GW. Mobius syndrome redefined: a syndrome of rhombencephalic maldevelopment. *Neurology.* 2003;61(3):327–333.

31. Nixon JN, Dempsey JC, Doherty D, Ishak GE. Temporal bone and cranial nerve findings in pontine tegmental cap dysplasia. *Neuroradiology.* 2016;58(2):179–187.

32. Leiva-Salinas C, Mukherjee S, Kesser BW, Deib G, Flors L, Raghavan P. Imaging case of the month: abnormalities of the cochlear nerves and internal auditory canals in pontine tegmental cap dysplasia. *Otol Neurotol.* 2012;33(9):e73–e74.

33. Du C, Korogi Y, Nagahiro S, et al. Hemifacial spasm: three-dimensional MR images in the evaluation of neurovascular compression. *Radiology.* 1995;197(1):227–231.

34. Ho SL, Cheng PW, Wong WC, et al. A case-controlled MRI/MRA study of neurovascular contact in hemifacial spasm. *Neurology.* 1999;53(9):2132–2139.

35. Naraghi R, Tanrikulu L, Troescher-Weber R, et al. Classification of neurovascular compression in typical hemifacial spasm: three-dimensional visualization of the facial and the vestibulocochlear nerves. *J Neurosurg.* 2007;107(6):1154–1163.

36. Palacios E, Kaplan J, Gordillo H, Rojas R. Facial nerve hemangioma. *Ear Nose Throat J.* 2003;82(11):836–837.

37. Zhi-yao S, Jian-dong L. Facial nerve hemangiomas: a review. *J Otol.* 2012;7(1):28–30.

38. Ross L, Drazin D, Eboli P, Lekovic GP. Atypical tumors of the facial nerve: case series and review of the literature. *Neurosurg Focus.* 2013;34(3):E2.

39. Benoit MM, North PE, McKenna MJ, Mihm MC, Johnson MM, Cunningham MJ. Facial nerve hemangiomas: vascular tumors or malformations? *Otolaryngol Head Neck Surg.* 2010;142(1):108–114.

40. Escada P, Capucho C, Silva JM, Ruah CB, Vital JP, Penha RS. Cavernous haemangioma of the facial nerve. *J Laryngol Otol.* 1997;111(9):858–861.

41. Mijangos SV, Meltzer DE. Case 171: facial nerve hemangioma. *Radiology.* 2011;260(1):296–301.

42. Eby TL, Fisch U, Makek MS. Facial nerve management in temporal bone hemangiomas. *Am J Otol.* 1992;13(3):223–232.

43. Davis RE, Telischi FF. Traumatic facial nerve injuries: review of diagnosis and treatment. *J Craniomaxillofac Trauma.* 1995;1(3):30–41.

44. Hato N, Nota J, Hakuba N, Gyo K, Yanagihara N. Facial nerve decompression surgery in patients with temporal bone trauma: analysis of 66 cases. *J Trauma.* 2011;71(6):1789–1792.

45. Phillips CD, Bubash LA. The facial nerve: anatomy and common pathology. *Semin Ultrasound CT MR.* 2002;23(3):202–217.

46. Sartoretti-Schefer S, Scherler M, Wichmann W, Valavanis A. Contrast-enhanced MR of the facial nerve in patients with posttraumatic peripheral facial nerve palsy. *AJNR Am J Neuroradiol.* 1997;18(6):1115–1125.

47. Darrouzet V, Duclos JY, Liguoro D, Truilhe Y, De Bonfils C, Bebear JP. Management of facial paralysis resulting from temporal bone fractures: our experience in 115 cases. *Otolaryngol Head Neck Surg.* 2001;125(1):77–84.

48. Croxson G. The assessment of facial nerve dysfunction. *J Otolaryngal Soc Aust.* 1990;4:252–263.

49. Eviston TJ, Croxson GR, Kennedy PGE, Hadlock T, Krishnan AV. Bell's palsy: aetiology, clinical features and multidisciplinary care. *J Neurol Neurosurg Psychiatry.* 2015;86(12):1356–1361.

50. Fukazawa T, Moriwaka F, Hamada K, Hamada T, Tashiro K. Facial palsy in multiple sclerosis. *J Neurol.* 1997;244(10):631–633.

51. Nemzek W, Swartz J. Temporal bone: inflammatory disease. In: Som PM, Curtin HD, eds. *Head and Neck Imaging.* St Louis, MO: Mosby; 2003.

52. Daniels DL, Czervionke LF, Millen SJ, et al. MR imaging of facial nerve enhancement in Bell palsy or after temporal bone surgery. *Radiology.* 1989;171(3):807–809.

53. Tien R, Dillon WP, Jackler RK. Contrast-enhanced MR imaging of the facial nerve in 11 patients with Bell's palsy. *AJR Am J Roentgenol.* 1990;155(3):573–579.

54. Beal M, Hauser S. Trigeminal neuralgia, Bell's palsy, and other cranial nerve disorders. In: *Harrison's Principles of Internal Medicine.* New York: McGraw Hill; 2005.

55. Iwasaki H, Toda N, Takahashi M, et al. Vestibular and cochlear neuritis in patients with Ramsay Hunt syndrome: a Gd-enhanced MRI study. *Acta Otolaryngol (Stockh).* 2013;133(4):373–377.

56. Sartoretti-Schefer S, Kollias S, Valavanis A. Ramsay Hunt syndrome associated with brain stem enhancement. *AJNR Am J Neuroradiol.* 1999;20(2):278–280.

57. Chung MS, Lee JH, Kim DY, et al. The clinical significance of findings obtained on 3D-FLAIR MR imaging in patients with Ramsay-Hunt syndrome. *Laryngoscope.* 2015;125(4):950–955.

58. Gaio E, Marioni G, de Filippis C, Tregnaghi A, Caltran S, Staffieri A. Facial nerve paralysis secondary to acute otitis media in infants and children. *J Paediatr Child Health.* 2004;40(8):483–486.

59. Schwarz J, Harnsberger H. The middle ear and mastoid. In: Swartz JD, Harnsberger HR, eds. *Imaging of the Temporal Bone.* 3rd ed. New York: Thieme Medical Publishers; 1998.

60. Gross BC, Carlson ML, Moore EJ, Driscoll CL, Olsen KD. The intraparotid facial nerve schwannoma: a diagnostic and management conundrum. *Am J Otolaryngol.* 2012;33(5):497–504.

61. Mundada P, Purohit BS, Kumar TS, Tan TY. Imaging of facial nerve schwannomas: diagnostic pearls and potential pitfalls. *Diagn Interv Radiol Ank Turk.* 2016;22(1):40–46.

62. Salzman KL, Davidson HC, Harnsberger HR, et al. Dumbbell schwannomas of the internal auditory canal. *AJNR Am J Neuroradiol.* 2001;22(7):1368–1376.

63. Wiggins 3rd RH, Harnsberger HR, Salzman KL, Shelton C, Kertesz TR, Glastonbury CM. The many faces of facial nerve schwannoma. *AJNR Am J Neuroradiol.* 2006;27(3):694–699.

64. Shimizu K, Iwai H, Ikeda K, Sakaida N, Sawada S. Intraparotid facial nerve schwannoma: a report of five cases and an analysis of MR imaging results. *AJNR Am J Neuroradiol.* 2005;26(6):1328–1330.

65. Liu R, Fagan P. Facial nerve schwannoma: surgical excision versus conservative management. *Ann Otol Rhinol Laryngol.* 2001;110(11):1025–1029.

66. Smith MM, Thompson JE, Thomas D, et al. Choristomas of the seventh and eighth cranial nerves. *AJNR Am J Neuroradiol.* 1997;18(2):327–329.

67. Ginsberg L. Imaging of perineural tumor spread in head and neck cancer. In: Som PM, Curtin HD, eds. *Head and Neck Imaging.* St Louis, MO: Mosby; 2003.

68. Shang J, Sheng L, Wang K, Shui Y, Wei Q. Expression of neural cell adhesion molecule in salivary adenoid cystic carcinoma and its correlation with perineural invasion. *Oncol Rep.* 2007;18(6):1413–1416.

69. Schmalfuss IM, Tart RP, Mukherji S, Mancuso AA. Perineural tumor spread along the auriculotemporal nerve. *AJNR Am J Neuroradiol.* 2002;23(2):303–311.

70. Penn R, Abemayor E, Nabili V, Bhuta S, Kirsch C. Perineural invasion detected by high-field 3.0-T magnetic resonance imaging. *Am J Otolaryngol.* 2010;31(6):482–484.

71. Kirsch CFE. Advances in magnetic resonance imaging of the skull base. *Int Arch Otorhinolaryngol.* 2014;18(suppl 2):S127–S135.

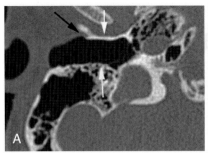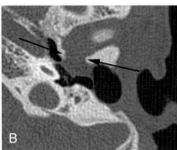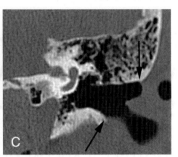

FIG. 10.1 Postoperative appearance of the external auditory canal (EAC). **(A)** Axial CT with absence of the normal bony isthmus (*white arrows*) and a foreshortened anterior wall (*black arrow*) from bone drilling. **(B)** Axial CT, defect in the anterior wall of the EAC (between *black arrows*) is covered by scar. **(C)** Coronal CT, flaring of the EAC from medial to lateral, which appears patulous laterally (between *black arrows*) after combined meatoplasty/canaloplasty.

the EAC is common; this "acute" angle is formed by the TM and the adjacent anterior wall of the EAC.

## Tympanoplasty

Although tympanoplasty and myringoplasty seem to be synonymous, the term "tympanoplasty" may include surgery involving the TM, ossicles, and associated ME disease.[4]

A tympanoplasty classification developed by Wullstein in 1956 included five types.[5]

Type 1—Tympanoplasty with intact ossicular chain.

Type 2—Malleus partially eroded.

Type 3—Malleus and incus eroded, TM/graft extends to the intact stapes.

Type 4—Stapes superstructure eroded but footplate is mobile.

Type 5—Reconstruction with a fixed stapes footplate, a graft extending to a horizontal semicircular canal fenestration.

With the advancement of surgical techniques/instruments and development of ossicular prosthesis, the classification has been modified over the years. For example, the Type 5 tympanoplasty is now of historical interest only (Fig. 10.2).

Although Wullstein's classification describes the anatomic situation, there have been attempts to modify it with regards to prognosis and functional results. In 1971, Austin included the status of the ossicular chain as a prognostic factor for hearing results.[6] In 1973, Belluci proposed a dual classification, also taking into consideration the presence or absence of ME disease; the spectrum extended from Group 1, a disease-free dry ear, through Group 4, a draining ear with nasopharyngeal malformation (cleft palate, choanal atresia).[7] In 1994, Kartush described the Middle Ear Risk Index, which combines the Belluci and Austin schemes with

additional prognostic factors, including the status of the TM, presence/absence of cholesteatoma, ME effusion/granulation tissue, history of prior surgery, and smoking status.[8]

## Ossiculoplasty

Ossiculoplasty reconstructs a sound-conducting mechanism between the TM/graft and oval window.[9] The surgery performed is dependent on the ossicular deficit. Variations include the use of a prosthesis, autologous ossicle (most commonly the incus), bone cement, cartilage, etc.

In general terms, a partial ossicular replacement prosthesis extends from the TM, malleus, or incus to an intact stapes with mobile footplate. A total ossicular replacement prosthesis (TORP) extends to the footplate, a term used even if other ossicles and the stapes superstructure are present.[9-11] A stapes prosthesis is a form of TORP but is often referred to as a "stapes prosthesis." Because of the wide variety of ossicular and prosthesis combinations, it is best to describe the actual anatomic situation (Fig. 10.2).

The prosthesis and materials used are numerous and are in general made from calcified particles or hydroxyapatite, metal (e.g., titanium), or plastic (e.g., plastipore). Stacked cartilage and bone cement may also be used with or without a prosthesis.[12-14] Specific prostheses are not discussed here because they are numerous and in constant evolution. It is helpful to become familiar with the techniques and prosthesis used locally by your surgeons.

There are two important points regarding ossiculoplasty. First, look for continuity of the ossicular chainprosthesis from the TM/graft to the stapes or footplate (Fig. 10.3). Off-axis reformatted images are often valuable for this purpose.[15,16] The ossicular reconstructions

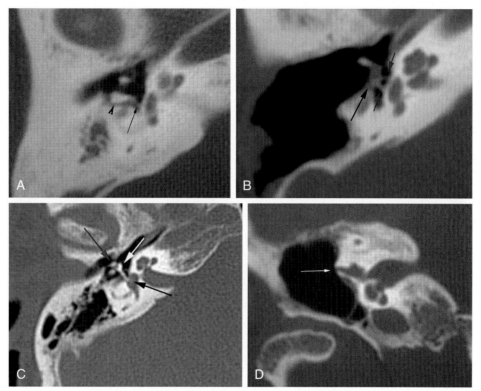

FIG. 10.2 Tympanoplasty types. **(A)** Type 2—axial CT, incus interposition (*arrowhead*) to intact stapes (*arrow*). **(B)** Type 3—axial CT, tympanic membrane (TM)/graft (*black arrow*) in contact with intact stapes (*red arrows*). **(C)** Type 4—axial CT, absent stapes superstructure, mobile footplate. Prosthesis cupped laterally (*white arrow*) around malleus remnant (*red arrow*) to stapes footplate (*black arrow*). **(D)** Type 5—coronal CT, patient post bilateral type 5 tympanoplasty in the late 1950s, right side shown. Fenestration of the horizontal canal (*white arrow*), TM/graft applied against the fenestration is thin and not well seen by CT.

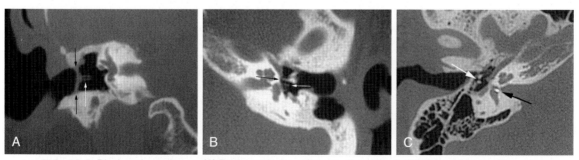

FIG. 10.3 Displaced prostheses. **(A)** Partial ossicular replacement prosthesis (PORP) (*white arrow*) based on the deep margin of the thickened tympanic membrane/graft (*black arrows*) is lateralized with the graft; tip of the PORP is well away from the oval window/stapes. **(B)** Tip of an incus interposition (*black arrow*) is displaced anterior to the stapes capitulum (*white arrow*). **(C)** Piston-type prosthesis after stapedectomy is displaced deep into the vestibule, the tip against the medial margin (black arrows). There was no identifiable connection to the incus (white arrow) by CT.

used are quite variable and not always a "straight line" or centered on the footplate (Fig. 10.2C). The prosthesis may extend just deep to the footplate but should not extend into the medial half of the vestibule (Fig. 10.3C). It is important to remember that the apparent penetration below the footplate estimated by CT may be more or less than the actual penetration anatomically, particularly in the case of a metallic prosthesis with streak artifact.[17] Second, audiometry trumps imaging. That is to say, if there is significant conductive hearing loss (CHL), even with a "satisfactory" imaging appearance, the patient will need revision surgery.

### Imaging After Stapedectomy

Stapes surgery is performed most commonly for otosclerosis with an intact ossicular chain but with stapes footplate fixation. The role of preoperative imaging is to confirm the diagnosis and exclude a third window that may be the actual cause of hearing loss. The extent of stapes resection is variable, and the footplate may remain in place. A stapedotomy is a small hole drilled and/or lasered in the footplate to facilitate placement of a prosthesis through the footplate. Surgery is considered successful if the air-bone gap is closed to 10 dB or less. In a large series with mobile malleus and incus, this was achieved in 94.2% of patients.[18]

In the typical case of otosclerosis, the malleus and incus remain, with a prosthesis attached to the long process of the incus extending medially through a stapedotomy. Penetration into the vestibule is variable, typically less than 50% of the width of the vestibule. Pneumolabyrinth is common in the first week after surgery. Beyond a week, a perilymphatic fistula should be suspected.[19]

In broad terms, over time patients may require revision surgery for recurrent CHL, sensorineural hearing loss (SNHL), vestibular symptoms, or mixed hearing loss. High-resolution CT may be useful in defining the etiology and for surgical planning purposes. In a study of patients undergoing revision stapes surgery, the authors were able to prospectively identify all cases of oval window dislocation, incus erosion with lateralized prosthesis, and short piston. Most but not all cases of obliterative otosclerosis were identified. CT was less accurate in cases of long pistons. Surgical findings in patients undergoing revision surgery without CT findings included a nonmobile piston encased in scar or new bone formation and prosthesis uncrimping.[20]

CHL after stapes surgery most frequently occurs on a delayed basis. In 80% of cases this results from prosthesis migration or dislocation. Lagleyre et al. in reporting their series of 119 revision surgeries for CHL described a "lateralized piston syndrome" in 18.5% of those revisions. Preoperative CT demonstrated a lateralized piston in 81% of cases touching the TM. In 54.5% there was closure of the stapedotomy with incus necrosis in 77%.[21] In a separate study of 201 revision stapes surgeries, prosthesis lateralization occurred in 53%, incus necrosis in 33%, reossification of the footplate in 31%, and uncrimping of the prosthesis to the incus in 9%.[22] Ossicular necrosis after stapes surgery most commonly involves the long process of the incus at the point of prosthesis attachment. There are rare reports of ossicular necrosis unrelated to ME disease or surgery.[23]

Vestibular symptoms and/or progressive SNHL occur in 0.6%–3% of patients after initial surgery and up to 14% of patients after revision surgery.[24] Etiologies include serous or infectious labyrinthitis, reparative granuloma, labyrinthine fistula, or intravestibular foreign body. Progressive otosclerosis may lead to CHL or SNHL and may be seen many years after the initial surgery. In a Swedish study evaluating patients 30 years after stapedectomy, patients demonstrated primarily progression of SNHL, which could not be explained by age alone.[25]

### Mastoidectomy

The term "mastoidectomy" is a general term referring to removal of a segment of the mastoid cortex and subjacent air cells to deal with disease, for access to the ME, inner ear (e.g., cochlear implantation), or endolymphatic sac (for shunting), or for the repair of superior canal dehiscence, etc.[26] Anterior and superiorly, the surgery may extend to the epitympanum and the anterior attic region, with the geniculate ganglion the anteriormost landmark. The size of the mastoidectomy defect is quite variable and depends on the degree of mastoid pneumatization, extent of disease, and procedures performed. The smallest defects are in patients with no mastoid disease, and the surgery is performed for the placement of an endolymphatic shunt (Fig. 10.4B). Large defects are seen in patients with well-pneumatized mastoids with extensive disease, and they require complete air cell exenteration. Rarely, patients may present after automastoidectomy; the CT appearance mimics a mastoid surgical defect (Fig. 10.4A).

Preoperatively, radiologists should make note of very sclerotic mastoids, especially those with almost no aeration of the mastoid antrum and a low-lying tegmen. In these patients, the transmastoid approach can be dangerous because it is difficult to delineate the lateral semicircular canal and second genu of the facial nerve, both of which may be injured at the time

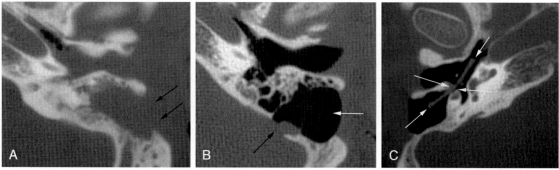

FIG. 10.4 Mastoid defects with intact posterior canal wall. **(A)** Axial CT, patient with history of radiation therapy and ear drainage, automastoidectomy (*black arrows*) with no history of surgery. **(B)** Small well-aerated mastoid defect (*white arrow*) after endolymphatic surgery. The shunt is superficial to the defect in the sinodural plate (*black arrow*). **(C)** Mastoid defect with extension through the facial recess (between *yellow arrows*), silastic extending through the defect into the middle ear (between *white arrows*) to prevent scarring of the tympanic membrane against the promontory before ossiculoplasty.

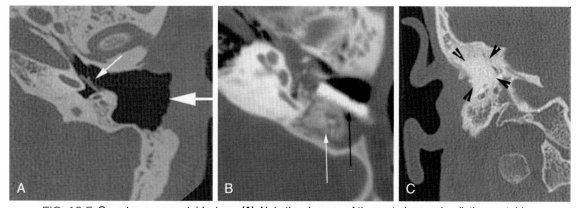

FIG. 10.5 Open tympanomastoidectomy **(A)**. Note the absence of the posterior canal wall; the mastoid is well aerated (*large white arrow*). Silastic in the middle ear to prevent scarring (*small white arrow*) before staged reconstruction. **(B)** "Open-closed" mastoidectomy with reconstruction of the posterior canal wall with hydroxyapatite sheets (*black arrow*) held in position by bone pate (*white arrow*). **(C)** Open mastoid, partial obliteration of the cavity with injectable hydroxyapatite (HydroSet, Stryker). Note lack of normal bone architecture in the uniformly dense HydroSet (*black arrowheads*).

of surgery. On postoperative scans in these patients it is common to see thinning of bone or small surgical defects in the mastoid tegmen, mastoid segment of cranial nerve (CN) 7, or sinodural plate.

The posterior wall of the EAC may be left intact or resected. When intact, this is commonly referred to as a "closed" mastoidectomy or mastoidectomy with intact posterior canal wall (Fig. 10.4C). If the posterior canal wall is removed, this is referred to as mastoidectomy with takedown of the posterior canal wall or "open" mastoidectomy (Fig. 10.5A). The posterior canal wall may be removed, allowing wider access to the ME and

mastoid, and then replaced or reconstructed immediately or at a later date (Fig. 10.5B). Materials used include the original canal wall, autologous bone, bone substitutes, or a prosthesis.[27–29] This reconstruction may be combined with mastoid "obliteration" to reduce the size of the mastoid defect for quality-of-life issues to include elimination of malodorous drainage, caloric-effect vertigo, and lifelong water precautions and for improved cosmesis, ease of care, and facilitating placement of a hearing aid (Fig. 10.5C).[30,31]

In the case of cholesteatoma, with the canal wall down mastoidectomy and meatoplasty, additional surgery is required in approximately 10% of patients.[31] With the intact canal wall mastoidectomy for cholesteatoma, historically a "second-look" surgery was often required, as residual/recurrent cholesteatoma was seen in a significant number of patients, even if the surgeon believes all cholesteatoma was removed grossly during the initial operation. A common site for recurrent cholesteatoma is around the oval window because complete surgical removal of the cholesteatoma around the facial nerve or that adherent to the mobile stapes footplate can result in facial nerve paralysis or SNHL, tinnitus, or dizziness with vertigo.

## FACIAL RECESS APPROACH

This approach is performed with an intact canal wall mastoidectomy with an opening made just medial to the chordal eminence and lateral to the mastoid segment of the facial nerve. This approach is used for cochlear implant surgery and as a means for removal of disease in the facial recess and ME (Fig. 10.4C).

### Atticotomy

An atticotomy refers to removal of the lateral wall of the epitympanum. This is not typically described separately for a patient after mastoidectomy, as the lateral wall may be removed as part of the mastoid procedure. On occasion, however, atticotomy alone is performed with variable absence of the scutum and lateral attic wall. The mastoid cortex and posterior canal wall appear normal. An isolated atticotomy is best visualized on coronal images.

## IMAGING THE POSTOPERATIVE MASTOID

Patients are not typically imaged immediately unless complications are suspected. Immediately after surgery, it is normal to see soft tissue swelling, absorbable gelatin sponge, mastoid cell opacification, and fluid levels. For intracranial complications, such as stroke, dural sinus thrombosis, abscess, or cerebritis, MR of the brain, MRA, and MRV are preferred. CT has a limited role but may be useful if there is clinical concern for cerebrospinal fluid (CSF) leak, facial nerve injury, or labyrinthine fistula.

In the more typical case, patients are imaged months or years after surgery for progressive hearing loss, drainage, or cholesteatoma. Postoperative CT imaging after mastoidectomy for inflammatory disease or cholesteatoma is challenging with regard to differentiating acute disease from chronic, nonactive disease or intentional mastoid obliteration. Mild flat smooth soft tissue thickening with otherwise good aeration is commonly seen and represents scar or granulation tissue. More extensive thickening, especially when accompanied by fluid or complete opacification of the ME and mastoid, is more likely to represent active disease. It is common to see soft tissue opacification of residual mastoid air cells and around the margins of the mastoid defect, especially if the margins are irregular with "overhanging" edges.[32] Patients with Eustachian tube dysfunction often have retained fluid.

Hazy ill-defined new bone formation is occasionally seen about the margins of the mastoid and ME. When seen, this should suggest active inflammation (Fig. 10.6A and B).

Tympanosclerosis (myringosclerosis if confined to the TM) refers to fibrous tissue, calcification, or new bone formation in response to chronic otitis media (Fig. 10.6D).[32]

It is important to note the presence and extent of tympanosclerosis. It is a cause of CHL poorly visualized by the surgeon. Tympanosclerotic fixation of the malleus and incus most commonly occurs in the lateral epitympanum or involves the stapes footplate. The scarring obliterates normal ME landmarks that the surgeon relies on for orientation. This increases morbidity and results in longer operative times.

Recurrent cholesteatoma may be difficult to diagnose with certainty by CT, especially when it is surrounded by inflammatory disease or fluid. Cholesteatoma may recur in the EAC, TM, ME, or mastoid. Progressive bone erosion should always raise concern, but this requires a baseline postoperative examination (rarely indicated) to be differentiated from preoperative erosion or operative drilling. A focal round soft tissue mass is suspicious but nonspecific and indicates differential considerations other than cholesteatoma, including encephalocele-meningocele and cholesterol granuloma (Fig. 10.6C and E). It is important to inspect the tegmen to be sure it is intact. On occasion, a mass will have irregular air-filled interstices from shedding of keratin debris (Fig. 10.6C). Rarely, the cholesteatoma contents are shed or removed, with only the peripheral matrix remaining, a so-called thin-walled or mural cholesteatoma. These cholesteatomas are very slow growing and may not be detectible by CT or MR.

### MR Diffusion Imaging for Cholesteatoma

The incidence of residual/recurrent cholesteatoma has been reported to be 9%–70% after intact canal wall surgery versus 4%–17% for canal wall down mastoidectomy.[33] For this reason, the historical standard of

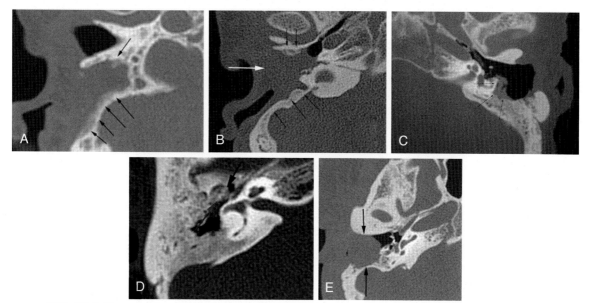

**FIG. 10.6** Signs of active disease. **(A)** Patient with drainage after open mastoidectomy. Hazy new bone formation is consistent with osteitis present about the periphery of the mastoid cavity (*black arrows*). **(B)** Three years after **(A)**, the bone has evolved/matured into more normal-appearing bone (*black arrows*). Interval conversion to an open mastoid with partial obliteration of the mastoid and EAC, the canal is over-sewn (*white arrow*) after **(A)** to control drainage. **(C)** There is irregular soft tissue in the deep aspect of the open mastoid (*black arrows*); air-filled crevices are nonspecific but suspicious for cholesteatoma. **(D)** Tympanosclerosis surrounds the ossicles in the epitympanum; the head of the malleus (*black arrow*) and incus body (*red arrow*) are barely discernable within the surrounding calcification. **(E)** Round soft tissue density (between *arrows*) in an open cavity is a nonspecific finding on CT. Primary considerations are cholesteatoma, encephalocele, or cholesterol granuloma.

care has been a second-look surgery, particularly with an intact canal wall. Historically, MR was infrequently performed because it seldom altered traditional surgical management.

Numerous articles over the past 10+years have explored the use of MR diffusion-weighted imaging (DWI), initially echo planar (EP), subsequently non-echo planar (NEP), for the detection of cholesteatoma.[34–37] Using the NEP-DWI, cholesteatomas as small as 2 mm have been reported.[38] In the context of the postoperative patient, this has resulted in a potential paradigm shift emphasizing MR over CT or second-look surgery for the detection of residual/recurrent cholesteatoma.[39,40]

On MR imaging, a cholesteatoma demonstrates T1 hypointense and T2 hyperintense signal. Post-Gd, there is usually a rim of enhancing tissue around the nonenhancing cholesteatoma (Fig. 10.7). Early reports described the benefit of delayed imaging after contrast administration; more recent reports suggest gadolinium is unnecessary unless otherwise indicated.

False positives in early reports included skull base artifact with EP-DWI; this is less of an issue with NEP-DWI. Other false positives have been from cartilage or bone dust (used in reconstruction), wax/cerumen, and mastoid abscess (usually evident clinically).[41,42] False negatives have occurred from tiny (less than 2 mm) or "mural" (thin-walled) cholesteatomas.[43] Improper technique and patient motion may also result in false negatives.

In one series, 31% of patients with a negative initial postoperative NEP-DWI study subsequently demonstrated DWI evidence for cholesteatoma.[44] In another study, 12 patients were followed up clinically without surgery, 7 of whom showed regression in size or absence of a persistent DWI finding on follow-up imaging.[45] The appropriate scanning interval and number of scans following surgery remains to be determined. Although these reports suggest imaging may be sufficient to exclude significant residual/recurrent disease, it will take time for otologists in general to abandon the concept of second-look surgery.

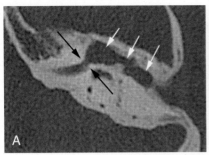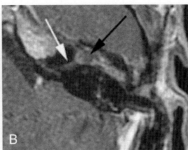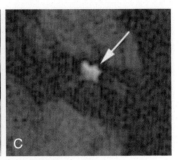

**FIG. 10.7** Patient with remote history of cholesteatoma surgery, negative interval imaging studies, and new-onset facial paresis. **(A)** Axial CT, nonspecific soft tissue opacification of the mastoid (*white arrows*) with subtle widening of the labyrinthine segment of the facial nerve (between *black arrows*). **(B)** Axial MR, T1 post-Gd, small focus of intermediate signal (*black arrow*) with surrounding enhancement along the course of the facial nerve (*white arrow*). **(C)** Non-echo-planar diffusion-weighted imaging (PROPELLER) sequence confirms the suspicion for recurrent cholesteatoma (*white arrow*).

## Superior Canal Dehiscence—Postoperative Imaging

Superior semicircular canal dehiscence (SSCD) syndrome was first reported by Dr. Minor in 1998.[46] The most common location for labyrinthine dehiscence (third window) is the arcuate eminence of the superior semicircular canal (SSC). Less common locations include between a superior petrosal sinus and the SSC, the posterior semicircular canal (spontaneous or from jugular vein enlargement/diverticulum), cochlear carotid interval, between the facial nerve and basal turn of the cochlea, or from a subarcuate vessel with the third window the undersurface of the SSC.[47-49] There have been reports of a similar third window phenomenon with lesions of the temporal bone, including meningioma, fibrous dysplasia, cavitary otosclerosis, and Paget disease.[50-52]

There is evidence that SSCD is part of a more general process of acquired skull base thinning that includes the temporal bone tegmen and geniculate ganglion, and the incidence increases with age.[53-58] An association with obesity and obstructive sleep apnea has been described, with or without CSF leak.[59]

Patients with SSCD are offered surgery if they fulfill three criteria. First, classic symptoms (pressure or sound-induced vertigo, oscillopsia, hyperacusis, autophony, aural fullness, hearing loss, and tinnitus). Second, evidence of a third window with absence of other findings that might explain the presenting symptoms such as otosclerosis. Third, testing results that support the diagnosis (audiometry, vestibular symptoms, vestibular evoked myogenic potential (ocular and cervical, oVEMP and cVEMP respectively) air-bone gap). Because the spectrum of defects ranges from "near

dehiscence" to "wide dehiscence," there is some basis to suggest that symptoms and test results will vary as well.[60-63] The final decision to perform surgery is the judgment of an experienced surgeon.

Surgery is performed via a middle cranial fossa or transmastoid approach.[61,62] The transmastoid approach has the advantage of avoiding a craniotomy with temporal lobe elevation but may be precluded by a low-lying tegmen. The surgical goal is to plug the superior canal on either side of the dehiscence with or without resurfacing of the defect.[64-69] In theory, both the plugging material and dehiscence covering should protect the remaining inner ear structures from CSF pulsations. This would favor "hard" (bone dust/chips/grafts, bone cement) over "soft" (fascia, bone wax) plugging and covering materials. An analysis of reported outcomes suggested the transmastoid approach has a lower complication and revision rate, with a shorter hospital stay.[70]

Imaging is typically reserved for persistent or recurrent symptoms. The postoperative imaging results may be quite variable depending on the site of the third window and the material used for plugging/resurfacing. In a report on revision surgery for failed initial surgery, the authors noted a variety of materials used for resurfacing, including fascia, bone chips, bone dust, bone wax, fibrin glue, injectable hydroxyapatite, a stapes piston, and bone grafts. In that series, 80% of patients had undergone both resurfacing of the dehiscence and plugging of the superior canal on both sides of the dehiscence.[71] In patients undergoing surgery for SSCD, it is common to see postsurgical changes involving a tegmen repair as well. Repair of a tegmen defect with little apparent surgical change by CT imaging at

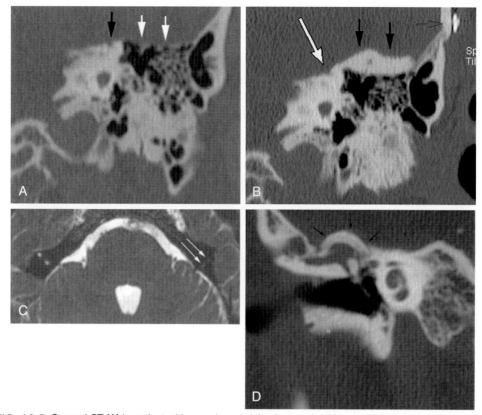

FIG. 10.8 Coronal CT **(A)** in patient with superior semicircular canal dehiscence (*black arrow*). The tegmen is thin (*white arrows*) at this level and dehiscent further anteriorly. **(B)** After repair via a middle cranial fossa approach (*red arrow*), the tegmen has been reinforced with HydroSet and is intact (*black arrows*). Note the indistinct lumen of the superior semicircular canal after plugging (*white arrow*), with no evidence of a "hard" cover. **(C)** Axial T2* FIESTA image confirms plugging of the canal on both sides of the dehiscence, with lack of normal labyrinthine fluid signal (*white arrows*). **(D)** Coronal CT in patient after the repair of a tegmen defect with cadaver sclera (*black arrows*), which was used in otologic surgery in the pre-HIV era.

the site of SSCD should not be mistaken for "wrong site" surgery or lateral migration of a "hard" cover (Fig. 10.8A,B, and D).

CT is typically the first-order technique used to evaluate persistent or recurrent symptoms. MRI may also be useful in select cases to confirm adequate plugging of the superior canal on both sides of the dehiscence by showing lack of fluid signal at the plug sites (Fig. 10.8C).

## Imaging of the Postoperative Internal Auditory Canal and Cerebellopontine Angle

Vestibular schwannomas (VSs) are the most commonly encountered internal auditory canal (IAC)-cerebellopontine angle (CPA) tumors followed in frequency by meningiomas. These lesions along with epidermoids account for over 90% of CPA tumors. Over 60 other

tumors account for the other 10%, most commonly facial schwannoma, lipochoristoma, and hemangioma. Tumors may present as a purely intracanalicular lesion (VS, meningioma, facial neuroma, hemangioma, lipoma, and so forth), within the CPA or in both regions.[72-74]

Once the tumors are diagnosed, the options include observation, surgery, radiotherapy, or a combination of all three. This chapter will not discuss radiotherapy or imaging algorithms for observation. There are three standard approaches to the IAC-CPA region with variations described in the literature. In general, the approach used depends more on the presence or absence of residual hearing and the expertise of the surgeons rather than the size or location of the lesion.

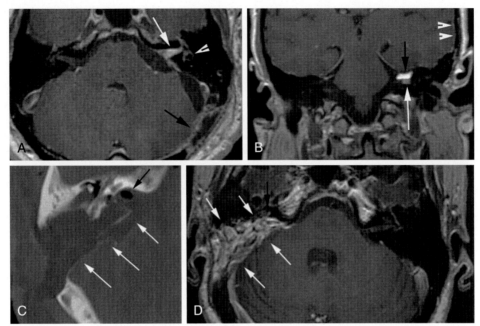

FIG. 10.9 Imaging after vestibular schwannoma (VS) surgery. **(A)** Baseline study after VS surgery via the retrosigmoid approach, axial T1 post-Gd. Enhancing scar tissue and fluid are present deep to the craniotomy (*black arrow*). There is scalloped widening of the cerebrospinal fluid cistern between the cerebellum and temporal bone. Enhancement in the internal auditory canal (IAC) (*white arrow*) is nonspecific and needs correlation with (1) precontrast T1 images, (2) the extent of tumor preoperatively, and (3) soft tissue that may have been placed at the time of surgery. Note an increased T1 signal in the labyrinth (*white arrowhead*) related to drilling of the posterior semicircular canal during surgery (blood versus granulation tissue). **(B)** Coronal T1 post-Gd image after VS surgery via a middle cranial fossa approach. Note subtle dural enhancement deep to the craniotomy (*white arrowheads*). The surgical defect in the roof of the IAC is filled with fat (*black arrow*). Enhancement in the IAC (*white arrow*) is nonspecific on this baseline postoperative scan. **(C)** Axial CT demonstrates fat filling the translabyrinthine surgical defect extending from the mastoid cortex to the IAC. Note the broad exposure to the posterior fossa (*white arrows*) and small volume of gas in the IAC (*black arrow*) on this CT performed the day after surgery. **(D)** Axial MR in a similar patient; fat and fascia fill the surgical defect (*white arrows*), including the IAC. Note preservation of the cochlea (*black arrow*).

## RETROSIGMOID APPROACH

The retrosigmoid approach typically involves a neurosurgeon performing a craniotomy with cerebellar retraction and the neurotologist performing any required drilling around the IAC with subsequent tumor removal. Advantages are that tumors of any size can be removed. There is excellent exposure to the CPA, lower cranial nerves, brainstem, and cerebellum. The cisternal segments of CN7 and CN8 are easily identified. After drilling of the IAC, the most difficult part of the surgery is the removal of the tumor around the porous acousticus, as the facial nerve is often splayed and adherent to the capsule of the tumor anteriorly.[75,76]

Monitoring of the facial nerve (CN7) significantly reduces the risk of facial paresis and paralysis. The use of intraoperative auditory nerve monitoring also reduces the risk of hearing loss caused by small tumors, usually those confined in the IAC.[77–79]

A weakness of this approach is that the lateral 2–3 mm of the IAC cannot be exposed without potential hearing loss from drilling into the posterior semicircular canal or into the vestibule, both of which could result in significant SNHL (Fig. 10.9A). If hearing is to be spared, then the lateral 2–3 mm of the IAC is not drilled and tumor may be left in this area. If the labyrinth is violated, preservation of the lateral semicircular canal is most critical. Careful removal of the superior and posterior semicircular canals can be performed without significant loss of hearing over 80% of the time (transcrusal approach to the petrous apex).[80,81]

## TRANSLABYRINTHINE APPROACH

This approach is used if there is no useful hearing on the side of the tumor. After an extended mastoid-ectomy, the labyrinth is drilled away with removal of all three of the semicircular canals and opening into the vestibule. The facial nerve can be followed directly from the second genu in the mastoid to the geniculate and points the way into the IAC. This approach was developed by Drs. William House and William Hitsel-berger for identification of the facial nerve.[82] When this approach was developed, there was no intraoperative facial nerve monitoring available. Bone over the sigmoid sinus is removed to allow placement of a retractor for better exposure of the CPA. Subsequently, the posterior wall of the IAC is removed and the tumor in the IAC and CPA is exposed and resected. The size of the defect depends on the exposure required. The cochlea is spared if the patient is a candidate for a cochlear implant (Fig. 10.9C and D).

This approach may be used for tumors of all sizes, with exposure facilitated by extensive drilling of bone lateral to the tumor. Wide access nearly to the midline can be achieved, extending anteriorly to the carotid and posteriorly to the sinodural plate. After tumor removal, the medial defect is covered with fascia and then filled laterally with fat. There is complete hearing loss after surgery. Advantages include early identification of CN7 lateral to the tumor (in the case of VS) and low incidence of tumor recurrence.[83] The incidence of headache is low, and the incidence of CSF leak is similar to that of the posterior fossa approach (about 5%). Disadvantages include lack of visualization of the brainstem until the tumor is resected and limited familiarity of the approach to neurosurgeons should complications arise.

## MIDDLE CRANIAL FOSSA APPROACH

After a subtemporal craniotomy, the dura along the floor of the middle cranial fossa is elevated along with the temporal lobe extradurally. The dura covering the middle cranial fossa floor is elevated medially to the petrous ridge, usually from a posterior to anterior direction, with the superior petrosal sinus as the medial landmark. The anterior limit is the middle meningeal artery.

Care is taken during dural elevation from posterior to anterior to look for dehiscence of the greater superficial petrosal nerve (40%–50%) or the SSC (5% or more). This method could result in facial nerve injury or hearing loss.[2,83] The location of the IAC can be found by locating the arcuate eminence or by locating the superior

petrosal nerve, which leads to the geniculate ganglion of the facial nerve. Imaging guidance can facilitate localization of both the SSC and IAC. The IAC superiorly is drilled from medial to lateral with special care laterally so as not to violate the SSC, labyrinthine portion of the facial nerve, and the basal turn of the cochlea.[84,85] These structures are the lateral limits of the exposure and are within 2–3 mm of each other. The labyrinthine portion of the facial nerve comes laterally from the lateral end of the IAC to the geniculate ganglion at a 45-degree angle, is not covered by dura, and is quite small. This is the portion of the facial nerve most commonly injured during middle fossa removal of a VS (Fig. 10.9B).

Advantages include better hearing preservation, low incidence of CSF leak and headache, excellent exposure to the lateral portion of the IAC, and less meningeal irritation. The dura does not need to be opened, and this protects the temporal lobe from further injury. Disadvantages are a higher incidence of CN7 injury, occasional memory disturbances, aphasia, and seizures.[86,87]

## TWO-STAGE SURGERY FOR VS

For so-called giant VS with the CPA component larger than 3 cm, there is support in the literature for a staged or less-than-complete resection of the tumor.[88,89] In one report, the first stage was performed via a retrosigmoid approach, with the CPA component debulked to relieve brainstem compression. The IAC was not drilled. During surgery, if there was cerebellar or brainstem edema, excessive adherence of tumor to the brainstem or CN7, a poorly stimulating facial nerve, or a thinned/splayed facial nerve, the remainder of the tumor was resected at a later date.[90] The second surgery is often translabyrinthine, as the facial nerve can be readily identified and followed to the tumor, facilitating preservation of function, and the tissue planes have not been disturbed by the earlier surgery (Fig. 10.10). There was better preservation of facial nerve function with the staged approach without a significant increase in morbidity. A second study comparing two-stage surgery with single-stage surgery with or without radiosurgery noted similar results.[89]

## COMPLICATIONS

Complications related to VS resection are uncommon but include hemorrhage, stroke, vascular injury, infection and meningitis, brainstem and cranial nerve injury, CSF leak, and death.[91–95] The incidence of cranial nerve injury has diminished with the availability of real-time monitoring. CN7 in particular can be difficult to identify

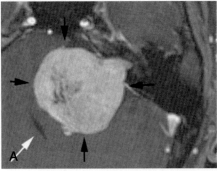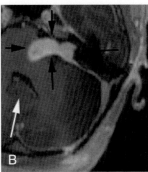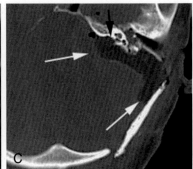

FIG. 10.10 Staged surgery for "giant" vestibular schwannoma (VS). **(A)** Axial T1 post-Gd preoperatively demonstrates a 4-cm VS (*black arrows*). Note the marked compression of the fourth ventricle (*white arrow*). **(B)** Axial T1 post-Gd MR after the first stage via a retrosigmoid approach. Note the residual tumor (*black arrows*) with diminished mass effect on the fourth ventricle (*white arrow*). **(C)** Axial CT 1 day after translabyrinthine resection of the residual tumor. Fat fills the surgical defect (*white arrows*) and the internal auditory canal (*black arrow*) to the level of the fundus.

secondary to displacement and effacement, adhesions, or involvement by the tumor. Transient pneumocephalis in the immediate postoperative period is expected but should not persist. CSF leaks may occur with all three approaches, especially if a combined approach is used. Air cells opened during the craniotomy or drilling around the IAC need to be sealed by bone wax, fascia, or resorbable mesh.[96,97] Leaks may resolve with conservative measures, such as elevation of the head and lumbar drains. Occasionally surgery is required, especially if the patient experiences meningitis. Over a 2- to 3-month basis, in patients with CSF leak, meningitis occurs 50% of the time.[91] Perioperative meningeal irritation is common and managed conservatively. A multiinstitutional review of all three approaches suggested the complication rates of each were comparable.[98]

## POSTOPERATIVE IMAGING

The need for postoperative imaging is dictated by the tumor pathology and completeness of resection. For benign lesions, such as VS, a baseline postoperative MR 6–12 months after surgery is helpful. If imaging is performed well beyond 12 months post surgery, it may be difficult to differentiate postoperative change from recurrent or residual disease without the baseline examination. This may lead to multiple unnecessary additional follow-up examinations to clarify. A baseline examination after uncomplicated surgery may be confined to the posterior fossa (unless otherwise indicated) and typically consists of thin T1 axial images pre-/post-Gd and thin T2* images (fast imaging employing steady-state acquisition [FIESTA], constructive interference in steady state).

CT is less useful for tumor exclusion after surgery but excludes larger tumors in patients in whom MR imaging is contraindicated. For bone-destroying or matrix-producing tumors, subtle destruction/creation of additional bone demonstrated by CT is more sensitive for detection of disease progression than is change of tumor size detected by MR imaging.

After translabyrinthine surgery, there is a triangular defect in the mastoid extending anteriorly through the labyrinth, the apex directed toward the IAC.[99,100] The vestibule and cochlea typically remain anteriorly. Signal in the residual labyrinth may be altered by blood, fibrosis, or ossification. On MR imaging, the fat graft filling the defect is the predominant feature early on but will resorb or atrophy over time and be replaced by air, fluid, or scar tissue (Fig. 10.10C). Fascia closing the dural defect is typically poorly visualized as is the resorbable is helpful. mesh used to prevent CSF leak.[96]

After a middle fossa approach, postoperative changes may be minimal and missed on axial images if the craniotomy is not noted.[99] Coronal imaging facilitates visualization of the surgical approach and postoperative alterations to the temporal lobe and roof of the IAC (Fig. 10.9B). There is typically a small volume of fat/fascia filling the defect in the roof of the IAC, which may partially protrude into the IAC. The IAC-CPA may look normal. Dural thickening or hyperemia may be seen in the portion of the dura elevated along the approach. The CPA may appear widened, especially if the tumor was large and the brainstem compressed.[101] Gliosis involving the inferior aspect of the temporal lobe will be missed unless sagittal or coronal FLAIR images are obtained.

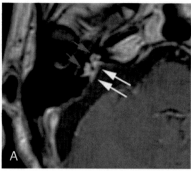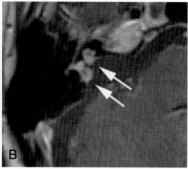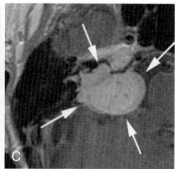

FIG. 10.11 Baseline axial T1 post-Gd image **(A)** after resection of a large vestibular schwannoma with labyrinthine extension (*red arrows*). Note the flat/concave medial contours to the residual enhancing tissue (*white arrows*). **(B)** One year later, there is a change with enhancing tissue now subtly convex medially in two locations (*white arrows*). Patient was lost to follow-up and returned 10 years later. **(C)** Note the large tumor (*white arrows*) now contacting the cerebellum and lateral margin of the brainstem.

After the retrosigmoid approach, the craniotomy defect will become subtler over time. The cerebellum commonly demonstrates variable encephalomalacia from retraction-infarction but may appear normal.[101] The CPA appears wide, especially if the tumor was large and the brainstem compressed. If the posterior wall of the IAC was drilled, there is a widened appearance to the porous acousticus. Alteration of the labyrinthine signal (blood, fibrosis, ossification, granulation tissue) indicates transgression of the semicircular canals, usually the posterior semicircular canal (Figs. 10.9A and 10.10B).

With all three approaches, scar, fascia, and dura may be rather unapparent or enhance in a linear or "whorled" fashion, the extent depending on the tumor size, dural repair, and so forth.[102–104] This is commonly confined to the region of the IAC but may be found anywhere along the surgical approach to the tumor. The prominence of enhancement decreases over time and then stabilizes after 12–24 months. Round or globular enhancement in the region of the original tumor should be viewed with suspicion (Fig. 10.11). For benign tumors, enhancement not in the original tumor bed should be considered scar/granulation tissue. Similarly, nodular enhancement in the fundus of the IAC is less concerning if the tumor did not originally extend there.[105,106] If muscle or other tissue was used to fill a defect, this may mimic enhancing tumor and should be correlated clinically. On follow-up imaging it should remain stable or atrophy.

The tumor may be incompletely removed for clinical reasons. With "near-total" resection, the residual tumor may be devitalized by laser or cautery. If the tumor is not resected in a second-stage surgery, patients are followed up with more frequent imaging after the 6-month baseline examination for evaluation of the growth potential (if any) of the residua. On rare occasions patients will have progressive disease after both surgery and radiotherapy.

In all the three approaches, bone wax may be used to control bleeding or to seal air cells exposed at the time of surgery. With the retrosigmoid and translabyrinthine approaches, wax may migrate into the sigmoid sinus, mimicking a thrombosis.[107]

The appearance of CN7 after surgery is quite variable (authors' observations). With small tumors, CN7 appears normal and can be traced from the brainstem to at least the porous. With larger tumors, CN7 is stretched and displaced, typically anteriorly and either superiorly or inferiorly depending on the nerve of origin. In the CPA, the nerve may have a bowed appearance, concave posteriorly (Fig. 10.12B). It may appear relatively normal in thickness or be obscured either from adhesions or residual tumor (Fig. 10.12A). After removing a large tumor, it is unusual for the nerve to be fully visualized. This makes evaluation of CN7 difficult in those patients who have postoperative facial paralysis or paresis because lack of definitive visualization of CN7 is common and does not necessarily indicate injury or transection.

## SUMMARY

Interpreting CT and MR images in patients who have undergone surgery in the ME, mastoid, or CPA-IAC can be challenging. Understanding the surgical options and typical/atypical postoperative appearance in these regions facilitates rendering interpretations that are both succinct and accurate.

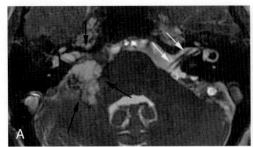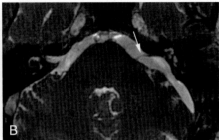

FIG. 10.12 Postoperative facial nerve evaluation. **(A)** Axial T2* FIESTA. After partial resection of a large vestibular schwannoma, there is a complex combination of fluid, scar, and tumor (*black arrows*), which precludes identification of the facial nerve as a discrete structure. Note the normal CN7 on the left (*white arrows*). **(B)** Axial T2* FIESTA. Probable identification of CN7, displaced anteriorly through the cerebellopontine angle (*white arrow*), poorly seen laterally through the surgically widened internal auditory canal.

# REFERENCES

1. Mingkwansook V, Curtin HD, Kelly HR. CT findings in the external auditory canal after transcanal surgery. *AJNR Am J Neuroradiol.* 2015;36:982–986.
2. Jackler RK, Brackman DE. *Neurotology.* Philadelphia: Elsevier/Mosby; 2005.
3. Fisch U. Myringoplasty. In: *Tympanoplasty, Mastoidectomy and Stapes Surgery.* New York: Thieme; 1994:10–40.
4. Fisch U. Tympanoplasty. In: *Tympanoplasty, Mastoidectomy and Stapes Surgery.* New York: Thieme; 1994:2–7.
5. Wullstein H. Theory and practice of tympanoplasty. *Laryngoscope.* 1956;66:1076–1093.
6. Austin DF. Ossicular reconstruction. *Arch Otolaryngol.* 1971;94:525–535.
7. Belluci RJ. Dual classification of tympanoplasty. *Laryngoscope.* 1973;83:1754–1758.
8. Kartush JM. Ossicular chain reconstruction: capitulum to malleus. *Otolaryngol Clin N Am.* 1994;27:689–715.
9. Fisch U. Ossiculoplasty. In: *Tympanoplasty, Mastoidectomy and Stapes Surgery.* New York: Thieme; 1994:44–116.
10. Stone JA, Mukherji SK, Jewett BS, et al. CT evaluation of prosthetic ossicular reconstruction procedures. *Radiographics.* 2000;20:593–605.
11. Baker AB, O'Connell BP, Nguyen SA, Lambert PR. Ossiculoplasty with titanium prosthesis in patients with intact stapes: comparison of TORP versus PORP. *Otol Neurotol.* 2015;36:1676–1682.
12. Hudson SK, Gurgel RK, Shelton C. Revision stapedectomy with bone cement: are results comparable to those of standard techniques? *Otol Neurotol.* 2014;35:1501–1503.
13. House JW, Lupo JE, Goddard JC. Management of incus necrosis in revision stapedectomy using hydroxyapatite bone cement. *Otol Neurotol.* 2014;35:1312–1316.
14. Mangham Jr CA. Long term impact of incus necrosis on revision stapes surgery: incus versus malleus reconstruction. *Otol Neurotol.* 2009;30:1145–1151.
15. Lane JI, Witte RJ, Driscoll CL, et al. Imaging microscopy of the middle and inner ear: CT microscopy. *Clin Anat.* 2004;17:607–612.
16. Fatterpekar GM, Doshi AH, Dugar M, et al. Role of 3D CT in the evaluation of the temporal bone. *Radiographics.* 2006;26:S117–S132.
17. Hahn Y, Diaz R, Hartman J, et al. Assessing stapes piston position using computed tomography: a cadaveric study. *Otol Neurotol.* 2009;30:223–230.
18. Vincent R, Sperling N, Oates J, et al. Surgical findings and long-term hearing results in 3,050 stapedotomies for primary otosclerosis: a prospective study with the otology-neurotology database. *Otol Neurotol.* 2006;27:S25–S47.
19. Bajin MD, Mocan BO, Sarac S, Sennaroglu L. Early computed tomography findings in the inner ear after stapes surgery and its clinical correlations. *Otol Neurotol.* 2013;34:639–643.
20. Whetstone J, Nguyen A, Nguyen-Huynh A, Hamilton BE. Surgical and clinical confirmation of temporal bone CT findings in patients with otosclerosis with failed stapes surgery. *AJNR Am J Neuroradiol.* 2014;35:1195–1201.
21. Lagleyre S, Calmels MN, Escude B, et al. Revision stapes surgery: the "lateralized piston syndrome". *Otol Neurotol.* 2009;30:1138–1144.
22. Schmid P, Hausler R. Revision stapedectomy: an analysis of 201 operations. *Otol Neurotol.* 2009;30:1092–1100.
23. Choudhury N, Kumar G, Krishnan M, et al. Atypical incus necrosis: a case report and literature review. *J Laryngol Otol.* 2008;122:1124–1126.
24. Yehudai N, Luntz M. Resolution of delayed sudden sensorineural hearing loss after stapedectomy: a case report and review of the literature. *Med J Otol.* 2006;3:156–160.
25. Redfors YD, Moller C. Otosclerosis: thirty-year follow-up after surgery. *Ann Otol Rhinol Laryngol.* 2011;120:608–614.
26. Fisch U. Mastoidectomy. In: *Tympanoplasty, Mastoidectomy and Stapes Surgery.* New York: Thieme; 1994:146–197.
27. Walker PC, Mowry SE, Hansen MR, Gantz BJ. Long-term results of canal wall reconstruction tympanomastoidectomy. *Otol Neurotol.* 2013;35:e24–e30.
28. Deveze A, Rameh C, Puchol MS, et al. Rehabilitation of canal wall down mastoidectomy using a titanium ear canal implant. *Otol Neurotol.* 2010;31:220–224.

29. Schwager K, Zirkler J. Reconstruction of the mastoid using a titanium cage. *Otol Neurotol.* 2014;35:1463–1465.

30. Cox MD, Dunlap QA, Trinidade A, Dornhoffer JL. Long-term outcomes after secondary mastoid obliteration. *Otol Neurotol.* 2016;37:1358–1365.

31. Harun A, Clark J, Semenov YR, Francis HW. The role of obliteration in the achievement of a dry mastoid bowl. *Otol Neurotol.* 2015;36:1510–1517.

32. Schuknecht HF. *Pathology of the Ear.* Malvern, PA: Lea and Febiger; 1993:563–574.

33. Tomlin J, Chang D, McCutcheon B, Harris J. Surgical technique and recurrence in cholesteatoma: a meta-analysis. *Audiol Neurootol.* 2013;18:135–142.

34. Venail F, Bonafe A, Poirrier V, Mondain M, Uziel A. Comparison of echo-planar diffusion-weighted imaging and delayed postcontrast T1-weighted MR imaging for the detection of residual cholesteatoma. *AJNR Am J Neuroradiol.* 2008;29:1363–1368.

35. Schwartz KM, Lane JI, Bolster Jr BD, Neff BA. The utility of diffusion-weighted imaging for cholesteatoma evaluation. *AJNR Am J Neuroradiol.* 2011;32:430–436.

36. Mudit J, Riskalla A, Jiang D, et al. A systematic review of diffusion-weighted magnetic resonance imaging in the assessment of postoperative cholesteatoma. *Otol Neurotol.* 2011;32:1243–1249.

37. Mas-Estelles F, Mateos-Fernandez M, Carrascosa-Bisquert B, et al. Contemporary non-echo-planar diffusion-weighted imaging of middle ear cholesteatomas. *Radiographics.* 2012;32:1197–1213.

38. De Foer B, Vercruysse JP, Pilet J, et al. Single-shot, turbo spin-echo, diffusion-weighted imaging versus spin-echo-planar, diffusion weighted imaging in the detection of acquired middle ear cholesteatoma. *AJNR Am J Neuroradiol.* 2006;27:1480–1482.

39. Migirov L, Tal S, Eyal A, Kronenberg J. MRI, not CT, to rule out recurrent cholesteatoma and avoid unnecessary second-look mastoidectomy. *Isr Med Assoc J.* 2009;11:144–146.

40. Lingam RK, Nash R, Majithia A, et al. Non-echoplanar diffusion weighted imaging in the detection of postoperative middle ear cholesteatoma: navigating beyond the pitfalls to find the pearl. *Insights Imaging.* 2016;7(5):669–678.

41. Karandikar A, Loke SC, Goh J, et al. Evaluation of cholesteatoma: our experience with DW propeller imaging. *Acta Radiol.* 2015;56(9):1108–1112.

42. Migirov L, Wolf M, Greenberg G, Eyal A. Non-EPI DW in planning the surgical approach to primary and recurrent cholesteatoma. *Otol Neurotol.* 2013;35:121–125.

43. Barath K, Huber AM, Stampfli P, Varga Z, Kollias S. Neuroradiology of cholesteatomas. *AJNR Am J Neuroradiol.* 2011;32:221–229.

44. Steens S, Venderink W, Kunst D, et al. Repeated postoperative follow-up diffusion-weighted magnetic resonance imaging to detect residual or recurrent cholesteatoma. *Otol Neurotol.* 2016;37:356–361.

45. Wong PY, Lingam RK, Pal S, et al. Monitoring progression of 12 cases of non-operated middle ear cholesteatoma with non-echoplanar diffusion weighted magnetic resonance imaging: our experience. *Otol Neurotol.* 2016;37:1573–1576.

46. Minor LZB, Solomon D, Zinreich JS, Zee DS. Sound-and/or-pressure induced vertigo due to bone dehiscence of the superior semicircular canal. *Arch Otolaryngol Head Neck Surg.* 1998;124(3):249–258.

47. Gopen QG, Zhou G, Poe D, Kenna M, Jones D. Posterior semicircular canal dehiscence: first reported case series. *Otol Neurotol.* 2010;31(2):339–344.

48. McCall AA, McKenna MJ, Merchant SN, Curtin HD, Lee DJ. Superior canal dehiscence syndrome associated with the superior petrosal sinus in pediatric and adult patients. *Otol Neurotol.* 2011;32:1312–1319.

49. Fang CH, Chung SY, Blake DM, et al. Prevalence of cochlear-facial dehiscence in a study of 1,020 temporal bone specimens. *Otol Neurotol.* 2016;37(7):967–972.

50. McCall AA, Curtin HD, McKenna MJ. Posterior semicircular canal dehiscence arising from temporal bone fibrous dysplasia. *Otol Neurotol.* 2010;31:1516–1517.

51. Crane BT, Carey JP, McMenomey S, Minor LB. Meningioma causing superior canal dehiscence syndrome. *Otol Neurotol.* 2010;31:1009–1010.

52. Makerem AO, Hoang TA, Lo WWM, Linthicum FH, Fayad JN. Cavitating otosclerosis: clinical, radiologic and histopathologic correlations. *Otol Neurotol.* 2010;31:381–384.

53. Whyte J, Tejedor MT, Faile JJ, et al. Association between tegmen tympani status and superior semicircular canal pattern. *Otol Neurotol.* 2015;36:66–69.

54. Nadaraja GS, Gurgel RK, Fischbein NJ, et al. Radiographic evaluation of the tegmen in patients with superior semicircular canal dehiscence. *Otol Neurotol.* 2012;33:1245–1250.

55. Nelson RF, Hansen KR, Gantz BJ, Hansen MR. Calvarium thinning in patients with spontaneous cerebrospinal fluid leak. *Otol Neurotol.* 2014;36:481–485.

56. Isaacson B, Vrabec JT. The radiographic prevalence of geniculate ganglion dehiscence in normal and congenitally thin temporal bones. *Otol Neurotol.* 2007;28:107–110.

57. Nadgir RN, Ozonoff A, Devaiah AK, et al. Superior semicircular canal dehiscence: congenital or acquired condition? *AJNR Am J Neuroradiol.* 2011;32:947–949.

58. Lookabaugh S, Kelly HR, Carter MS, et al. Radiologic classification of superior canal dehiscence: implications for surgical repair. *Otol Neurotol.* 2015;36:118–125.

59. Schutt CA, Neubauer P, Samy RN, et al. The correlation between obesity, obstructive sleep apnea and superior semicircular canal dehiscence: a new explanation for an increasingly common problem. *Otol Neurotol.* 2014;36:551–554.

60. Pfammatter A, Darrouzet V, Gartner M, et al. A superior semicircular canal dehiscence syndrome multicenter study: is there an association between size and symptoms? *Otol Neurotol.* 2010;31:447–454.

61. Yuen HW, Boeddinghaus R, Eikelboom RH, et al. The relationship between the air-bone gap and the size of superior semi-circular canal dehiscence. *Otolaryngol Head Neck Surg.* 2009;141:689–694.

62. Lookabaugh S, Niesten MEF, Owoc M, et al. Audiologic, cVEMP and radiologic progression in superior canal dehiscence syndrome. *Otol Neurotol.* 2016;37:1393–1398.

63. Ward BK, Wenzel A, Ritzl EK, et al. Near-dehiscence: clinical findings in patients with thin bone over the superior semicircular canal. *Otol Neurotol.* 2013;34:1421–1428.

64. Beyea JA, Agrawal SK, Parnes LS. Transmastoid semicircular canal occlusion: a safe and highly effective treatment for benign paroxysmal positional vertigo and superior canal dehiscence. *Laryngoscope.* 2012;122:1862–1866.

65. Shaia WT, Diaz RC. Evolution in surgical management of superior canal dehiscence syndrome. *Curr Opin Otolaryngol Head Neck Surg.* 2013;21:497–502.

66. Phillips DJ, Souter MA, Vitkovic J, Briggs RJ. Diagnosis and outcomes of middle cranial fossa repair for patients with superior semicircular canal dehiscence syndrome. *J Clin Neurosci.* 2010;17:339–341.

67. Lundy L, Zapala D, Moushey J. Cartilage cap occlusion technique for dehiscent superior semicircular canals. *Otol Neurotol.* 2011;32:1281–1284.

68. Teixido M, Seymour PE, Kung B, Sabra O. Transmastoid middle fossa craniotomy repair of superior semicircular canal dehiscence using a soft tissue graft. *Otol Neurotol.* 2011;32:877–881.

69. Powell HRF, Khalil SS, Saeed SR. Outcomes of transmastoid surgery for superior semicircular canal dehiscence syndrome. *Otol Neurotol.* 2016;37(7):e228–e233.

70. Ziylan F, Kinaci A, Beynon AJ, Kunst HPM. A comparison of surgical treatments for superior semicircular canal dehiscence: a systematic review. *Otol Neurotol.* 2017;38:1–10.

71. Sharon JD, Pross SE, Ward BK, Carey JP. Revision surgery for superior canal dehiscence syndrome. *Otol Neurotol.* 2016;37:1096–1103.

72. Calzada AP, Go JL, Tschirhart DL, Brackmann DE, Schwartz MS. Cerebellopontine angle and intracanalicular masses mimicking vestibular schwannomas. *Otol Neurotol.* 2014;36:491–497.

73. Schuknecht HF. *Pathology of the Ear.* 2nd ed. Malvern, PA: Lea and Febiger; 1993:210–211.

74. Eisenman D, Voight EP, Selesnick SH. Unusual tumors of the internal auditory canal and cerebellopontine angle. In: Jackler RK, Driscoll CLW, eds. *Tumors of the Ear and Temporal Bone.* Philadelphia, PA: Lippincott Williams and Wilkins; 2000:236–275.

75. Driscoll CLW. Vestibular schwannoma (acoustic neuroma). In: Jackler RK, Driscoll CLW, eds. *Tumors of the Ear and Temporal Bone.* Philadelphia, PA: Lippincott Williams and Wilkins; 2000:172–218.

76. Mazzoni A, Calabrese V, Danesi G. A modified retrosigmoid approach for direct exposure of the fundus of the internal auditory canal for hearing preservation in acoustic neuroma surgery. *Am J Otol.* 2000;21(1):98–109.

77. Bennett M, Haynes D. Surgical approaches and complications in the removal of vestibular schwannomas. *Otolaryngol Clin N Am.* 2007;40:589–609.

78. Moriyama T, Fukushima T, Asaoka K, et al. Hearing preservation in acoustic neuroma surgery: importance of adhesions between the cochlear nerve and the tumor. *J Neurosurg.* 2002;97(2):337–340.

79. Yingling CD, Gardi JN. Intraoperative monitoring of facial and cochlear nerves during acoustic neuroma surgery. *Otolaryngol Clin N Am.* 1992;25(2):413–448.

80. Horgan MA, Delashaw JB, Schwartz MS, et al. Transcrusal approach to the petroclival region with hearing preservation. *J Neurosurg.* 2001;94:660–666.

81. Kaylie DM, Horgan MA, Delashaw JB, McMenomey SO. Hearing preservation with the transcrusal approach to the petroclival region. *Otol Neurotol.* 2004;25:594–598.

82. House WF, Luetje CM. Management. In: *Acoustic Tumors.* vol. II. Baltimore: Univ Park Press; 1979:43–88.

83. Schmerber S, Palombi O, Boubagra K, et al. Long-term control of vestibular schwannoma after a translabyrinthine complete removal. *Neurosurgery.* 2005;57(4):693–698.

84. House WF, Luetje CM. Management. In: *Acoustic Tumors.* vol. II. Baltimore: Univ Park Press; 1979:15–42.

85. Driscoll CL, Jackler RK, Pitts LH, et al. Is the entire fundus of the internal auditory canal visible during the middle fossa approach for acoustic neuroma? *Am J Otol.* 2000;21(3):382–388.

86. Schick B, Greess H, Gill S, et al. Magnetic resonance imaging and neuropsychological testing after middle fossa vestibular schwannoma surgery. *Otol Neurotol.* 2008;29(1):39–45.

87. Bryce GE, Nedzelski JM, Rowed DW, et al. Cerebrospinal fluid leaks and meningitis in acoustic neuroma surgery. *Otolaryngol Head Neck Surg.* 1991;104(1):81–87.

88. Schwartz MS, Kari E, Strickland BM, et al. Evaluation of the increased use of partial resection of large vestibular schwannomas: facial nerve outcomes and recurrence/regrowth rates. *Otol Neurotol.* 2013;34:1456–1464.

89. Porter RG, LaRouere MJ, Kartush JM, et al. Improved facial nerve outcomes using an evolving treatment method for large acoustic neuromas. *Otol Neurotol.* 2013;34:304–310.

90. Raslan AM, Liu JK, McMenomey SO, Delashaw Jr MD. Staged resection of large vestibular schwannomas. *J Neurosurg.* 2012;116(5):1126–1133.

91. Ross D, Rosegay H, Pons V. Differentiation of aseptic and bacterial meningitis in postoperative neurosurgical patients. *J Neurosurg.* 1988;69(5):669–674.

92. Hegarty JL, Jackler RK, Rigby PL, et al. Distal anterior inferior cerebellar artery syndrome after acoustic neuroma surgery. *Otol Neurotol.* 2002;23(4):560–571.

93. Mass SC, Wiet RJ, Dinces E. Complications of the translabyrinthine approach for the removal of acoustic neuromas. *Arch Otolaryngol Head Neck Surg.* 1999;125(7):801–804.

94. Ajolloveyan M, Doust B, Atlas MD, et al. Pneumocephalus after acoustic neuroma surgery. *Am J Otol.* 1998;19(6):824–827.
95. Falcioni M, Romano G, Aggarwal N, et al. Cerebrospinal fluid leak after retrosigmoid excision of vestibular schwannomas. *Otol Neurotol.* 2008;29:384–386.
96. Hunter JB, Sweeney AD, Carlson ML, et al. Prevention of postoperative cerebral fluid leaks after translabyrinthine tumor resection with resorbable mesh cranioplasty. *Otol Neurotol.* 2015;36:1537–1542.
97. Gal TJ, Bartels LJ. Use of bone wax in the prevention of cerebrospinal fluid fistula in acoustic neuroma surgery. *Laryngoscope.* 1999;109(1):167–169.
98. Tolisano AM, Littlefield PD. *Adverse Events Following Vestibular Schwannoma Surgery: A Comparison of Surgical Approach. Otol Neurotol.* 2017;38:551–554.
99. Brors D, Schafers M, Bodmer D, et al. Postoperative magnetic resonance imaging findings after transtemporal and translabyrinthine vestibular schwannoma resection. *Laryngoscope.* 2003;113:420–426.
100. Silk PS, Lane JL, Driscoll CL. Surgical approaches to vestibular schwannomas: what the radiologist needs to know. *Radiographics.* 2009;29:1955–1970.
101. Bordure P, O'Donoghue GM, Jaspan T, et al. Cerebellar encephalomalacia after removal of acoustic tumor. *Otolaryngol Head Neck Surg.* 1999;121(1):144–149.
102. Weissman JL, Hirsch BE, Fukui MD, et al. The evolving MR appearance of structures in the internal auditory canal after removal of an acoustic neuroma. *AJNR Am J Neuroradiol.* 1997;18(3):313–323.
103. Umezu H, Seki Y. Postoperative magnetic resonance imaging after acoustic neuroma surgery: influence of packing material in the drilled internal auditory canal on assessment of residual tumor. *Neurol Med Chiro (Tokyo).* 1999;39(2):141–147.
104. Bennett ML, Jackson CG, Kaufmann R, et al. Postoperative imaging of vestibular schwannomas. *Otolaryngol Head Neck Surg.* 2008;138:667–671.
105. Carlson ML, Van Abel KM, Schmitt WR, et al. Nodular enhancement within the internal auditory canal following retrosigmoid vestibular schwannoma resection: a unique radiologic pattern. *J Neurosurg.* 2011;115:835–841.
106. Vorasubin N, Miller ME, Mastrodimos B, Cueva RA. Enhancing tissue in the internal auditory canal after retrosigmoid vestibular schwannoma resection. *Otol Neurotol.* 2016;37:e178–e179.
107. Byrns K, Khasgiwala A, Patel S. Migration of bone wax into the sigmoid sinus after posterior fossa surgery. *AJNR Am J Neuroradiol.* 2016;37:2129–2133.

## FURTHER READING

1. Brackman DE, Shelton C, Arriaga MA. *Otologic Surgery.* 3rd ed. Philadelphia: Saunders Elsevier.

# CHAPTER 11

# Petrous Apex

ILONA M. SCHMALFUSS, MD

## INTRODUCTION

The petrous apex is the most medial portion of the temporal bone. Its deep location precludes direct clinical examination and safe percutaneous biopsy. In addition, many of the petrous apex lesions are asymptomatic or present with nonspecific symptoms such as headache, making it harder to justify an invasive procedure for diagnostic purposes. Therefore, the referring physician primarily relies upon imaging for the evaluation of petrous apex abnormalities. Fortunately, many of the petrous apex lesions have characteristic imaging features that allow for correct diagnosis. However, anatomic variations of the petrous apex may mimic an underlying pathology. Hence, the radiologist is required to be familiar with the petrous apex anatomy, normal anatomic variations, and imaging features of the different disease processes to facilitate accurate image interpretation with high degree of confidence.

## ANATOMY

The petrous apex forms the medial temporal bone and resembles a pyramid, with its tip pointing anteromedially and its base posterolaterally. Its roof forms the floor of the middle cranial fossa and its posterior border constitutes the anterior wall of the posterior cranial fossa. It is separated by the petrosphenoidal fissure from the greater sphenoid wing, the petrooccipital synchondrosis from the occipital bone, and by the petroclival suture from the clivus.[1]

The petrous apex is subdivided into a larger anterior and a smaller posterior portion by the internal auditory canal (Fig. 11.1).[1] The anterior portion usually contains bone marrow, whereas the posterior portion is very dense in appearance, as it derives from the otic capsule (Fig. 11.1).[1] In 30% of patients, the petrous apex is pneumatized via tracts that directly communicate with the middle ear cavity or mastoid air cells. These tracts provide direct "pathways" for spread of diseases from the otomastoid region to the petrous apex and vice versa.[1,2]

The petrous apex contains a few important neurovascular structures:[3,4]

- The horizontal carotid canal runs within the anterior petrous bone (Fig. 11.2). It houses the petrous internal carotid artery (ICA) (C2 segment) and the sympathetic plexus. It is separated from the middle ear cavity by a thin, bony lamella that is often demineralized and dehiscent in older patients (Fig. 11.2).[5]
- The internal auditory canal (IAC) extends in coronal plane in relationship to the skull. It houses the facial nerve (cranial nerve [CN] VII) in the anterosuperior quadrant, the cochlear nerve in the anteroinferior quadrant, and the superior and inferior divisions of the vestibular nerve in the posterior quadrants. All four nerves are present only within the lateral IAC, as the different branches of the vestibulocochlear nerve (CN VIII) separate in the mid portion of the IAC. Therefore, only two nerves are typically identified in the medial IAC and in the cerebellopontine (CP) cistern.[6] In addition, the inferior vestibular nerve subdivides into the saccular and singular nerves. The singular nerve extends posterolaterally to the vestibule within the singular canal, which is consistently visible on temporal bone CT studies and should not be mistaken for a fracture.[7]
- The Dorello canal courses through the petrous apex tip along the petroclival suture. It is bounded by the petrosphenoidal ligament (aka Gruber ligament) superiorly and a small bony notch inferiorly. It houses the abducens nerve (CN VI), which is surrounded by a small venous plexus and a dural sleeve in the posterior canal.[3] Only the bony notch is usually seen on high-resolution CT studies (Fig. 11.2). On MRI, the cerebrospinal fluid-filled dural sleeve may be identified on high-resolution T2 sequences. Occasionally, faint enhancement of the venous plexus is noted, which should not be mistaken for pathology in an asymptomatic patient.[3]
- The arcuate canal (aka petromastoid canal) contains the arcuate vessels and courses between the crura of

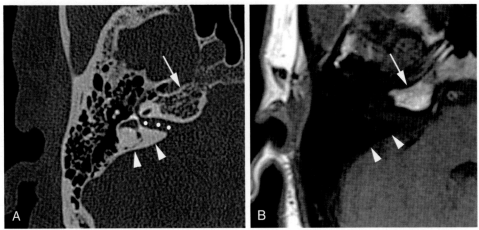

FIG. 11.1 **Subdivisions of the Petrous Apex and Their Imaging Appearance.** Axial CT image displayed in bone window **(A)** demonstrates the internal auditory canal (*dots*) subdividing the petrous apex into a larger, bone marrow-containing anterior part (*arrow*) and a smaller, dense-appearing posterior portion (*arrowheads*). On the T1-weighted image without contrast **(B)**, these exhibit different signal intensities, with the posterior petrous apex assuming very low signal intensity (*arrowheads*) because of the increased mineralization and the anterior part showing T1 hyperintensity (*arrow*) related to fatty bone marrow replacement in older patient. In younger patients, intermediate signal intensity of the still active bone marrow would be expected.

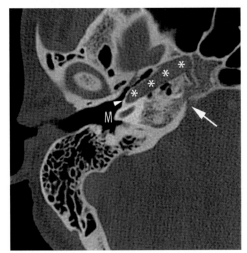

FIG. 11.2 **Location of Neurovascular Channels Within the Petrous Apex.** The axial CT image displayed in bone window shows the horizontal carotid canal (*asterisks*) that is located in the anterior petrous apex. It is separated from the middle ear cavity (M) by a thin bony lamella (*arrowhead*) that can get demineralized and partially dehiscent with aging. Notice also the bony notch (*arrow*) along the posterior petrous apex leading to the Dorello canal.

the superior semicircular canal (Fig. 11.3). Owing to its very small size, it is inconsistently visible on imaging and might be mistaken for a fracture.

- The Meckel cave, a dural-lined, cerebrospinal fluid-filled pocket within the posterior cavernous sinus, forms a marked depression in the anterosuperior petrous apex. It houses the rootlets of the trigeminal nerve and the trigeminal ganglion (aka Gasserian ganglion) along its inferior boundary.[3]

## CLINICAL PRESENTATIONS

Patients with petrous apex lesions are typically asymptomatic or present with nonspecific symptoms, e.g., headache or ear pain. As lesions enlarge, they might involve adjacent anatomic structures such as the cavernous sinuses or posterior cranial fossa and present with cranial neuropathies leading to sensorineural hearing loss, vertigo, double vision, facial pain, or facial weakness.

## ANATOMIC VARIATIONS AND PATHOLOGIC ENTITIES OF THE PETROUS APEX

Petrous apex abnormalities can be grouped into five categories based on origin, petrous apex size, and aggressiveness: (1) lesions related to neurovascular channels,

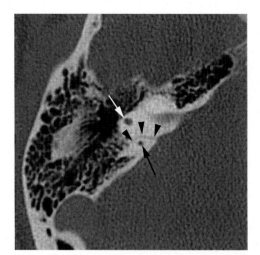

**FIG. 11.3 The Arcuate Canal.** Axial CT image displayed in bone window reveals a thin, lucent line (*arrowheads*) between the crura of the superior semicircular canal (*arrows*). This is the characteristic location for the arcuate canal that is inconsistently seen, even on high-resolution CT studies. Therefore, it is sometimes mistaken for a fracture. Petrous apex fractures, however, have a tendency to extend perpendicular to the long axis of the temporal bone and involve the internal auditory canal and/or cochlea (see Fig. 11.8 for comparison).

(2) intrinsic lesions without petrous apex enlargement, (3) intrinsic lesions with petrous apex enlargement and nonaggressive appearance, (4) intrinsic lesions with aggressive features, and (5) extrinsic petrous apex lesions. Even though some aggressive diseases might manifest without enlargement or destructive features in the early stages of disease, such classification provides a reasonable approach to generate a list of differential diagnostic considerations.

## Petrous Apex Lesions Related to Neurovascular Channels

### Absence and hypoplasia of the internal carotid artery

Congenital absence or hypoplasia of the ICA is exceedingly rare.[8,9] Patients are typically asymptomatic because a well-established collateral flow is present through the circle of Willis and more rarely through persistent fetal or extracranial collaterals (Fig. 11.4).[8,9] The diagnosis is usually made when the patient undergoes vascular imaging for other reasons and confirmed with CT displaying absent or hypoplastic carotid canal (Fig. 11.4). Occasionally, patients present with transient ischemic attacks or congenital, ipsilateral Horner syndrome.[9]

Development of intracranial aneurysms, in particular of the anterior communicating artery, is a frequent complication.[9] In addition, patients with intercavernous collaterals are predisposed to catastrophic complications during transphenoidal hypophyseal surgery. Therefore, it is critical for the radiologist to report absent or hypoplastic petrous carotid canal on imaging performed for operative guidance purposes.

### Aberrant internal carotid artery

Aberrant ICA is also a very uncommon congenital anomaly related to in utero involution of the cervical ICA and compensatory enlargement of the inferior tympanic and caroticotympanic arteries that connect to the petrous ICA. On imaging, the petrous carotid canal extends posterolaterally into the middle ear cavity to the cochlear promontory.[4,10] These features are easily identified on axial images. However, in the coronal plane, the lesion at the cochlear promontory might be mistaken for a glomus tumor, as the connection to the petrous segment of the ICA is more difficult to appreciate. Such misinterpretation may lead to uncontrollable bleeding or brain infarction when removal of the aberrant ICA is attempted.[11] Therefore, the radiologist is required to confirm the appropriate position and intactness of the ICA canal when a middle ear cavity mass is present.[11]

### Petrous segment internal carotid artery aneurysm

Petrous segment ICA aneurysms are rare, usually asymptomatic, and, hence, typically incidentally detected on imaging for other indications.[12] Occasionally, they cause pulsatile tinnitus, cranial neuropathies, or Horner syndrome.[12] On CT, petrous segment ICA aneurysms manifest as well-defined lytic lesions with variable expansion of the anterior petrous apex. They are often mistaken for a cholesterol granuloma or petrous apex mucocele on CT, with contrasted CT leading to the correct diagnosis unless the aneurysm is thrombosed. On MRI, the aneurysms demonstrate mixed signal intensity and heterogeneous enhancement related to the turbulent flow or thrombus. Characteristic pulsation artifacts in the phase-encoding direction are seen with nonthrombosed aneurysms. MR angiography typically underestimates the size of the aneurysm because of the turbulent flow or thrombus.

### Narrow internal auditory canal syndrome

Narrow IAC syndrome is a rare, unilateral temporal bone abnormality that causes congenital sensorineural

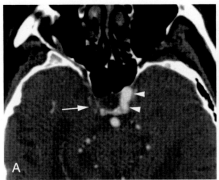
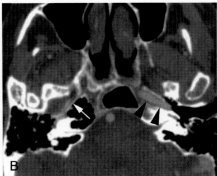
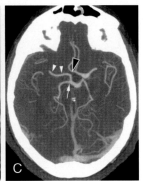

FIG. 11.4 **Congenital Aplasia of the Internal Carotid Artery (ICA).** A 67-year-old man undergoes stroke workup. The axial CT angiography source image **(A)** shows absence of the right ICA within the right cavernous sinus (*arrow* in **A**), with normal caliber of the ICA on the left side (*arrowheads* in **A**). A CT angiography image performed more inferiorly **(B)** reveals the absence of the petrous carotid canal on the right (*arrow* in **B**) with normal appearance on the left (*arrowhead* in **B**), consistent with congenital aplasia of the ICA. In complete occlusion of the ICA, a normal petrous carotid bony canal that shows lack of vascular contrast enhancement is seen. The maximum intensity projection image **(C)** maps out the collateral flow, with the middle cerebral artery (*white arrowheads* in **C**) arising from the posterior cerebral artery (*arrow* in **C**), which is an exceedingly rare abnormality of the circle of Willis. Collateral flow to the right ACA is provided via a robust anterior communicating artery (*black arrowhead*), which is a common anatomic variation.

hearing loss as a result of aplasia or hypoplasia of CN VIII. It represents a relative contraindication to cochlear implantation. CN VII function is typically preserved. On imaging, a small (<2 mm in vertical diameter) duplicated IAC is seen, with one canal containing CN VII and the second canal being empty or housing the hypoplastic CN VIII.[13]

### Schwannoma

In the petrous apex region, schwannomas may arise from CN V through VIII, with the vestibular division of CN VIII being most commonly affected.[14] CN VII and VIII abnormalities are discussed in Chapters 7 and 6, respectively.

CN V schwannomas are rare and frequently originate from the main trunk or within Meckel cave causing indentation along the superomedial petrous apex.[15] They grow along the nerve and its branches to involve the infratemporal and pterygopalatine fossae and expand the according neural foramina. CN V schwannomas are usually more heterogeneous on imaging than other cranial nerve schwannomas because of their propensity for cystic degeneration.[15]

CN VI schwannomas usually affect the cisternal segment and are exceptionally rare.[16] Preoperatively, they are often misdiagnosed as CN V schwannomas because of their rarity, similar course as CN V schwannomas in the prepontine cistern, and similar imaging features.[16]

## Intrinsic Petrous Apex Lesions Without Petrous Apex Enlargement
### Asymmetric pneumatization

The petrous apex is typically nonaerated, with physiologic pneumatization occurring in about 30% of individuals. In less than 10% of patients, such pneumatization is asymmetric, which is easily recognized with CT.[3] On MRI, however, the nonpneumatized petrous apex is often misinterpreted as cholesterol granuloma in older adults because of the inherent T1 hyperintensity of the fatty bone marrow (Fig. 11.5). Lack of mass effect, striation of the high T1 signal related to preserved bony trabeculae, lower-than-fluid T2 signal intensity on the fast spin echo T2 sequences, and suppression of signal on fat-suppressed T1 weighted images (Fig. 11.5) usually lead to the correct diagnosis.[17] In younger patients, the intermediate T1 and T2 signal intensity of red bone marrow is less likely to be mistaken for a petrous apex lesion.

### Petrous apex effusion

Petrous apex effusion (aka trapped fluid) represents fluid accumulation within a pneumatized petrous apex.[17,18] Often these are asymptomatic and do not require treatment. However, in some patients, this is a manifestation of an indolent infection causing hearing loss, facial spasm, or positional vertigo.[18] Imaging usually reveals fluid attenuation with preservation of the air cell trabeculations (Fig. 11.6). Confusion with a cholesterol granuloma occurs when the trapped fluid is

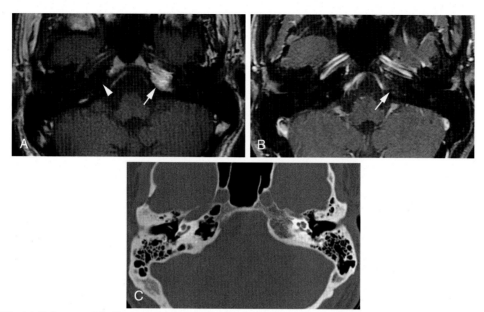

FIG. 11.5 **Asymmetric Pneumatization of the Petrous Apex Mimicking Pathology.** A 45-year-old woman undergoes MRI for migraines. The axial, T1-weighted image without contrast **(A)** reveals a hyperintense left petrous apex (*arrow*) that was initially mistaken for a cholesterol granuloma. The left petrous apex exhibited T2 hyperintensity (not shown) and was barely visible (*arrow*) on the fat-suppressed, contrast-enhanced T1 weighted image **(B)**. Such imaging appearance is consistent with fatty bone marrow within the left petrous apex that can mimic a lesion when the contralateral petrous apex is pneumatized (*arrow-head*), as this was the case in this patient. Axial CT displayed in bone window **(C)** confirms this normal anatomic variation.

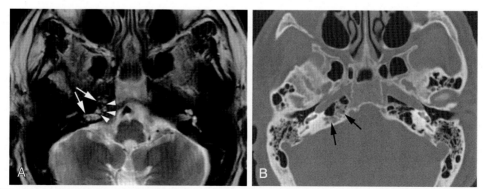

FIG. 11.6 **Petrous Apex Effusion.** Axial T2 image **(A)** of a 65-year-old-man undergoing workup for headaches reveals T2 hyperintensity (*arrows*) in the posteromedial portion of the right petrous apex that showed fluid attenuation on the T1 images (not shown) and lack of enhancement after gadolinium administration (not shown). Notice the preservation of focal septations (*arrowheads*) within the T2 hyperintensity, indicative of petrous apex effusion. Cholesteatoma and mucocele would lead to absence of the air cell septations. In contrast, early petrous apicitis usually shows marked enhancement after contrast administration and is associated with otomastoiditis that is not seen in this patient. Petrous apex effusion (*arrows*) within a pneumatized petrous apex is confirmed on an axial CT image displayed in bone window **(B)**.

proteinaceous and exhibits T1 hyperintensity. In those instances, the intact air cell septations indicate petrous apex effusion, whereas their absence is more consistent with cholesterol granuloma.

### Giant air cell

A petrous apex air cell larger than 1.5 cm represents a giant air cell.[19] When it is filled with fluid, it might be mistaken for a petrous apex mucocele or meningocele. However, the lack of petrous apex expansion and connection to intracranial structures, respectively, usually lead to the correct diagnosis of opacified giant air cell.

### Petrous apex cephaloceles

Petrous apex cephaloceles are posterolateral outpouchings of the Meckel cave into the petrous apex.[20] They follow fluid attenuation with possible mild rim enhancement.[20] They are rare and usually asymptomatic, with bilateral involvement in 30% of patients.[20] Surgical intervention is reserved for symptomatic patients who may present with CN III, V, or VI palsy, cerebrospinal fluid leak, or meningitis.[20]

### Arachnoid granulations

Arachnoid granulations are small outpouchings of the pia-arachnoid that typically protrude into the venous sinuses or inner table of the skull along the high convexities.[22] They can, however, affect any part of the skull or skull base and mimic an epidermoid cyst or

metastasis.[21–23] On imaging, they are multilobulated, exhibit fluid attenuation, and lack complete disruption of the cortex (Fig. 11.7). They show no or minimal capsule-like enhancement, in contrast to metastasis, and lack restricted diffusion as seen with epidermoid cysts. Occasionally, they protrude into a pneumatized petrous apex and cause a cerebrospinal fluid leak or meningitis.[24]

### Trauma

Temporal bone fractures are subdivided into petrous apex and non-petrous apex fractures. Petrous apex fractures tend to involve the IAC and cochlea, explaining the higher prevalence of CN VII and VIII dysfunction than with non-petrous apex fractures (Fig. 11.8).[25] The petrous carotid canal may also be affected in petrous apex fractures, requiring further evaluation with CT or MR angiography to exclude traumatic ICA injury (Fig. 11.8). Occasionally, the singular and arcuate canals are misinterpreted as temporal bone fractures. However, their characteristic location and preservation of the cortex should lead to the correct diagnosis.[26]

## Intrinsic Petrous Apex Lesions With Enlargement of the Petrous Apex and Nonaggressive Appearance
### Cholesterol granulomas

Cholesterol granulomas represent the most frequent expansile lesions of the petrous apex. Their etiology is still unclear. One theory is that negative pressure in

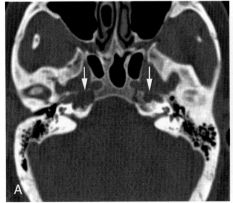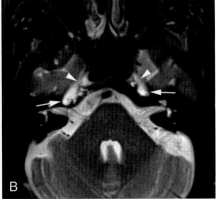

FIG. 11.7 **Arachnoid Granulations Affecting the Petrous Apices.** Axial CT image displayed in bone window **(A)** of a 60 year old patient undergoing imaging for headaches shows multilobulated lesions (*arrows*) in the anterior petrous apices bilaterally, right greater than left, without aggressive behavior. The subsequently performed T2-weighted image with fat suppression **(B)** reveals fluid attenuation in both lesions (*arrows*). The multilobulated nature of the lesions that contain fluid is most consistent with arachnoid granulations. Notice the stalk of the lesion (*arrowheads*) toward the intracranial structures confirming the diagnosis. Such arachnoid granulation may eventually develop into meningoceles potentially causing cerebrospinal fluid leakage and/or meningitis.

the pneumatized petrous apex causes reabsorption of air, mucosal edema, and hemorrhage, leading to tissue breakdown, cholesterol accumulation, and foreign body reaction.[27] The other, newer theory hypothesizes that the aggressive pneumatization of the petrous apex

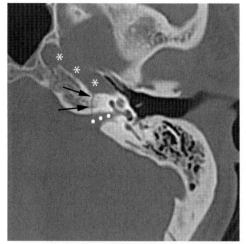

FIG. 11.8 **Transverse Petrous Apex Fracture.** Axial CT image displayed in bone window demonstrates a thin, lucent line (*arrows*) in the medial petrous apex that is oriented almost perpendicular to the long axis of the temporal bone and consistent with a transverse, petrous apex fracture. Notice the extension into the internal auditory canal (*dots*), placing the patient at risk for CN VII and VIII injury, and into the petrous carotid canal (*asterisk*). CT or MR angiography is warranted in this patient to exclude an underlying internal carotid artery injury.

leads to exposed bone marrow, subsequent hemorrhage, cholesterol accumulation, and foreign body reaction that obstructs the outflow tract and forms a cyst with eventual petrous apex expansion.[28] Both theories agree on the presence of blood products and cholesterol, which exhibit characteristic hyperintensity on T1 and T2 sequences (Fig. 11.9),[29] a hallmark of cholesterol. A hypointense rind is typically observed corresponding to the surrounding fibrous capsule and hemosiderin.

Many cholesterol granulomas are incidentally detected on imaging performed for other reasons.[3] On CT, an expansile, smooth, lytic lesion is seen within the petrous apex. Without contrast, it may be mistaken for a petrous apex aneurysm, a differential diagnosis that the radiologist should always consider to avoid catastrophic hemorrhage during biopsy or surgical resection. On MRI, the nonpneumatized petrous apex is often mistaken for a cholesterol granuloma, in particular when the contralateral petrous apex is pneumatized (Fig. 11.5). As stated earlier, the lack of expansion and preservation of the bony trabeculae should lead to the correct diagnosis. Occasionally, large cholesterol granulomas show a hematocrit level in their dependent portion (Fig. 11.9).

### Petrous apex mucoceles

Petrous apex mucoceles are related to postinflammatory obstruction. They mimic cholesterol granulomas on CT but exhibit low to intermediate signal intensity on T1 sequences in contrast to the characteristic T1 hyperintensity of cholesterol granulomas (Fig. 11.10).[30]

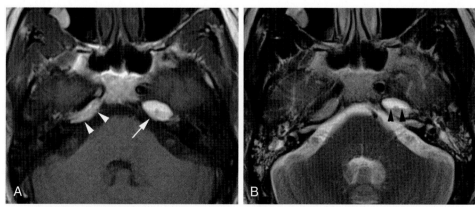

FIG. 11.9 **Cholesterol Granuloma With a Hematocrit Level.** Axial T1-weighted image **(A)** shows a well-defined expansile mass in the left petrous apex (*arrow*) when compared with the normal size of the right petrous apex (*white arrowheads*). The markedly hyperintense nature of the lesion is most consistent with cholesterol granuloma. The axial T2-weighted image **(B)** reveals a hematocrit level (*black arrowheads*) within the dependent lesion that can sometimes be observed in cholesterol granulomas.

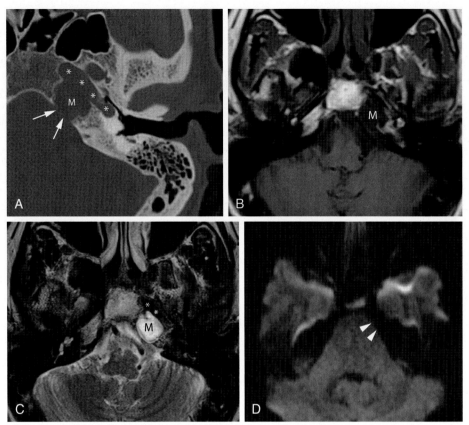

**FIG. 11.10** **Petrous Apex Mucocele.** Axial CT displayed in bone window **(A)** demonstrates an expansile mass (M) in the petrous apex causing marked thinning and partial dehiscence toward the posterior cranial fossa (*arrows*) and petrous carotid canal (*asterisks*). The differential diagnosis for such an appearance includes cholesterol granuloma, mucocele, and cholesteatoma. Petrous carotid artery aneurysm is unlikely, as the mass is centered in the posterior petrous apex. On the T1-weighted **(B)** and fat-suppressed T2-weighted **(C)** images the mass (M) shows fluid attenuation that is located posterior to the flow void created by the petrous segment of the internal carotid artery (*asterisks*), narrowing the differential diagnosis to mucocele and cholesteatoma. The lack of restricted diffusion in the expected location of the mass (*arrowheads*) on the diffusion-weighted image **(D)** established the final diagnosis of petrous apex mucocele.

### Fibrous dysplasia

Fibrous dysplasia is a congenital disorder caused by incorrect transformation of immature woven to mature lamellar bone, leading to disorganized bony trabeculae intermixed with well-vascularized fibrous stroma and fluid-filled cysts. Although the disease is benign, the lesions continue to grow until skeletal maturity is achieved. Craniofacial involvement is seen in up to 25% of patients with monostotic fibrous dysplasia.[31]

Fibrous dysplasia is usually incidentally discovered on imaging. Symptomatic patients may present with cranial neuropathy or ischemia related to foraminal narrowing. On CT, fibrous dysplasia usually shows the classic "ground-glass" matrix (Fig. 11.11). However, sometimes the cystic components predominate,

resulting in a more lytic appearance. On MRI, fibrous dysplasia can assume any signal intensity or enhancement, reflecting the different degrees of fibrous and cystic components. Hence, it is often mistaken for other benign or malignant lesions. Clues to the correct diagnosis on MRI include low attenuation on all sequences reflecting the high degree of mineralization, bony expansion with cortical preservation, and involvement of multiple adjacent skull base bones, as fibrous dysplasia tends to ignore suture lines (Fig. 11.11).[31]

### Paget disease

Paget disease is a disorder of osteoclastic overactivity causing excessive bone resorption (lytic phase) followed by compensatory, exuberant bone formation

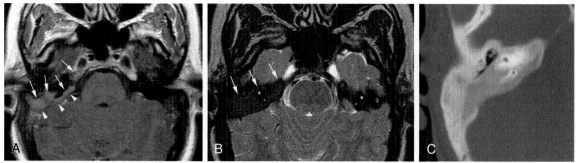

FIG. 11.11 **Fibrous Dysplasia of the Temporal Bone.** A 72-year-old woman undergoes MRI examination for staging of breast cancer. The axial, contrast-enhanced T1-weighted image **(A)** shows an enhancing lesion (*arrows*) in the petrous apex that extends laterally to involve the mastoid bone. Notice the preserved posterior cortical margin (*arrowheads*). The lesion (*arrows*) is of very low attenuation on the axial, T2-weighted image **(B)** and shows mild expansion of the affected temporal bone. The constellation of findings is most consistent with fibrous dysplasia, which was confirmed through the characteristic ground-glass appearance on CT displayed in bone window **(C)**.

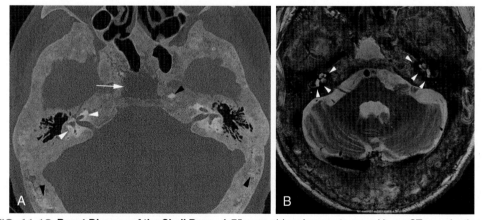

FIG. 11.12 **Paget Disease of the Skull Base.** A 75-year-old undergoes temporal bone CT examination for hearing loss and tinnitus. The axial CT image displayed in bone window **(A)** shows marked thickening of the skull and sclerosis of the skull base with areas of lysis (*arrow*) and sclerosis (*black arrowheads*). The imaging appearance is consistent with advanced Paget disease. On MRI, Paget disease demonstrates heterogeneous signal within the expanded bone marrow as illustrated on the axial T2-weighted image **(B)** in the presented patient. Notice the preservation of the otic capsule immediately adjacent to the vestibulo-cochlear apparatus (*white arrowheads*).

(mixed and subsequent sclerotic phase) leading to larger but mechanically weaker and less compact bone. Paget disease most commonly affects elderly males. Patients may present with deafness, vertigo, and tinnitus when the petrous apex is affected, with demineralization of the otic capsule, obliteration of the cochlear venous outflow, and stapes footplate fixation or fracture reported as possible etiologies.[32,33] Depending on the phase of the disease, variable degrees of lysis and sclerosis, often intermixed, will be seen on CT, with thickened and dense-appearing bone

in advanced stages (Fig. 11.12A). Heterogeneous T1 and T2 signal with variable enhancement is observed on MRI (Fig. 11.12B).[26]

### Intrinsic Petrous Apex Lesions With Aggressive Appearance
#### Petrous apicitis
Petrous apicitis (aka apical petrositis) is a rare infection of the pneumatized petrous apex caused by the antero-medial extension of an acute otomastoiditis. Therefore, opacification of the petrous air cells in combination

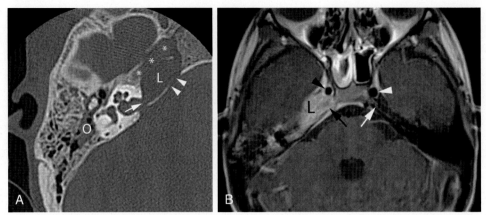

**FIG. 11.13 Petrous Apicitis Causing Gradenigo Triad.** An 8-year-old undergoes workup for fever, facial pain, and diplopia. The axial CT image displayed in bone window **(A)** reveals nonaggressive otomastoiditis (O) and an aggressive lesion in the petrous apex (L) with focal areas of bony destruction toward the posterior fossa (*arrowheads* in **A**) and internal auditory canal (*arrow* in **A**). There is also lack of bony coverage of the petrous carotid canal (*asterisks*). The subsequently performed gadolinium-enhanced T1 image **(B)** reveals an enhancing lesion (L) centered in the right petrous apex with extension into the cavernous sinus where the Meckel cave is completely obliterated (*black arrow* in **B**) when compared with the normal left side (*white arrow* in **B**). There is also mild narrowing of the internal carotid artery on the right (*black arrowhead* in **B**) when compared with the left (*white arrowhead* in **B**). The constellation of findings is most consistent with petrous apicitis, with cavernous sinus involvement causing the classic symptoms of Gradenigo syndrome. Restricted diffusion was seen on the diffusion-weighted images (not shown), confirming the diagnosis.

with otomastoid disease is usually seen on imaging in the early stages, with development of bony destruction with progressive disease (Fig. 11.13).[34] Gradenigo triad with ipsilateral CN VI palsy, severe facial pain, and otomastoiditis has been associated with petrous apicitis. However, only a minority of patients exhibit all three symptoms.[35] Potentially lethal intracranial complications may occur, including meningitis, abscess formation, or thrombophlebitis and require imaging with contrast, preferably with MRI (Fig. 11.13). Gallium single-photon emission computed tomography (SPECT) is helpful for monitoring the response to antibiotic therapy.[34]

### Petrous apex osteomyelitis

Petrous apex osteomyelitis is also an aggressive infection usually presenting with severe, deep ear pain that is out of proportion to clinical examination.[36] It has two features distinct from petrous apicitis: (1) it affects the nonpneumatized petrous apex and therefore reveals petrous apex fragmentation early in the disease[1]; (2) it has a different etiology, as it is often caused by direct extension of the necrotizing otitis externa into the petrous apex. MRI is the preferred imaging method because it better demonstrates the bone marrow involvement in early disease and possible subsequent

intracranial complications. Technetium-99 bone SPECT scan is also highly sensitive in the detection of petrous apex osteomyelitis. In addition, it can predict patient's long-term outcome, with spread across midline indicating least favorable prognosis.[36] In contrast, gallium SPECT imaging is preferred to monitor the response to antibiotic therapy, as other imaging lags behind in normalization of tissue planes.

### Petrous apex cholesteatomas

Petrous apex cholesteatomas (aka epidermoid cysts) typically originate in persistent, ectopic ectoderm and cause accumulation of desquamated tissue.[37] These most commonly affect children and young adults. On CT, they present as expansile, lytic lesions with variable borders ranging from well defined to destructive. When well defined, they may be misinterpreted as cholesterol granuloma or mucocele on CT. On MRI, cholesteatomas mimic mucoceles, as they are T1 hypointense and T2 hyperintense and lack intrinsic enhancement. In contrast to mucoceles, however, petrous apex cholesteatomas exhibit diffusion restriction.[3,37] Therefore, a diffusion-weighted sequence should always be included in the workup of petrous apex masses. It is also the critical sequence for detection of recurrent cholesteatoma after surgical resection.[38]

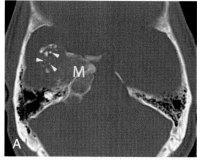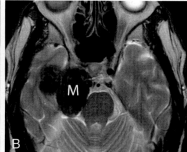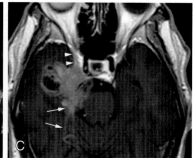

**FIG. 11.14 Petroclival Meningioma Mimicking Chondrosarcoma on CT.** A 76-year-old man undergoes head CT examination for mental status changes. The axial CT displayed in bone window **(A)** reveals a mass (M) arising from the superior aspect of the right petrous apex, with focal areas of ring and arcs (*arrowheads* in **A**) suggestive of a chondroid matrix tumor such as chondrosarcoma. On the subsequently performed MRI, the mass (M) exhibits very low T2 **(B)** signal intensity that is not consistent with a chondrosarcoma, leading to the correct diagnosis of partially calcified petroclival meningioma with its characteristic growth pattern along the lateral wall of the cavernous sinus (*arrowheads* in **C**) and along the tentorial edge (*arrows* in C) as best seen on the contrast-enhanced T1-weighted image **(C)**.

### Langerhans cell histiocytosis

Langerhans cell histiocytosis is a collection of idiopathic, pediatric neoplasms characterized by the proliferation of mature eosinophils and bone marrow-derived Langerhans cells[39] consisting of an infantile form (Letterer-Siwe disease), Hand-Schüller-Christian disease, and eosinophilic granuloma.[39] Eosinophic granuloma is the localized form of Langerhans cell histiocytosis that is most commonly encountered by radiologists, with preferential involvement of the frontal and temporal bones in the head.[39,40] It manifests on CT as a round to oval, punched-out, markedly enhancing lytic lesion without sclerosis of the bony margins. Extensive, ill-defined, perilesional bone marrow and soft tissue edema with enhancement is seen on MRI, which might be mistaken for aggressive osteomyelitis or neoplasm.[41,42] Therefore, the radiologist should always consider the diagnosis of eosinophilic granuloma in a pediatric patient with an aggressive bone lesion, as isolated lesions are often cured with surgical resection.[39]

### Chondrosarcoma

Petrous apex chondrosarcomas are malignant cartilaginous tumors arising from the petrooccipital fissure.[3] They can be subdivided into classic, myxoid, and mesenchymal types. The classic variant is most common, affects elderly patients, and is the least aggressive with slow growth, minimal risk of metastatic disease, and best prognosis.[43] In contrast, the mesenchymal type occurs in young adults and is the most aggressive with rapid growth and worst prognosis.[44] Headache, CN VI palsy, and hearing loss are the leading symptoms.

On CT, an expansile to destructive petrous apex mass is seen depending on tumor subtype that often contains "ring and arcs" reflecting the chondroid origin of the tumor (Fig. 11.14A). On MRI, chondrosarcomas are T1 hypointense and strongly T2 hyperintense.[45] Variable enhancement is seen, with some tumors showing mild "honeycomb" enhancement and others exhibiting profound enhancement that mimics a vascular tumor such as hemangiopericytoma.[44] Chordomas assume similar imaging characteristics as chondrosarcomas. However, they are typically centered in the clivus.

### Endolymphatic sac tumor

Endolymphatic sac tumors are low-grade adenocarcinomas arising from the endolymphatic sac within the posterior petrous apex.[46] They are very rare and can be sporadic or associated with von Hippel-Lindau disease. Bilateral involvement is seen in 30% of patients with von Hippel-Lindau disease.[46] Hearing loss and tinnitus are the leading symptoms. On CT, an erosive mass with internal bony speculations is seen in the posteromedial petrous apex. On MRI, endolymphatic sac tumors show heterogeneous appearance with foci of T1 and T2 hyperintensity related to blood products and cholesterol accumulation[46] intermixed with low signal intensity related to calcifications and hemosiderin.

### Metastatic disease

The skull base is commonly affected by metastatic disease with preferential involvement of the petrous apex within the temporal bone.[3,26] Breast cancer is the most frequent metastasis, followed by lung and prostate cancer.[3,26] As in other locations, bony metastases manifest with initial bone marrow infiltration that is best appreciated on MRI and subsequent destructive, enhancing masses. Observation of additional sites of bony involvement usually leads to the correct diagnosis.

### Plasmocytoma/multiple myeloma

Plasmocytoma and multiple myeloma refer to a localized or multifocal neoplastic proliferation of monoclonal plasma cells, respectively.[3] They show similar imaging characteristics as metastatic disease, with isolated involvement observed with plasmocytomas. The clinical history and presentation usually help to differentiate multiple myeloma from metastatic disease, with anemia, bone pain, and renal failure being the most common initial symptoms of multiple myeloma.[47]

### Lymphoma

Isolated lymphoma of the petrous apex is exceedingly rare. More often, the petrous apex is affected in association with diffuse disease of the skull base. The imaging appearance ranges from diffuse replacement of the fatty bone marrow to frank destructive lesions, depending on the lymphoma type. In general, lymphoma exhibits slight T2 hypointensity and restricted diffusion related to its high cellularity.[26]

## Extrinsic Petrous Apex Lesions
### Meningioma

Meningioma of the petrous apex can be subdivided into CP angle and petroclival meningiomas. The CP angle meningiomas arise from the dura along the posterior petrous apex and tend to grow into the IAC, where they can mimic a vestibular schwannoma (Fig. 11.15). Close inspection of the lesion for a dural tail and analysis of the growth vector usually lead to the correct diagnosis (Fig. 11.15). In contrast, the petroclival meningiomas like to drape over the petrous apex, involve the Dorello canal, and extend inferiorly along the clivus or anteriorly into the ipsilateral cavernous sinus to cause various cranial neuropathies (Fig. 11.14).[3,26]

As with other meningiomas, a dural-based, slightly hyperdense mass is seen on CT, with T1 hypointensity and T2 iso- to hyperintensity observed on MRI.[3,26] Homogenous enhancement is usually noted after contrast administration. Associated hyperostosis of the petrous apex manifests as low T1 and T2 signal intensity and may mimic blastic metastasis or lymphoma.

### Paraganglioma

Occasionally, glomus jugulare or jugulotympanic tumors extend superomedially and erode the posteromedial

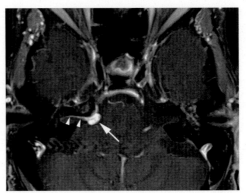

**FIG. 11.15 Cerebellopontine (CP) Angle Meningioma.** Axial T1-weighted images with fat suppression after gadolinium administration reveal a small enhancing mass (*arrow*) in the right CP angle. The lesion extends into the right internal auditory canal and shows a long dural tail (*arrowheads*) consistent with a meningioma.

petrous apex (Fig. 11.16A). Their origin in the jugular foramen and their characteristic imaging appearance with an aggressive, hypervascular mass on CT and "salt and pepper" appearance on MRI usually lead to the correct diagnosis (Fig. 11.16).[3]

### Nasopharyngeal carcinoma

Nasopharyngeal carcinoma may secondarily affect the petrous apex via direct invasion or growth through the foramen lacerum into the petrous carotid canal.[48] Direct invasion is usually best visualized with CT or noncontrasted T1 images, whereas involvement along the ICA is more challenging to diagnose and might manifest as erosions of the petrous carotid canal on CT, ICA narrowing on CT or MR angiography, or soft tissue attenuation around the ICA on MRI.[48] Petrous apex involvement by nasopharyngeal cancer might present with the Gradenigo triad and mimic petrous apicitis.[26,35] Therefore, the radiologists need to carefully evaluate the nasopharynx in every patient with a petrous apex mass.

In summary, the radiologist plays a vital role in the workup of petrous apex abnormalities, as this area is not accessible for direct clinical examination or percutaneous biopsy and is often affected by anatomic variations. Therefore, the radiologist is required to have in-depth knowledge of the anatomy, normal anatomic variations, and imaging features of the different diseases of the petrous apex to facilitate correct image interpretation with high degree of confidence and to avoid misinterpretation of an anatomic variation or "do-not-touch" lesion for a disease process requiring surgical treatment.

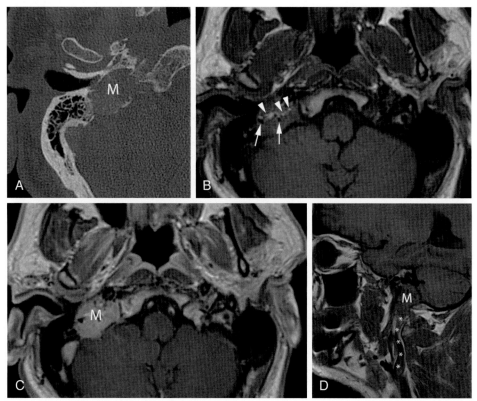

**FIG. 11.16 Glomus Jugulare Extending Into the Petrous Apex.** Axial CT displayed in bone window **(A)** demonstrates a destructive mass (M) affecting the medial inferior aspect of the petrous apex. This is a nonspecific pattern and can be observed with metastatic disease, lymphoma, plasmocytoma, chondrosarcoma, and glomus jugulare. Axial T1-weighted image **(B)** reveals "salt (*arrowheads*) and pepper (*arrows*)" appearance within the mass, a characteristic MR feature of paragangliomas, with dark areas (*arrows*) corresponding to flow voids. The marked enhancement on the contrast-enhanced T1-weighted image **(C)** and the growth of the mass (M) below the skull base along the jugular vein (*asterisks*) as best seen on the sagittal T1-weighted image **(D)** support the diagnosis of glomus jugulare.

## REFERENCES

1. Connor SEJ, Leung R, Natas S. Imaging of the petrous apex: a pictorial review. *Br J Radiol.* 2008;81(965):427–435.
2. Virapongse C, Sarwar M, Bhimani S, et al. Computed tomography of temporal bone pneumatization: 1. Normal pattern and morphology. *AJR Am J Roentgenol.* 1985;145(3):473–481.
3. Chapman PR, Shah R, Curé JK, et al. Petrous apex lesions: pictorial review. *AJR Am J Roentgenol.* 2011;196:WS26–WS37.
4. Koesling S, Kunkel P, Schul T. Vascular anomalies, sutures and small canals of the temporal bone on axial CT. *Eur J Radiol.* 2005;54(3):335–343.
5. Tauber M, Van Loveren HR, Jallo G, et al. The enigmatic foramen lacerum. *Neurosurgery.* 1999;44(2):386–391.
6. Rubinstein D, Sandberg EJ, Cajade-Law AG. Anatomy of the facial and vestibulocochlear nerves in the internal auditory canal. *AJNR Am J Neuroradiol.* 1996;17(6):1099–1105.
7. Muren C, Wadin K, Dimopoulos P. Radioanatomy of the singular nerve canal. *Eur Radiol.* 1991;1:65–69.
8. Midkiff RB, Boykin MW, McFarland DR, et al. Agenesis of the internal carotid artery with intercavernous anastomosis. *AJNR Am J Neuroradiol.* 1995;16:1356–1359.
9. Given CA, Huang-Hellinger F, Baker MD, et al. Congenital absence of the internal carotid artery: case reports and review of collateral circulation. *AJNR Am J Neuroradiol.* 2001;22:1953–1959.
10. Ginsberg LE, Pruett SW, Chen MYM, et al. Skull-base foramina of the middle cranial fossa: reassessment of normal variations with high-resolution CT. *AJNR Am J Neuroradiol.* 1994;15(2):283–291.
11. Sauvaget E, Paris J, Kici S, et al. Aberrant internal carotid artery in the temporal bone: imaging findings and management. *Arch Otolaryngol Head Neck Surg.* 2006;132(1):86–91.

12. Liu JK, Gottfried ON, Amini A, et al. Aneurysms of the petrous internal carotid artery: anatomy, origins, and treatment. *Neurosurg Focus.* 2004;17(5):1–9.

13. Cho Y-S, Na DG, Jung JY, et al. Narrow internal auditory canal syndrome: parasagittal reconstruction. *J Laryngol Otol.* 2000;114(5):392–394.

14. Consensus Development Panel. National Institutes of Health consensus development conference statement on acoustic neuroma. December 11-13, 1991. *Arch Neurol.* 1994;51:201–207.

15. Mehra S, Garg UC. Radiological imaging in trigeminal nerve schwannoma: a case report and review of literature. *JIMSA.* 2013;26(2):117–119.

16. Li X, Li J, Li J, Wu Z. Schwannoma of the 6th nerve: case report and review of the literature. *Chin Neurosurg J.* 2015;1:1–7.

17. Moore KR, Harnsberger HR, Shelton C, Davidson C. 'Leave me alone' lesions of the petrous apex. *AJMR Am J Neuroradiol.* 1998;19:733–738.

18. Arriaga MA. Petrous apex effusion: a clinical disorder. *Laryngoscope.* 2006;116(8):1349–1356.

19. Dubois PJ, Roub LW. Giant air cells of the petrous apex: tomographic features. *Radiology.* 1978;129(1):103–109.

20. Moore KR, Fischbein NJ, Harnsberger HR, et al. Petrous apex cepholoceles. *AJNR Am J Neuroradiol.* 2001;22(10):1867–1871.

21. Kuroiwa T, Kajimoto Y, Ohta T, et al. Symptomatic hypertrophic pacchionian granulation mimicking bone tumor: case report. *Neurosurgery.* 1996;39(4):860–862.

22. Lee MH, Kim HJ, Lee IH, et al. Prevalence and appearance of the posterior wall defects of the temporal bone caused by presumed arachnoid granulations and their clinical significance: CT findings. *AJNR Am J Neuroradiol.* 2008;29:1704–1707.

23. Okamoto K, Ito J, Tokiguchi S, et al. Arachnoid granulations of the posterior fossa: CT and MR findings. *Clin Imaging.* 1997;21(1):1–5.

24. Perry BP, Rubinstein JT. Meningitis due to acute otitis media and arachnoid granulations. *Ann Otol Rhinol Laryngol.* 2000;109(9):877–879.

25. Ishman SL, Friedland DR. Temporal bone fractures: traditional classification and clinical relevance. *Laryngoscope.* 2004;114(10):1734–1741.

26. Razek AA, Huang BY. Lesions of the petrous apex: classification and findings on CT and MR imaging. *Radiographics.* 2012;32:151–173.

27. Farrior B, Kampsen E, Farrior JB. The positive pressure of cholesterol granuloma idiopathic blue eardrum. Differential diagnosis. *Laryngoscope.* 1981;91(8):1286–1296.

28. Jackler RK, Cho M. A new theory to explain the genesis of petrous apex cholesterol granuloma. *Otol Neurotol.* 2003;24(1):96–106.

29. Chaljub G, Vrabec J, Hollingsworth C, et al. Magnetic resonance imaging of petrous tip lesions. *Am J Otolaryngol.* 1999;20(5):304–313.

30. Muckle RP, De la Cruz A, Lo WM. Petrous apex lesions. *Am J Otol.* 1998;19(2):219–225.

31. Utz JA, Krandorf MJ, Jelinek JS, et al. MR appearance of fibrous dysplasia. *J Comput Assist Tomogr.* 1989;13(5):845–851.

32. Monsell EM, Cody DD, Bone HG, et al. Hearing loss as a complication of Paget's disease of bone. *J Bone Miner Res.* 1999;2:92–95.

33. Dimitriadis PA, Bamiou DE, Bibas AG. Hearing loss in Paget's disease: a temporal bone histopathology study. *Otol Neurotol.* 2012;33(2):142–146.

34. Lee YH, Lee NJ, Kim JH, et al. CT, MRI and gallium SPECT in the diagnosis and treatment of petrous apicitis presenting as multiple cranial neuropathies. *Br J Radiol.* 2005;78:948–951.

35. Gradenigo G. Sulla leptomeningite circonscritta e sulla paralisi dell' abducenta di origine otitica. *Giornale dell'Accademia di medicina di Torino.* 1904;10:59–84.

36. Lee S, Hooper R, Fuller A, et al. Otogenic cranial base osteomyelitis: a proposed prognosis-based system for disease classification. *Otol Neurotol.* 2008;29(5):666–672.

37. Robert Y, Carcasset S, Rocourt N, et al. Congenital cholesteatoma of the temporal bone: MR findings and comparison with CT. *AJNR Am J Neuroradiol.* 1995;16(4):755–761.

38. Aikele P, Kittner T, Offergeld C, et al. Diffusion-weighted MR imaging of cholesteatoma in pediatric and adult patients who have undergone middle ear surgery. *AJR Am J Roentgenol.* 2003;181(1):261–265.

39. Howarth DM, Gilchrist GS, Mullan BP, et al. Langerhans cell histocytosis: diagnosis, natural history, management, and outcome. *Cancer.* 1999;85(10):2278–2290.

40. Miller C, Lloyd TV, Johnson JC, et al. Eosinophilic granuloma of the base of the skull. Case report. *J Neurosurg.* 1978;49(3):464–466.

41. DiNardo LJ, Wetmore RF. Head and neck manifestations of histocytosis-X in children. *Laryngoscope.* 1989;99(7 Pt 1):721–724.

42. Beltran J, Aparisi F, Bonmati LM, et al. Eosinophic granuloma: MRI manifestations. *Skelet Radiol.* 1993;22(3):157–161.

43. Evans HL, Ayala AG, Romsdahl MM. Prognostic factors in chondrosarcoma of bone. A clinicopathologic analysis with emphasis on histologic grading. *Cancer.* 1977;40(2):818–831.

44. Maslehaty H, Petrides AK, Kinzel A, et al. Chondrosarcoma of the petrous bone: a challenging clinical entity. *Head Neck Oncol.* 2013;5(2):13–20.

45. Bourgouin PM, Tampieri D, Robitaille Y, et al. Low-grade myxoid chondrosarcoma of the base of the skull: CT, MRI, and histopathology. *J Comput Assist Tomogr.* 1992;16(2):268–273.

46. Ferri E, Amadori M, Armato E, et al. A rare case of endolymphatic sac tumours: clinicopathologic study and surgical management. *Case Rep Otolaryngol.* 2014;2014:376761.

47. Agarwal A, Chirindel A, Shah BA, et al. Evolving role of FDG PET/CT in multiple myeloma imaging and management. *AJR Am J Roentgenol.* 2013;200:884–890.

48. King AD, Bhatia KSS. Magnetic resonance imaging staging of nasopharyngeal carcinoma in the head and neck. *World J Radiol.* 2010;2(5):159–165.

# CHAPTER 12

# Imaging of the Cerebellopontine Angle

MARGARET N. CHAPMAN, MD • OSAMU SAKAI, MD, PHD, FACR

## INTRODUCTION

The cerebellopontine angle (CPA) cistern is a subarachnoid space within the posterior cranial fossa. About 6%–10% of all intracranial masses are found in this location.[1–6] Vestibular schwannomas (VSs) are the most commonly encountered lesion in the CPA, followed by meningiomas. Together these masses account for 85%–90% of all CPA tumors. Other less common entities comprise the remaining 15% of lesions, and although encountered less frequently, these are also readily identified by imaging.[2] The clinical presentation of the various lesions depends on the location and the associated mass effect on adjacent structures. The purpose of this chapter is to review the imaging features of common and uncommon CPA lesions.

## ANATOMY

The CPA is a triangular subarachnoid space located within the posterior cranial fossa and centered at the level of the internal auditory canal (IAC). The apex of the space is medially positioned within the prepontine cistern. The petrous temporal bone forms the anterolateral border, and the cerebellum forms the posteromedial border. The space extends craniocaudally from the cranial nerve V to the cranial nerve IX-X-XI complex.[1,5]

The contents of the CPA therefore include the cerebrospinal fluid (CSF) and cranial nerves and vessels. Lesions occurring within this region may originate from any of these structures, from the meninges lining the petrous temporal bone, or from extension of lesions arising from the adjacent temporal bone, brainstem, or cerebellum. The clinical presentation and symptoms associated with the various lesions may be nonspecific clinically and vary depending on where the lesion arises and if there is involvement or compression of adjacent structures.

## IMAGING TECHNIQUES
### Magnetic Resonance Imaging
MRI has excellent soft tissue contrast resolution and is the preferred imaging modality for differentiation and characterization of various soft tissues and fluids. In addition to conventional MR sequences of the brain, current imaging evaluation of the CPA includes high-resolution heavily T2-weighted imaging, such as constructive interference in steady-state (CISS), driven equilibrium (DRIVE), fast imaging employing steady-state acquisition (FIESTA), with submillimeter slice thickness, allowing evaluation of the cranial nerves and surrounding CSF without intravenous contrast administration. High-resolution pre- and postcontrast T1-weighted images through the CPA and IAC are also routinely obtained for complete characterization.

Diffusion-weighted imaging (DWI) has been utilized for temporal bone and CPA imaging, particularly when abscesses or epidermoid/cholesteatoma are suspected. Diffusion restriction is seen with these pathologies and this specific sequence can be helpful in differentiation from other conditions (described in greater detail later).

If there is suspicion for a vascular lesion as the etiology of a CPA "mass," two or three-dimensional time-of-flight techniques may be performed for arterial imaging without intravenous contrast administration. Phase-contrast MR angiography is another technique to demonstrate vascular structures without intravenous contrast administration, which enables the quantitative analysis of flow as well as the visualization of arterial and venous structures.[7] Dynamic contrast-enhanced MR angiography can also be performed as clinically required.[8]

### Computed Tomography
CT is often performed for the evaluation of nonspecific clinical symptoms related to the CPA and posterior fossa and may initially identify culprit lesions. CT provides excellent definition of bone and air-filled spaces. However, fluid, nerves, and tumors are similar in density. Therefore, CT usually has difficulty differentiating fluids from soft tissues without contrast. Fat is substantially lower in density and darker than other soft tissues on CT, and fat-containing lesions are readily identified.

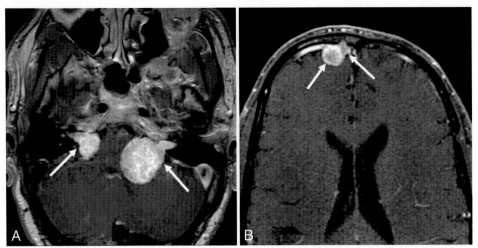

FIG. 12.1 **Neurofibromatosis Type II (NF II) With Bilateral Vestibular Schwannomas and Menin-gioma. (A)** Axial postcontrast T1-weighted image shows lobulated masses located within the bilateral cerebellopontine angles with extension into the internal auditory canals (IACs) (*arrows*). Note the "ice cream cone" appearance with the rounded cisternal "ice cream" component and the canalicular "cone" within the IAC. **(B)** Axial postcontrast fat-suppressed T1-weighted image through the cerebral hemispheres demon-strates a dural-based homogeneously enhancing mass (*arrow*) consistent with a meningioma.

The administration of intravenous iodinated contrast enables the identification of enhancing lesions and ves-sels and may increase lesion conspicuity.[8]

Currently, most CT examinations are performed with multidetector-row CT with submillimeter slice thickness through regions of interest. At our institution, temporal bone and CPA imaging is performed with slices of 0.625 mm thickness, which are reconstructed with 0.3 mm interval, with high-quality multiplanar reformatted images obtained from the axially acquired "volume data." Axial and coronal are the primary planes utilized for imaging evaluation.[8]

## EXTRAAXIAL LESIONS

Extraaxial lesions are often readily identified as sepa-rate and distinct from brain parenchyma on CT and MRI. In some cases, differentiation may be difficult and secondary signs of the extraaxial location (including the identification of a CSF cleft between the lesion and the parenchyma and enlargement of the cisterns) may help in localization. Extraaxial lesions may also "push away" cranial nerves and adjacent structures.[2,9]

### Vestibular Schwannoma

VSs are by far the most commonly encountered lesion in the CPA, comprising 70%–80% of the lesions in this location.[1] Most of these lesions develop from the Schwann cell within the IAC and as they grow extend

out of the porus acousticus into the CPA.[10] There are no Schwann cells associated with the cisternal segment of the cranial nerve VIII, thus precluding primary ori-gin of the lesion within the segment of the nerve in the CPA.[5]

Aside from symptoms related to cranial nerve VIII origin, additional clinical symptoms caused by VS may be related to the mass effect imposed on adja-cent structures in the posterior fossa, more often seen with larger and purely cisternal lesions. Bilateral VSs are a diagnostic feature of neurofibromatosis type II (Figs. 12.1 and 12.2).[5,11]

On CT examinations, VSs are often isodense to brain parenchyma. Erosion or remodeling of the adjacent temporal bone is often present, although often very subtle.[1,5]

On MRI, VSs demonstrate isointense signal on T1-weighted images, intermediate to hyperintense signal on T2-weighted images, and avid enhance-ment, although heterogeneity and cystic degenera-tion is commonly seen with an increase in size. The presence of foci of susceptibility caused by intratu-moral microhemorrhage is characteristic and helpful to differentiate from other lesions such as meningi-oma (Figs. 12.3 and 12.4).[12] VSs may appear as a "fill-ing defect" within the CPA on heavily T2-weighted images or MR cisternography (Fig. 12.5).[1,5,8]

Three enhancement patterns have been identi-fied[13,14]: homogeneous enhancement (50%–60% of

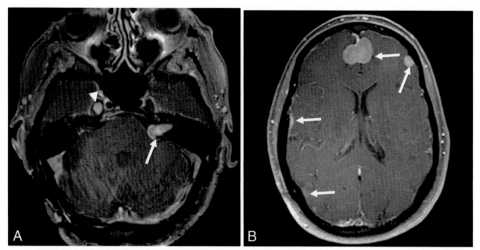

FIG. 12.2 **Neurofibromatosis Type II (NF II) With Unilateral Vestibular Schwannoma, Trigeminal Schwannoma, and Multiple Meningiomas.** **(A)** Axial postcontrast fat-suppressed T1-weighted image shows a lobulated mass located within the left cerebellopontine angle with extension into the left internal auditory canal (*arrow*). There is an additional cranial nerve V schwannoma located within the right Meckel cave (*arrowhead*). **(B)** Axial postcontrast T1-weighted image through the cerebral hemispheres demonstrates multiple homogeneously enhancing dural-based masses, consistent with multiple meningiomas in this patient with known NF II.

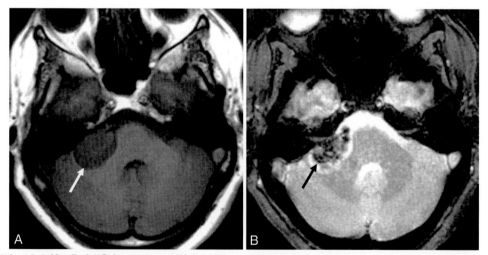

FIG. 12.3 **Vestibular Schwannoma.** **(A)** Axial T1-weighted image demonstrates a hypointense mass centered in the right cerebellopontine angle (*arrow*). There is associated mass effect on the right lateral cerebellum and middle cerebellar peduncle without apparent signal abnormality. **(B)** Axial gradient echo image demonstrates susceptibility artifact within the lesion because of hemosiderin deposit from microhemorrhage (*arrow*).

cases), heterogeneous enhancement (30%–40% of cases), and central cystic change without enhancement (5%–15% of cases).[1,13–16] Studies suggest that the enhancement characteristics may be related to the tumor size and Antoni cell type. Small VSs often comprise Antoni type A cells and demonstrate homogeneous enhancement. Larger lesions (greater than 2.5 cm) often demonstrate heterogeneous enhancement and are more often Antoni type B cells or a mix of Antoni type A and type B cells.[14,17]

T2 hyperintense signal in the dorsal brainstem is another imaging feature that can be seen with VS and may be related to degeneration of the vestibular nucleus.[1,18]

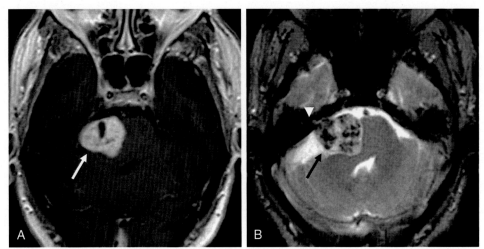

FIG. 12.4 **Vestibular Schwannoma. (A)** Axial postcontrast T1-weighted image demonstrates a hetero-geneously enhancing extraaxial mass with a central nonenhancing region located in the right aspect of the prepontine cistern (*arrow*). There is associated mass effect upon the right pons and middle cerebellar peduncle with distortion of the fourth ventricle. **(B)** Axial gradient echo image demonstrates heterogeneous signal within the mass with multiple regions of susceptibility artifact from hemosiderin deposit secondary to prior microhemorrhage (*arrow*). Note the mass widens the right porus acousticus and extends into the right internal auditory canal (*arrowhead*).

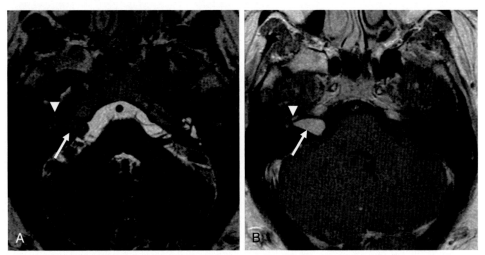

FIG. 12.5 **Cochlear Schwannoma. (A)** Axial high-resolution 3D T2-weighted image demonstrates a lobulated hypointense "filling defect" within the right CPA with extension into the widened right IAC (*arrow*). There is also asymmetric loss of the usual fluid signal within the right cochlea (*arrowhead*). **(B)** Axial postcontrast T1-weighted image demonstrates homogeneous enhancement of the mass (*arrow*) and of the basal turn of the cochlea (*arrowhead*).

Advanced MRI techniques have been utilized to evaluate for imaging characteristics unique to VS. DWI has not shown reliability in differentiating VS from meningioma, although studies suggest that apparent diffusion coefficient (ADC) values are higher in VS when compared with meningioma and that higher ADC values may be related to VS rich in Antoni type B cells.[1,19,20] MR perfusion has shown that relative tumor blood volume may be lower in VS compared with meningioma.[1,21] MR spectroscopy demonstrates a myoinositol peak at 3.55 ppm. Furthermore, the alanine peak seen in meningioma is absent in the setting of VS.[1,22]

## Other Schwannomas

Schwannoma arising from other cranial nerves may also extend into the CPA and may mimic VS. CN V, VII, and IX–XI can be involved. The imaging features of these schwannoma are similar to those of VS, and distinction is made on the basis of clinical symptoms and on the mass following the trajectory of a specific nerve, enlargement of specific skull base foramina, and possible denervation changes of corresponding muscles. For instance, trigeminal nerve (CN V) schwannoma are located cranial to VS, are oriented in a more anteroposterior axis (relative to VS), and may extend into Meckel cave (Fig. 12.1). CN IX–XI schwannomas are located caudal to the CPA and may extend through the jugular foramen.[1,2,5]

Facial nerve (CN VII) schwannoma may be difficult to distinguish from VS because of similar lesion location and similar trajectory of the cranial nerve through the IAC.[23] However, facial nerve schwannoma are located superiorly and anteriorly within the IAC and may extend into the temporal bone along the course of the facial nerve canal.[1,24,25]

## Meningioma

Meningiomas are the most common intracranial extraaxial mass and are the second most common mass found in the CPA (after VS), accounting for 10%–15% of all tumors in this location.[1,8] Ten percent of meningiomas occur in the CPA.[6]

Given their location in the CPA, symptoms related to CN VIII may be encountered. Facial pain, less common with VS, can occur in up to 30% of patients with CPA meningiomas.[6]

Histopathologically, meningiomas are derived from arachnoid meningoepithelial cells. Within the CPA, meningiomas most often arise from the posterior petrous dura. Meningiomas extend into, but do not enlarge, the porus acousticus, a subtle but important imaging feature. Hyperostosis is more common than bone erosion.[1,6]

CT usually demonstrates a hyperdense mass with occasional calcification in the CPA, although not necessarily centered at the IAC. Evaluation for subtle hyperostosis of the petrous temporal bone may aid in diagnosis (Fig. 12.6). MRI demonstrates a dural-based extraaxial lesion, isointense to cortex on T1-weighted imaging with intense enhancement (Figs. 12.6–12.8).[1,5,6,8] Enhancing dural tails are a frequent imaging feature, although they are nonspecific and may be related to reactive change as opposed to a neoplastic process.[26]

Meningiomas and VSs may appear similar by imaging, and several studies have utilized advanced MRI techniques for potential differentiation between the two. DWI characteristics of meningioma and VS have been compared, but the ADC values have not shown reliability in distinction between these two lesions.[1,19,20] Relative tumor blood volume has also been shown to be higher in meningiomas than in VS.[1,21] An alanine peak and elevated glutamate/glutamine peak is seen with meningioma with MR spectroscopy.[22] Microhemorrhage on gradient echo sequences has been shown to have high sensitivity and specificity in distinguishing VS from meningioma.[12]

## Hemangiopericytoma

Hemangiopericytomas, which are currently accepted as a cellular variant of solitary fibrous tumor,[27] are rare hypervascular lesions that are infrequently encountered in the CPA. These lesions are similar in imaging appearance to meningioma, often with more aggressive features and a much greater risk for recurrence and metastases.[6,28,29]

## Epidermoid Cysts

Epidermoid cysts are the third most common tumor of the CPA, accounting for 5% of all lesions in this location and 1% of all intracranial tumors.[1,6,9] These are congenital lesions arising from the inclusion of ectodermal epithelial tissue during neural tube closure. About 50% of intracranial epidermoid cysts are located in the CPA.[9,30]

Epidermoid cysts enlarge over time because of the accumulation of keratin and cholesterol produced by the desquamation of the squamous epithelium. These lesions tend to encase and surround (and not displace) adjacent structures, such as cranial nerves and vessels in the CPA.[6,9,31–33] Clinical symptoms therefore tend to arise when the lesions become large. A unique clinical presentation of epidermoid cysts is recurrent episodes of aseptic meningitis related to inflammation induced by the keratin debris.[6,34]

Epidermoid cysts are hypodense and almost isoattenuating to CSF in the CPA on CT examinations (Fig. 12.9), although marginal calcifications may be seen.[2,5] These lesions also demonstrate imaging characteristics and a signal intensity similar to that of CSF on conventional MRI whereby they are hypointense in signal on T1 and hyperintense in signal on T2. Fluid-attenuated inversion recovery (FLAIR) images are useful in distinguishing these lesions from the CSF normally located in the CPA, as signal is incompletely suppressed in an epidermoid cyst (Fig. 12.9).[5,6,9] Furthermore, the characteristic imaging feature associated with this lesion is the presence of restricted diffusion, not only useful in initial evaluation but also of high utility in the postoperative

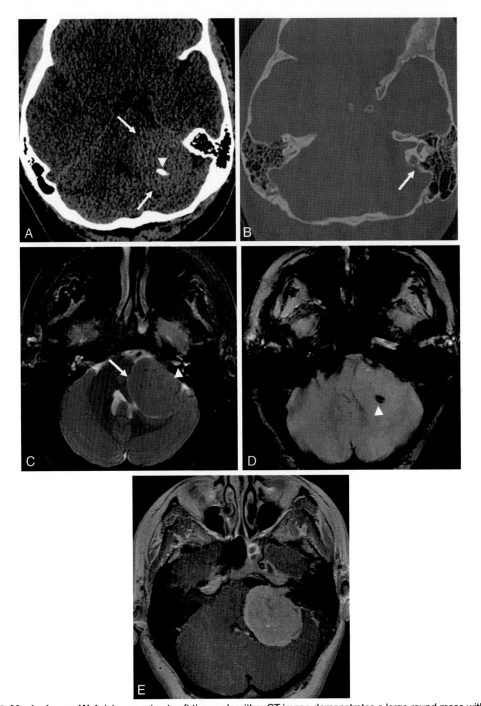

FIG. 12.6 **Meningioma.** **(A)** Axial noncontrast soft tissue algorithm CT image demonstrates a large round mass within the left aspect of the posterior fossa (*arrows*). Note the central coarse calcification (*arrowhead*). The mass is isodense to slightly hyperdense to the adjacent brain parenchyma. There is mass effect on the left aspect of the pons, middle cerebellar peduncle, and cerebellum, with partial effacement of the fourth ventricle. **(B)** Axial bone algorithm CT image at the level of the left internal auditory canal (IAC) demonstrates subtle hyperostosis of the temporal bone posterior to the IAC (*arrow*). **(C)** Axial fat-suppressed T2-weighted image demonstrates the large mass predominantly located in the left cerebellopontine angle (*arrow*). Note the increased soft tissue contrast of MR allowing for more accurate depiction of the mass and distinction from the adjacent brainstem and cerebellum. Extension of the mass through the left porus acousticus into the IAC is seen. The mass does not reach the fundus of the IAC, as shown by preservation of the cerebrospinal fluid within this region (*arrowhead*). **(D)** Axial gradient echo image shows the focal region of susceptibility (*arrowhead*) corresponding to the coarse calcification seen on CT. **(E)** Axial postcontrast T1-weighted image shows near-homogeneous enhancement of the mass (cisternal and canalicular components).

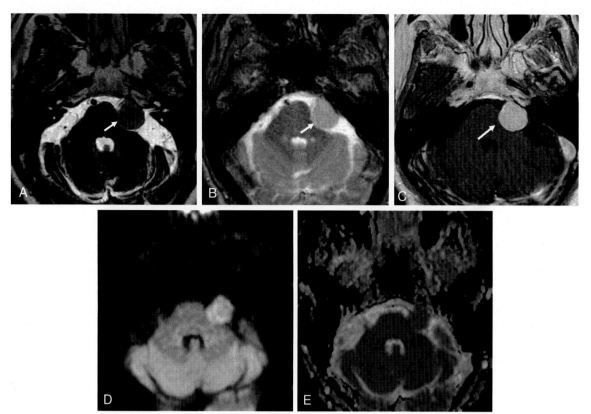

FIG. 12.7 **Meningioma. (A)** Axial high-resolution 3D T2-weighted image demonstrates a round hypointense mass centered within the left cerebellopontine angle and along the left petrous apex (*arrow*). **(B)** Axial gradient echo image demonstrates no susceptibility artifact within the lesion (*arrow*). **(C)** Axial postcontrast T1-weighted image demonstrates homogeneous enhancement of the lesion with a broad base dural attachment (*arrow*). Note that the lesion does not extend into the internal auditory canal. Axial diffusion-weighted image **(D)** and the corresponding apparent diffusion coefficient (ADC) map **(E)** show associated restricted diffusion.

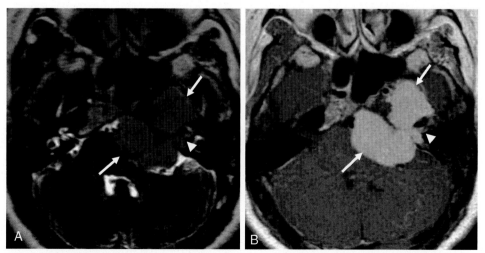

FIG. 12.8 **Meningioma. (A)** Axial high-resolution 3D T2-weighted image demonstrates a multilobulated hypointense mass centered within the left cerebellopontine angle (*arrows*). Note the mass effect on the left aspect of the pons and middle cerebellar peduncle with associated hyperintense signal consistent with edema. There is extension of the tumor into the middle cranial fossa and into the left internal auditory canal (*arrowhead*). **(B)** Axial postcontrast T1-weighted image demonstrates homogeneous enhancement of the lesion (*arrows*) including the portion within the IAC (*arrowhead*).

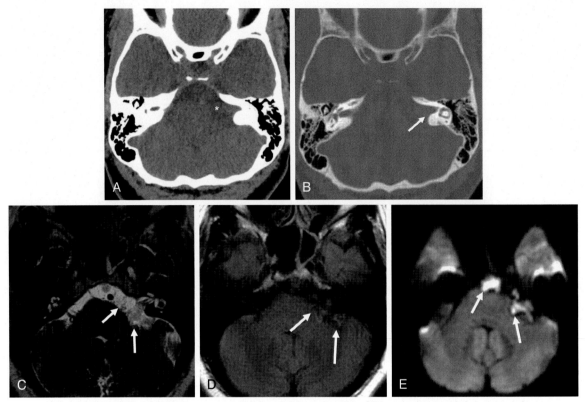

**FIG. 12.9 Epidermoid. (A)** Axial unenhanced soft tissue algorithm CT image shows subtle asymmetric widening of the left cerebellopontine angle (CPA) cistern (*asterisk*) and mild mass effect on the left aspect of the pons. **(B)** Corresponding bone algorithm CT image shows subtle asymmetric widening of the left porus acousticus (*arrow*). **(C)** Axial high-resolution 3D T2-weighted image demonstrates the asymmetric expansion of the left aspect of the CPA cistern and flattening of the pons (*arrows*). **(D)** Axial fluid-attenuated inversion recovery image demonstrates heterogeneously increased signal within the CPA cistern and prepontine cistern (*arrows*). There is subtle extension into the porus acousticus. **(E)** Axial diffusion-weighted image shows the characteristic restricted diffusion of these lesions (*arrows*).

patient for the evaluation of residual tumor (Figs. 12.9 and 12.10).[9,35–37] An elevated lactate peak is seen with this lesion if evaluated by MR spectroscopy.[9,38]

Arachnoid cysts (described in greater detail later) may appear quite similar to epidermoid cysts on imaging. An epidermoid cyst can be differentiated from arachnoid cysts on the basis of incomplete suppression of signal on FLAIR images, the presence of diffusion restriction, and the absence of scalloping or erosion of the adjacent temporal bone.[2,39]

### Arachnoid Cysts

Arachnoid cysts account for less than 1% of lesions in the CPA. These are usually found in the supratentorial location, most commonly in the middle cranial fossa (70% of lesions). Seven percent of all arachnoid

cysts are located in the CPA, and of these, 15% develop symptoms, usually related to mass effect.[6,9,40]

Arachnoid cysts are CSF-filled masses of uncertain etiology, although they are thought to be congenital lesions. These are usually incidentally found on imaging but can be associated with cranial nerve symptoms caused by mass effect.[2,5,9] Posterior fossa and CPA arachnoid cysts may also result in brainstem and cerebellar compression, suboccipital headaches, tonsillar descent, and syringomyelia.[6,41]

On imaging, these are smooth lesions that displace adjacent structures (such as cranial nerves and vessels in the CPA) and scallop adjacent bones.[2,9] They are isoattenuating to CSF on CT but can be identified by asymmetric enlargement of a CSF space. Arachnoid cysts follow CSF intensity on all MR sequences, including complete suppression of signal on FLAIR.

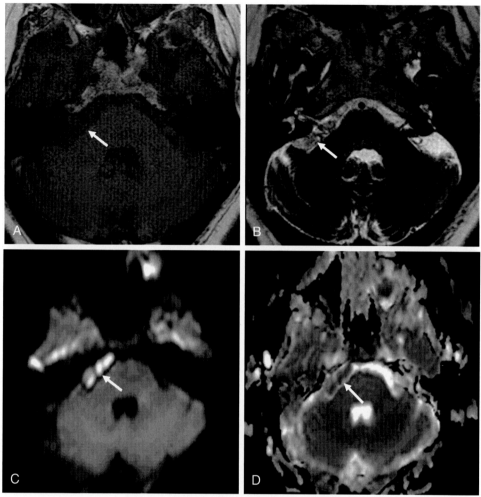

FIG. 12.10 **Epidermoid. (A)** Axial T1-weighted image demonstrates faint isointense signal in the mildly expanded right cerebellopontine angle (CPA). Note the asymmetry in signal intensity in comparison with cerebrospinal fluid within the left CPA cistern and the slight contour abnormality with flattening of the right lateral pons and cerebellum (*arrow*). **(B)** Axial high-resolution 3D T2-weighted image better depicts the margins of the lobulated hypointense lesion (*arrow*). Axial diffusion-weighted **(C)** and ADC **(D)** images show the characteristic diffusion restriction (*arrows*) and very clearly define the margins of the lesion, a useful technique for pre- and postoperative evaluation.

Differentiation from epidermoid cysts is made by the complete absence of signal on FLAIR images and by lack of diffusion restriction on DWI (Fig. 12.11).[2,6,9]

### Dermoid Cysts
Dermoid cysts may rarely involve the CPA, as these are usually midline lesions, formed from the congenital inclusion of the cutaneous ectoderm. As such, these lesions are fat attenuation on CT and may be heterogeneous with calcifications caused by the inclusion of all elements of the skin. Dermoid cysts also demonstrate fat signal intensity on MRI, with hyperintense signal on T1-weighted images and a characteristic fat fluid level.[2,9,39]

### Lipomas
Lipomas are congenital masses arising from the abnormal differentiation of meninges. These are uncommon in the CPA, accounting for less than 1% of all lesions in this location, and are more commonly located near the corpus callosum.[6,9]

Lipomas appear identical to fat on CT and MRI. They are homogeneous fatty lesions, encasing and surrounding adjacent structures, hypodense on CT, and hyperintense in signal on T1 and T2-weighted images (Fig. 12.12). There is complete suppression of signal with fat-suppression techniques. Lipomas do not enhance.[2,6,9] In a series of 100 cases, lipomas were found to encase adjacent neurovascular structures with dense adhesions.[9] Symptoms are related to compression of adjacent structures, including cranial nerves.[6]

## Neurenteric Cysts

Neurenteric cysts are congenital cysts that may result from dysgenesis of the neurenteric canal during embryogenesis. These cysts are lined by mucin-producing epithelium of endodermal origin, closely resembling the gastrointestinal tract mucosa. These are rarely encountered in the CPA and, when found in the neuraxis, are usually located in the spinal canal. However, when involving the posterior fossa, the CPA is the most common location.[2,9,42–44]

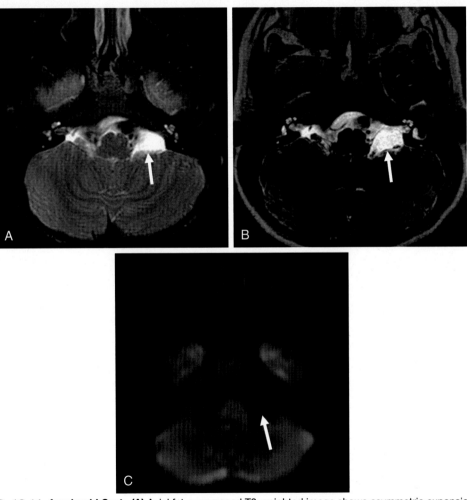

**FIG. 12.11 Arachnoid Cyst. (A)** Axial fat-suppressed T2-weighted image shows asymmetric expansion of the left cerebellopontine angle cistern (*arrow*). Note the absence of signal loss from cerebrospinal fluid pulsation. There is mild mass effect with displacement of the anterior lateral margin of the left cerebellum without associated parenchymal signal abnormality. **(B)** Axial high-resolution 3D T2-weighted image better depicts the lesion (*arrow*). There is anterior displacement of the VII-VIII cranial nerve complex. **(C)** Diffusion-weighted image demonstrates no diffusion signal abnormality (*arrow*), a helpful feature in distinguishing from an epidermoid.

Imaging characteristics depend on the protein content of the cyst. Lesions are usually round and smoothly marginated and may demonstrate rare peripheral enhancement.[2,9,42,44,45]

## Metastases

Metastases involving the CPA should be considered in patients with a known primary malignancy presenting with posterior fossa or cranial nerve symptoms.[1] Metastatic lesions may arise from the brain parenchyma, temporal bone, or meninges. Metastatic involvement of the CPA accounts for less than 1% of tumors in this location. The most common primary malignancies to involve this region include breast, lung, melanoma, thyroid, renal, and prostate cancers (Fig. 12.13).[6]

## INFECTIOUS/INFLAMMATORY LESIONS

Infectious, inflammatory, and granulomatous involvement of the leptomeninges near the skull base and involvement of the CPA may be responsible for posterior fossa and cranial nerve symptoms associated with the CPA region (Fig. 12.14).

### Neurosarcoidosis

Sarcoidosis involves the central nervous system in 5% of cases and most often presents as leptomeningeal and dural involvement.[46] Although meningeal enhancement usually involves the suprasellar and frontal regions, involvement of the CPA can also be seen.[1,46] Presenting symptoms can include headache and symptoms related to cranial nerve involvement. Imaging can reveal diffuse dural thickening or focal dural masses as T1 isointense on precontrast MR images, with homogeneous enhancement on postcontrast T1-weighted images (Fig. 12.15). Typically, there is associated T2

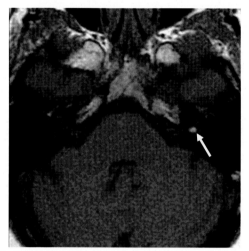

FIG. 12.12 **Lipoma.** Axial unenhanced T1-weighted image shows a hyperintense nodule at the fundus of the left internal auditory canal, consistent with a lipoma (*arrow*).

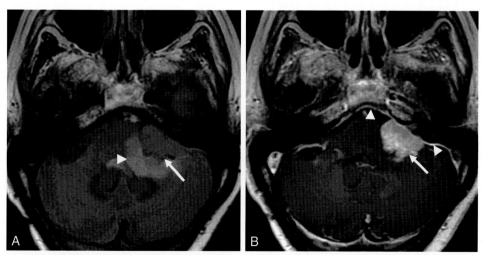

FIG. 12.13 **Dural Metastasis From Lung Cancer. (A)** Axial fluid-attenuated inversion recovery image demonstrates a slightly hyperintense mass centered in the left cerebellopontine angle (*arrows*). Note the significant mass effect on the left brainstem and cerebellum, with associated hyperintense signal related to edema (*arrowhead*). **(B)** Axial postcontrast T1-weighted image demonstrates homogeneous enhancement of the mass (*arrow*) and associated extension of the dural enhancement (*arrowheads*).

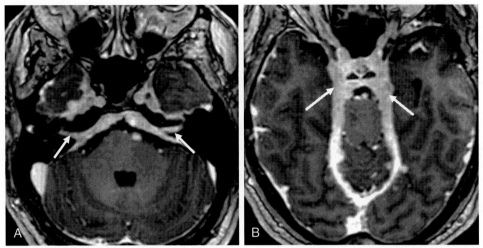

FIG. 12.14 **Idiopathic Hypertrophic Pachymeningitis.** **(A)** Axial postcontrast T1-weighted image demonstrates thickening and enhancement of the dura with extension into the bilateral internal auditory canal (*arrows*). **(B)** Axial postcontrast T1-weighted image through the middle cranial fossa and cerebellar vermis shows extensive thick dural enhancement along the tentorium and along the temporal convexities. Note the thick dural enhancement in the parasellar region and along the right optic nerve sheaths (*arrows*).

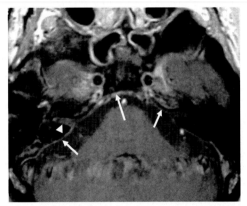

FIG. 12.15 **Sarcoidosis.** Axial postcontrast T1-weighted image demonstrates dural enhancement involving the bilateral cerebellopontine angles (*arrows*). There is also enhancement of the intracanalicular segment of the right cranial nerve VII-VIII complex (*arrowhead*).

hypointensity, which may help to differentiate sarcoidosis from other differential considerations, although this feature is nonspecific.[46,47]

## Tuberculosis

Central nervous system tuberculosis most often manifests with basilar (leptomeningeal) enhancement. Involvement of the CPA is rare.[1,48] As with neurosarcoidosis, clinical presentation and imaging features are nonspecific, and the diagnosis should be considered in patients with risk factors for the disease.

## Neurocysticercosis

Neurocysticercosis, an infectious disease caused by the parasite *Taenia solium*, most commonly affects the cerebral cortex as multifocal cystic lesions presenting clinically with seizures. In its racemose form, multiple nonenhancing cysts can be seen, sometimes in the CPA.[9] Imaging may show multiple lobulated cysts without associated mural nodules or enhancement. Lesions in this form may appear similar to arachnoid cysts. As the lesions are of CSF signal intensity, they are often difficult to appreciate and diagnose but should be considered in the setting of a single enlarged cistern in a patient from an endemic area.[9,49,50] The lack of adjacent osseous erosion and absence of diffusion restriction may help to distinguish neurocysticercosis from arachnoid cysts and epidermoid cysts, respectively.[9,49]

## SKULL BASE LESIONS
### Cholesterol Granuloma

Cholesterol granulomas are expansile lesions of the petrous apex that may grow large enough to affect adjacent structures in the CPA.[9] These result from the obstruction of petrous apex air cells with resultant repeated hemorrhage and inflammation, leading to gradual lesion expansion with bone remodeling and resorption.[51]

On CT, cholesterol granulomas are sharply marginated lesions with bone remodeling occurring in the temporal bone with density similar to that of brain parenchyma. MRI shows central heterogeneous hyperintensity on T1- and T2-weighted images within lesions caused by repeated hemorrhage, with peripheral hypointense signal.[2,9,51]

## Paraganglioma (Glomus Tumors)

Paragangliomas, also known as glomus tumors, are highly vascular benign but locally aggressive neuroendocrine tumors often seen in the head and neck. Paragangliomas that affect the CPA most often arise from the CN X at the jugular foramen (glomus jugulare) or from Jacobson nerve (tympanic branch of the CN IX) or Arnold nerve (auricular branch of the CN X) within the middle ear (glomus tympanicum).[2,9] Of these, glomus jugulares more commonly affect the CPA.[6]

CT demonstrates permeative or infiltrative osseous changes with loss of the cortex of the jugular foramen or temporal bone and avid enhancement after contrast administration. MRI also shows hypervascular soft tissue masses with a "salt-and-pepper" appearance related to linear and serpinginous flow voids and regions of T1 hyperintensity from intralesional hemorrhage, often with prominent draining veins (Fig. 12.16).[2,9,52,53]

## Chondromas and Chondrosarcomas

Chondromas and chondrosarcomas develop from embryologic cartilaginous remnants of bone. Lesions that may affect the CPA arise from the petroclival and sphenooccipital synchondroses.[2,9,51] On CT, chondromas and chondrosarcomas are usually hypodense because of hyaline cartilaginous components and often have internal calcifications. There may also be associated destruction of adjacent bone. MRI characteristics are also related to the hyaline cartilage within these lesions, with hyperintense signal on T2-weighted images and hypointense signal on T1-weighted images. There is relatively little enhancement due to the hypovascularity of these lesions.[2,9,51,54]

## Chordoma

Chordoma are thought to arise from primitive notochord remnants and usually occur at the midline near the dorsum sellae. They rarely extend into the CPA cistern.[2,9] Chordoma appears as a well-circumscribed centrally located expansile soft tissue mass associated with the destruction of the clivus and possible peripheral calcifications. On MRI, the lesions demonstrate T2 hyperintensity with lobulated margins. Internal septations are considered a characteristic imaging feature.[51,55] The T1 signal can be low to intermediate due to regions of residual bone, protein, or hemorrhage. There may be mild enhancement.[2,9,51,55]

## Endolymphatic Sac Tumors

Endolymphatic sac tumors (ELSTs) are papillary adenomatous tumors that arise from the endolymphatic sac. Twenty percent of the cases arise from sporadic mutations, although they are associated with von Hippel-Lindau (VHL) disease. On CT, ELSTs appear as destructive osseous lesions of the retrolabyrinthine petrous temporal bone with possible internal spiculations of bone. They demonstrate heterogeneous signal intensity on MR images because of the presence of intratumoral hemorrhage and avid enhancement.[2,6,9,51]

## Petrous Apicitis

Petrous apicitis refers to an inflammatory process centered in the petrous apex of the temporal bone, often resulting as sequelae of otitis media and otomastoiditis. Cranial neuropathy is often clinically present. Gradenigo syndrome refers to the presence of fifth and sixth cranial neuropathies in the setting of petrous apicitis.[51,56]

CT may demonstrate destructive changes of the petrous apex with imaging features of otitis media, such as a middle ear effusion[2,51]; however, changes in the petrous apex may be subtle on CT. MRI demonstrates edema and inflammatory changes and enhancement in the petrous apex, which may or may not be pneumatized. Careful evaluation of the cavernous sinus is necessary to evaluate for the extension of the inflammatory process and resultant complications such as cavernous sinus thrombosis.[56] Enhancement may also be seen along the fifth and sixth cranial nerves in the clinical setting of Gradenigo syndrome.[2,51,56]

# INTRAAXIAL LESIONS
## Glioma

Brainstem gliomas may asymmetrically expand the brainstem and extend into the region of the CPA cistern, sometimes with a pedicle. The imaging features are relatively nonspecific. A hypodense mass with variable enhancement can be seen on CT. MRI shows a T2 hyperintense intraaxial lesion often with surrounding edema. Enhancement is variable depending on the grade of the tumor.[2,9]

## Choroid Plexus Papilloma

Choroid plexus papillomas arise from the neuroepithelial cells of the choroid plexus. Although they are most often found in the pediatric population, they may also be seen in adults, where they most commonly arise from the fourth ventricle and extend through foramen of Luschka.[2,6,9]

Choroid plexus papillomas are hyperdense on CT, with possible cysts and associated calcifications. They appear as irregular T2 hyperintense and T1 isointense masses with

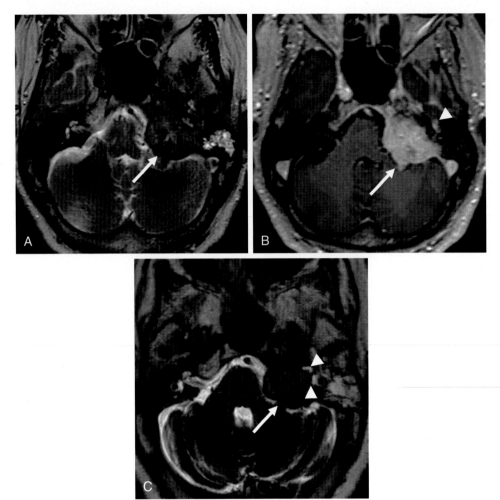

**FIG. 12.16 Glomus Jugulotympanicum. (A)** Axial T2-weighted image demonstrates a heterogeneous, mostly hypointense mass within the left cerebellopontine angle (CPA) (*arrow*) with associated mass effect on the left pontomedullary region and left cerebellum. There is fluid opacification of the left mastoid air cells. **(B)** Axial postcontrast T1-weighted image demonstrates avid enhancement of the lesion (*arrow*). Note also the enhancement within the left middle ear cavity (*arrowhead*). **(C)** Axial high-resolution 3D T2-weighted image demonstrates the mass as a large hypointense filling defect in the left CPA cistern (*arrow*). Note the preserved fluid signal in the cochlea and vestibule (*arrowheads*), although fluid signal in completely lost in the left internal auditory canal.

intense enhancement. Hydrocephalus may be seen on both CT and MRI because of CSF production from the tumor and from obstruction of the fourth ventricle.[9,57]

## Lymphoma

Lymphoma may be either intra- or extraaxial in the CPA region and may also present as leptomeningeal disease.[2,9,58] Parenchymal lymphoma usually demonstrates iso- to hyperattenuation on CT with enhancement. On MRI, lesions are T1 hypointense with enhancement.[2] Seventy-five percent of lesions demonstrate a T2-hypointense

signal because of the high cellularity of the tumor. Restricted diffusion is also often seen because of the high cellularity.[9,59–61] MR perfusion shows low cerebral blood volume because of the low vascularity of lesions.[21]

## Hemangioblastoma

Hemangioblastomas are benign vascular intraaxial lesions often located in the cerebellum. These lesions are often associated with VHL but are sporadic 25% of the time.[2,6,9] On CT, a well-circumscribed homogeneous hypodense cystic mass with an enhancing mural nodule is most

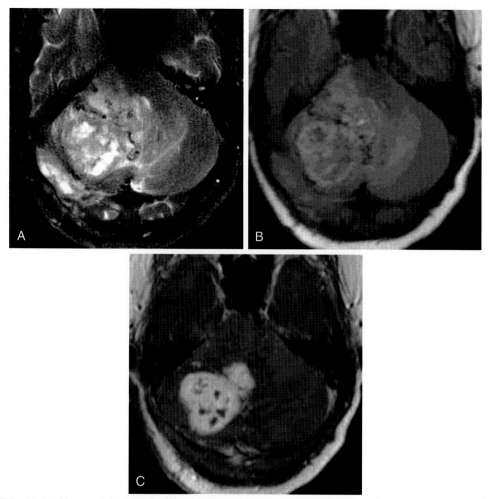

FIG. 12.17 **Hemangioblastoma. (A)** Axial T2-weighted image with fat suppression shows a heterogeneous T2 hyperintense mass centered in the right cerebellum. Note the linear T2 hypointense foci consistent with flow voids. **(B)** Axial fluid-attenuated inversion recovery image shows the extensive edema extending into the right pons. There is mass effect in the right cerebellum and brainstem with effacement of the CPA cistern. **(C)** Axial postcontrast T1-weighted images show the large heterogeneously enhancing mass.

often seen (60% of cases). Hemangioblastomas can also appear as a solid mass without a cystic component.[2,9] On MRI, the cystic component is similar in intensity to CSF, although it demonstrates slightly increased signal and incomplete signal suppression on the FLAIR images. The nodule is hypointense on T1-weighted images, is hyperintense on T2-weighted images, and demonstrates intense enhancement (Fig. 12.17). The highly vascular nature of this mass is readily identified on angiography with the demonstration of a tumoral blush.[9,62,63]

## Ependymoma

Ependymomas are tumors that arise from ependymal cells or ependymal rests. They are found along the neuraxis,

although two-thirds of tumors are found in the posterior fossa. Ependymomas usually arise in the fourth ventricle and extend into the CPA, although they can arise directly from within the CPA. Extension of a fourth ventricular ependymoma through the foramen of Luschka is seen more commonly than with choroid plexus papilloma.[2,9]

Ependymomas appear as irregular lobulated masses on imaging that conform to the shape of the ventricles and cisterns. They may have a cystic component with regions of necrosis and calcifications on CT. They are iso- to hypointense on T1-weighted images and hyperintense on T2-weighted images and demonstrate irregular enhancement. Hydrocephalus is commonly seen with these lesions.[2,5,6,9]

## Medulloblastoma

Medulloblastomas are primary neuroepithelial tumors that can occur at midline in the posterior fossa in children. Medulloblastomas may be seen as a part of Gorlin (nevoid basal-cell carcinoma) syndrome.[27] The adult form occurs in the third or fourth decade of life and is more common in the cerebellar hemispheres than in the vermis. There may be an exophytic component that extends into the CPA cistern. Medulloblastomas are associated with CSF seeding, and imaging of the entire neuraxis is essential to evaluate for dissemination.[2,9,64]

CT imaging of medulloblastoma demonstrates a hyperdense mass because of the high cellularity of the lesions. Calcifications are uncommonly seen. Medulloblastomas are hypointense on T1-weighted images and iso- to hyperintense on T2-weighted images, with cystic and necrotic components and enhancement.[2,9] DWI shows low ADC values.[65] Evaluation of medulloblastoma with MR spectroscopy reveals elevated taurine and choline peaks.[66]

## Metastases

Metastases to the cerebellum and brainstem may result in parenchymal edema that effaces the CPA cistern (Fig. 12.18). As described earlier, metastases to the CPA region may arise from the brain parenchyma, temporal bone, or meninges. The imaging features of metastatic parenchymal lesions are nonspecific but should be strongly considered in a patient with a known primary malignancy and multiple intracranial lesions.[6,9]

## VASCULAR LESIONS

Various abnormalities related to the intracranial vessels in the posterior fossa may compress structures and produce symptoms that correlate clinically with a CPA process. Aneurysms, vascular malformations, and tortuosity (dolichoectasia) of the vertebral, posterior inferior cerebellar, anterior inferior cerebellar, and basilar arteries may be seen.[1]

Enlargement and tortuosity of the vessels are easily identified on angiographic imaging of the intracranial vessels, either with CT or MR angiography (Fig. 12.19). Aneurysms may be seen on CT or MRI of the brain as a well-defined round or oval lesion (Fig. 12.20). In the absence of significant central thrombosis, the aneurysm may be associated with significant signal void and pulsation artifacts on MRI. If there is intraluminal thrombus, heterogeneous iso- to hyperintense signal on T1-weighted images with variable enhancement may be seen.[1,2,8,67]

## Cavernoma

Cavernomas (cavernous malformations) are benign vascular hemartomas composed of closely apposed immature blood vessels. These lesions are most commonly located in the pons, although they are often found in the cerebellum. Cavernomas rarely arise in the extraaxial location in the CPA from cranial nerves.[1]

Cavernomas are well characterized on MRI, which reveals a lobulated lesion with heterogeneous signal on T1-weighted images corresponding to blood products of various ages. There is often central T1 hyperintense signal and T2 hyperintense signal. A hypointense hemosiderin rim is seen on all imaging sequences. CT may demonstrate a rounded hyperdense lesion with possible calcifications.[1,68]

## OSSEOUS LESIONS

Osseous lesions of the temporal bone may also extend into the CPA cistern and result in a mass effect upon the CPA structures. The petrous apex is the most commonly affected part of the temporal bone, thought to result from slow blood flow through the relatively large marrow space.[69] The most common tumors to involve the petrous apex are breast, lung, prostate, and renal cell carcinomas.[70] Significant bone destruction may be seen on CT. MRI more clearly depicts the soft tissue component, including involvement of the CPA.[69] Neoplastic involvement from lymphoma and multiple myeloma (plasmacytoma) may also affect the petrous apex and CPA.[69]

Systemic bone disorders, such as Paget disease, may also affect the temporal bone. Paget disease, or osteitis deformans, is a disorder of bone remodeling, characterized by excessive bone resorption and disordered bone formation. The temporal bone is affected in 65%–70% of patients.[71] Patients usually present with hearing loss. On imaging, thickened bone with a "cotton wool" appearance is often seen. MRI features of Paget disease vary depending on the phase of disease, ranging from signal characteristics similar to fat (most common) and heterogeneous T1 and high T2 signal intensity "speckled" appearance (Fig. 12.21) to T1 and T2 hypointense signal (least common).[72]

## CONCLUSION

A number of common and uncommon lesions can be found in the CPA on imaging evaluation of the region. Although the most commonly encountered lesions are VS and meningioma, lesions that arise from the CPA cranial nerves, vessels, or adjacent structures can be found.

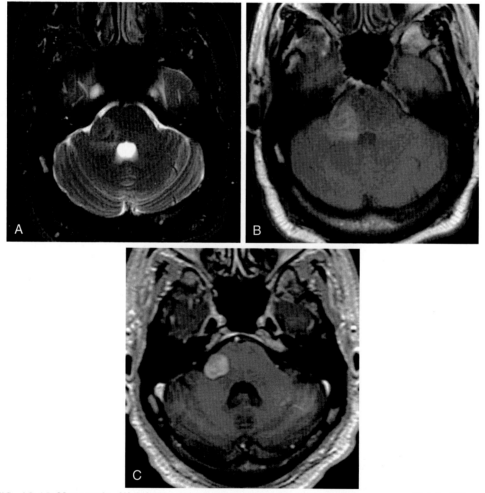

FIG. 12.18 **Metastasis.** **(A)** Axial T2-weighted image with fat suppression shows a round faintly T2 hyperintense mass centered in the right middle cerebellar peduncle. Note the subtle expansion into the right cerebellopontine angle cistern. **(B)** Axial fluid-attenuated inversion recovery image shows the edema within the right pons. **(C)** Axial postcontrast T1-weighted images show the homogeneously enhancing parenchymal mass from metastatic carcinoid (primary mass involving the ileocecal valve).

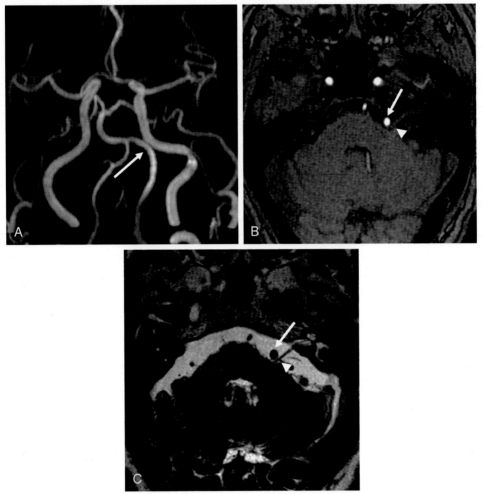

FIG. 12.19 **Neurovascular Compression. (A)** 3D time-of-flight MR angiography (MRA) maximum intensity projection image demonstrates tortuous basilar artery and left vertebral artery (*arrow*). **(B)** Axial MRA source image demonstrates proximity of the left vertebral artery (*arrow*) to the origin of the left cranial nerve (CN) VII-VIII complex (*arrowhead*). **(C)** Axial high-resolution 3D T2-weighted image better delineates the compression of the CN VII-VIII complex (*arrowhead*) by the tortuous left vertebral artery (*arrow*).

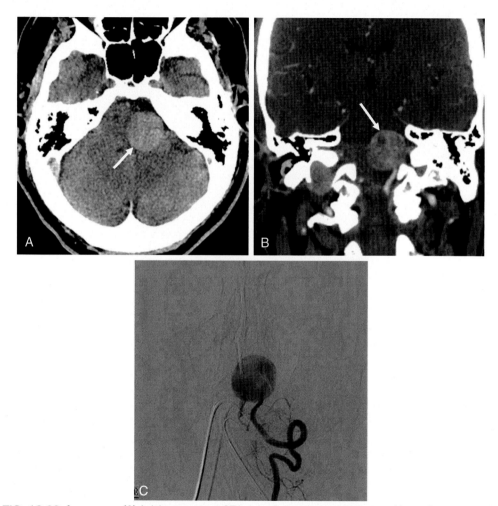

FIG. 12.20 **Aneurysm. (A)** Axial noncontrast CT image demonstrates a large round hyperdense mass in the left cerebellopontine angle (CPA) cistern (*arrow*) with mass effect on the adjacent pons and middle cerebellar peduncle. There is also partial effacement of the fourth ventricle. **(B)** Coronal postcontrast CT image demonstrates heterogeneous but early enhancement of the lesion (*arrow*), located close to the left vertebral artery. **(C)** Digital subtraction image of conventional left vertebral angiography shows vertebral origin of this large left CPA aneurysm.

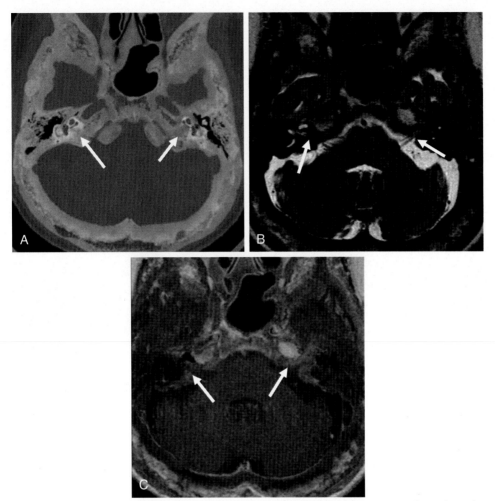

**FIG. 12.21** **Paget Disease. (A)** Axial CT image demonstrates expansile heterogeneous bone throughout the skull base, including the temporal bones. Note the near-complete obliteration of the internal auditory canals (IACs) (*arrows*). **(B)** Axial high-resolution 3D T2-weighted image demonstrates effacement of the cerebrospinal fluid signal in the IACs (*arrows*). **(C)** Axial postcontrast T1-weighted images show heterogeneous enhancement of the bone surrounding the IACs (*arrows*), reflecting hypervascularity of the lesions.

# REFERENCES

1. Bonneville F, Savatovsky J, Chiras J. Imaging of cerebello-pontine angle lesions: an update. Part 1: enhancing extra-axial lesions. *Eur Radiol.* 2007;17(10):2472–2482.
2. Bonneville F, Sarrazin JL, Marsot-Dupuch K, et al. Unusual lesions of the cerebellopontine angle: a segmental approach. *Radiographics.* 2001;21(2):419–438.
3. Brunori A, Scarano P, Chiappetta F. Non-acoustic neuroma tumor (NANT) of the cerebello-pontine angle: a 15-year experience. *J Neurosurg Sci.* 1997;41(2):159–168.
4. Moffat DA, Ballagh RH. Rare tumours of the cerebello-pontine angle. *Clin Oncol.* 1995;7(1):28–41.
5. Smirniotopoulos JG, Yue NC, Rushing EJ. Cerebellopontine angle masses: radiologic-pathologic correlation. *Radiographics.* 1993;13(5):1131–1147.
6. Friedmann DR, Grobelny B, Golfinos JG, Roland Jr JT. Nonschwannoma tumors of the cerebellopontine angle. *Otolaryngol Clin N Am.* 2015;48(3):461–475.
7. Turski PSA, Hartman E, Clark Z, et al. Neurovascular 4DFlow MRI (Phase Contrast MRA): emerging clinical applications. *Neurovascular Imaging.* 2016;2(8):11.
8. Sakai O, Nadgir RN, Fujita A, El Beltagi AH. Imaging of the temporal bone. In: Kirtane MV, De Souza K, Sanna M, Devaiah AK, eds. *Otology and Neurotology (Otorhinolaryngology – Head and Neck Surgery).* Noida: Theme; 2013.

9. Bonneville F, Savatovsky J, Chiras J. Imaging of cerebellopontine angle lesions: an update. Part 2: intra-axial lesions, skull base lesions that may invade the CPA region, and non-enhancing extra-axial lesions. *Eur Radiol.* 2007;17(11):2908–2920.

10. Khrais T, Romano G, Sanna M. Nerve origin of vestibular schwannoma: a prospective study. *J Laryngol Otol.* 2008;122(2):128–131.

11. Bonneville F, Cattin F, Czorny A, Bonneville JF. Hypervascular intracisternal acoustic neuroma. *J Neuroradiol.* 2002;29(2):128–131.

12. Thamburaj K, Radhakrishnan VV, Thomas B, Nair S, Menon G. Intratumoral microhemorrhages on T2*-weighted gradient-echo imaging helps differentiate vestibular schwannoma from meningioma. *AJNR Am J Neuroradiol.* 2008;29(3):552–557.

13. Charabi S, Tos M, Thomsen J, Rygaard J, Fundova P, Charabi B. Cystic vestibular schwannoma–clinical and experimental studies. *Acta Otolaryngol Suppl.* 2000; 543:11–13.

14. Gomez-Brouchet A, Delisle MB, Cognard C, et al. Vestibular schwannomas: correlations between magnetic resonance imaging and histopathologic appearance. *Otol Neurotol.* 2001;22(1):79–86.

15. Delsanti C, Regis J. Cystic vestibular schwannomas. *Neurochirurgie.* 2004;50(2–3 Pt 2):401–406.

16. Fundova P, Charabi S, Tos M, Thomsen J. Cystic vestibular schwannoma: surgical outcome. *J Laryngol Otol.* 2000;114(12):935–939.

17. Duvoisin B, Fernandes J, Doyon D, Denys A, Sterkers JM, Bobin S. Magnetic resonance findings in 92 acoustic neuromas. *Eur J Radiol.* 1991;13(2):96–102.

18. Okamoto K, Furusawa T, Ishikawa K, Sasai K, Tokiguchi S. Focal T2 hyperintensity in the dorsal brain stem in patients with vestibular schwannoma. *AJNR Am J Neuroradiol.* 2006;27(6):1307–1311.

19. Sener RN. Diffusion magnetic resonance imaging of solid vestibular schwannomas. *J Comput Assist Tomogr.* 2003;27(2):249–252.

20. Yamasaki F, Kurisu K, Satoh K, et al. Apparent diffusion coefficient of human brain tumors at MR imaging. *Radiology.* 2005;235(3):985–991.

21. Hakyemez B, Erdogan C, Bolca N, Yildirim N, Gokalp G, Parlak M. Evaluation of different cerebral mass lesions by perfusion-weighted MR imaging. *J Magn Reson Imaging.* 2006;24(4):817–824.

22. Cho YD, Choi GH, Lee SP, Kim JK. (1)H-MRS metabolic patterns for distinguishing between meningiomas and other brain tumors. *Magn Reson Imaging.* 2003;21(6):663–672.

23. Jacob JT, Driscoll CL, Link MJ. Facial nerve schwannomas of the cerebellopontine angle: the mayo clinic experience. *J Neurol Surg B Skull Base.* 2012;73(4):230–235.

24. Wiggins 3rd RH, Harnsberger HR, Salzman KL, Shelton C, Kertesz TR, Glastonbury CM. The many faces of facial nerve schwannoma. *AJNR Am J Neuroradiol.* 2006;27(3):694–699.

25. Xu F, Pan S, Bambakidis NC. Intracranial facial nerve schwannomas: current management and review of the literature. *World Neurosurg.* 2016;100: 444–449.

26. Guermazi A, Lafitte F, Miaux Y, Adem C, Bonneville JF, Chiras J. The dural tail sign–beyond meningioma. *Clin Radiol.* 2005;60(2):171–188.

27. Bonfioli AA, Orefice F. Sarcoidosis. *Semin Ophthalmol.* 2005;20(3):177–182.

28. Tashjian VS, Khanlou N, Vinters HV, Canalis RF, Becker DP. Hemangiopericytoma of the cerebellopontine angle: a case report and review of the literature. *Surg Neurol.* 2009;72(3):290–295.

29. Ben Nsir A, Badri M, Kassar AZ, Hammouda KB, Jemel H. Hemangiopericytoma of the cerebellopontine angle: a wolf in sheep's clothing. *Brain Tumor Res Treat.* 2016;4(1):8–12.

30. Hasegawa M, Nouri M, Nagahisa S, et al. Cerebellopontine angle epidermoid cysts: clinical presentations and surgical outcome. *Neurosurg Rev.* 2016;39(2):259–266. Discussion 266–257.

31. Osborn AG, Preece MT. Intracranial cysts: radiologic-pathologic correlation and imaging approach. *Radiology.* 2006;239(3):650–664.

32. Springborg JB, Poulsgaard L, Thomsen J. Nonvestibular schwannoma tumors in the cerebellopontine angle: a structured approach and management guidelines. *Skull Base.* 2008;18(4):217–227.

33. Gao PY, Osborn AG, Smirniotopoulos JG, Harris CP. Radiologic-pathologic correlation. Epidermoid tumor of the cerebellopontine angle. *AJNR Am J Neuroradiol.* 1992;13(3):863–872.

34. Mallucci CL, Ward V, Carney AS, O'Donoghue GM, Robertson I. Clinical features and outcomes in patients with non-acoustic cerebellopontine angle tumours. *J Neurol Neurosurg Psychiatry.* 1999;66(6):768–771.

35. Liu P, Saida Y, Yoshioka H, Itai Y. MR imaging of epidermoids at the cerebellopontine angle. *Magn Reson Med Sci.* 2003;2(3):109–115.

36. Murakami N, Matsushima T, Kuba H, et al. Combining steady-state constructive interference and diffusion-weighted magnetic resonance imaging in the surgical treatment of epidermoid tumors. *Neurosurg Rev.* 1999;22(2–3):159–162.

37. Annet L, Duprez T, Grandin C, Dooms G, Collard A, Cosnard G. Apparent diffusion coefficient measurements within intracranial epidermoid cysts in six patients. *Neuroradiology.* 2002;44(4):326–328.

38. Nguyen JB, Ahktar N, Delgado PN, Lowe LH. Magnetic resonance imaging and proton magnetic resonance spectroscopy of intracranial epidermoid tumors. *Crit Rev Comput Tomogr.* 2004;45(5–6):389–427.

39. Smirniotopoulos JG, Chiechi MV. Teratomas, dermoids, and epidermoids of the head and neck. *Radiographics.* 1995;15(6):1437–1455.

40. Helland CA, Lund-Johansen M, Wester K. Location, sidedness, and sex distribution of intracranial arachnoid cysts in a population-based sample. *J Neurosurg.* 2010;113(5):934–939.

41. Jallo GI, Woo HH, Meshki C, Epstein FJ, Wisoff JH. Arachnoid cysts of the cerebellopontine angle: diagnosis and surgery. *Neurosurgery.* 1997;40(1):31–37. Discussion 37–38.

42. Preece MT, Osborn AG, Chin SS, Smirniotopoulos JG. Intracranial neurenteric cysts: imaging and pathology spectrum. *AJNR Am J Neuroradiol.* 2006;27(6): 1211–1216.

43. Shin JH, Byun BJ, Kim DW, Choi DL. Neurenteric cyst in the cerebellopontine angle with xanthogranulomatous changes: serial MR findings with pathologic correlation. *AJNR Am J Neuroradiol.* 2002;23(4):663–665.

44. Brooks BS, Duvall ER, el Gammal T, Garcia JH, Gupta KL, Kapila A. Neuroimaging features of neurenteric cysts: analysis of nine cases and review of the literature. *AJNR Am J Neuroradiol.* 1993;14(3):735–746.

45. Chaynes P, Thorn-Kany M, Sol JC, Arrue P, Lagarrigue J, Manelfe C. Imaging in neurenteric cysts of the posterior cranial fossa. *Neuroradiology.* 1998;40(6):374–376.

46. Chapman MN, Fujita A, Sung EK, et al. Sarcoidosis in the head and neck: an illustrative review of clinical presentations and imaging findings. *AJR Am J Roentgenol.* 2017;208(1):66–75.

47. Christoforidis G, Spickler EM, Recio MV, Mehta BM. MR of CNS sarcoidosis: correlation of imaging features to clinical features and response to treatment. *AJNR Am J Neuroradiol.* 1999;20:655–669.

48. Goyal M, Sharma A, Mishra NK, Gaikwad SB, Sharma MC. Imaging appearance of pachymeningeal tuberculosis. *AJR Am J Roentgenol.* 1997;169(5):1421–1424.

49. Duchene M, Benoudiba F, Iffenecker C, Hadj-Rabia M, Caldas J, Doyon D. Neurocysticercosis. *J Radiol.* 1999;80(12):1623–1627.

50. Razek AA, Castillo M. Imaging lesions of the cavernous sinus. *AJNR Am J Neuroradiol.* 2009;30(3):444–452.

51. Chapman PR, Shah R, Cure JK, Bag AK. Petrous apex lesions: pictorial review. *AJR Am J Roentgenol.* 2011;196 (3 suppl):WS26–37. Quiz S40–23.

52. Olsen WL, Dillon WP, Kelly WM, Norman D, Brant-Zawadzki M, Newton TH. MR imaging of paragangliomas. *AJR Am J Roentgenol.* 1987;148(1):201–204.

53. Lee KY, Oh YW, Noh HJ, et al. Extraadrenal paragangliomas of the body: imaging features. *AJR Am J Roentgenol.* 2006;187(2):492–504.

54. Brownlee RD, Sevick RJ, Rewcastle NB, Tranmer BI. Intracranial chondroma. *AJNR Am J Neuroradiol.* 1997; 18(5):889–893.

55. Erdem E, Angtuaco EC, Van Hemert R, Park JS, Al-Mefty O. Comprehensive review of intracranial chordoma. *Radiographics.* 2003;23(4):995–1009.

56. Thayll N, Chapman MN, Saito N, Fujita A, Sakai O. Magnetic resonance imaging of acute head and neck infections. *Magn Reson Imaging Clin N Am.* 2016;24(2): 345–367.

57. Shin JH, Lee HK, Jeong AK, Park SH, Choi CG, Suh DC. Choroid plexus papilloma in the posterior cranial fossa: MR, CT, and angiographic findings. *Clin Imaging.* 2001;25(3):154–162.

58. Nishimura T, Uchida Y, Fukuoka M, Ono Y, Kurisaka M, Mori K. Cerebellopontine angle lymphoma: a case report and review of the literature. *Surg Neurol.* 1998;50(5):480–485. Discussion 485–486.

59. Cotton F, Ongolo-Zogo P, Louis-Tisserand G, et al. Diffusion and perfusion MR imaging in cerebral lymphomas. *J Neuroradiol.* 2006;33(4):220–228.

60. Yang PJ, Seeger JF, Carmody RF, Mehta BA. Cerebellopontine angle lymphoma. *AJNR Am J Neuroradiol.* 1987;8(2): 368–369.

61. Kariya S, Nishizaki K, Aoji K, Akagi H. Primary malignant lymphoma in the cerebellopontine angle. *J Laryngol Otol.* 1998;112(5):476–479.

62. Quadery FA, Okamoto K. Diffusion-weighted MRI of haemangioblastomas and other cerebellar tumours. *Neuroradiology.* 2003;45(4):212–219.

63. Abo-Al Hassan A, Ismail M, Panda SM. Pre-operative endovascular embolization of a cerebellar haemangioblastoma. A case report. *Med Princ Pract.* 2006;15(6):459–462.

64. Pant I, Chaturvedi S, Gautam VK, Pandey P, Kumari R. Extra-axial medulloblastoma in the cerebellopontine angle: report of a rare entity with review of literature. *J Pediatr Neurosci.* 2016;11(4):331–334.

65. Rodallec M, Colombat M, Krainik A, Kalamarides M, Redondo A, Feydy A. Diffusion-weighted MR imaging and pathologic findings in adult cerebellar medulloblastoma. *J Neuroradiol.* 2004;31(3):234–237.

66. Moreno-Torres A, Martinez-Perez I, Baquero M, et al. Taurine detection by proton magnetic resonance spectroscopy in medulloblastoma: contribution to noninvasive differential diagnosis with cerebellar astrocytoma. *Neurosurgery.* 2004;55(4):824–829. Discussion 829.

67. Papanagiotou P, Grunwald IQ, Politi M, Struffert T, Ahlhelm F, Reith W. Vascular anomalies of the cerebellopontine angle. *Radiology.* 2006;46(3):216–222.

68. Kim M, Rowed DW, Chueng G, Ang L. Cavernous malformation presenting as an extra-axial cerebellopontine angle mass: case report. *Neurosurgery.* 1997;40(1):187–190.

69. Razek AA, Huang BY. Lesions of the petrous apex: classification and findings at CT and MR imaging. *Radiographics.* 2012;32(1):151–173.

70. Isaacson B, Kutz JW, Roland PS. Lesions of the petrous apex: diagnosis and management. *Otolaryngol Clin N Am.* 2007;40(3). 479–519, viii.

71. Shonka Jr DC, Kesser BW. Paget's disease of the temporal bone. *Otol Neurotol.* 2006;27(8):1199–1200.

72. Theodorou DJ, Theodorou SJ, Kakitsubata Y. Imaging of Paget disease of bone and its musculoskeletal complications: self-assessment module. *AJR Am J Roentgenol.* 2011;196(6 suppl):WS53–56.

# CHAPTER 13

# Jugular Foramen

CHIH CHING CHOONG, MBCHB, FRCR •
ERIC T.Y. TING, MBBS (HONS), FRANZCR •
VINCENT CHONG, MD, MBA, MHPE, FRCR

The jugular foramen is a complex bony canal containing neurovascular structures deep in the skull base. It is inaccessible to direct clinical examination and difficult to access surgically because of the surrounding critical structures. Radiology plays a central role in the diagnostic evaluation and management planning of jugular foramen lesions. Consequently, it is important to comprehend the normal anatomy of the jugular foramen, as well as to recognize the anatomical variants and imaging artifacts, which are potential diagnostic pitfalls that may mimic pathology and lead to inappropriate intervention.

Lesions affecting the jugular foramen may arise from its intrinsic contents or from invasion by adjacent contiguous structures. Primary jugular foraminal tumors expand the canal and may extend intracranially, presenting as a posterior fossa or cerebellopontine angle mass, whereas distal lesions that extend extracranially result in a cervical or carotid space mass. Patients often present with otologic symptoms, such as hearing loss and tinnitus, as well as vertigo or ataxia, pain, and lower cranial nerve palsies. Owing to the small caliber of the jugular foramen and close proximity of the nerves within, a space-occupying lesion is likely to impinge on more than one cranial nerve to produce a combination of cranial nerve palsies, which include Vernet syndrome, Tapia syndrome, Schmidt syndrome, Avellis syndrome, Collet-Sicard syndrome, Villaret syndrome, and Jackson syndrome.[1]

Advances in microsurgical techniques have allowed for the resection of jugular foraminal lesions, with improved morbidity and mortality rates. Optimal assessment of jugular foramen diseases preoperatively requires both magnetic resonance imaging (MRI) and computed tomography (CT) with thin-section bone algorithm. MRI shows the exact soft tissue extent of lesions, whereas CT allows precise evaluation of the surrounding bone changes. Angiography may be useful to outline the vascular road map for surgeons or in preoperative embolization for certain hypervascular tumors. This chapter presents an overview of the anatomy of the jugular foramen, including its variants and anomalies, and illustrates the pathologic processes that may involve this foramen.

## APPLIED ANATOMY OF THE JUGULAR FORAMEN

The jugular foramen is an irregular-shaped recess with endocranial and exocranial openings (Fig. 13.1). Embryologically, the jugular foramen is established from the union of the otic capsule and the basioccipital plate, forming a canal-like aperture between reciprocal depressions of the petrous temporal bone and occipital bone.[2] It has a complex oblique course running anteriorly, then laterally, and eventually inferiorly through the skull base into the carotid space.[3] The petrous segment of the temporal bone forms the anterior wall and dome, whereas the jugular process and condylar portions of the occipital bone form the posteromedial margins of the jugular foramen.

There are several important surface landmarks and structures surrounding the jugular foramen. The entry point of the carotid canal is anteromedial to the jugular foramen, separated by the carotid ridge (Fig. 13.1A). Lateral to the carotid ridge is a tiny opening, the inferior tympanic canaliculus, where the tympanic nerve courses into the middle ear. Medially, the carotid ridge is contiguous with the jugular spine of the temporal bone. The hypoglossal canal is just inferomedial to the jugular foramen, located above the occipital condyle (Fig. 13.1B). Lateral to the jugular foramen is the styloid process, which separates it from the temporomandibular joint. The stylomastoid foramen, where the facial nerve exits, is located just posterior to the base of the styloid process and a few millimeters posterolateral to the jugular foramen.

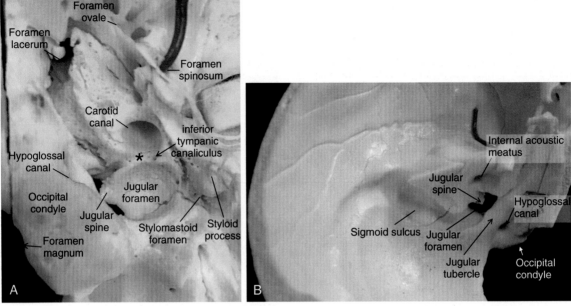

**FIG. 13.1 Jugular Foramen Anatomy on Skull Specimen. (A)** Exocranial view of the left skull base shows the opening of the jugular foramen in relation to the carotid canal (anteriorly), hypoglossal canal (inferomedially), and stylomastoid foramen (posterolaterally). The carotid and jugular openings are separated by the carotid ridge (*asterisk*). Lateral to the carotid ridge is a tiny opening, the inferior tympanic canaliculus, whereas medially it is contiguous with the jugular spine of the temporal bone. **(B)** Endocranial view of the right posterior skull base shows the termination of the sigmoid sulcus into the jugular foramen. The jugular spine demarcates the location of the intrajugular compartment. Medially, the opening of the hypoglossal canal where cranial nerve XII enters is located between the jugular tubercle and occipital condyle.

The cranial nerves within the jugular foramen are difficult to visualize using the conventional MRI protocols. They are best seen on contrast-enhanced three-dimensional fast imaging employing steady-state acquisition and high-resolution contrast-enhanced sequences such as gradient-echo MR angiography (MRA).[4] The steady-state sequence provides high contrast and spatial resolutions using a refocused gradient-echo sequence, whereas enhancement of the jugular vein and venous plexuses further increases the contrast between the hypointense cranial nerves and their surrounding hyperintense venous compartments.

The jugular foramen is divided into three compartments, consisting of two venous (petrous and sigmoid) and a neural (intrajugular) component.[5] The larger posterolateral sigmoid venous compartment drains the sigmoid sinus, whereas the smaller anteromedial petrosal compartment contains the inferior petrosal sinus. The inferior petrosal sinus is the main drainage outlet of the cavernous sinus. It runs along the petroclival fissure into the petrosal compartment of

the jugular foramen, where it forms a multichanneled confluence that receives tributaries from the hypoglossal and vertebral venous plexuses. This confluence then empties into the jugular bulb, or less commonly into the internal jugular vein, through openings between the glossopharyngeal (cranial nerve [CN] IX) and vagus (CN X) nerves in the medial wall of the jugular bulb (Fig. 13.2A). The posterior meningeal artery also traverses the jugular foramen adjacent to the vagus and accessory (CN XI) nerves to supply the posterior fossa meninges. It is usually a branch of the ascending pharyngeal artery, although it may occasionally arise from the anterior inferior cerebellar artery.

The two venous compartments are separated by a fibrous or bony septum between the jugular spine of the temporal bone and jugular process of the occipital bone (Fig. 13.2A). Occasionally, this septum may be completely ossified. The glossopharyngeal, vagus, and accessory nerves exit the cranium through the intrajugular compartment, which is located between the two venous compartments. There are two characteristic

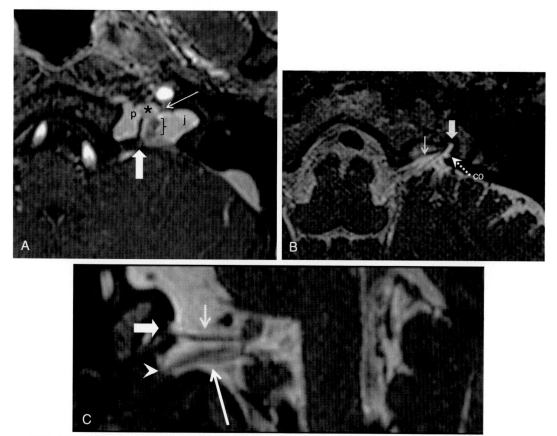

**FIG. 13.2** **Jugular Foramen Anatomy on MRI. (A)** Axial contrast-enhanced T1-weighted VIBE image demonstrating the three compartments of the jugular foramen: the jugular bulb (j) is separated from the inferior petrosal sinus (p) by a dural septum, which is a linear hypointense structure attached to the inter-jugular process (*thick arrow*). The intrajugular compartment in the middle contains cranial nerve (CN) IX (*thin arrow*) anterolaterally and the CNX/XI complex (*bracket*) posteromedially. The inferior petrosal sinus empties into the jugular bulb via perforations in the dural septum (*asterisk*). **(B)** Axial and **(C)** oblique sagittal FIESTA images. The intracranial segment of the glossopharyngeal nerve (*short arrow*) pierces the dura at the glossopharyngeal meatus (*solid arrow*) to enter the jugular foramen. The cochlear aqueduct (co) opens just above the glossopharyngeal meatus. The vagus nerve (*long arrow*) enters the vagus meatus (*arrowhead*) more inferiorly.

perforations in the dural roof of the jugular foramen: the glossopharyngeal meatus where CN IX enters, and inferiorly the vagal meatus through which CN X and XI penetrate (Fig. 13.2B and C). The two meatuses are separated by a dural septum.[5,6]

Upon entering the jugular foramen, CN IX turns forward and downward, forming a genu that is lodged at or near the external opening of the cochlear aqueduct, before coursing inferiorly into the carotid sheath. Extreme care is essential during translabyrinthine surgery to avoid injuring the CN IX genu.[6,7] The CN IX forms a superior and inferior ganglion within the jugular foramen, with

the tympanic branch (Jacobson nerve) arising from the latter. The Jacobson nerve enters the inferior tympanic canaliculus, coursing into the hypotympanum where it forms the tympanic plexus over the cochlear promontory. CN IX is situated anterosuperolateral to CNs X and XI. Upon exiting the jugular foramen, CN IX runs between the carotid artery and the internal jugular vein.

The CNs X and XI complex pierce the dura inferior to the glossopharyngeal nerve. CN X also forms a superior and inferior ganglion within the jugular foramen, with the auricular branch (Arnold nerve) arising from the superior ganglion. This nerve passes through the mastoid

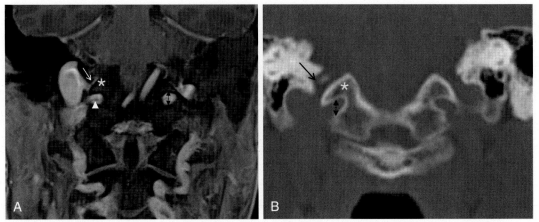

**FIG. 13.3 Imaging of the Jugular Foramen and Hypoglossal Canal. (A)** Coronal contrast-enhanced T1-weighted MR with fat saturation and **(B)** coronal CT bone window images demonstrating the classic "eagle's head" configuration of the jugular tubercle, which resembles the eagle's head (*asterisk*). This is a useful landmark in locating the jugular foramen (*long arrow*) and the hypoglossal canal (*double arrows*). The normal hypoglossal nerve (*arrowhead*) can be seen on MR because of the background hyperintensity of the contrast-enhanced anterior condylar vein.

canaliculus into the facial nerve canal (mastoid segment) before exiting via the tympanomastoid fissure into the external auditory canal. The CN X and XI nerve fibers intermingle throughout the jugular foramen and are inseparable by microdissection.[8] Within the intrajugular compartment, CN IX is located anterolaterally, whereas the CN X/XI complex is seen posterolaterally (Fig. 13.2A).

The hypoglossal canal is inferomedial to the jugular foramen, located between the occipital condyle and jugular tubercle (Fig. 13.1B). On coronal images, the jugular tubercle has a characteristic "eagle's head" configuration, which is an important anatomic landmark in locating and separating the hypoglossal canal from the jugular foramen superolaterally (Fig. 13.3). The venous plexus within the hypoglossal canal is referred to as the anterior condylar vein, which joins the inferomedial margin of the inferior petrosal sinus. The hypoglossal canal also contains the neuromeningeal branch of the ascending pharyngeal artery and the hypoglossal nerve (CN CXII). The hypoglossal nerve may consist of one or two trunks, which penetrate the dura to exit the cranium via a single or duplicated hypoglossal canal located above the occipital condyle.[9] CN XII then descends in the carotid sheath together with the glossopharyngeal, vagus, and accessory nerves.

## JUGULAR BULB VARIANTS AND ANOMALIES

Upon entering the jugular foramen, the sigmoid sinus turns laterally and expands into the jugular bulb. The

jugular bulb is usually larger on the right side in up to 75% of individuals.[10] There are a number of important jugular bulb variants and anomalies that should be recognized.

### High-Riding and Dehiscent Jugular Bulb

Conventionally, a high-riding jugular bulb is defined as a jugular bulb with its roof or dome extending above the inferior tympanic annulus[11] or floor of the internal acoustic canal. Some authors used the inferior margin of the basal turn of cochlea as the criterion[12] (Fig. 13.4). High-riding jugular bulbs are more common on the right side, with an incidence of 4%–24%.[11,12] This is an important variant to be mentioned if found incidentally during the evaluation of cerebellopontine angle lesions, as its presence compromises the operative window during a translabyrinthine surgery and precludes adequate exposure of the inferior compartment of the inner ear and the cerebellopontine angle.[13] Modified surgical techniques may be required, such as transotic or retrosigmoid approaches.[14,15]

A high jugular bulb may be associated with focal dehiscence of the jugular (sigmoid) plate, allowing protrusion of the bulb superolaterally into the posterior hypotympanum (Fig. 13.5A). When this occurs, the dehiscent jugular bulb is seen as a bluish posteroinferior retrotympanic mass on otoscopic examination. These patients are asymptomatic, although some may experience pulsatile tinnitus or conductive hearing loss secondary to obliteration of the round window niche

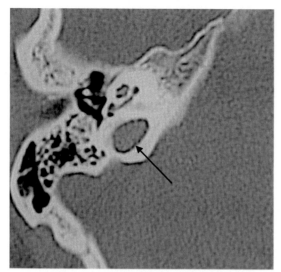

FIG. 13.4 **Normal Variant: High-Riding Jugular Bulb.**
Axial right temporal bone CT shows a high-riding jugular bulb
(*arrow*) with its roof extending above the level of basal turn of
cochlea.

or impingement of the ossicular chain[16] (Fig. 13.5B).
More importantly, it is imperative that surgeons are
alerted to this anatomic variant, in view of the high risk
of torrential bleeding should a myringotomy or exploratory tympanotomy be performed in these patients.[17]

### Jugular Bulb Diverticulum

Jugular bulb diverticula are thought to be more common than previously reported in English literature.[18]
The diverticulum is an out-pouching that is often, but
not always, from a high-riding jugular bulb. It most
commonly extends superomedially into the petrous
temporal bone medial to the labyrinth and may be
in close relationship with the internal acoustic canal,
endolymphatic duct or sac, or the posterior semicircular canal.[16] Some authors believe that it represents
a variant or medially located high-riding jugular bulb,
which has extended into the petrous temporal bone
but is partly hindered by the dense otic capsule. Others
considered this to be a true venous anomaly that has
enlarged over time.[19,20]

Jugular bulb diverticulum is usually an incidental finding on imaging for unrelated reasons. However, individuals may present with an air-bone gap or
sensorineural hearing loss caused by dehiscence into
the posterior semicircular canal or internal acoustic
canal, or Meniere syndrome secondary to encroachment of the endolymphatic sac.[21] Jugular bulb diverticula are not visible on otoscopic examination; thus

this is essentially a radiologic diagnosis. It is best demonstrated on high-resolution temporal bone CT as a
well-corticated polypoid projection extending from the
jugular bulb margin (Fig. 13.6).

### Jugular Bulb Pseudolesion

It is common knowledge that both turbulent and
slow flow within venous structures result in increased
signal intensity on MRI. This is frequently detected
in the jugular bulb, especially on the right side in an
asymmetrically large and often high jugular bulb.
The flow phenomenon results in high or intermediate signal intensity particularly on the T1-weighted
images (Fig. 13.7A and B), simulating an intraluminal thrombus or tumor. This potential imaging pitfall
should be recognized and avoided by radiologists,
sparing patients from unnecessary treatment and risk.

By definition, jugular bulb pseudolesions are asymptomatic and found incidentally during MRI. Careful
scrutiny of the pseudolesion usually reveals that the flow
phenomenon does not hold up on all MR sequences.
Further assessment with phase contrast MR venogram or
a contrast-enhanced CT or MR is also useful in demonstrating a patent jugular bulb with normal flow enhancement (Fig. 13.7C and D), thus excluding an intraluminal
lesion or thrombus.[22] On high-resolution CT of the
temporal bone, the normal smooth cortical margins of
the jugular foramen are preserved with an intact jugular
spine.

## VASCULAR CONDITIONS OR LESIONS
### Dural Arterial Venous Fistula

Intracranial dural arteriovenous fistulas (DAVFs) have
a direct communication between meningeal arteries
and dural veins or venous sinuses. DAVFs in the posterior fossa are more common in the region of the
transverse and sigmoid sinuses and rarely around the
jugular foramen, with predominantly case reports in
the literature.[23–26] The arterial supply may be provided
by branches of the vertebral or external carotid arteries,
most commonly the occipital and ascending pharyngeal arteries.

Patients may present with a myriad of clinical signs
and symptoms, depending on the location and venous
drainage pattern, including the presence of venous
reflux. The common symptoms are often nonspecific,
such as headache and pulsatile tinnitus. Conventional
MRI and CT may show intracranial hemorrhage, venous
congestion and edema, parenchymal or leptomeningeal
enhancement, and tortuous vascular flow voids. There
may be a shaggy appearance of the bony margins on CT

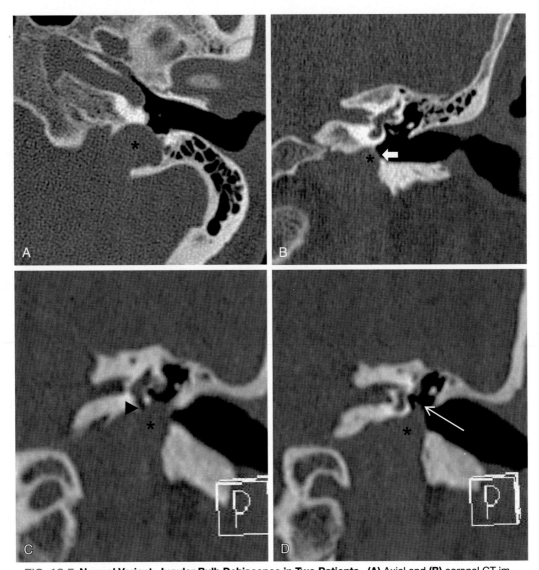

FIG. 13.5 **Normal Variant: Jugular Bulb Dehiscence in Two Patients. (A)** Axial and **(B)** coronal CT images of the left temporal bone in one patient demonstrating focal dehiscence of the jugular plate (*asterisk*) into the hypotympanum (*short arrow*). In another patient, coronal CT images **(C)** and **(D)** of the left temporal bone show a dehiscent jugular plate (*asterisk*). The jugular bulb covers the round window (*arrowhead*) and abuts the incudostapedial joint (*long arrow*).

bone algorithm because of transcalvarial venous channels (Fig. 13.8B). CT or MR angiogram may be used to show enlarged feeding arteries and prominent draining veins with early venous enhancement (Fig. 13.8A and C). More recently, time-resolved dynamic MRA techniques have been shown to be more sensitive than time-of-flight MRA in the detection of DAVFs, including in the posterior fossa.[27] However, imaging studies are often unremarkable for small or benign DAVFs. Catheter angiogram remains

the gold standard for the definitive diagnosis and assessment of DAVFs.

Treatment options include endovascular, surgical (including stereotactic radiosurgery), or combined management, mainly determined by the location and accessibility of the lesion and skill of the neurosurgeon and interventional radiologist. Management decisions are also influenced by patient characteristics, presence of aggressive features such as venous

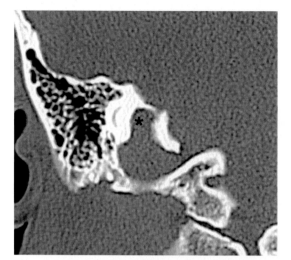

**FIG. 13.6 Normal Variant: Jugular Bulb Diverticulum.**
Coronal right temporal bone CT shows a jugular bulb diverticulum (*asterisk*) as a well-corticated thumb-like projection extending superiorly from the roof of the jugular bulb.

congestion or hemorrhage, and ultimately the estimated risk of hemorrhage from an untreated DAVF compared with morbidity and mortality from treatment complications.

### Jugular Vein Thrombosis

Venous thrombosis of the jugular or cerebral veins is difficult to diagnose clinically and may be missed on initial imaging by the unsuspecting radiologist. The presenting clinical symptoms are usually nonspecific, such as headache or neck pain, seizures, and fever. Risk factors may be present, such as dehydration, coagulopathies, peripartum state, or infection. Thrombophlebitis of the internal jugular vein may occur secondary to local infection (e.g., mastoiditis) or in Lemierre syndrome as a result of hematogenous seeding from bacterial pharyngitis (*Fusobacterium necrophorum*). This in turn may lead to thrombosis of the internal jugular vein and septic embolism.

The appearance on nonenhanced MR or CT depends on the age of the thrombus. In acute thrombosis, a

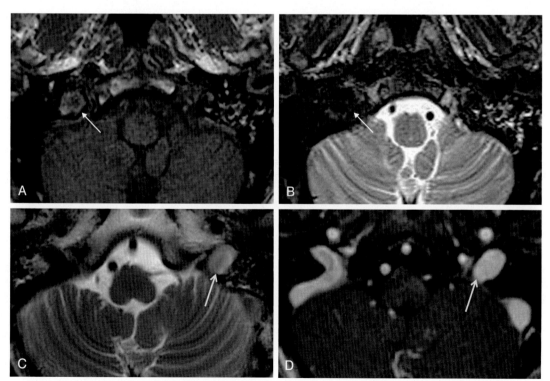

**FIG. 13.7 Jugular Bulb Pseudolesion in Two Patients. (A)** Axial T1-weighted MR image in patient A shows mildly heterogeneous intermediate signal intensity in an asymmetrically larger right jugular bulb (*arrow*), simulating a mass. **(B)** Axial T2-weighted MR image with fat saturation in the same patient demonstrates normal flow void in the right jugular foramen (*arrow*), consistent with a jugular foramen pseudolesion. **(C)** Axial T2-weighted MR image in patient B shows hyperintense signal in the left jugular bulb (*arrow*), simulating a thrombus or mass. **(D)** Axial contrast-enhanced T1-weighted image shows the normal enhancement of the jugular bulb (*arrow*).

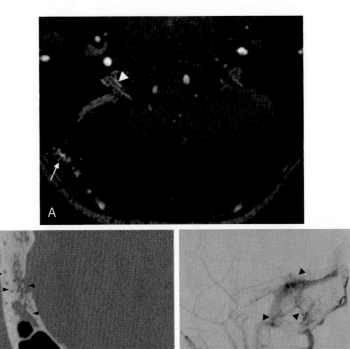

**FIG. 13.8 Dural Arteriovenous Fistula (DAVF) of the Transverse Sinus. (A)** Time-of-flight MR angiography source image shows hypertrophied branches of the posterior meningeal artery ascending within the right jugular foramen (*white arrowhead*), as well as vascular channels (*long arrow*) around the right transverse sinus with arterialized flow signal within the sigmoid sinus. **(B)** Coronal CT bone algorithm shows focal erosions in the inner table and multiple tortuous linear lucencies within the diploë because of transcalvarial venous channels (*arrowheads*). **(C)** Catheter angiogram: lateral injection of the right external carotid artery confirms a right transverse sinus DAVF supplied by branches of the right internal maxillary, ascending pharyngeal and occipital branches (*arrowheads*).

hyperdense clot is seen on nonenhanced CT. Following intravenous contrast administration, there is enhancement surrounding the hypoattenuating thrombus on CT (Fig. 13.9).

On MRI, when normal venous flow void is absent on routine spin-echo sequences, the vein has to be carefully scrutinized for the possibility of thrombosis. This may warrant further evaluation with a contrast-enhanced study or venogram. MR venogram techniques include two-dimensional time-of-flight or phase-contrast study. Slow flow or hypoplasia of the jugular vein can be easily mistaken as thrombosis. In the latter, there is associated hypoplasia of the ipsilateral transverse sinus and usually homogenous enhancement of

the veins when contrast is administered. Occasionally, heterogeneous enhancement of the vein on contrast-enhanced T1-weighted images caused by turbulence may resemble central thrombus. As a result of MRI pitfalls, CT venogram is generally regarded as a more reliable modality because it is easy to interpret and is less subject to false diagnosis from the flow-related artifacts on MRI.

## PRIMARY NEOPLASMS OF THE JUGULAR FORAMEN

Primary neoplasms arising from the intrinsic structures of the jugular foramen include paragangliomas,

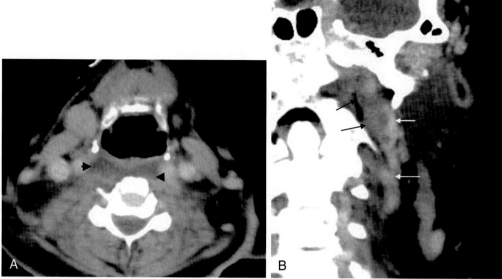

**FIG. 13.9 Lemierre Syndrome.** On contrast-enhanced CT of the neck, **(A)** axial image shows a retropharyngeal abscess (*arrowheads*), whereas **(B)** coronal image shows hypodense thrombus (*black arrows*) within the contrast-enhancing left internal jugular vein (*white arrows*).

which are by far the most common, followed by schwannomas and meningiomas. Rare cases of primary peripheral primitive neuroectodermal tumor and neuroendocrine carcinoma of the jugular foramen have also been reported.[28,29]

### Paragangliomas (Glomus Jugulare and Jugulotympanicum)

Paragangliomas account for up to 80% of primary neoplasms of the jugular foramen.[30] They arise from glomus tissue in the adventitia of the jugular bulb, the superior ganglion of CN X, or along Jacobson and Arnold nerves.[31] Histologically, they exhibit a characteristic biphenotypic cell pattern, consisting of chief cells aggregated into compact cell nests (termed "zellballen" by Kohn) surrounded by flattened sustentacular cells. Most paragangliomas are benign but locally aggressive. Malignant degeneration occurs in approximately 3%–4% of cases.[32] They may be multicentric in 5%–10% of patients, with the incidence rising to 25%–50% in familial paragangliomas.[33,34] Association with multiple endocrine neoplasia syndrome type 1 and neurofibromatosis (NF) type 1 is well recognized.

Paragangliomas of the jugular foramen most frequently occur in women (female: male ratio, 3–5:1) in their fifth and sixth decades.[34] They present initially with pulsatile tinnitus and conductive hearing loss and a vascular retrotympanic mass on otoscopic examination.

With disease progression, they may develop jugular foramen or Horner syndrome.[35] This tumor is typically nonsecretory, with only 1%–3% of patients showing clinical features of excessive catecholamine release.[32]

Paragangliomas have a relatively predictable vector of spread along the paths of least resistance.[36] They typically extend superolaterally, eroding through the jugular plate into the middle ear and ossicles, so-called glomus jugulotympanicum paraganglioma. They may also extend into the mastoid air cell tracts and the Eustachian tube or invade the jugular bulb and sigmoid sinus. On bone algorithm CT, paragangliomas produce characteristic "moth-eaten" permeative destructive bone changes around the jugular foramen (Fig. 13.10D and E) as a result of tumor infiltration through the Haversian canal system. MRI delineates the exact soft tissue extent of these tumors, which enhance intensely following intravenous contrast administration. Larger lesions may demonstrate the characteristic "salt and pepper" appearance on T1-weighted images. The hypointense "pepper" may also be evident on T2-weighted images, representing high-velocity flow voids of feeding arterial branches within the tumors (Fig. 13.10A–C). The less commonly seen hyperintense "salt" is due to underlying foci of subacute hemorrhage. However, this feature is not pathognomonic for paragangliomas, as it has been reported in hypervascular metastases and plasmacytoma of the jugular foramen.

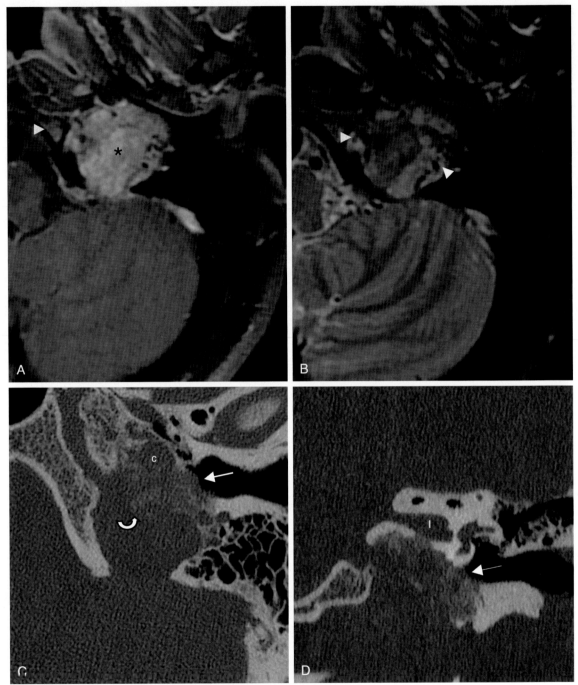

**FIG. 13.10 Jugular Foramen Paraganglioma. (A)** Post-contrast T1-weighted MR of the left jugular foramen reveals an avidly enhancing intraforaminal mass (*). **(B)** T2-weighted image shows multiple punctate
high velocity flow voids (*arrowheads*), characteristic of a paraganglioma. **(C)** Axial and **(D)** coronal CT bone
algorithm images demonstrate permeative bone destruction (*curved arrow*), with the mass eroding through
the jugular plate laterally into the hypotympanum (*straight arrows*), superiorly into the floor of the internal
auditory canal (I), and anteriorly into the posterior wall of the carotid canal (c).

Conventional angiography is often performed to provide a vascular road map for surgeons, and preoperative endovascular embolization has been shown to reduce the vascular volume of the tumor mass and decrease intraoperative bleeding.[37] Most paragangliomas of the jugular foramen involve multiple arterial territories, and hence, vascular supply is classically divided into inferomedial, posterolateral, anterior, and superior compartments.[38] The ascending pharyngeal artery (via the inferior tympanic artery) is the most common arterial feeder and supplies the inferomedial territory. The stylomastoid artery primarily supplies the posterolateral compartment, with possible contributions from posterior auricular and occipital arteries. The anterior tympanic artery supplies the anterior compartment, whereas the middle meningeal and accessory meningeal arteries supply the superior compartment. Larger paragangliomas may derive further feeding vessels from branches of the internal maxillary, internal carotid, or vertebral arteries via meningeal or pial arterial branches, with pial artery supply indicating transdural spread.[39]

Surgery for glomus jugulare was revolutionized by the introduction of the infratemporal fossa approach by Ugo Fisch in 1978.[40] Different surgical techniques have since been proposed with the ultimate goal for complete surgical resection of tumors with preservation of cranial nerve functions. However, this is not always possible because the lower cranial nerves are frequently engulfed by the tumors. Radiation therapy is advocated as the alternative primary treatment for selected patients in whom surgery is contraindicated. Essentially, treatment should be individualized based on patient's age and comorbidities, the tumor extent, and the preoperative status of the lower cranial nerve functions.

### Jugular Foramen Schwannoma
Schwannomas of the jugular foramen are benign encapsulated tumors arising from Schwann cells of the cranial nerve sheaths encasing CNs IX, X, and XI. The glossopharyngeal nerve is most commonly involved, or less frequently the Jacobson and Arnold nerves.[41] Schwannomas most often arise from the glial-Schwann cell junction of cranial nerves, and it is believed that the Schwann cells around the ganglia of CNs IX and X within the jugular foramen are particularly susceptible to tumor development.[42] In the absence of NF type 2, involvement of the jugular foramen is rare and constitutes only 3% of all intracranial schwannomas. Histologically, schwannomas typically have a biphasic pattern, with areas of compacted elongated spindle cells (Antoni type A) and hypocellular regions of

loosely arranged myxoid matrix with lipid-laden cells and occasional cyst formation (Antoni type B). Malignant schwannomas are exceedingly rare but have been previously reported.[43]

Schwannomas typically grow along the course of the cranial nerves. The Kaye and Pellet surgical classification groups jugular foraminal schwannomas into four types: type A: tumors with intracranial extension (Fig. 13.12); type B: tumors confined within the jugular foramen (Fig. 13.11); type C: tumors with extracranial extension; type D: dumb-bell tumors saddled across the jugular foramen with intracranial and extracranial components.[44,45] Intraforaminal or intracranial types are more common and manifest upon reaching large sizes because of their slow insidious growth pattern. Clinical signs and symptoms are most commonly associated with otolaryngologic deficits (hearing loss, tinnitus, hoarseness, vertigo, and swallowing difficulties) and cerebellar disturbances (such as ataxia, nystagmus, and dizziness).[46] Lower cranial neuropathies occur late and do not necessarily correlate with the nerves of origin.[47] Large cerebellopontine angle mass in type A lesions may present with unilateral hearing loss and should not be confused with vestibular schwannomas, which primarily involve the internal acoustic canal.[48]

Schwannomas may be isodense to brain parenchyma or hypodense because of their rich lipid content. The low-density (near water) appearance on CT is particularly characteristic.[49] Bone algorithm CT shows smooth and sharply marginated scalloping or enlargement of the jugular foramen (Fig. 13.11D). On MRI, schwannomas demonstrate low and high signal intensity on T1- and T2-weighted images, respectively, with moderate or marked contrast enhancement. Smaller lesions tend to enhance homogenously, whereas larger lesions may be heterogeneous because of degenerative changes, more commonly cyst formation, which may be present in up to 25% of the tumors (Fig. 13.11A–C).[50] Rarely there may be intratumoral hemorrhage or calcification (Fig. 13.12), resulting in an acute presentation with pain and cranial nerve palsies. Surgical resection, stereotatic radiosurgery, or combinations of both are the treatments of choice, with delayed lower cranial neuropathies as the main therapeutic complication.

### Primary Jugular Foramen Meningioma
The jugular foramen is an unusual location for this common intracranial tumor and constitutes one of the smallest subgroups of meningiomas.[51] Primary meningiomas of the jugular foramen arise intrinsically from arachnoidal meningothelial cap cells (leptomeninges) found along CNs IX, X, and XI, whereas

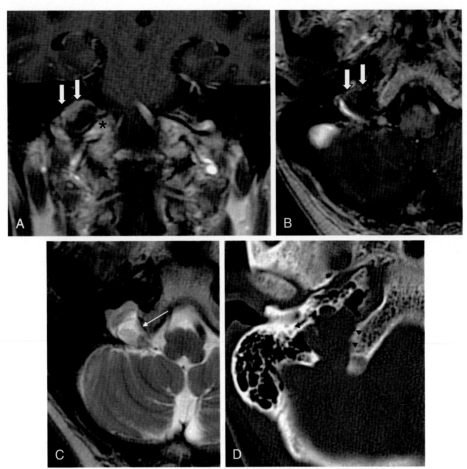

FIG. 13.11 **Kaye and Pellet Type B Jugular Foramen Schwannoma (A)** Coronal and **(B)** axial contrast-enhanced T1-weighted images of an intraforaminal cystic-solid lesion superolateral to the occipital condyle (*asterisk*). **(C)** Axial T2-weighted image shows the hyperintense cystic component (*thin arrow*), whereas the enhancing solid component is seen on the contrast-enhanced sequences (*thick arrows*). **(D)** Axial bone algorithm CT shows right jugular foramen enlargement with smooth, sharply defined margins (*arrowheads*) in contrast with that in a paraganglioma.

secondary lesions extend from the posterior fossa into the jugular foramen. The typical patient is a 40- to 60-year-old female who presents with hearing loss, tinnitus, and progressive lower cranial neuropathies. In NF type 2, there may be multiple meningiomas or schwannomas.

Typically, meningiomas appear hyperdense on CT, isointense on T1-weighted, and hypointense on T2-weighted MR images because of their increased cellularity and diffuse microcalcification. In addition, the extracranial component of jugular foraminal meningiomas shows significantly lower signal intensity than the intracranial component on T1-, T2-, and postcontrast T1-weighted images, possibly related to its increased fibrosis and collagen content.[52]

Primary meningiomas of the jugular foramen behave differently from the typical intracranial meningiomas, including those that involve the jugular foramen secondarily from the posterior cranial fossa. They are characterized by centrifugal spread in all directions from the jugular foramen. Most commonly, the tumor extends along the basal cistern dural reflection, resulting in enhancing "dural tails." There is often extensive intraosseous infiltration (Fig. 13.13), with hyperostosis and permeative-sclerotic changes in the surrounding skull base.[53] They may also invade the middle ear, the jugular bulb, and dural sinus or grow inferiorly into the carotid space.

Single-stage complete tumor removal is the ultimate goal, but surgery often results in multiple lower cranial neuropathies.[54,55] In contrast to paragangliomas, there

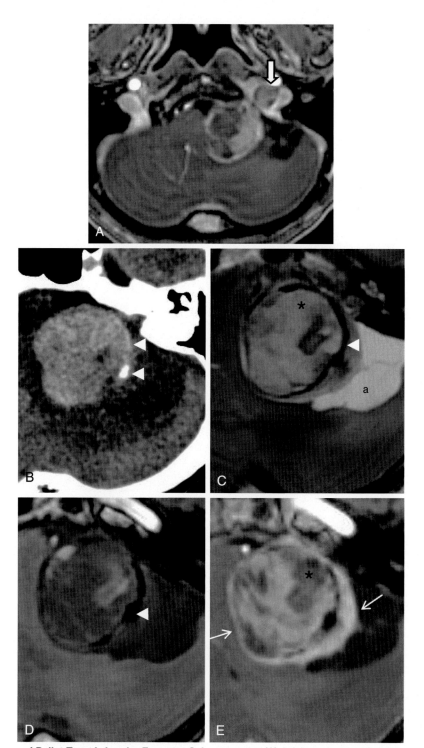

FIG. 13.12 **Kaye and Pellet Type A Jugular Foramen Schwannoma. (A)** Axial postcontrast T1-weighted MR image shows a heterogeneously enhancing large mass in the cerebellopontine cistern with a smaller intrajugular component (*block arrow*). **(B)** Axial noncontrast CT shows a hyperdense lesion caused by intratumoral hemorrhage, with a peripheral rim of calcification (*arrowheads*). **(C)** Axial T2-weighted and **(D)** pre- and **(E)** postcontrast T1-weighted images show the heterogenous signal characteristics of the large degenerative central component of the tumor (*asterisk*) with peripheral enhancement in the peridegenerative areas and fibrous capsule (*thin arrows*). On MRI, the calcifications are markedly hypointense (*arrowheads*). In contrast to paragangliomas, there are no intratumoral flow voids in schwannomas. Apart from cystic degeneration within schwannomas, there is also a known association with extramural or arachnoid cysts (a) as seen in this patient.

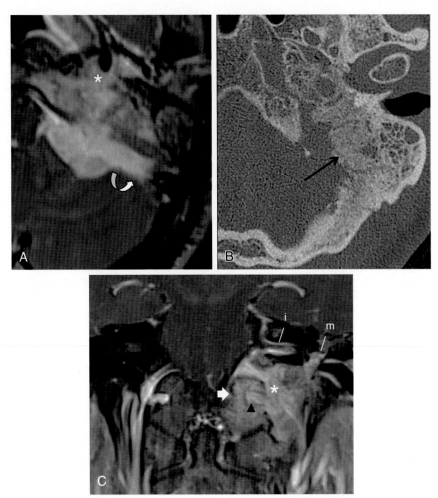

**FIG. 13.13 Jugular Foramen Meningioma. (A)** On axial contrast-enhanced fat-saturated T1-weighted sequence, there is an enhancing mass within the jugular foramen extending extracranially (*asterisk*) into the carotid space and intracranially (*curved arrow*) in the retromastoid region **(B)** Axial CT bone window shows bony hyperostosis (*long arrow*) of the mastoid temporal bone. **(C)** Coronal postcontrast image shows dural enhancement within the internal auditory canal (i) and enhancement in the skull base marrow (*short arrow*), hypoglossal canal (*arrowhead*), and middle ear (m) due to tumor infiltration.

is no conclusive evidence to support preoperative embolization of jugular foraminal meningiomas.[41] Radiation therapy is an alternative for elderly patients with high operative risk, patients with tumor volume of less than 20 mL, or those who decline surgery.[56]

## SECONDARY JUGULAR FORAMEN NEOPLASMS

The jugular foramen may be involved secondarily by tumors arising from adjacent structures and infiltrating the foramen or from metastatic disease.

## Metastatic Disease to Skull Base or Dura

It has previously been reported that metastasis may be more common than primary tumor as the cause of jugular foramen syndrome.[48] The rapid onset of complex lower cranial neuropathy in patients with a known primary malignancy should raise this possibility.[57] The most common primary malignancies that metastasize to the skull base include breast, lung, and prostate cancer. Unlike primary jugular foramina lesions where complete or partial surgical resection may be achieved, skull base metastases have an ominous prognosis and are managed with palliative radiotherapy.

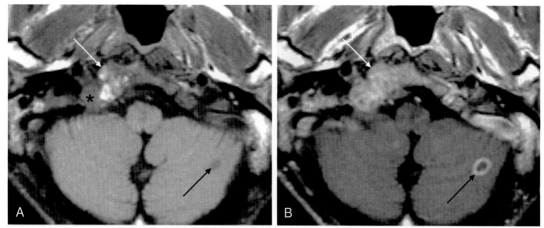

FIG. 13.14 **Metastatic Renal Cell Carcinoma.** **(A)** Axial T1-weighted MR image shows a heterogeneous tumor in the right petroclival region with areas of hyperintensity consistent with intratumoral hemorrhage (*white arrow*). The tumor has infiltrated the right jugular foramen (*asterisk*). A small hypointense lesion is also seen in the left cerebellar hemisphere (*black arrow*). **(B)** Axial postcontrast T1-weighted MR image demonstrates avid enhancement of the hypervascular metastasis (*white arrow*). The left cerebellar deposit is more conspicuous, with a characteristic rim enhancement (*black arrow*).

On CT bone algorithm, the appearance of skull base metastases varies depending on the primary disease, which may produce lytic lesions, such as in thyroid or renal cell carcinoma; mixed lytic-sclerotic lesions such as in lung and breast cancer; or purely sclerotic appearance as seen in breast, prostate cancer, or carcinoid. MRI shows marrow infiltration, which is hypointense on non-fat saturation T1-weighted images and enhances after contrast administration. MRI is superior in depicting the soft tissue extent of metastatic deposits and invasion of skull base foramina, leading to compression or infiltration along the cranial nerves (perineural disease) before bone changes are evident on CT.[58] Hypervascular metastases from melanoma, renal, or thyroid carcinomas may contain intratumoral flow voids or hemorrhage, thus mimicking paragangliomas (Fig. 13.14).

Intracranial metastasis such as in lymphoma or leukemia may lead to cerebrospinal fluid dissemination of malignant cells, with tumor infiltration along the meninges surrounding the cranial nerves. On MRI, this is best seen on contrast-enhanced T1-weighted and contrast-enhanced fluid-attenuated inversion recovery sequences as an enhancing dural-based mass (Fig. 13.15) or nodular leptomeningeal enhancement along the intracisternal segments of the cranial nerves.

## Skull Base Tumors

Skull base tumors are rare but should also be considered in the differential diagnosis of a large base of

skull mass invading the jugular foramen. These include chondrosarcoma, chordoma, plasmacytoma, temporal bone giant cell tumors, and Langerhans cell histiocytosis. Although these are uncommon, several primary skull base tumors should also be considered in the differential diagnosis of jugular foramen masses.

The skull base develops by endochondral ossification, in contrast to the vault, which develops by intramembranous ossification. Primary skull base chondrosarcomas arise de novo from embryonal remnants of cartilage, most commonly in the petrooccipital fissure just anteromedial to the jugular foramen.[59] Secondary chondrosarcomas are known to develop in preexisting cartilaginous tumors or abnormalities, such as in Paget disease, Ollier disease, and Maffucci syndrome. The principal presenting symptoms are headache and diplopia caused by tumor involvement of the abducens nerve (CN VI) in the Dorello canal. CT shows lytic destructive bone changes with a sharp transition zone. The characteristic chondroid calcification within the tumor matrix is seen in 50% of the cases. These tumors are hypo- to isointense on T1-weighted images and hyperintense on T2-weighted images, in keeping with the underlying chondroid matrix. They are typically avascular or hypovascular on MR or conventional angiography.[60]

Chordomas, which arise from the embryologic notochord, share similar imaging features with chondrosarcomas. The key differentiating finding is their midline clival origin when compared with chondrosarcomas, which

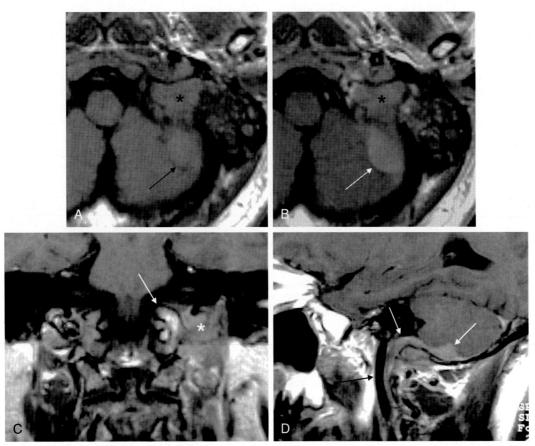

FIG. 13.15 **Pachymeningeal Leukemia. (A)** Axial pre-contrast T1-weighted MR image shows a posterior cranial fossa lesion of intermediate signal intensity (*black arrow*) which shows mild enhancement on the **(B)** post-contrast image (*white arrow*), with the lesion extending into the left jugular foramen (*). **(C)** Coronal postcontrast T1-weighted MR image shows mildly enhancing left jugular foramen tumor (*asterisk*) with infiltration of the jugular tubercle marrow (*arrow*). **(D)** Sagittal postcontrast T1-weighted MR image demonstrates thickened meninges along the floor of the posterior cranial fossa extending to the jugular foramen (*white arrows*). Note the normal internal carotid artery with flow voids (*black arrow*).

are usually off-midline in the petrooccipital fissure.[48] However, chordomas may rarely originate from ectopic notochordal remnants in the petrous apex and invade the jugular foramen secondarily, hence becoming virtually indistinguishable from chondrosarcomas.[61]

Although diffuse involvement of the skull is common in multiple myeloma, solitary skull base plasmacytomas are rare. In the temporal bone, they may arise as solitary intraosseous plasmacytomas from the marrow-rich petrous temporal bone or extramedullary plasmacytomas from the mucosal lining of the middle ear and mastoid air cells with subsequent jugular foramen invasion.[62] Otologic complaints and abducens palsy are the main presenting features.[63] They appear as osteolytic lesions without sclerotic rims on CT. They show low to intermediate signal on T1-weighted sequence and are relatively isointense on T2-weighted MRI because of their high nuclear to cytoplasmic ratio. Plasmacytomas are hypervascular lesions with marked postcontrast enhancement and possible intratumoral flow voids, which mimic paragangliomas.[64]

Temporal bone giant cell tumors with jugular foramen involvement are very rare. Patients usually present with local pain, facial weakness, and hearing loss.[65] CT shows a nonspecific expansile lytic lesion. MRI may reveal a hypointense rim or occasionally diffuse T2 hypointensity because of intratumoral hemosiderin from prior hemorrhage in these hypervascular tumors.[66]

Langerhans cell histiocytosis involving the temporal bone usually presents in the first two decades of life. Up to 30% of patients may have bilateral disease.[67] Otologic symptoms are typical, although seventh and eighth nerve palsies may also occur.[68] CT demonstrates a large lytic lesion centering in the mastoid air cells with secondary involvement of the jugular foramen. It is iso- to hypointense and iso- to hyperintense on T1- and T2-weighted MRI, respectively, with marked postcontrast enhancement. Although the imaging features are nonspecific, Langerhans cell histiocytosis should be considered in a young patient who presents with soft tissue masses associated with extensive bony destruction in the mastoid complexes bilaterally.

### Infiltration by Other Adjacent Tumors

The jugular foramen may be invaded by contiguous spread of temporal bone carcinomas arising from the external auditory canal or endolymphatic sac.[69,70] Endolymphatic sac tumors are very rare tumors that may occur sporadically or in von Hippel-Lindau disease. Despite their benign histopathologic appearance, endolymphatic sac tumors are locally aggressive and frequently invade the labyrinth, mastoid and petrous temporal bone, cerebellopontine angle, and adjacent skull base foramina, including the jugular foramen and internal acoustic canal. Otologic symptoms such as tinnitus and hearing loss are the prominent features in these patients. CT usually shows expansile lytic temporal bone or "moth-eaten" destruction. MRI may demonstrate a heterogeneous mass with cystic areas that may be hyperintense on both T1- and T2-weighted sequences and mild to moderate postcontrast enhancement.[48]

Certain head and neck tumors may also ascend into the jugular foramen via retrograde perineural spread or invasion along the internal jugular vein (Fig. 13.16). Posterolateral extension of locally invasive nasopharyngeal carcinoma arising from the fossa of Rosenmüller may infiltrate the carotid space and jugular foramen (Fig. 13.17) with resultant lower cranial nerve palsies.[71]

## INFECTIVE AND INFLAMMATORY LESIONS

Temporal bone osteomyelitis may occur as a complication of mastoiditis or severe otitis media or externa, with subsequent involvement of the jugular foramen and resultant lower cranial neuropathies.[72] Elderly diabetic patients are particularly susceptible. In the early stage of the disease, CT often shows no evidence of bony destruction. There may be intravenous gas pockets in the jugular foramina readily seen on CT (Fig. 13.18). Thrombophlebitis may occur, leading to thrombosis of the internal jugular vein or sigmoid sinus. Delayed diagnosis and treatment may lead to jugular foramen abscess formation, which appears as a rim-enhancing lesion associated with irregular cortical erosion.[73]

Varicella zoster virus has a high affinity for nerve ganglia. In addition to the well-known Ramsay-Hunt syndrome, there may be CN IX-XI neuropathies caused by the virus. High-resolution MRI demonstrates marked swelling of the nerves with postcontrast enhancement due to breakdown of the blood-nerve barrier.[74] The diagnosis is confirmed by the presence of anti-varicella zoster antibodies or varicella zoster DNA in cerebrospinal fluid.[75]

## CONCLUSION

The jugular foramen is a fascinating and complex skull base foramina because of the intricate nature of its neurovascular organization and difficult accessibility, which poses a major challenge to surgeons. A thorough understanding of its anatomy, anatomic variants, and imaging artifacts is important to avoid unnecessary intervention. Apart from primary tumors that arise from the structures within the jugular foramen, there are a large variety of other pathologies that may involve this foramen secondarily. Although no imaging feature is pathognomonic, meticulous preoperative radiologic evaluation and correlation with the patient's clinical presentation can often lead to a specific diagnosis.

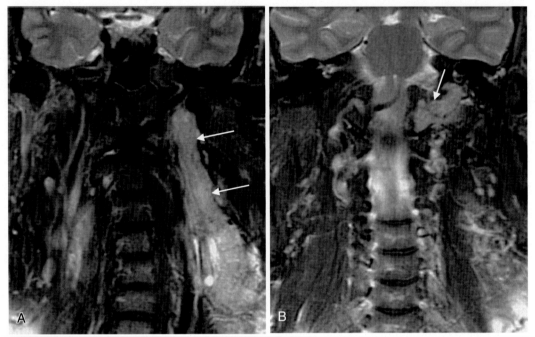

FIG. 13.16 **Papillary Carcinoma of the Thyroid Gland.** **(A)** Coronal postcontrast T1-weighted MR images show enhancing tumour thrombus (*arrows*) along the left internal jugular vein in figure **(A)** extending up to the jugular foramen in **(B)**.

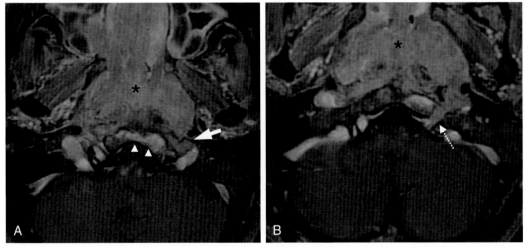

FIG. 13.17 **Nasopharyngeal Carcinoma With Perineural Invasion.** Contrast enhanced T1-weighted fat saturated axial images at the level of the jugular foramen **(A)** and hypoglossal canal **(B)** show a large nasopharyngeal carcinoma (*) with skull base invasion (*arrowheads*). Posteriorly, there is tumour invading the left jugular foramen (*solid arrow*) and the hypoglossal canal (*dashed arrow*).

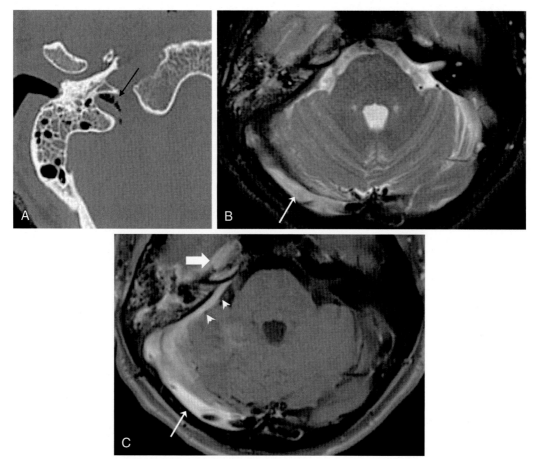

**FIG. 13.18 Complications of Acute Mastoiditis. (A)** Axial CT bone window image in a patient with right mastoiditis shows gas in the jugular vein (*black arrow*). **(B)** Axial T2-weighted MR image shows abnormal flow signal of the sigmoid sinus (*arrow*), which enhances homogenously on the **(C)** contrast-enhanced T1-weighted image (*arrow*), representing thrombophlebitis. There is also diffusely thickened dural enhancement (*arrowheads*) adjacent to the enhancing marrow of the petrous apex (*block arrow*) because of temporal bone osteomyelitis.

## REFERENCES

1. Svien HJ, Baker HL, Rivers MH. Jugular foramen syndrome and allied syndromes. *Neurology.* 1963;13:797–809.
2. Ayeni SA, Ohata K, Tanaka K, Hakuba A. The microsurgical anatomy of the jugular foramen. *J Neurosurg.* 1995;83:903–909.
3. Lo WWM, Solti-Bohman LG. High-resolution CT of the jugular foramen: anatomy and vascular variants and anomalies. *Radiology.* 1984;150:743–747.
4. Linn J, Peters F, Moriggl B, Naidich TP, Bruckmann H, Yousry I. The jugular foramen: imaging strategy and detailed anatomy at 3T. *AJNR Am J Neuroradiol.* 2009;30:34–41.
5. Rhoton AL. Jugular foramen. *Neurosurgery.* 2007;61. S4-S229–S4-S250.
6. Tekdemir I, Tuccar E, Aslan A, et al. The jugular foramen: a comparative radioanatomic study. *Surg Neurol.* 1998;50(6):557–562.
7. Aslan A, Falcioni M, Baylan FR, et al. The cochlear aqueduct: an important landmark in lateral skull base surgery. *Otolaryngol Head Neck Surg.* 1998;118:532–536.
8. Tummala RP, Coscarella E, Morcos JJ. Surgical anatomy of the jugular foramen. *Oper Tech Neurosurg.* 2005;8: 2–5.
9. Naidich TP, Duvernoy HM, Delman BN, Sorensen AG, Kollias SS, Haacke EM. *Duvernoy's atlas of the human brain stem and cerebellum: high-field MRI: surface anatomy, internal structure, vascularization and 3D sectional anatomy;* 2009:p147.

10. Tekdemir I, Tuccar E, Asian A, Elhan A, Ersoy M, Deda H. Comprehensive microsurgical anatomy of the jugular foramen and review of terminology. *J Clin Neurosci.* 2001;8:351–356.

11. Overton SB, Ritter FN. A high placed jugular bulb in the middle ear: a clinical and temporal bone study. *Laryngoscope.* 1986;83:1986–1991.

12. Kawano H, Tono T, Schachern PA, Paparella MM, Komune S. Petrous high jugular bulb: a histological study. *Am J Otolaryngol.* 2000;21:161–168.

13. Dai PD, Zhang HQ, Wang ZM, Sha Y, Wang KQ, Zhang TY. Morphological and positional relationships between the sigmoid sinus and the jugular bulb. *Surg Radiol Anat.* 2007;29:643–651.

14. Shao KN, Tatagiba M, Samii M. Surgical management of high jugular bulb in acoustic neurinoma via rectosigmoid approach. *Neurosurgery.* 1993;32:32–37.

15. Roche PH, Moriyama T, Thomassin JM, Pellet W. High jugular bulb in the translabyrinthine approach to the cerebellopontine angle: anatomical considerations and surgical management. *Acta Neurochir.* 2006;148:415–420.

16. Merchant SN, Nadol JB. Jugular bulb. In: *Schuknecht's Pathology of the Ear.* 3rd ed. 2010:237–241.

17. Tomura N, Sashi R, Kobayashi M, Hirano H, Hashimoto M, Watarai J. Normal variations of the temporal bone on high resolution CT: their incidence and clinical significance. *Clin Radiol.* 1995;50:144–148.

18. Bilgen C, Kirazli T, Ogut F, Totan S. Jugular bulb diverticula: clinical and radiologic aspects. *Otolaryngol Head Neck Surg.* 2003;128:382–386.

19. Kobanawa S, Atsuchi M, Tanaka J, Shigeno T. Jugular bulb diverticulum associated with lower cranial nerve palsy and multiple aneurysms. *Surg Neurol.* 2000;53:559–562.

20. Koesling S, Kunkel P, Schul T. Vascular anomalies, sutures and small canals of the temporal bone on axial CT. *Eur J Radiol.* 2005;54:335–343.

21. Schmerber S, Lefournier V, Lavieille JP, Boubagra K. Endolymphatic duct obstruction related to a jugular bulb diverticulum: high resolution CT and MR imaging findings. *Clin Radiol.* 2002;57:424–428.

22. Widick MH, Haynes DS, Jackson G, Patterson K, Glasscock ME, Macias JD. Slow-flow phenomenon in magnetic resonance imaging of the jugular bulb masquerading as skull base neoplasms. *Am J Otol.* 1996;17:648–652.

23. Ernst R, Bulas R, Tomsick T, van Loveren H, Aziz KA. Three cases of dural arteriovenous fistula of the anterior condylar vein within the hypoglossal canal. *AJNR Am J Neuroradiol.* 1999;20:2016–2020.

24. Byun JS, Hwang SN, Park SW, Nam TK. Dural arteriovenous fistula of jugular foramen with subarachnoid haemorrhage: selective transarterial embolization. *J Korean Neurosurg Soc.* 2009;45(3):199–202.

25. Kiyosue H, Hori Y, Okahara M, et al. Treatment of intracranial dural arteriovenous fistulas: current strategies based on location and hemodynamics, and alternative techniques of transcatheter embolization. *Radiographics.* 2004;24(6):1637–1653.

26. Miller T, Gandhi D. Intracranial dural arteriovenous fistulae; clinical presentation and management strategies. *Stroke.* 2015;46:2017–2025.

27. Pekkola J, Kangasniemi M. Posterior fossa dural arteriovenous fistulas: diagnosis and follow-up with time-resolved imaging of contrast kinetics (TRICKS) at 1.5T. *Acta Radiol.* 2011;52:442–447.

28. Yamazaki T, Kuroki T, Katsume M, Kameda N. Peripheral primitive neuroectodermal tumor of jugular foramen: case report. *Neurosurgery.* 2002;51:1286–1289.

29. Leonetti JP, Shirazi MA, Marzo S, Anderson D. Neuroendocrine carcinoma of the jugular foramen. *Ear Nose Throat J.* 2008;87(86):88–91.

30. Megerian CA, McKenna MJ, Nodal JB. Non-paraganglioma jugular foramen lesions masquerading as glomus jugulare tumors. *Am J Otol.* 1995;16:94–98.

31. Robertson JH, Gardner G, Cocke EW. Glomus jugulare tumors. *Clin Neurosurg.* 1994;41:39–61.

32. Caldemeyer KS, Mathews VP, Azzarelli B, Smith RR. The jugular foramen: a review of anatomy, masses, and imaging characteristics. *Radiographics.* 1997;17:1123–1139.

33. Wharton SM, Davis A. Familial paraganglioma. *J Laryngol Otol.* 1996;110:688–690.

34. Jackson CG. Glomus tympanicum and glomus jugulare tumors. *Otolaryngol Clin N Am.* 2001;34:941–970.

35. Lustrin ES, Palestro C, Vaheesan K. Radiographic evaluation and assessment of paragangliomas. *Otolaryngol Clin N Am.* 2001;34:881–906.

36. Weber PC, Patel S. Jugulotympanic paragangliomas. *Otolaryngol Clin N Am.* 2001;34:1231–1240.

37. Noonan PT, Choi IS. Diagnostic imaging, angiography, and interventional techniques for jugular foramen tumors. *Oper Tech Neurosurg.* 2005;8:13–18.

38. Rao AB, et al. Paragangliomas of the head and neck: radiologic-pathologic correlation1. *Radiographics.* 1999;19:1605–1632.

39. Vogl TJ, Bisdas S. Differential diagnosis of jugular foramen lesions. *Skull Base.* 2009;19(1):3–16.

40. Fisch U. Infratemporal fossa approach to tumors of the temporal bone and base of the skull. *J Laryngol Otol.* 1978;92:949–967.

41. Quaranta N, Cassano M, Del Giudice AM, Quaranta A. A rare case of jugular foramen schwannoma arising from Jacobsen nerve. *Acta Otolaryngol.* 2007;127:667–672.

42. Song MH, Lee HY, Jeon JS, Lee JD, Lee HK, Lee WS. Jugular foramen schwannoma: analysis on its origin and location. *Otol Neurotol.* 2008;29:387–391.

43. Balasubramaniam C. A case of malignant tumor of the jugular foramen in a young infant. *Childs Nerv Syst.* 1999;15:347–350.

44. Kaye AH, Hahn JF, Kinney SE, Hardy RW, Bay JW. Jugular foramen schwannomas. *J Neurosurg.* 1984;60:1045–1053.

45. Pellet W, Cannoni M, Pech A. The widened transcochlear approach to jugular foramen tumors. *J Neurosurg.* 1988;69:887–894.

46. Bakar B. Jugular foramen schwannomas: review of the large surgical series. *J Korean Neurosurg Soc.* 2008;44(5): 285–294.

47. Lustig LR, Jackler RK. The variable relationship between the lower cranial nerves and jugular foramen tumors: implications for neural preservation. *Am J Otol.* 1996;17: 658–668.

48. Lowenheim H, Koerbel A, Ebner FH, Kumagami H, Ernemann U, Tatagiba M. Differentiating imaging findings in primary and secondary tumors of the jugular foramen. *Neurosurg Rev.* 2006;29:1–11.

49. Chong VFH, Fan YF. Pictorial review: radiology of the jugular foramen. *Clin Radiol.* 1998;53:405–416.

50. Carvalho GA, Tatagiba M, Samii M. Cystic schwannomas of the jugular foramen: clinical and surgical remarks. *Neurosurgery.* 2000;46:560–566.

51. Amautovic K, Al-Mefty O. Primary meningiomas of jugular fossa. *J Neurosurg.* 2002;97:12–20.

52. Shimono T, Akai F, Yamamoto A, et al. Different signal intensities between intra- and extracranial components in jugular foramen meningioma: an enigma. *AJNR Am J Neuroradiol.* 2005;26:1122–1127.

53. MacDonald AJ, Salzman KL, Harnsberger HR, Gilbert E, Shelton C. Primary jugular foramen meningioma: imaging appearance and differentiating features. *AJR Am J Roentgenol.* 2004;182:373–377.

54. Ramina R, Neto MC, Fernandes YB, Aguiar PH, de Meneses MS, Torres LF. Meningiomas of the jugular foramen. *Neurosurg Rev.* 2006;29:55–60.

55. Sanna M, Bacciu A, Falcioni M, Taibah A, Piazza P. Surgical management of jugular foramen meningiomas: a series of 13 cases and review of the literature. *Laryngoscope.* 2007;117:1710–1719.

56. Nicollato A, Foroni R, Pellegrino M, Ferraresi P, Alessandrini F, Gerosa M. Gamma knife radiosurgery in meningiomas of the posterior fossa: experience with 62 treated lesions. *Minim Invasive Neurosurg.* 2001;44: 211–217.

57. Chacon G, Alexandraki I, Palacio C. Collet-Sicard syndrome: an uncommon manifestation of metastatic prostate cancer. *South Med J.* 2006;99:898–899.

58. Schweinfurth JM, Johnson JT, Weissman J. Jugular foramen syndrome as a complication of metastatic melanoma. *Am J Otolaryngol.* 1993;14:168–174.

59. Neff B, Sataloff RT, Storey L, Hawkshaw M, Speigel JR. Chondrosarcoma of the skull base. *Laryngoscope.* 2002;112:134–139.

60. Schmidinger A, Rosahl SK, Vorkapic P, Samii M. Natural history of chondroid skull base lesions – case report and review. *Neuroradiology.* 2002;44:268–271.

61. Itoh T, Harada M, Ichikawa T, Shimoyamada K, Katayama N, Tsukune Y. A case of jugular foramen chordomas with extension to the neck: CT and MR findings. *Radiat Med.* 2000;18:63–65.

62. Nofsinger YC, Mirza N, Rowan P, Lanza D, Weinstein G. Head and neck manifestations of plasma cell neoplasms. *Laryngoscope.* 1997;107:741–746.

63. Solitary plasmacytomas of the skull base presenting with unilateral sensorineural hearing loss. *J Laryngol Otol.* 1999;113:164–166.

64. Solitary plasmacytomas of the occipital bone: a report of two cases. *Eur Radiol.* 1997;7:503–506.

65. Wang Y, Honda K, Suzuki S, Ishikawa K. Giant cell tumor at the lateral skull base. *Am J Otolaryngol.* 2006;27: 64–67.

66. Tang JY, Wang CK, Su YC, Yang SF, Huang MY, Huang CJ. MRI appearance of giant cell tumor of the lateral skull base. A case report. *Clin Imaging.* 2003;27:27–30.

67. Marioni G, De Filippis C, Stramare R, Carli M, Staffieri A. Langerhans' cell histiocytosis: temporal bone involvement. *J Laryngol Otol.* 2001;115:839–841.

68. Bonafe A, Joomye H, Jaeger P, Fraysse B, Manelfe C. Histiocytosis X of the petrous bone in the adult: MRI. *Head Neck Radiol.* 1994;36:330–333.

69. Ong CK, Pua U, Chong VF. Carcinoma of the external auditory canal: a pictorial essay. *ICIS Cancer Imaging.* 2008;8:191–198.

70. Megerian CA, McKenna MJ, Nuss RC, et al. Endolymphatic sac tumors: confirmation, clinical characterization and implication in von Hippel-Lindau disease. *Laryngoscope.* 1995;105:801–808.

71. Chong VF, Ong CK. Nasopharyngeal carcinoma. *Eur J Radiol.* 2008;66:437–447.

72. Rowlands RG, Lekakis GK, Hinton AE. Masked pseudomonal skull base osteomyelitis presenting with a bilateral Xth cranial nerve palsy. *J Laryngol Otol.* 2002;116:556–558.

73. Mirza S, Dutt SN, Irving RM. Jugular foramen abscess. *Otol Neurol.* 2001;22:973–974.

74. Adachi M. A case of varicella zoster virus polyneuropathy: involvement of the glossopharyngeal and vagus nerves mimicking a tumor. *AJNR Am J Neuroradiol.* 2008;29(9):1743–1745.

75. Kawabe K, Sekine T, Murata K, et al. A case of Vernet syndrome with varicella zoster virus infection. *J Neurol Sci.* 2008;270:209–210.

**TABLE 14.1**
**Measurements Commonly Used in Evaluating the Craniovertebral Junction (CVJ) on Lateral Projection or Sagittal View in Images**

| | Fig. 14.1 | Normal Range | Remarks |
|---|---|---|---|
| Chamberlain line (Palatooccipital line) | A to B | Dens apex < 5 mm above this line, anterior arch of C1 typically lies below | Diagnosis of basilar invagination. (Posterior rim of foramen magnum shows great anatomic variability and also it may be difficult to radiologically pinpoint opisthion) |
| McGregor line (Palatosuboccipital line) | A to C | Dens apex < 7 mm above this line, anterior arch of C1 typically lies below | Diagnosis of basilar invagination |
| McRae line (Foramen magnum line) | B to D | Tip of dens below this line | Assess the decrease in content injury |
| Wackenheim line (craniovertebral or clivus-canal angle) | D to E | Line falls tangent to, or intersects, the posterior one-third of the odontoid | Assessment of CVJ traumatic injuries |
| Welcher basal angle | Angle D-F-G | < 140 degrees | Assessment of platybasia |

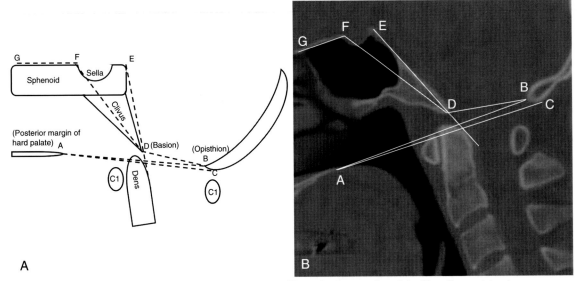

FIG. 14.1 **(A and B)** Measurements commonly used in evaluating craniovertebral junction on lateral projection. For the name of different lines, refer to Table 14.1. A, posterior margin of hard palate; B, opisthion; C, inferior margin of the posterior rim of foramen magnum; D, basion; E, dorsum sella; F, anterior clinoid process; G, floor of anterior cranial fossa.

developmental invagination, which is more common, and secondary or acquired invagination.

Developmental invagination is associated with atlantooccipital assimilation, hypoplasia of the basiooccipital or atlas, incomplete fusion of the posterior arch of the atlas, odontoid anomalies, Klippel-Feil syndrome, and vertebral artery anomalies. In about 25%–35% of cases, basilar invagination is associated with Arnold-Chiari malformation, syringomyelia, and hydrocephalus. The symptoms and signs of developmental basilar invagination usually occur in the second or third decade. The most common local finding

## BOX 14.1
## Congenital Malformations at the Craniovertebral Junction

Malformations of the occipital bone
1. Platybasia
2. Basilar invagination (basioccipital hypoplasia)
3. Condylar hypoplasia
4. Condylar dysplasia (condylus tertius, paracondyloid process, and basilar process)

Malformations of the atlas
1. Atlas assimilation
2. Aplasia and hypoplasia of the atlas
3. Atlas arch anomaly
4. Ponticulus posticus

Malformations of the axis and odontoid process
1. Aplasia or hypoplasia of the dens
2. Persistent ossiculum terminale
3. Os odontoideum
4. Klippel-Feil anomaly

Adapted from Chen YF, Liu HM. Imaging of craniovertebral junction. *Neuroimaging Clin N Am.* 2009;19(3):483–510.

is short neck and torticollis. The patients might have symptoms and signs of increased intracranial pressure because of blockage of cerebrospinal fluid (CSF) circulation or vertical or lateral nystagmus because of compression of the cerebellum and vestibular apparatus. Some patients present with vertebral artery insufficiency.

Our and previous observations[2,3] indicate there may be two different types of developmental basilar invaginations based on imaging findings. One group of patients had classical imaging findings (Fig. 14.2) of odontoid process protrusion into the foramen magnum in the cephalad direction, C1-2 dislocation or dens-clivus dislocation causing direct compression of the pontomedullary junction with violation of the Chamberlain, McRae, and Wackenheim lines, and listhesis of the oblique C1 and C2 facets. The other group of patients had imaging findings such as horizontal orientation of the clivus and anatomic alignment of the odontoid process and clivus despite the presence of basilar invagination, violation of the Chamberlain line but not the McRae and Wackenheim lines, and normal or fused horizontal C1-2 facet joints. This type of developmental basilar invagination is considered to be related to atlantoaxial dislocation stemming from aplasia and hypoplasia of the atlas. For details, please see the following section.

Acquired basilar invagination may be due to general osteopenia (Paget disease, osteomalacia, renal osteodystrophy, and hyperparathyroidism), local bone destruction (from a primary or secondary tumor or infection) (Fig. 14.3), trauma, and systematic diseases such as osteogenesis imperfecta, achondrodysplasia, osteopetrosis, mucopolysaccharidosis, and cretinism.

### Condylar Hypoplasia
In condylar hypoplasia, the occipital condyles are underdeveloped and have a flattened appearance; as a result, the skull base is flattened or even ascends medially, leading to basilar invagination and widening of the atlantooccipital joint axis angle. The lateral masses of the atlas may be fused to the hypoplastic condyles and further accentuate the basilar invagination.

Condylar hypoplasia restricts movement at the atlantooccipital joint and may lead to compression of the vertebral artery because of posterior sliding of the occiput in relation to the atlas.[4]

### Condylar Dysplasia (Condylus Tertius, Third Occipital Condyle)
Condylar dysplasia is characterized by persistence of the proatlas (the hypochordal bow of the fourth occipital sclerotome) or its failed integration into the occipital bone. This leads to an ossified remnant present at the distal end of the clivus.[5]

It is usually directly above and anterior to the arch of C1 and may form a joint or pseudojoint with the clivus, odontoid process, or anterior arch of C1 (Fig. 14.4). Occasionally, it can cause limitation in the range of motion of the CVJ.

## MALFORMATIONS OF THE ATLAS
### Atlas Assimilation (Atlantooccipital Assimilation, Occipitalization of the Atlas)
Atlas assimilation refers to complete or partial congenital fusion of C1 with the occiput. It results from failure of segmentation between the fourth occipital sclerotome and first spinal sclerotome.[6] The most common form of atlas abnormality is atlas assimilation, which is fusion of the anterior arch of C1 with the lowest end of the clivus (Fig. 14.2A and B). It may be unilateral (Fig. 14.5), segmental, focal, or bilateral. Bilateral atlas assimilation invariably leads to basilar invagination. It occurs commonly in conjunction with other abnormalities such as Klippel-Feil syndrome. When this is present, especially in the second and third cervical vertebrae (Fig. 14.6), there is a gradual loosening of the atlantoaxial joint, and the atlantoaxial subsequently becomes

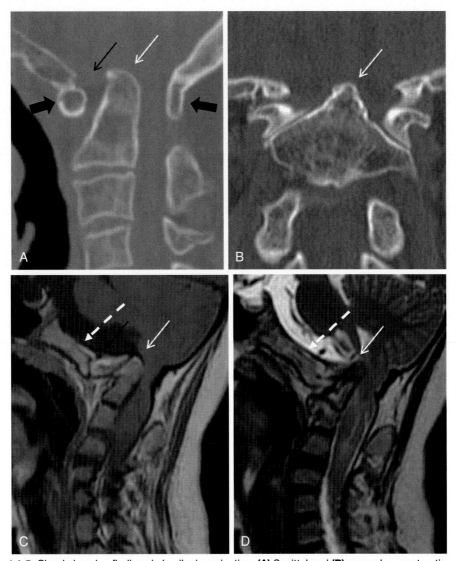

**FIG. 14.2** Classic imaging findings in basilar invagination. **(A)** Sagittal and **(B)** coronal reconstruction of CT scan. **(C)** Sagittal T1- and **(D)** sagittal T2-weighted images. Key findings are odontoid process cephalad protruding into the foramen magnum (*small white arrow*) and C1-2 dislocation or dens-clivus dislocation (*small black arrow*) directly compressing the pontomedullary. The upper row is a case associated with atlas assimilation (*large black arrow*) and agenesis of occipital condyle. The lower row is another case with dysplasia of clivus (*white dotted arrow*) and partial agenesis of atlas.

unstable. Sudden death has been reported in a patient with atlas assimilation.[7]

## Aplasia and Hypoplasia of the Atlas

Most isolated atlas anomalies are benign except the atlantal assimilations mentioned earlier. They produce no abnormal CVJ relationships and are not associated with basilar invagination. CT shows that several ossification centers participate in atlas development.[8] The lateral atlantal masses must be present at birth, and the neural ring must be formed by the age of 3 years. Abnormal atlantal development is observed in skeletal dysplasia syndromes (spondyloepiphyseal dysplasia, achondroplasia, Goldenhar syndrome) and in genetic abnormalities (Down syndrome).

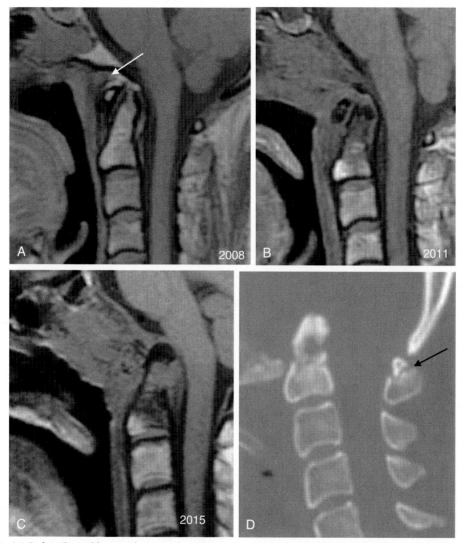

FIG. 14.3 A patient with nasopharyngeal carcinoma has secondary basilar invagination due to local bone destruction. Serial follow-up sagittal T1-weighted MR images **(A–C)** from 2008 to 2013. A subtle recurrent tumor was noted in the anterior supraodontal space (SOS) in 2008 (*white arrow*). In 2011, the tumor became obvious and invaded the SOS, prevertebral space, clivus, and upper C2. In 2013, the lesion converted to a diagnosis of recurrent cancer with basilar invagination. Sagittal CT reconstruction **(D)** shows upper displacement of the C2 and also posterior (*black arrow*).

A persistent bifid anterior and posterior arch of the atlas beyond the age of 3–4 years is observed in skeletal dysplasias, mucopolysaccharidosis, Down syndrome, Goldenhar syndrome, Conradi syndrome, Morquio syndrome, and atlas assimilation. The presentation is torticollis and plagiocephaly. Without proper management, this subsequently results in atlantoaxial subluxation (AAS). Down syndrome is associated with a 14%–20% incidence of atlantoaxial

dislocation.[9] This developmental and slow-in-coming acquired change may subsequently evolve into basilar invagination.

In the initial stage, atlantoaxial instability is reducible. The pannus, a prolific granulation tissue mass, surrounds the odontoid process providing protection and preventing the upward motion of the dens into the irreducible basilar invagination until the individual reaches the age of 14–15 years. However, compression

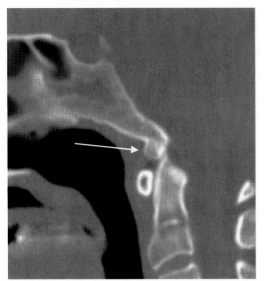

FIG. 14.4 Condylar dysplasia (condylus tertius). The ossified remnant (*white arrow*) is present at the distal end of the clivus, and it fuses to the lower end of the clivus.

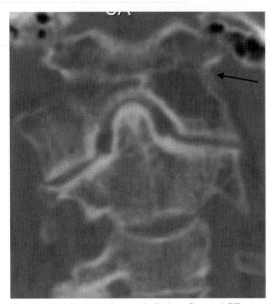

FIG. 14.5 Unilateral atlas assimilation. Coronal CT reconstruction, frontal view. In this case, the left lateral mass (*black arrow*) of C1 fuses with the occipital condyle but not the right side.

of the cervicomedullary junction may cause the clinical symptoms and signs.

In the irreducible basilar invagination (Fig. 14.7), the CVJ emerges from the abnormal groove behind the occipital condyles and pushes up into the cranial base, resulting in platybasia and a short horizontal clivus.[3] The upward excursion of the cranial base and the decrease of the vertical height of the posterior fossa leads to an acquired hindbrain herniation syndrome. The treatment of reducible, irreducible, and acquired hindbrain herniation syndrome are completely different.[3,8]

### Atlas Arch Anomaly

Total or partial aplasia of the posterior atlas arch is rare, but clefts in the atlas arches are much more common, with posterior clefts being the most common and apparent in 4% of adults. The majority of posterior atlas clefts (97%) are midline. Bilateral atlas posterior clefts may resemble the Jefferson fracture.[10,11] Anterior arch clefts are quite rare (0.1%) and usually associated with posterior clefts (split atlas). In Down syndrome, split atlas occurs frequently and is associated with os odontoideum and the subsequent formation of AAS.

On a lateral radiograph of the upper cervical spine, the predental space sits between the anterior arch of the atlas (which appears to be crescent, or half-moon, shaped) and the dens. In the anterior arch cleft, the predental space is obscured by the anterior arch, which becomes fatty and round and appears to overlap the dens.

Ponticulus posticus (Kimmerle deformity, sagittale foramen, atlantal posterior foramen, arcuate foramen, upper retroarticular foramen, canalis vertebralis, retroarticular vertebral artery ring, retroarticular canal, and retrocondilar vertebral artery) is a bony arch located between the posterior portion of the superior articular process and the posterolateral portion of the superior margin of the posterior arch of the atlas and is formed by ossification of a portion of the oblique atlantooccipital ligament.[12,13] It may be only a few millimeters long or if longer may produce a foramen through which the V3 portion of the vertebral artery passes. The incidence of ponticulus posticus is about 8% (range 2.6%–14.3%), and it is slightly more common in females. It can be complete, incomplete, or calcified and may be unilateral or bilateral (Fig. 14.8). Complete ponticulus posticus may cause chronic tension-type headache, orofacial pain, and migraine,[13] and its relationship to Bow hunter syndrome (BHS) is unclear.

## MALFORMATIONS OF THE AXIS AND ODONTOID PROCESS

### Aplasia or Hypoplasia of the Dens

Total aplasia of the odontoid process is extremely rare.[14] It can be identified as an extension of the dens to just above the lateral articular masses, with its tip lying below the level of the superior margin of the C1

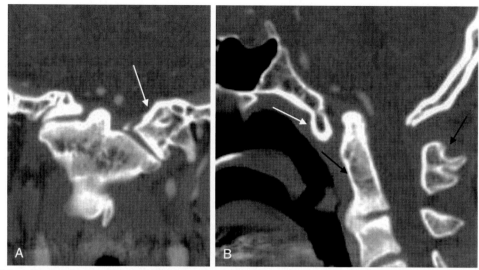

FIG. 14.6 A case (**A**, coronal and **B**, sagittal reconstruction CT) of right occipital condyle dysplasia, left lateral mass, and anterior C1 assimilation (*white arrows*) associated with Klippel-Feil anomaly (*black arrow*). Basilar invagination is evident on sagittal view.

anterior arch. The attachments for the apical and alar ligaments are absent in aplasia and hypoplasia of the odontoid and predisposing to atlantoaxial dislocation. Odontoid aplasia has been reported to have an association with a variety of congenital dysplastic syndromes such as Morquio syndrome, spondyloepiphyseal dysplasia, and metatrophic dwarfism.

## Persistent Ossiculum Terminale (Bergmann Ossicle)

Persistent ossiculum terminale results from nonfusion of the terminal ossification center with the remnant of the odontoid process (Fig. 14.9). It has to be differentiated from type I odontoid fracture (avulsion of the terminal ossicle).[15] The odontoid process is usually of normal height. This anomaly is stable when isolated and of little clinical significance.

## Ossiculum Odontoideum (Os Odontoideum)

Os odontoideum is an independent bone lying cranially to the C2 body in place of the dens. Radiographically, the os odontoideum has smooth borders and a small dens is always present. The anterior arch of C1 may appear rounded and hypertrophic. Os odontoideum is located in the same position as the dens near the clivus, with which it may fuse. The gap between the os odontoideum and the C2 usually extends above the level of the superior facets of the C2 (Fig. 14.10).

There are two types of os odontoideum. The first (type A, the orthotopic type) is defined by relocation of

the os odontoideum to the site of the dens and movement of the os odontoideum with the C1 and C2 vertebrae. The second (type B, the dystopic type) is defined by relocation of the os odontoideum to a site near the skull base and movement of the os odontoideum with the clivus. The entire complex leads to an incompetence of the cruciate ligament and, subsequently, to atlantoaxial instability.[16] In extreme cases, the os odontoideum may become fixed and associated with severe basilar invagination and compression of the cervicomedullary junction.

## Klippel-Feil Anomaly

Klippel-Feil anomaly is a congenital fusion or malsegmentation of the cervical spine. It is due to failure of normal segmentation of the cervical somites between the third and eighth weeks of gestation. Klippel-Feil anomaly can be localized, multisegmental, or diffuse. In the involved segment, the disk space may be absent or hypoplastic, and vertebral bodies become narrow or flat and wide (Figs. 14.6, 14.10, and 14.11). This finding is not obvious in infancy because of incomplete ossification. Klippel-Feil anomaly can occasionally involve posterior elements such as the lamina.

Less than 50% of cases present with the classic triad of short neck, webbed neck, and low hairline. Many associated symptoms and signs have been noted, including deafness, high arch palate, facial palsies, facial asymmetry, torticollis, ptosis of the eye, Duane eye contracture, abnormal rib fusion, scoliosis, syndactyly, hypoplastic

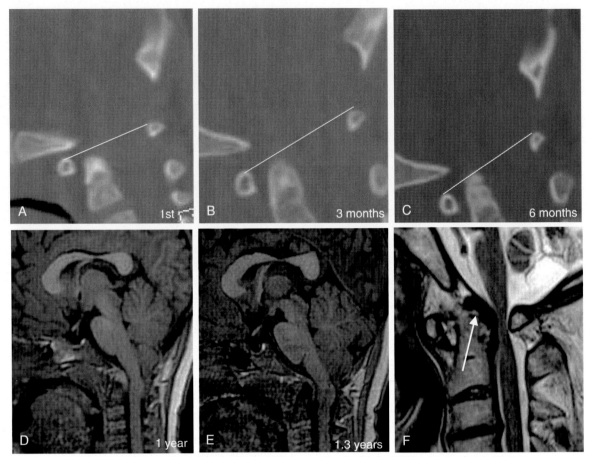

**FIG. 14.7** Dislocation of the atlantoaxial joint and stages of reducible instability progressing to irreducible and basilar invagination. **(A–C)** Serial follow-up sagittal reconstruction CT and **(D)** and **(E)** sagittal T1-weighted image after last CT of the same patient. From **(A)** to **(B)**, the dens moves posteriorly, increasing the distance of the atlantodental space; from **(B)** to **(C)**, the dens ascends into the foramen magnum; note the distance from the line between the upper margins of the anterior and posterior arches of C1. The distance from the tip of the dens is shortening between the serial studies. Compare **(D)** and **(E)**, there is more indentation of dens to the pontomedullary junction. **(F)** Another patient with atlantoaxial dislocation. Sagittal T2-weighted image shows granulation tissue formation at the top of the dens (*white arrow*). This can prevent the further upward movement of the dens.

thumb, supernumerary digits, hypoplasia of the upper extremity, genitourinary tract abnormalities, and cardiovascular abnormalities.

## FRACTURE

Basilar skull fractures are defined as linear fractures in the skull base, and are usually a part of multitude of facial fractures that extend to the skull base. CVJ fracture can occur in four major elements of its anatomic organization.

## Clivus Fracture

Clivus fractures are uncommon, with an incidence of 0.21%–0.56% among patients with head trauma, usually high-energy blunt head trauma.[17] The diagnosis of clivus fracture from plain radiographs is difficult because of the overlaying dense petrous temporal bones. In one study, high-resolution CT scanning with multiplanar reconstruction revealed clivus fracture in 9 (0.36%) of 2500 patients with head trauma.[18] Clivus fracture can be longitudinal, transverse, or oblique and result in cranial nerve deficits (cranial nerves VI and VII) and vascular complications.

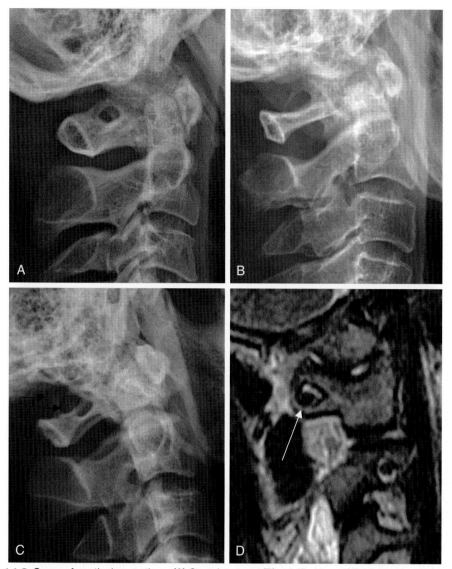

FIG. 14.8 Cases of ponticulus posticus. **(A)** Complete type; **(B)** calcified type; **(C)** bilateral involvement (*black arrows*); **(D)** the vertebral artery goes through the ponticulus posticus (*white arrow*).

Mortality is high (24%–31%) because of brain stem trauma and carotid or vertebrobasilar occlusion.[17] Transverse and diastatic fractures are associated with a higher mortality rate and worse outcome.

## Occipital Condyle Fracture

Occipital condylar fractures tend to be high-energy blunt traumas. Because occipital condylar fracture may be asymptomatic or masked by death or concomitant injuries or have delayed manifestations, the true incidence is difficult to determine. One report suggests that the incidence of craniocervical injury might be as high as 16%.[19]

Diagnosis of fracture of the occipital condyle requires a high index of suspicion and high-resolution tomography. Occipital condyle fracture should be suspected when paralysis of the 9th through the 12th nerves (Collet-Sicard syndrome) occurs after minor head trauma. These fractures are divided into three types (see Box 14.2).

It has been well established that conventional radiographs alone miss up to half of patients with acute

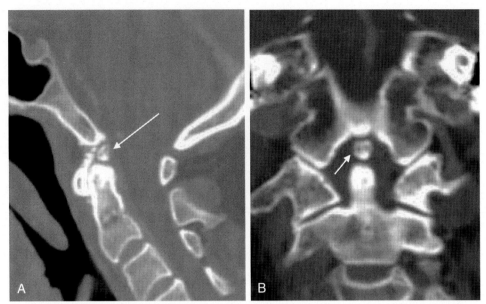

FIG. 14.9 Persistent ossiculum terminale (*white arrow*) (**A**, coronal; **B**, coronal reconstruction) located above the alignment of upper C1 and the dens, between the dens and the lowest end of the clivus.

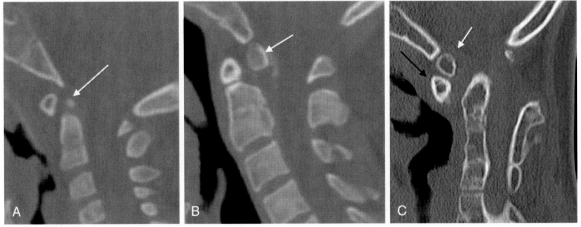

FIG. 14.10 Os odontoideum. Two types (**A**, orthotopic type and **B**, dystopic type) of os odontoideum are shown on the sagittal view of reconstruction CT. The os (*white arrow*) moves in different relationship to the clivus and the rest of C2. Please note the round or triangular shape of the anterior arch of C1 (*black arrow*). With associated Klippel-Feil anomaly basilar invagination resulted (**C**).

craniocervical instability.[19] Patients with occipital condyle fractures may have a wide variety of clinical outcomes and high incidence of additional cervical spine injuries affecting neurologic outcome.

## Atlas Fracture

Atlas fractures account for 2%–13% of acute injuries of the cervical spine (see Box 14.3), are due to a traumatic axial load, and are typically associated with other damage to the upper cervical spine. C1 anterior ring fractures are not an uncommon finding, and a prevertebral soft tissue thickness of >10 mm on radiography is highly suggestive of such a fracture. Definitive diagnosis of an isolated fracture often requires CT scans (Fig. 14.11), whereas ligamentous injury is most readily identified with MRI. The distance between the atlas and the dens (atlantodens interval, ADI) is a marker for ligamentous instability. Normally, ADI is <3 mm in adults (<5 mm

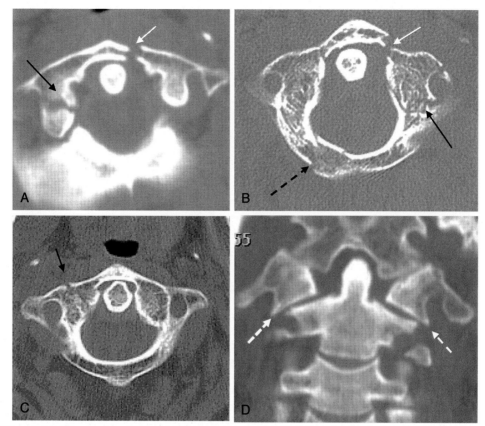

FIG. 14.11 Atlas fracture. (**A–C**, axial; **D**, coronal reconstruction). Anterior ring fracture (*white arrow*) is shown on (**A**) and (**B**). Lateral mass fracture (*black arrow*) is shown on (**A**), (**B**), and (**D**). Posterior arch fracture (*dash black arrow*) is shown on (**B**). Transverse foramen fracture is shown on (**B**), and vertebral artery (VA) injury is suspected. (**D**) shows lateral displacement of bilateral atlas lateral masses with the outer border (*dash white arrows*) sliding laterally on the C2, and fracture of both arches is highly suspected.

---

**BOX 14.2**
**Classification of Occipital Condyle Fracture**

Type 1 fractures result from axial compression with comminution of the occipital condyle, and the intact alar ligaments and tectorial membrane tend to stabilize the craniovertebral junction (CVJ).

Type 2 fractures result from a direct blow to the skull base and occipital condyle, and the intact alar ligaments tend to stabilize the CVJ.

Type 3 fractures result from avulsion, and the torn alar ligaments tend to destabilize the CVJ.

---

**BOX 14.3**
**Classification of Atlas Fractures by Fracture Pattern**

Type I—fractures that are limited to the anterior or posterior arch, with intact transverse ligament

Type II—fractures (also known as Jefferson fractures) that typically consist of bilateral burst fractures through the anterior and posterior arches of C1

Type III—fractures that involve the lateral mass

---

in children), but when it is 3–5 mm in adults, injury to the transverse ligament with intact alar and apical ligaments is suggested. ADI >5 mm in adults indicates serious injury to the transverse ligament, alar ligament, and tectorial membrane (atlantoaxial subluxation or

dislocation). In children, the C1 body may not be visualized radiographically until patients reach 1 year of age and does not fuse until they reach 4 years of age.

Jefferson fractures (type II) (Fig. 14.12) and lateral mass fractures (type III) may occur in isolation or in conjunction with significant ligamentous disruption.[20]

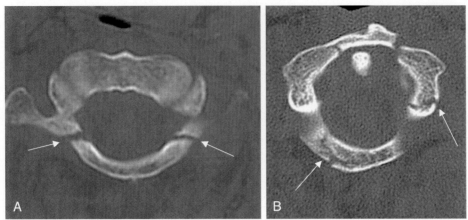

FIG. 14.12 Jefferson fracture involving the bilateral posterior arch (*white arrows*). (**A** and **B**) Axial CT. On (**B**), both anterior and posterior arches are fractured.

If the sum of lateral mass displacement is >7 mm, then a transverse ligament rupture is assured and the injury pattern is considered unstable. MRI is more sensitive at detecting injury to transverse ligaments. Vertebral artery injuries are assessable with neck computed tomography angiography (CTA) when atlas fracture is diagnosed. If a vertebral artery dissection is found, the patient will need anticoagulation with heparin and further evaluation by interventional radiology.

### Axis Fracture (Odontoid Fracture)

The incidence of odontoid fractures approaches 15% of all C-spine fractures (see Box 14.4). Usually, these fractures are secondary to motor vehicle accidents or falls. When an odontoid fracture is suspected, it is important to rule out concomitant associated C-spine injuries.

A type I fracture (less than 5% of cases) usually is stable if limited to an avulsion injury to the tip of the odontoid process. Occasionally, the apical and/or alar ligaments are injured as a result of traction forces and become unstable. More than 60% of odontoid fractures are type II fractures (Fig. 14.13). A type III fracture (30% of cases) can extend laterally to the superior articular facet of the atlas and develop vertically in the odontoid process and body of the axis (less than 5% of cases). An isolated C2 lateral mass fracture is extremely rare, and if found, other C-spine pathology must be sought.

Hangman fracture (Fig. 14.14 and Box 14.5) involves the pars interarticularis and adjacent structures and results from hyperextension injury.

## DEGENERATIVE LESIONS OF THE CVJ

The degenerative lesions in the CVJ include degenerative arthritis (osteoarthritis), ossification of the posterior longitudinal ligament, and diffuse idiopathic skeletal hyperostosis (DISH). The retroodontoid pseudotumor (ROP) (which might be associated with various kinds of degenerative or inflammatory arthritis in the CVJ region) is discussed herein.

### Degenerative Arthritis

Degenerative arthritis of the CVJ is not uncommon but is easily neglected because the lower cervical spine degeneration is more prevalent and causes more specific symptoms such as radiculopathy. Atlantoaxial osteoarthritis is an underrecognized source of neck pain, limitation of range of motion, and cervicogenic headaches.[21] The complex anatomy of the occiput-atlas-axis complex and the wide range of motion at the occipitocervical junction and atlantoaxial joints render them susceptible to multiple degenerative and traumatic processes.[22] The incidence of degenerative arthritis of the CVJ increases with age. An earlier

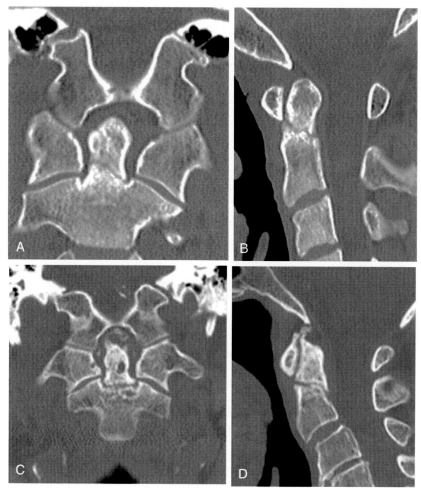

FIG. 14.13 Odontoid fracture. Type 2 fracture shows on **(A)** coronal and **(B)** sagittal reconstruction CT. Type 3 fracture shows on **(C)** coronal and **(D)** sagittal reconstruction CT. Note that on the sagittal view alone, sometimes, it is difficult to differentiate the types of fracture.

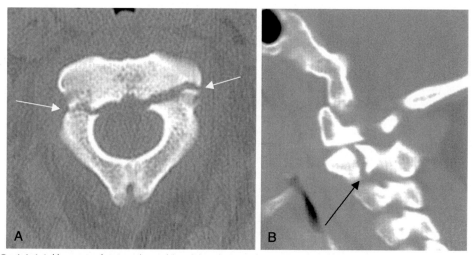

FIG. 14.14 Hangman fracture (*arrow*) involving the pars interarticularis. **(A)** Axial and **(B)** sagittal reconstruction CT.

study using radiographs reported that the prevalence of severe lateral atlantoaxial osteoarthritis ranges from 5.4% in the sixth to 18.2% in the ninth decade of life.[23] A more recent prevalence study using CT in a group of 1543 adult subjects (aged 18–103 years) found osteoarthritis of the anterior atlantodens joint in 44.6% and that with age, a significant increase occurs in the prevalence of degenerative changes at the atlantoaxial joint, ranging from 1.4% in the youngest group to 92.9% in the oldest group. They found that, with age, the ADI narrowed linearly, the prevalence of intraosseous cysts increased exponentially from 4.2% to 37.4%, and the prevalence of calcific synovitis increased from 0% to 11.1%.[24] Degenerative arthritis could be primary or secondary to trauma or even osteoradionecrosis (ORN) related to prior irradiation for head and neck cancer.[25] The degenerative arthritis at the CVJ may involve the lateral atlantoaxial joint (usually unilateral or bilateral asymmetric), the midline atlantoodontoid joint, and the occipitocervical joint. C1-C2 facet osteoarthritis is symptomatic in 4% of patients with known peripheral or spinal osteoarthritis, occurring in females at 74%, and presenting unilaterally in 76% in one large series.[26,27] Degenerative arthritis of the CVJ might also cause craniovertebral instability and resultant myelopathy. Surgical decompression and atlantoaxial fusion might be considered for managing refractory cases.

The imaging findings are similar to those seen in degenerative arthritis elsewhere in the body, including marginal osteophyte formation, joint space narrowing, subchondral sclerosis, and subchondral cyst formation[28] (Fig. 14.15). These findings are commonly associated with varying degrees of lateral mass collapse, ligamentous thickening, or calcification. Further radiologic features associated with craniovertebral instability include reduction in the height of the atlantoaxial lateral mass complex, mobile atlantoaxial dislocation, basilar invagination, and periodontoid degenerative tissue mass.[29]

## Ossification of the Posterior Longitudinal Ligament

The posterior longitudinal ligament extends from the tectorial membrane of the basion to the posterior surface of each vertebra and disc, down to the coccyx. Ossification of the posterior longitudinal ligament (OPLL) is commonly seen in oriental populations, and its cause remains obscure. OPLL occurs after the age of 50 years, and men are more frequently affected than women. The most commonly affected region is the cervical spine, usually at C4-5. But the ossification can extend from the C3 vertebra and lower levels to the posterior aspect of the C2 vertebra. Clinical presentations include neck pain, hand numbness, radicular pain, and myelopathy. The symptoms usually correlate with the thickness of ligament ossification and residual canal size,[30,31] and the location and extent of OPLL determine the type of neurologic symptoms. The occurrence of OPLL is highly associated with cervical spondylosis and DISH.[32]

CT is best at demonstrating ossification. On CT, OPLL characteristically appears as an "upside-down T" or "bowtie" posterior longitudinal ligament on axial views.[33] On MRI, detection depends on the morphology of the process and the presence or absence of bone marrow or calcium in the ligament. A hypertrophied OPLL usually appears as a hypointense structure on T1- and T2-weighted images (Fig. 14.16). Occasionally, a hyperintense signal (possibly representing fatty marrow within the bony component) is seen on T1-weighted images.[33] MRI may have difficulties in distinguishing ossification from ligament hypertrophy if the lesion appears as a dark signal on both T1- and T2-weighted images.

## Diffuse Idiopathic Skeletal Hyperostosis

DISH is a common ossifying diathesis in middle-aged and elderly patients characterized by bone proliferation along the anterior aspect of the spine and at extraspinal sites of ligament and tendon attachment to bone.[34] It involves the thoracic spine more than the cervical spine. DISH is usually an incidental finding but could be associated with symptoms such as neck stiffness or pain. Large lesions have also been reported to compress or obstruct the esophagus or airway.[35] The imaging pictures characteristically depict thick flowing ossification of the anterior longitudinal ligaments that are separated from their vertebral bodies by relatively normal intervertebral discs and facet joints. DISH is commonly associated with degenerative arthritis and OPLL, and it might be associated with AAS and ROP.[34,36]

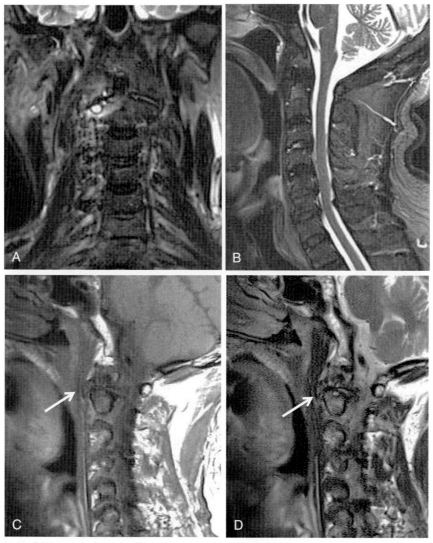

FIG. 14.15 C1-2 lateral atlantoaxial joint degenerative arthritis in a 74-year-old man presenting with nuchal pain and right occipital headache. **(A)** Coronal short-tau inversion recovery shows right facet joint space narrowing with subchondral cysts and bone marrow edema. **(B)** The midline joint is relatively spared. **(C)** Sagittal T1- and **(D)** T2-weighted images show marginal osteophytes around the narrowed facet joint space (*arrow*).

## Retroodontoid Pseudotumor

ROP is a nonneoplastic mass at the CVJ. It can be asymptomatic or cause cord compression and neurologic symptoms.[37,38] It is usually bony or cartilaginous and has been referred to as a pseudotumor, inflammatory granulation tissue, degenerative fibrochondral-like tissue, and cystic deterioration.[39] The pathology often reveals fibrous granulation tissue or fibrocartilaginous tissue. The underlying soft tissue usually elevates the posterior longitudinal ligament. It is more commonly seen in the elderly population and may be caused by atlantoaxial instability.[40] Goel suggested for the first time that retroodontoid tissue is a manifestation of atlantoaxial instability and proposed surgical procedures focused on atlantoaxial fixation to relieve this instability.[41] Subsequently, several authors performed atlantoaxial fixation for such lesions and demonstrated resolution of the retroodontoid mass.[42,43]

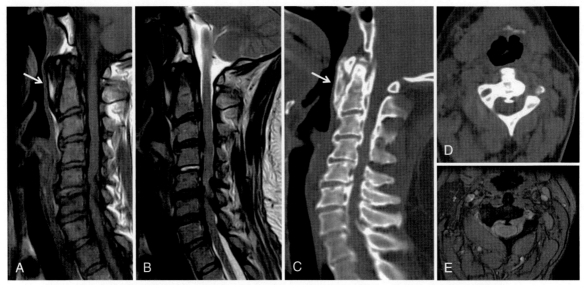

FIG. 14.16 Ossification of posterior longitudinal ligament (OPLL). **(A)** Sagittal T1-weighted, **(B)** T2-weighted, and **(C)** CT images in a 47-year-old woman presenting with myelopathy show long segmental OPLL from the C1-2 level down to C7. Also noted is ossification of the anterior longitudinal ligament, which shows signal of fat marrow (*arrow*). **(D)** Axial CT and **(E)** axial gradient echo show upside-down T appearance of the ossified posterior longitudinal ligament.

However, some of the lesions were not associated with instability.[38]

The ROP usually shows soft tissue density on CT. MRI shows hypointensity on both T1-weighted and T2-weighted images with peripheral enhancement (Fig. 14.17). The differential diagnosis of ROP includes rheumatoid arthritis (RA), calcium pyrophosphate dihydrate (CPPD) crystal deposition, and long-term hemodialysis (Figs. 14.18 and 14.19). However, these conditions in the differential diagnosis may share imaging features, making a definite diagnosis difficult. In RA of the CVJ (which is described later in this chapter), inflammation of the synovial membranes of the bursae, articular capsules, and tendon sheath and ligamentous insertion cause pannus and destroy the articular cartilage and subchondral bone in patients with long-standing disease. The pannus surrounding the odontoid process usually shows hypointensity on T2-weighted image with enhancement. There is usually AAS. CPPD crystal deposition disease or pseudogout is one of the most common forms of crystal-associated arthropathy in the elderly[44]; classically takes place within articular, hyaline, and fibrocartilaginous structures; and can also occur in periarticular structures such as the joint capsule, tendons, and ligaments. In cases of CPPD in the cervical spine, CT shows linear calcific deposits in the transverse ligament of the atlas and in other periodontoid structures, including alar ligaments, apical ligament,

and superior longitudinal fibers of the cruciate ligament. CPPD may also be present as a cystic retroodontoid mass.[45] The complications of long-term dialysis include β2-microglobulin–derived amyloid protein deposition in and around joints (resulting in bone erosion, subchondral cyst formation, and articular destruction) and ROPs (proliferative soft tissue lesions enveloping the odontoid process) caused by amyloid deposits and inflammatory cell infiltration of tissue surrounding the odontoid process.[46] The amyloid deposition may appear as a periodontoid soft tissue mass hypointense to muscle on both T1- and T2-weighted images.[47]

## INFECTIOUS/INFLAMMATORY LESIONS OF THE CVJ

The infectious/inflammatory lesions of the CVJ include inflammatory arthritis-like RA, ankylosing spondylitis (AS), CPPD disease, and infectious spondylodiscitis and can be pyogenic, nonpyogenic, or granulomatous. ORN, a serious complication of radiation therapy, may also cause inflammatory lesions at the CVJ.

### Rheumatoid Arthritis

Reports vary widely on the prevalence of cervical spine abnormality associated with RA and neurologic complications. According to one study, patients with RA

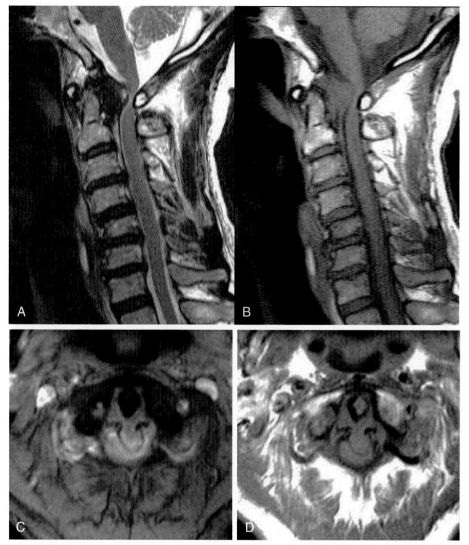

FIG. 14.17 Retroodontoid pseudotumor in a 76-year-old man who presented with myelopathy. There was no spinal stability before resection of the retroodontoid mass. **(A)** Sagittal T2-weighted (T2WI), **(B)** sagittal T1-weighted (T1WI), **(C)** axial gradient echo, and **(D)** axial T1W images show a retroodontoid mass that reveals dark signal on T2WI and isointensity on T1WI. The pathologic examination of the resected mass showed degenerative fibrocartilage and ligamentum with myxoid or edematous change.

for more than 7 years develop craniocervical complications in 30%–50% of cases, whereas patients with RA for more than 14 years develop AAS with myelopathy in 2.5% of cases.[48] RA occurs most commonly in middle age, more commonly in women, and usually involves the hands or feet if the spine is involved. The disease may affect the atlantoaxial joint, the occipital condyles and facets, and uncovertebral joints. These patients may present with morning pain and stiffness and

suboccipital pain related to AAS and C2 nerve compression. Inflammation of the synovial membranes of the bursae, articular capsules, and tendinous and ligamentous insertions causes pannus and destroys the articular cartilage and subchondral bone in patients with longstanding disease. The atlantoaxial joint is affected by the same mechanism, and erosion may give the dens of the atlantoaxial joint a "pencil-tip" appearance. Inflammation leads to weakening of the transverse and

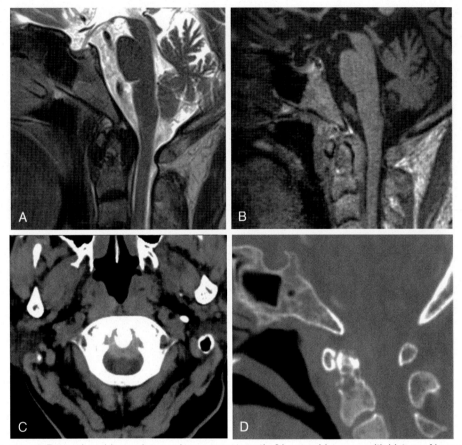

FIG. 14.18 Retroodontoid pseudotumor in an asymptomatic 61-year-old woman with history of hemo-dialysis for 20 years. **(A)** Sagittal T2-weighted (T2WI) and **(B)** T1-weighted (T1WI) images show soft tissue posterior to the dens, which is dark on T2WI and isointense on T1WI. **(C and D)** CT shows hyperdense soft tissue posterior to the dens with dens erosions.

alar ligaments, and AAS can occur. The histology of the patient with chronic rheumatoid disease indicates severe ligamentous and osseous destruction accompanied by fibrous tissue replacement of the rheumatoid synovium. Grossly, the osseous structures suggest severe destruction secondary to mechanical instability, rather than to an acute inflammatory process.[49] AAS with severe occipitalgia or high cervical myelopathy is the most common type of instability of the upper cervical spine in patients with RA. Lateral subluxation might also result in vertebral artery compression and then vertebrobasilar infarctions.[50]

On CT, an uncalcified pannus surrounds and erodes the dens. There are also erosions of the uncovertebral and facet joints. On MRI, the pannus shows low signal on T1-weighted image, heterogeneous signal on T2-weighted image (usually intermediate to low signal), and enhancement by injection of contrast medium (Fig. 14.19).

A retroodontoid mass should be differentiated from CPPD disease, amyloid arthropathy, and pseudotumors of the CVJ attributable to chronic mechanical instability.

### Ankylosing Spondylitis

AS is a seronegative spondyloarthropathy and a chronic inflammatory disease of unknown origin that affects the axial skeleton mostly. The best diagnostic clue is fusion between vertebral bodies. The majority of the patients have sacroiliitis and 90% of patients are HLA-B27 positive, which might help in the diagnosis.

The radiologic changes in the cervical spine in AS include vertebral squaring, syndesmophytes, ankylosis, ossification of the longitudinal ligaments, and AAS.[51]

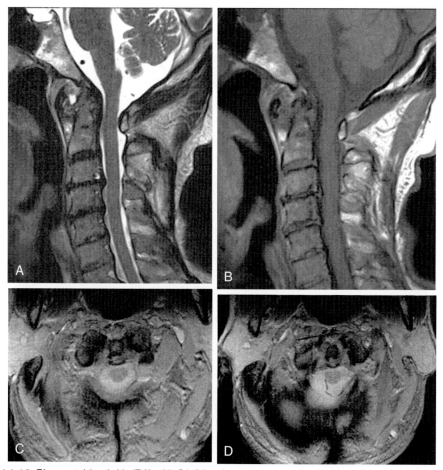

FIG. 14.19 Rheumatoid arthritis (RA) with C1-2 involvement in a 76-year-old man with a long history of RA. **(A)** Sagittal T2-weighted (T2WI), **(B)** T1-weighted (T1WI), and **(C** and **D)** axial gradient echo images show C1-2 subluxation with soft tissue lesions between C1 anterior arch and the dens and also the retroodontoid region. The soft tissue reveals heterogeneous hypo- to hyperintensity on T2WI and isointensity on T1WI, associated with dens erosions.

There may be erosions along the posterior dens margin, facet joint ankylosis, and an inflammatory retroodontoid fibrocartilaginous mass. AAS was found to be a frequent complication in 14.1% of patients with AS, regardless of cervical symptoms.[52] The pathophysiology of AAS in AS is likely secondary to subaxial fusion. The subaxial fusion places stress upon the atlantooccipital and atlantoaxial joints, predisposing them to dislocation and fracture.[53]

## Calcium Pyrophosphate Dihydrate Deposition Disease

CPPD disease is a pathologic process of crystal formation classically within articular, hyaline, and fibrocartilaginous structures and can also be found in periarticular structures, such as the joint capsule, tendons, and ligaments. CPPD disease can occur in the spine, sacroiliac joints, pubic symphysis, and peripheral skeleton (knees and wrists). CPPD disease is one of the most common forms of crystal-associated arthropathy in the elderly.[54] Spine involvement is often seen in the absence of peripheral skeleton involvement. It usually occurs in patients older than 50 years, and its incidence increases with age. The deposition of CPPD crystals can be asymptomatic but also lead to acute, subacute, or chronic inflammation of the joints. It can also cause more chronic arthritis that mimics osteoarthritis or RA. The relationship between degenerative arthritis and CPPD is unclear, and degenerative arthritis might be a risk factor of CPPD.

In cases of CPPD involving the C-spine, CT shows linear calcific deposits in the transverse ligament of the atlas and in other periodontoid structures, including alar ligaments, apical ligament, and superior longitudinal fibers of the cruciate ligament. There are also vertebral endplate erosions, odontoid subchondral cyst formation and erosions, and possibly AAS. Atlantoaxial CPPD deposition was initially described by Bouvet et al. as a "crowned dens" in 1985.[54] CT is the most sensitive modality of visualizing periodontoid calcifications, and the existing literature suggests that diagnosis of CPPD disease is largely radiographic, including the most comprehensive review by Goto et al.[55] Other than diffuse calcifications, CPPD in the atlantoaxial region may present as a cystic retroodontoidal mass and should be included in the differential list of ROP.[55] On MRI, the calcium deposition is often not visible, the intervertebral discs are narrow and of low signal on all sequences, the posterior longitudinal ligament and ligamentum flavum are thickened, the dens and vertebral endplates are eroded, and the soft tissue adjacent to the vertebra shows low to intermediate signal intensity on all sequences and minimal or peripheral enhancement with contrast medium.

### Pyogenic and Nonpyogenic Infection

Infection of the CVJ may result from inadequate treatment of a contiguous infection, such as otitis externa, paranasal sinusitis, or dental caries. Lymphatic channels play a role in the pathogenesis of any infective process at the CVJ. The synovial lining of the occipitoatlantoaxial joints receives afferents from the paranasal sinuses and nasopharyngeal and retropharyngeal areas. Retrograde infection may spread to the CVJ, resulting in instability or effusion as an inflammatory response. The clinical presentations are most commonly neck pain and limited range of motion. There may be associated medical conditions such as immunocompromised health status and previous surgical treatment or irradiation of adjacent areas. Pyogenic infection is more commonly seen in cases of contiguous infection, but fungal and tuberculosis (TB) infections of the CVJ are also reported. CVJ TB is a rare infection (occurring in only 0.3%–1% of spinal TB cases),[56] usually secondary to a primary focus, such as a bone elsewhere in the body. The ligaments are involved secondarily by displacement and disruption. The infection usually starts from the lateral joint and spreads to the midline and then to the contralateral joint in the late phase. Tissue biopsy is imperative to confirm the diagnosis and to obtain drug sensitivities.

The imaging findings of CVJ infection include bone erosion and ligament destruction leading to instability at the CVJ and phlegmon or abscess formation in the paravertebral and epidural regions (Fig. 14.20). The craniovertebral infection may extend to the skull base, clivus, and occipital condyles and usually crosses joint spaces. In evaluation of the disease extent, MRI is better since it is able to reveal osseous and soft tissue involvement and the spinal cord. The involved bone marrow shows hypointensity on T1-weighted image and hyperintensity on T2-weighted image, with variable enhancement on postcontrast images. The soft tissue component shows either heterogeneous enhancement (in phlegmons) or peripheral enhancement with central nonenhancing pus (in abscesses).

### Osteoradionecrosis

ORN is a serious complication of radiation therapy that occurs in patients treated for nasopharyngeal carcinoma (NPC) or other head and neck malignancies. Numerous factors are associated with the risk of developing ORN, including total radiation dose, fractionation, poor oral hygiene, alcohol and tobacco use, dental extractions, and tumor size, location, and staging. Radiation-induced endarteritis may injure the vasculature, causing bone and the overlying soft tissue to become hypovascular, hypocellular, and hypoxic.[57] Then tissue breaks down and nonhealing wounds develop. ORN is predisposing to bone and adjacent soft tissue inflammation. ORN related to head and neck cancer may occur in the mandible, maxillofacial bones, skull base, hyoid bone, laryngeal cartilage, external ear canal, and also the upper C-spine. The clinical presentations of ORN at the CVJ include neck pain, neurologic symptoms, epistaxis, and infectious symptoms.

Imaging of ORN of the CVJ usually reveals contiguous atlantoaxial or atlantooccipital bone involvement with intervening joint space changes caused by arthritis, collapse of the subchondral bone, reactive soft tissue swelling, and ulceration of the posterior pharyngeal mucosa.[58] The involved bone shows heterogeneous signal and enhancement on MRI (Fig. 14.21) and abnormal bone density with mixed osteolytic and osteosclerotic changes and cortical bone disruption on CT. On imaging, ORN may be hard to differentiate from local recurrent or metastatic tumors to the bone and soft tissue. However, compared with a tumor, CVJ ORN involvement tends to be more contiguous in bone and intervening joint space, more bilateral, and more destructive

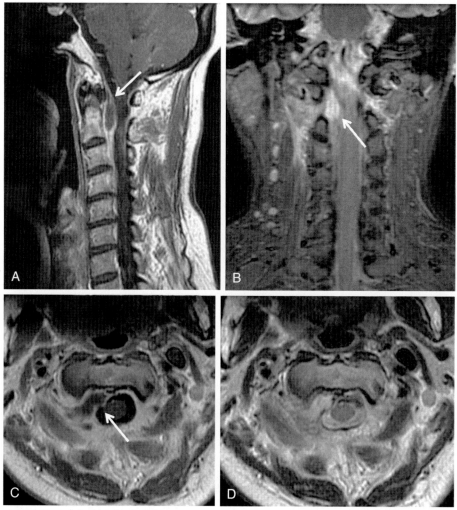

FIG. 14.20 Pyogenic infection at C1-2 epidural space in a 56-year-old woman presenting with neck pain and right occipital headache. **(A)** Sagittal and **(C)** axial T1-weighted images show a rim-enhancing collection (*arrows*) at C1-2 right anterior epidural space extending through the right neural foramen with C2 nerve root compression. **(B)** Coronal short-tau inversion recovery and **(D)** axial T2-weighted images show bright signal of the abscess.

of facet joints and subchondral bone. Tumor recurrence or metastasis at the CVJ tends to involve the posterior arch, tends to destroy lateral border bone, and tends to have extraosseous soft tissue mass (Fig. 14.22).

## TUMOR AND TUMOR-LIKE LESIONS

The tumor and tumor-like lesions at the CVJ include miscellaneous lesions arising from extradural structures, intradural extramedullary structures, and intramedullary structures. The largest group of lesions arises from the bone or adjacent extradural structures and includes chordoma, chondrasarcoma, bone origin tumors (such as fibrous dysplasia), hemangioma, aneurysmal bone cyst (ABC), osteoblastoma, bone metastasis, multiple myeloma, and lesions from adjacent pharyngeal mucosal malignancies. The intradural extramedullary tumors mainly include meningiomas, nerve sheath tumors, and some congenital cystic lesions. The intramedullary tumors mainly consist of intrinsic brainstem or

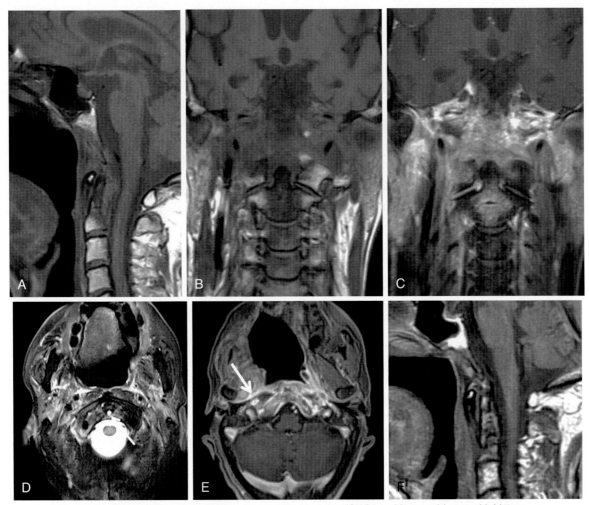

**FIG. 14.21** Osteoradionecrosis at the craniovertebral junction (CVJ) in a 66-year-old man with history of irradiated palatal cancer and diabetics who presented with neck pain. **(A)** Sagittal T1-weighted image (T1WI), **(B)** coronal precontrast T1WI, and **(C)** postcontrast T1WI show a wide area of signal change and enhancement involving the bone marrow, the occipitoatlas joints, and the right atlantoaxial joint. **(D)** Axial T2-weighted image and **(E)** postcontrast T1WI show a wide area of soft tissue edema and heterogeneous enhancement with focal soft tissue necrosis (*arrow*). After 1 year of conservative treatment, **(F)** sagittal T1WI shows partial resolution of the changes at CVJ, with mild C1-2 subluxation.

upper spinal cord tumors, which are not discussed here. The features of CVJ tumors on imaging are described in this section. The role of imaging is to determine the nature and resectability of the tumors. It is important in radiologic interpretation to evaluate the tumor extent, determine the direction of encroachment, determine whether the lesion has a vascular or intramedullary component, and evaluate craniovertebral stability.

## Extradural Tumors and Tumor-like Lesions
### Chordoma

Chordomas are locally aggressive tumors arising from primitive notochordal remnants. They occur along the vertebral axis with a propensity for the sphenooccipital region and the sacrum. The classic midline clival chordoma can spread inferiorly, thereby affecting the foramen magnum and nasopharynx, with erosion of the atlas and other cervical

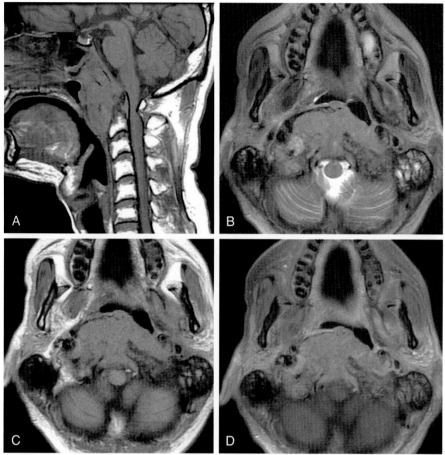

FIG. 14.22 A 35-year-old man with recurrent nasopharyngeal carcinoma (NPC) involving the craniovertebral junction (CVJ). **(A)** Sagittal T1-weighted image (T1WI) shows an infiltrative bulky soft tissue mass at the CVJ, with bone destruction of the clivus, C1, and C2. **(B)** Axial T2-weighted image (T2WI) and **(C)** precontrast and **(D)** postcontrast T1WIs show nasopharyngeal mucosal lesion with posterior and downward extension to involve the CVJ. The mass shows intermediate signal on T1WI and T2WI, with moderate enhancement after contrast injection typical of NPC.

vertebrae.[59] Generally, chordomas grow slowly and produce symptoms insidiously. Symptoms of intracranial chordomas vary with lesion location and proximity to critical structures.

The classic appearance of intracranial chordoma on CT is a well-defined expansile soft tissue mass that arises from the clivus with associated lytic bone change.[59] Intratumoral calcifications are common CT findings and are thought to represent either sequestra from bone destruction or calcifications within the chondroid matrix. On T1-weighted images, chordoma has an intermediate to low signal intensity and is easily recognized within the high-signal fatty marrow in the clivus. Small hyperintense foci can sometimes be visualized in the tumor on T1-weighted images because of intratumoral hemorrhage or mucous pools. Classic chordoma shows bright signal intensity on T2-weighted images, a finding that likely reflects the high fluid content of vacuolated cellular components (Fig. 14.23). The intratumoral area of calcification, hemorrhage, and a highly proteinaceous mucous pool usually appear as heterogeneous hypointensities on T2-weighted imaging. Most chordomas demonstrate moderate to marked enhancement after contrast material injection.

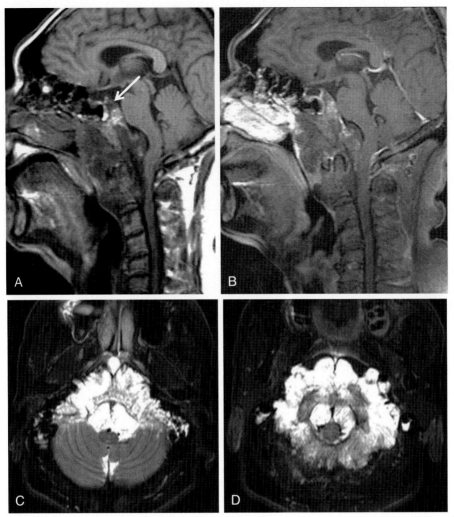

**FIG. 14.23** A huge craniovertebral junction chordoma in a 50-year-old man who presented with multiple lower cranial nerve palsy. **(A** and **B)** Pre- and postcontrast sagittal T1-weighted images (T1WI) show a huge lobulated mass with bone destruction of the clivus (*white arrow*), C1, and C2. The mass shows hypointensity on T1WI with some high signal foci inside. There is only mild enhancement after contrast injection. **(C** and **D)** Axial T2-weighted images show characteristic bright signal of the chordoma.

### Chondrosarcoma

The main differential diagnosis of skull base chordoma is chondrosarcoma, which, on imaging, may have an appearance similar to that of chordoma. The chondroid lesions are typically located in the paramedian petroclival synchondrosis, but they rarely occur in the midline associated with the sphenooccipital synchondrosis. The histopathologic findings of these two tumors may look similar, and the final diagnosis depends on immunohistochemical studies.

Lytic bone lesions with curvilinear calcifications indicative of chondroid matrix and presence of extraosseous soft tissue mass are evident on CT. On MRI, chondrosarcoma typically manifests as a destructive bone lesion with hypointense signal on T1-weighted images and bright signal on T2-weighted images. In some lesions, there may be marked signal inhomogeneity on T2-weighted images because of the presence of calcifications or hemorrhage. Heterogeneous ring and arc enhancement usually follows

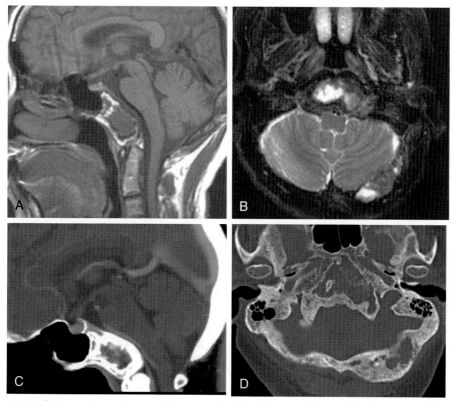

FIG. 14.24 Clivus and occipital bone fibrous dysplasia in a 62-year-old asymptomatic woman. Sagittal T1WI (A), axial T2WI (B), sagittal reconstruction CT (C), and axial CT (D) show expansile bone lesions without extraosseous mass or cortical destruction are seen. There are osseous, fibrous, and cystic components inside the masses.

contrast injection. Differentiation from chordomas is sometimes difficult based on conventional imaging, although an off-midline growth suggests chondrosarcoma. Diffusion-weighted imaging was reported to be a promising tool for the differentiation of chondrosarcoma from chordoma, with chondrosarcomas showing higher mean apparent diffusion coefficient values.[60,61]

### Miscellaneous benign bone tumors

A variety of benign bone tumors can occur at the CVJ. These include fibrous dysplasia, hemangioma, osteoid osteoma/osteoblastoma, ABC, eosinophilic granuloma, and osteochondroma. Fibrous dysplasia is a developmental disorder in which normal bone marrow is replaced by fibroosseous tissue. The involved bone is enlarged and shows abnormal mineralization. Fibrous dysplasia of the skull base usually involves the anterior cranial fossa and may involve the inferior clivus.[62] The MRI appearance

of fibrous dysplasia is variable. The lesions contain a mixture of fibrous tissue, cystic spaces, and cartilage (Fig. 14.24). The internal fibrous matrix may enlarge significantly and mimic a tumor. The typical "ground-glass" appearance on CT often makes the diagnosis more obvious.

Osteoblastomas are uncommon primary bone tumors that can occur in cervical vertebrae, mainly in the posterior elements of the cervical spine and rarely in the skull base. It most commonly affects males during the second decade. Osteoid osteomas and osteoblastomas differ only in size, potential for progression, and propensity to produce extreme pain. The CT appearance of osteoblastoma consists of a circumscribed lytic defect sometimes surrounded by a sclerotic rim. MRI usually reveals an aggressive appearance with heterogeneous enhancement and adjacent soft tissue swelling. Osteoblastoma is a rare benign tumor of bone that is known to incite a localized inflammatory response. These inflammatory features can simulate malignant behavior on MRI and can lead to misdiagnosis and unnecessarily aggressive resection unless one recognizes the classic benign features on CT.[63]

Hemangioma is a common benign venous malformation within vertebrae, which is usually intraosseous but may have an epidural component. The characteristic CT findings are well-defined lesions of fat density, with thickened trabeculae, but more aggressive lesions may contain ill-defined areas of bone destruction and have an extensive soft tissue component. The MRI may show hyperintensity or hypointensity on T1-weighted image, depending on the fat content, hyperintensity on T2-weighted image owing to vascular elements and variable enhancement.

About 10%–20% of ABCs occur in the spine, and 2% occur in the C-spine. ABC is an expansile benign bone neoplasm containing thin-walled, blood-filled cavities. ABCs in the spine tend to originate in the neural arch and extend to the vertebral body. About 80% of ABCs occur in young subjects (less than 20 years old).[64] Typical ABCs have an expansile cystic mass, a thin rim of calcification, bony trabeculae within the cyst on CT, and characteristic fluid-filled cysts on MRI. In addition, ABCs might be associated with pathologic fracture.

### Miscellaneous malignant bone tumors

Multiple myeloma/plasmacytoma and metastases are common malignant lesions found in the CVJ. Plasma cell myeloma occurs mainly in patients 40–80 years old. The axial bone is more likely involved than long bones. These tumors can be multifocal and diffuse or solitary plasmacytomas. Plasmacytomas in the CVJ can arise from nasopharyngeal submucosal tissue (extramedullary plasmacytoma) or the marrow space of the clivus or cervical vertebrae (solitary plasmacytoma of bone).[65] They have homogeneous signal intensity on T1- and T2-weighted images and usually lower signal intensity on T2-weighted images, reflecting the densely packed cells within the tumor (Fig. 14.25). The radiographic differential diagnosis for plasmacytoma includes lymphoma and metastasis. Pathologic examination is always necessary to establish the correct diagnosis.

Bone metastasis from malignancies in other areas of the body can occur anywhere, including the skull base and upper cervical vertebrae. The signal intensity and enhancement pattern on MRI may reflect the cell type of the original malignancy and be associated with necrosis or hemorrhage.

### Malignant lesions from adjacent soft tissue

NPC is a common primary head and neck malignancy in southern China and Southeast Asia. Skull base involvement is a common finding in patients who have NPC. Patients who have NPC can sometimes present with symptoms and imaging findings mimicking CVJ tumors when the invasive NPC extends directly. Imaging evaluation is thus important for the detection of possible mucosal malignancy. MR is better in demonstrating mucosal masses that vary in size, parapharyngeal fat involvement, and extent of skull base infiltration and intracranial involvement. The mucosal mass lesions show homogeneous intermediate signal intensity on T1-weighted images and T2-weighted images with moderate enhancement. NPC with skull base invasion is suggested by a focal or diffuse mucosal mass that is contiguous with the bone lesion (Fig. 14.25). On MRI, the signal intensity and enhancement pattern of tumor invasion from nasopharyngeal malignancies may mimic that of plasmacytoma or metastasis. In cases of CVJ bone lesion, the nasopharyngeal mucosa should always be carefully checked, because a small mucosal tumor could be overlooked.

Treatment of NPC may result in imaging changes of the CVJ, too. Normal postirradiation MRI shows increased fat marrow of the skull base and C-spine and disappearance of the nasopharyngeal mass. If the bone marrow is invaded by tumor before treatment, the bone marrow signal may gradually return to a normal fatty marrow signal years later. However, when ORN occurs, the signal and enhancement of the skull base or upper C-spine may be heterogeneous, which should differentiate it from a local recurrence.[58]

## Intradural Extramedullary Tumor and Tumor-like Lesions
### Meningioma

Meningiomas arise from arachnoid cap cells and are the most common primary nonglial intracranial tumors, and approximately 3% of all meningiomas occur at the foramen magnum. Nevertheless, meningiomas are the most common tumors (and 70% of all benign tumors) occurring at the foramen magnum. Like meningiomas at other locations, approximately two-thirds occur in women, who usually become symptomatic between the ages of 35 and 60 years. Meningiomas at the foramen magnum may present with sensory and motor deficits, gait disturbance, headache, or local pain.

Most foramen magnum meningiomas are strictly intradural. Ten percent have extradural extensions. The lesions typically are attached at the anterior rim of the foramen magnum and may invade the region

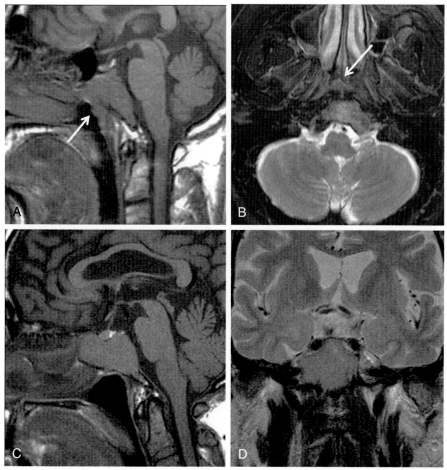

FIG. 14.25 **(A)** Sagittal T1-weighted (T1WI) and **(B)** axial T2-weighted (T2WI) images in a case of nasopharyngeal carcinoma shows a small nasopharyngeal mucosal tumor (*arrows*) with bone invasion and complete marrow replacement of the clivus. **(C)** Sagittal T1WI and **(D)** coronal T2WI in a case of plasmacytoma involving the clivus, with complete marrow replacement of the clivus and intermediate signal on T1WI and T2WI but without mucosal tumor.

surrounding the entrance to the vertebral artery and the exit of the cranial and cervical nerve roots.[66,67] This explains the higher incidence of incomplete removal of extradural meningiomas as compared with intradural meningiomas.

On MRI, the meningiomas usually appear rather homogeneous, have intermediate signal intensity on T1-weighted images and T2-weighted images, and show marked enhancement after contrast injection. Gadolinium-enhanced sequences help to delineate the dural attachment zone, the tumor, and its relation to neural and vascular structures (Fig. 14.26). The major imaging differential diagnosis is nerve sheath tumors, which usually show higher signal intensity on

T2-weighted image and are more likely to show heterogeneous enhancement, hemorrhage or cystic change, and neuroforaminal enlargement.

Tumors with adherence to the brainstem, encasement of the vertebral arteries and/or cranial nerves, en plaque growth pattern, high tumor grade, and high mitotic activity have been associated with an increased rate of incomplete resection and/or tumor recurrence. Radiosurgery is an alternative treatment in patients with advanced age and high operative risks and in those who refuse surgery or have residual or recurrent tumors. In a select group of patients with small lesions diagnosed by imaging as meningiomas, radiation may be used as a primary treatment option.[68]

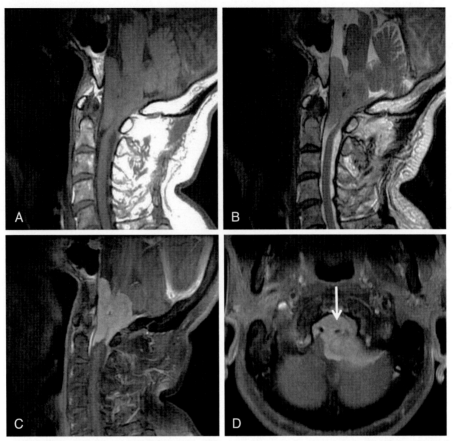

FIG. 14.26 Foramen magnum meningioma in a 66-year-old man who presented with left hemiparesis and numbness. **(A)** Sagittal T1-weighted image (T1WI), **(B)** sagittal T2-weighted image (T2WI), and **(C** and **D)** postcontrast T1WI show a large dura-based mass at the anterior and left lateral aspect of the foramen magnum with isointensity on T1WI and T2WI and strong enhancement after contrast injection. Note tumor encasement of left vertebral artery (*arrow*).

### Nerve sheath tumors

Nerve sheath tumors are the most common intradural extramedullary spinal tumors. Moreover, 70% of cases are intradural extramedullary, 15% are completely extradural, and 10% are transforaminal. Nerve sheath tumors of the CVJ include those arising from lower cranial nerves and those from upper cervical roots.[69] Most of them are schwannomas. They are the second most common nonosseous tumors of the CVJ. Schwannomas show markedly increased signal intensity on T2-weighted imaging and frequent central areas of hypointensity, which may represent denser areas of collagen and Schwann cells. These tumors usually show intense fairly homogeneous enhancement, except in areas of cystic degeneration or hemorrhage (Fig. 14.27). A solitary neurofibroma is difficult to distinguish from a schwannoma by imaging, but neurofibromas are more likely to show the target sign and less likely to have hemorrhage and cystic change than schwannomas.

### Congenital Cystic Lesions

Congenital cystic lesions of the CVJ include arachnoid, epidermoid, and neurenteric cysts. Arachnoid cysts are rare lesions in the CVJ. On MRI, the cysts have signal characteristics of CSF on all pulse sequences and may exert a mass effect on adjacent brain or bone. Epidermoid cysts are congenital lesions of ectodermal origin. The cysts grow by progressive desquamation of epithelial cells. The intradural lesions most commonly occupy the cistern of the cerebellopontine angle and,

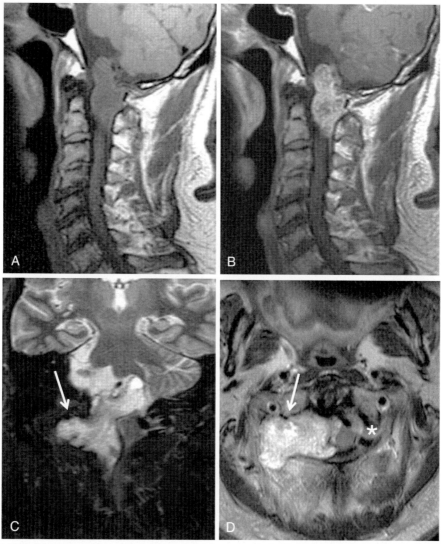

FIG. 14.27 A C1 neuroma in a 63-year-old man who presented with intermittent headache and progressive weakness in the four limbs. **(A** and **B)** Sagittal pre- and postcontrast T21-weighted images show a lobulated mass centered at the foramen magnum, with heterogeneous enhancement after contrast administration. **(C)** Coronal short-tau inversion recovery and **(D)** axial T2-weighted images show bright signal of the mass, which extends through the enlarged dural foramen (*arrow*) along the C1 root. On the opposite side is the normal dural entry of the vertebral artery and C1 root (*asterisk*).

less commonly, suprasellar areas, the middle cranial fossa, and the cisterna magnum. The lesions are lobulated in outline and slightly hyperintense to CSF on T1- and T2-weighted images. Diffusion-weighted imaging demonstrates restricted diffusion within epidermoid cysts, simplifying the diagnosis and aiding visualization. Neurenteric cysts are enteric-lined cysts within the spinal canal and usually exhibit spinal cord or vertebrae attachment. Most CVJ neurenteric cysts are located ventrally in the midline, anterior to the brainstem. Neurenteric cysts are usually isointense to hyperintense to CSF on T1-weighted images and show variable signal on T2-weighted images (usually hyperintense to CSF) and no enhancement after contrast injection.[70]

## VASCULAR LESIONS

This section discusses osseous-dural lesions, such as dural arteriovenous fistula (DAVF), and vertebral artery (VA) lesions, such as BHS, aneurysms, and vertebral artery arteriovenous fistula (VAVF), but does not discuss intraparenchymal lesions, such as arteriovenous malformation and arterial dissection.

### Bow Hunter Syndrome

BHS is a rare disorder resulting from mechanical occlusion or stenosis of VAs during head and neck rotation or extension. It is also known as rotational VA occlusion syndrome, for it is a mechanical occlusion of the vertebral artery that leads to a reduction in blood flow in the posterior cerebral circulation resulting in transient reversible symptomatic vertebrobasilar insufficiency. The exact incidence of BHS is still unknown. The underlying pathophysiology is dynamic stenosis (primary) or compression of the VA by abnormal bony structures (secondary) with neck rotation or extension. In the primary BHS the underlying pathogenesis is hemodynamic stress leading to endothelial damage and thromboembolic consequences. During head and neck rotation, the contralateral atlantoaxial joint rotates asymmetrically forward and downward.[71] This motion may lead to the lengthening of the VA, causing its thinning or occlusion.[72] And repetitive shear stress within the VA can damage its endothelial lining. At the atlantoaxial joint, the VA is relatively immobilized at the transverse foramen and the ponticulus posticus, thus making it prone to injury.[73,74]

In secondary BHS, stenosis or compression of the VA is caused by abnormal structures such as osteophytes, idiopathic skeletal hyperostosis, disc herniation, muscle hypertrophy, cervical spondylosis, tendinous bands, or tumors. Compression in BHS has been most commonly observed at or above the C2 level, so another classification divides BHS into atlantoaxial or subaxial types. In the atlantoaxial type, the VA is compressed or occluded by an ossified or thickened atlantooccipital membrane, a dural fold in the foramen magnum, an assimilated posterior ring of the atlas, an accessory ossicle behind the atlantoodontoid junction, erosive RA of C1-C2, C1-C2 facet hypertrophy, etc.[73,74]

There are still no diagnostic guidelines for BHS. Provocative DSA showing that the arteries are patent in the neutral position and stenotic with head rotation is the gold standard diagnostic method (Fig. 14.28). CT and MR can detect abnormal bony structures, infarction lesions, or stenotic arteries and are useful for individual management.

### Vertebral Artery Aneurysm at the Foramen Magnum

The huge saccular or fusiform aneurysms of the posterior circulation can manifest with varying neurologic signs that are the direct result of cranial nerve, cerebellum, or brainstem compression by these space-occupying lesions.[75,76] Such an aneurysm developing at the CVJ can compress the CVJ, causing "hemiplegia cruciata."[26] Occasionally, a giant aneurysm mimics a tumor and causes erosion of the adjacent foramen magnum (Fig. 14.29).

### Vertebral Artery Arteriovenous Fistula

A rare type of extradural arteriovenous fistula, the VAVF, is a simple or complex direct communication connecting the extracranial portion of the vertebral artery (truncal type) or one of its muscular or radicular branches (nontruncal type) to the neighboring venous plexus (epidural and paravertebral veins) most prominently at the C1-C2 and C6C7 levels. VAVFs occur spontaneously in association with connective tissue diseases, including fibromuscular dysplasia, neurofibromatosis, Ehlers-Danlos syndrome, and Marfan syndrome. In about 56%–68% of cases, VAVFs are secondary to posttraumatic and/or iatrogenic arteriovenous injury, and they can become symptomatic several weeks after an injury of known cause.

In a review of 47 cases reported by Kondoh et al.,[75] VAVFs were classified into three types based on their hemodynamic features (see Box 14.6).

In patients with type 1 VAVFs, 30% of patients are symptom-free, but the most common finding is pulsatile bruit over the neck with tinnitus. Type 2 and type 3 VAVFs can be associated with steal phenomenon and vertebrobasilar insufficiency resulting in transient ischemic attacks of diplopia, vertigo, and ataxia.[76] MRI may show an epidural flow void lesion in the CVJ region, extending from C2 to C8 level depending on the flow pattern. Differentiating this lesion from other vascular lesions depends on the results of catheter angiography (Fig. 14.30).

### Dural Arteriovenous Fistulas

DAVFs are shunts between the meningeal arteries and intracranial dural sinus, subarachnoid veins, or cortical veins. The incidence of DAVF is 0.16 per 100,000 persons per year in the adult population. According to an indirect comparison meta-analysis,[77] both CT and MRI had good diagnostic performance, but the performance of MRI was slightly better than that of CT ($P = .02$). Contrast medium use and time-resolved MR

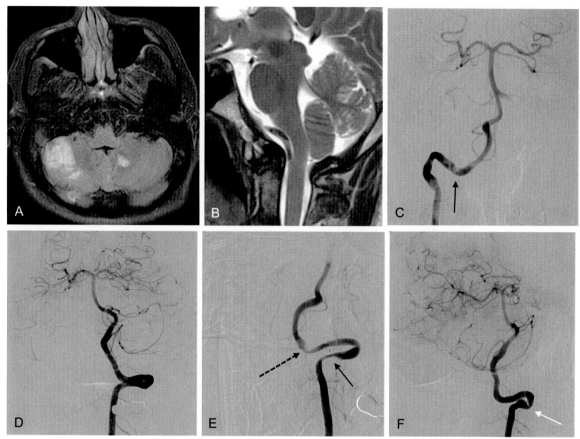

FIG. 14.28 A 28-year-old man with multiple episodic posterior circulation stroke was finally diagnosed with Bow Hunter syndrome. **(A)** Axial T2 fluid-attenuated inversion recovery shows multiple bright signals in bilateral cerebellum, thalamus, and occipital lobe (not shown). **(B)** Sagittal T2 shows atlas assimilation, Klippel-Feil anomaly in C2-3, and basilar invagination. Frontal views of right **(C)** and left **(D)** vertebral artery (VA) angiographies show abnormal pathway at the craniovertebral junction with mild stenosis at the right C1-2 level (*black arrow*). Right **(E)** and left **(F)** VA angiographies taken during left head turn depict two stenoses at the level of the right C1-2 (*black arrow*) and foramen magnum (*black dotted arrow*). Mild stenosis is noted at the left C1-2 level (*white arrow*).

angiography did not improve MRI diagnostic performance. A DAVF without cortical venous reflux usually has a benign course, but those with reflux into the cortical vein or perimedullary venous plexus are considered aggressive lesions because they might give rise to clinical features such as focal neurologic deficit, intracranial hemorrhage, myelopathy, or dementia. The CTA signs of cortical venous reflux include abnormal dilatation, early enhancement, and presence of a medullary or pial vein.[78] The MRI signs of corticovenous reflux include abnormal dilation, flow-related enhancement, cluster of flow void, early enhancement, and presence of a medullary or pial vein.[79,80] Two types of DAVFs at the

CVJ (the foramen magnum DAVF and anterior condylar DAVF) are discussed in detail.

### DAVF at the foramen magnum

Although foramen magnum DAVFs (Fig. 14.31) are rare, they have been associated with subarachnoid hemorrhage in 34%–45% of cases[81,82] and with the presence of varices of the draining veins and cephalad or intracranially directed venous drainage.[81] Most DAVFs at the foramen magnum are supplied by the vertebral artery or the occipital artery and ascending pharyngeal artery.[83] The complex anastomosis of the meningeal artery supply around the foramen magnum indicates

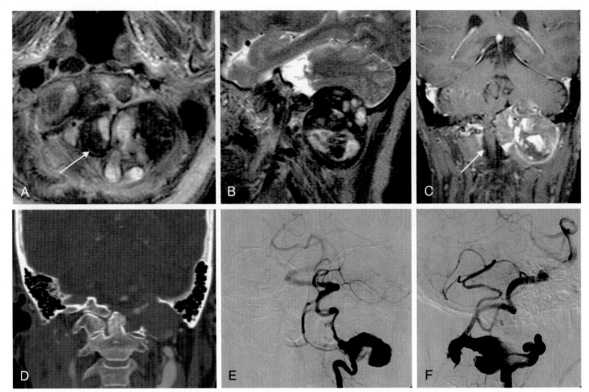

FIG. 14.29 A 60-year-old woman has left hemiparesis for 3 years. **(A)** Axial T2-weighted image (T2WI), **(B)** sagittal T2WI, and **(C)** coronal postcontrast T1-weighted image show enhancing mass lesion with mixed signal at the left craniovertebral junction with compression of the brainstem (*white arrow*). **(D)** Coronal CT depicts erosion of the left lateral mass of C1 and foramen magnum. **(E)** Frontal and **(F)** lateral views of left vertebral artery angiography show irregular, extraluminal contrast medium retention locally. Partial thrombotic aneurysm is diagnosed.

---

**BOX 14.6**
**Classification of Vertebral Artery Arteriovenous Fistula by Kondoh et al.**

Type 1 lesions receive retrograde flow from the parent vertebral artery.

Type 2 lesions receive retrograde flow from the contralateral vertebral artery.

Type 3 lesions are supplied from the contralateral vertebral artery and concurrent steal from the internal carotid arteries via basilar artery retrograde flow into the parent vertebral artery.

---

that treatment by direct microsurgery interruption of the arterialized venous circulation may be preferable to arterial embolization. The venous drainage pattern is the most important factor that influences the clinical presentation.[83]

### Anterior condylar DAVF (hypoglossal-clival DAVF)

In a review of 14 anterior condylar DAVFs treated successfully by intravascular coiling,[84] all the coils were found at the anterior condylar veins inside the hypoglossal canal, 54.2% at the lateral lower clivus, and only 14.2% at the anterior condylar confluence, which is ventrolateral to the anterior orifice of the hypoglossal canal. Anterior condylar DAVF involves mainly the epidural space and the adjacent osseous structures (clivus). Usually, anterior condylar veins have no primary role in the drainage of the central nervous system, but reflux to the cavernous sinus can occur once the venous outlet to the internal jugular vein is obstructed. In such a scenario, the patient might have a clinical presentation mimicking the carotid-cavernous fistula. It is difficult to detect the signal change in routine T1- and T2-weighted images, but the fast flow has a bright signal intensity on MRA, highlighting the lesion well (Fig. 14.32).

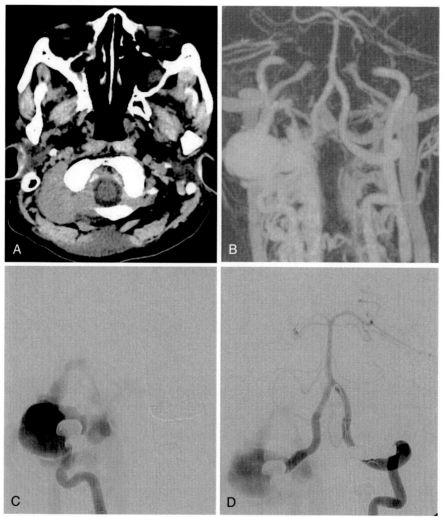

FIG. 14.30  A 34-year-old woman has a pulsatile mass in her right neck for years and it has progressed recently. **(A)** Axial CT shows a well-defined soft tissue mass at the level of C1-2 with intra- and extraspinal involvement. **(B)** Coronal reconstruction CT depicts abnormal vascular tuft with early venous shunting. **(C)** Right vertebral artery (VA) frontal view shows large vertebral artery arteriovenous fistula at the C1-2 level with complete steal. **(D)** Left VA frontal view shows a type 2 lesion.

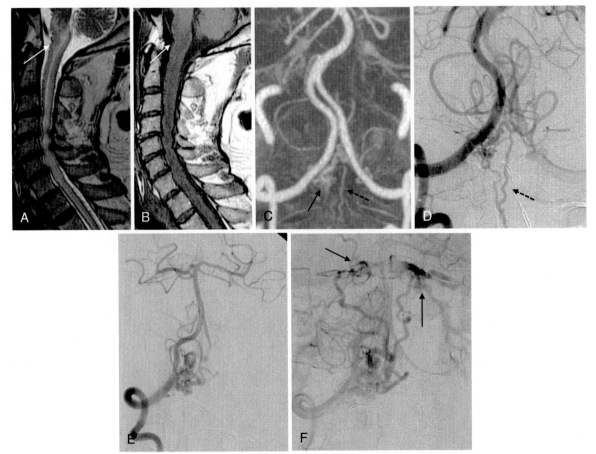

FIG. 14.31 A 68-year-old man **(A–D)** with exophthalmos and sudden onset of headache, nausea, and vomiting. **(A)** Sagittal T2-weighted and **(B)** postcontrast T1-weighted images show serpentine vascularity on the pial surface of lower medulla and upper cervical cord (*white arrows*). The cord is edematous and enlarged. **(C)** Coronal maximum intensity projection view of CT angiography shows abnormal vasculature (*black arrow*) at the foramen magnum with prominent venous drainage to the perimedullary veins (*black dotted arrows*), and dural arteriovenous fistula (DAVF) is confirmed by VA angiography **(D)**. Another patient with DAVF at the foramen magnum **(E)** with drainage upward to cavernous sinuses (**F**, *black arrows*).

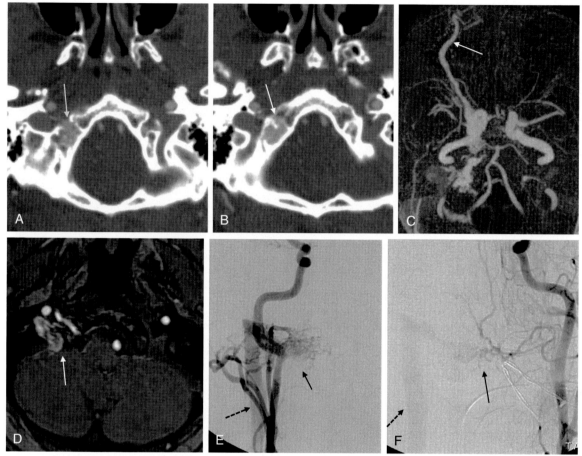

FIG. 14.32 A 43-year-old man **(A–C)** has right exophthalmos, chemosis, and vascular tinnitus for 3 months. **(A and B)** Axial CT angiography source images show abnormal enhancement in the right hypoglossal canal and basiocciput (*white arrows*). **(C)** Collapsed maximum intensity projection view shows abnormal contrast enhancement in the right hypoglossal canal extending to the cavernous sinus and the dilated superior ophthalmic vein (*white arrow*). A 50-year-old woman has vascular tinnitus for years. **(D)** MR angiography source image depicts high signal in the hypoglossal canal (*white arrow*) and adjacent bones. **(E)** Right and **(F)** left common carotid artery angiography shows dural arteriovenous fistula at the right hypoglossal canal with early drainage to the right internal jugular vein (*black dotted arrow*) supplied by bilateral ascending pharyngeal arteries (*black arrows*).

## REFERENCES

1. Chen YF, Liu HM. Imaging of craniovertebral junction. *Neuroimaging Clin N Am.* 2009;19(3):483–510.
2. Goel A. Basilar invagination, Chiari malformation, syringomyelia: a review. *Neurol India.* 2009;57(3):235–246.
3. Menezes AH. Evaluation and treatment of congenital and developmental anomalies of the cervical spine. *J Neurosurg.* 2004;2:188–197.
4. Bernini FP, Elefante R, Smaltino F, et al. Angiographic study on the vertebral artery in cases of deformities of the occipitocervical joint. *AJR Am J Roentgenol.* 1969;107:526–529.
5. Rao PV. Median (third) occipital condyle. *Clin Anat.* 2002;15(2):148–151.
6. Gehweiler J, Daffner R, Roberts LJ. Malformations of the atlas vertebra simulating the Jefferson fracture. *AJR Am J Roentgenol.* 1983;149:1083–1086.
7. Vakili ST, Aguilar JC, Muller J. Sudden unexpected death associated with atlanto-occipital fusion. *Am J Forensic Med Pathol.* 1985;6:39–43.
8. Menezes AH. Primary craniovertebral anomalies and the hindbrain herniation syndrome (Chiari I): data base analysis. *Pediatr Neurosurg.* 1995;23:260–269.
9. Taggard DA, Menezes AH, Ryken TC. Instability of the craniovertebral junction and treatment outcomes in patients with Down's syndrome. *Neurosurg Focus.* 1999;6(6). Article 3.

10. Gehweiler JA, Daffner RH, Robert SL. Malformations of the atlas vertebra simulating the Jefferson fracture. *AJNR Am J Neuroradiol.* 1983;4:187–190.

11. Dome HL, Just N, Lander PH. CT recognition of anomalies of the posterior arch of the atlas vertebra: differentiation from fracture. *AJNR Am J Neuroradiol.* 1986;7:176–177.

12. Schilling J, Schilling A, Suazo GI. Ponticulus posticus on the posterior arch of atlas, prevalence analysis in asymptomatic patients. *Int J Morphol.* 2010;28(1):317–322.

13. Chitroda PK, Katti G, Baba IA, et al. Ponticulus posticus on the posterior arch of atlas, prevalence analysis in symptomatic and asymptomatic patients of Gulbarga population. *J Clin Diagn Res.* 2013;7(12):3044–3047.

14. Gillman EL. Congenital absence of the odontoid process of the axis: report of a case. *J Bone Jt Surg Am.* 1959;41:345–348.

15. Anderson LD, D'Alonzo RT. Fracture of the odontoid process of the axis. *J Bone Jt Surg Am.* 1974;56:1663–1674.

16. Shirasaki N, Okada K, Oka S, et al. Os odontoideum with posterior atlantoaxial instability. *Spine.* 1992;16:706–715.

17. Winkler-Schwartz A, Correa JA, Marcoux J. Clival fractures in a level I trauma center. *J Neurosurg.* 2015;122:227–235.

18. Menku A, Koc RK, Tucer B, et al. Clivus fractures: clinical presentations and courses. *Neurosurg Rev.* 2004;27(3):194–198.

19. Hanson JA, Deliganis AV, Baxter AB, et al. Radiologic and clinical spectrum of occipital condyle fractures: retrospective review of 107 consecutive fractures in 95 patients. *AJR Am J Roentgenol.* 2002;178:1261–1268.

20. Mead II LB, Millhouse PW, Krystal J, et al. C1 fractures: a review of diagnoses, management options, and outcomes. *Curr Rev Musculoskelet Med.* 2016;9:255–262.

21. Elliott RE, Tanweer O, Smith ML, et al. Outcomes of fusion for lateral atlantoaxial osteoarthritis: meta-analysis and review of literature. *World Neurosurg.* 2013;80:e337–e346.

22. Grob D, Luca A, Mannion AF. An observational study of patient-rated outcome after atlantoaxial fusion in patients with rheumatoid arthritis and osteoarthritis. *Clin Orthop Relat Res.* 2011;469:702–707.

23. Zapletal J, de Valois JC. Radiologic prevalence of advanced lateral C1-C2 osteoarthritis. *Spine.* 1997;22:2511–2513.

24. Betsch MW, Blizzard SR, Shinseki MS, et al. Prevalence of degenerative changes of the atlanto-axial joints. *Spine J.* 2015;15:275–280.

25. Raza A, Islam M, Lakshmanan P. Secondary atlanto-odontoid osteoarthritis with osteoradionecrosis of upper cervical spine mimicking metastasis. *BMJ Case Rep.* 2013:2013.

26. Halla JT, Hardin Jr JG. Atlantoaxial (C1-C2) facet joint osteoarthritis: a distinctive clinical syndrome. *Arthritis Rheum.* 1987;30:577–582.

27. Guha D, Mohanty C, Tator CH, et al. Occipital neuralgia secondary to unilateral atlantoaxial osteoarthritis: case report and review of the literature. *Surg Neurol Int.* 2015;6:186.

28. Genez BM, Willis JJ, Lowrey CE, et al. CT findings of degenerative arthritis of the atlantoodontoid joint. *AJR Am J Roentgenol.* 1990;154:315–318.

29. Goel A, Shah A, Gupta SR. Craniovertebral instability due to degenerative osteoarthritis of the atlantoaxial joints: analysis of the management of 108 cases. *J Neurosurg Spine.* 2010;12:592–601.

30. Kwon JW, Choi JA, Kwack KS, et al. Myxoid chondrosarcoma in the calcaneus: a case report with MR imaging findings. *Skelet Radiol.* 2007;36(suppl 1):S82–S85.

31. Seo GS, Aoki J, Fujioka F, et al. MR appearance of periosteal chondrosarcoma of the foot. *J Comput Assist Tomogr.* 1995;19:106–110.

32. Bourgouin PM, Tampieri D, Robitaille Y, et al. Low-grade myxoid chondrosarcoma of the base of the skull: CT, MR, and histopathology. *J Comput Assist Tomogr.* 1992;16:268–273.

33. Kondziolka D, Lunsford LD, Flickinger JC. The role of radiosurgery in the management of chordoma and chondrosarcoma of the cranial base. *Neurosurgery.* 1991;29:38–45. Discussion 45–36.

34. Resnick D, Guerra Jr J, Robinson CA, et al. Association of diffuse idiopathic skeletal hyperostosis (DISH) and calcification and ossification of the posterior longitudinal ligament. *AJR Am J Roentgenol.* 1978;131:1049–1053.

35. Verlaan JJ, Boswijk PF, de Ru JA, et al. Diffuse idiopathic skeletal hyperostosis of the cervical spine: an underestimated cause of dysphagia and airway obstruction. *Spine J.* 2011;11:1058–1067.

36. Jun BY, Yoon KJ, Crockard A. Retro-odontoid pseudotumor in diffuse idiopathic skeletal hyperostosis. *Spine.* 2002;27:E266–E270.

37. Larsson EM, Holtas S, Zygmunt S. Pre- and postoperative MR imaging of the craniocervical junction in rheumatoid arthritis. *AJR Am J Roentgenol.* 1989;152:561–566.

38. Tanaka S, Nakada M, Hayashi Y, et al. Retro-odontoid pseudotumor without atlantoaxial subluxation. *J Clin Neurosci.* 2010;17:649–652.

39. Goel A. Retro-odontoid mass: an evidence of craniovertebral instability. *J Craniovertebr Junction Spine.* 2015;6:6–7.

40. Sze G, Brant-Zawadzki MN, Wilson CR, et al. Pseudotumor of the craniovertebral junction associated with chronic subluxation: MR imaging studies. *Radiology.* 1986;161:391–394.

41. Goel A, Phalke U, Cacciola F, et al. Atlantoaxial instability and retroodontoid mass–two case reports. *Neurol Med Chir.* 2004;44:603–606.

42. Barbagallo GM, Certo F, Visocchi M, et al. Disappearance of degenerative, non-inflammatory, retro-odontoid pseudotumor following posterior C1-C2 fixation: case series and review of the literature. *Eur Spine J.* 2013;22(suppl 6). S879–S888.23.

43. Yamaguchi I, Shibuya S, Arima N, et al. Remarkable reduction or disappearance of retroodontoid pseudotumors after occipitocervical fusion. Report of three cases. *J Neurosurg Spine.* 2006;5:156–160.

44. Sekijima Y, Yoshida T, Ikeda S. CPPD crystal deposition disease of the cervical spine: a common cause of acute neck pain encountered in the neurology department. *J Neurol Sci.* 2010;296:79–82.

45. Yoo HJ, Hong SH, Choi JY, et al. Differentiating high-grade from low-grade chondrosarcoma with MR imaging. *Eur Radiol.* 2009;19:3008–3014.

46. Vignes JR, Eimer S, Dupuy R, et al. Beta(2)-microglobulin amyloidosis caused spinal cord compression in a long-term haemodialysis patient. *Spinal Cord.* 2007;45:322–326.

47. Moonis G, Savolaine ER, Anvar SA, et al. MRI findings of isolated beta-2 microglobulin amyloidosis presenting as a cervical spine mass. Case report and review of literature. *Clin Imaging.* 1999;23:11–14.

48. Byers PD. A study of histological features distinguishing chordoma from chondrosarcoma. *Br J Cancer.* 1981;43:229–232.

49. O'Brien MF, Casey AT, Crockard A, et al. Histology of the craniocervical junction in chronic rheumatoid arthritis: a clinicopathologic analysis of 33 operative cases. *Spine.* 2002;27:2245–2254.

50. Takeshima Y, Matsuda R, Hironaka Y, et al. Rheumatoid arthritis-induced lateral atlantoaxial subluxation with multiple vertebrobasilar infarctions. *Spine.* 2015;40:E186–E189.

51. Lee HS, Kim TH, Yun HR, et al. Radiologic changes of cervical spine in ankylosing spondylitis. *Clin Rheumatol.* 2001;20:262–266.

52. Lee JS, Lee S, Bang SY, et al. Prevalence and risk factors of anterior atlantoaxial subluxation in ankylosing spondylitis. *J Rheumatol.* 2012;39:2321–2326.

53. Albert GW, Menezes AH. Ankylosing spondylitis of the craniovertebral junction: a single surgeon's experience. *J Neurosurg Spine.* 2011;14:429–436.

54. Becker GW, Battersby RD. Spinal neurenteric cyst presenting as recurrent midline sebaceous cysts. *Ann R Coll Surg Engl.* 2005;87:W1–W4.

55. Owosho AA, Tsai CJ, Lee RS, et al. The prevalence and risk factors associated with osteoradionecrosis of the jaw in oral and oropharyngeal cancer patients treated with intensity-modulated radiation therapy (IMRT): the Memorial Sloan Kettering Cancer Center experience. *Oral Oncol.* 2017;64:44–51.

56. Chatterjee S, Das A. Craniovertebral tuberculosis in children: experience of 23 cases and proposal for a new classification. *Childs Nerv Syst.* 2015;31:1341–1345.

57. Marx RE. Osteoradionecrosis: a new concept of its pathophysiology. *J Oral Maxillofac Surg.* 1983;41:283–288.

58. Wu LA, Liu HM, Wang CW, et al. Osteoradionecrosis of the upper cervical spine after radiation therapy for head and neck cancer: differentiation from recurrent or metastatic disease with MR imaging. *Radiology.* 2012;264:136–145.

59. Erdem E, Angtuaco EC, Van Hemert R, et al. Comprehensive review of intracranial chordoma. *Radiographics.* 2003;23:995–1009.

60. Yeom KW, Lober RM, Mobley BC, et al. Diffusion-weighted MRI: distinction of skull base chordoma from chondrosarcoma. *AJNR Am J Neuroradiol.* 2013;34:1056–1061. S1051.

61. Muller U, Kubik-Huch RA, Ares C, et al. Is there a role for conventional MRI and MR diffusion-weighted imaging for distinction of skull base chordoma and chondrosarcoma? *Acta Radiol.* 2016;57:225–232.

62. Adada B, Al-Mefty O. Fibrous dysplasia of the clivus. *Neurosurgery.* 2003;52:318–322. Discussion 323.

63. Chakrapani SD, Grim K, Kaimaktchiev V, et al. Osteoblastoma of the spine with discordant magnetic resonance imaging and computed tomography imaging features in a child. *Spine.* 2008;33:E968–E970.

64. Novais EN, Rose PS, Yaszemski MJ, et al. Aneurysmal bone cyst of the cervical spine in children. *J Bone Jt Surg Am.* 2011;93:1534–1543.

65. Wein RO, Popat SR, Doerr TD, et al. Plasma cell tumors of the skull base: four case reports and literature review. *Skull Base.* 2002;12:77–86.

66. Kano T, Kawase T, Horiguchi T, et al. Meningiomas of the ventral foramen magnum and lower clivus: factors influencing surgical morbidity, the extent of tumour resection, and tumour recurrence. *Acta Neurochir.* 2010;152:79–86. Discussion 86.

67. Talacchi A, Biroli A, Soda C, et al. Surgical management of ventral and ventrolateral foramen magnum meningiomas: report on a 64-case series and review of the literature. *Neurosurg Rev.* 2012;35:359–367. Discussion 367–358.

68. Starke RM, Nguyen JH, Reames DL, et al. Gamma knife radiosurgery of meningiomas involving the foramen magnum. *J Craniovertebr Junction Spine.* 2010;1:23–28.

69. George B, Lot G. Neurinomas of the first two cervical nerve roots: a series of 42 cases. *J Neurosurg.* 1995;82:917–923.

70. Preece MT, Osborn AG, Chin SS, et al. Intracranial neurenteric cysts: imaging and pathology spectrum. *AJNR Am J Neuroradiol.* 2006;27:1211–1216.

71. Toole JF, Tucker SH. Influence of head position upon cerebral circulation. Studies on blood flow in cadavers. *Arch Neurol.* 1960;2:616–623.

72. Barton JW, Margolis MT. Rotational obstructions of the vertebral artery at the atlantoaxial joint. *Neuroradiology.* 1975;9:117–120.

73. Rastogi V, Rawls A, Moore O, et al. Rare etiology of bow hunter's syndrome and systematic review of literature. *J Vasc Interv Neurol.* 2015;8:7–16.

74. Duan G, Xu J, Shi J, et al. Advances in the pathogenesis, diagnosis and treatment of bow hunter's syndrome: a comprehensive review of the literature. *Interv Neurol.* 2016;5:29–38.

75. Kondoh T, Tamaki N, Takeda N, et al. Fatal intracranial hemorrhage after balloon occlusion of an extracranial vertebral arteriovenous fistula. Case report. *J Neurosurg.* 1988;69:945–948.

76. Panagiotopoulos VE, Zampakis PE, Konstantinou DT, et al. Selective endovascular occlusion of a high-flow cervical direct vertebro-vertebral arteriovenous fistula maintaining vertebral artery patency. *EJMINT Tech Note.* 2014:1438000174.

77. Lin YH, Lin HH, Liu HM, et al. Diagnostic performance of CT and MRI on the detection of symptomatic intracranial dural arteriovenous fistula: a meta-analysis with indirect comparison. *Neuroradiology.* 2016;58(8):753–763.

78. Lee CW, Huang A, Wang YH, et al. Intracranial dural arteriovenous fistulas: diagnosis and evaluation with 64-detector row CT angiography. *Radiology.* 2010;256:219–228.

79. Willinsky R, Goyal M, terBrugge K, et al. Tortuous, engorged pial veins in intracranial dural arteriovenous fistulas: correlations with presentation, location, and MR findings in 122 patients. *AJNR Am J Neuroradiol.* 1999;20:1031–1036.

80. Kwon BJ, Han MH, Kang HS, et al. MR imaging findings of intracranial dural arteriovenous fistulas: relations with venous drainage patterns. *AJNR Am J Neuroradiol.* 2005;26:2500–2507.

81. Aviv RI, Shad A, Tomlinson G, et al. Cervical dural arteriovenous fistulae manifesting as subarachnoid hemorrhage: report of two cases and literature review. *AJNR Am J Neuroradiol.* 2004;25:854–858.

82. Kai Y, Hamada J, Morioka M, et al. Arteriovenous fistulas at the cervicomedullary junction presenting with subarachnoid hemorrhage: six case reports with special reference to the angiographic pattern of venous drainage. *AJNR Am J Neuroradiol.* 2005;26:1949–1954.

83. Takami T, Ohata K, Nishio A, et al. Microsurgical interruption of dural arteriovenous fistula at the foramen magnum. *J Clin Neurosci.* 2005;12:580–583.

84. Hsu YH, Lee CW, Liu HM, et al. Endovascular treatment and computed imaging follow-up of 14 anterior condylar dural arteriovenous fistulas. *Interv Neuroradiol.* 2014;20:368–377.

# CHAPTER 15

# Skull Base Bone Lesions I: Imaging Technique, Developmental and Diffuse Bone Lesions

ALEXANDRA BORGES, MD

## INTRODUCTION

The skull base is a bony-cartilaginous structure, oriented in the axial plane, providing a barrier between the intracranial compartment and the extracranial head and neck. It is pierced by several neurovascular foramina, which provide a crossroad for disease to spread between these two compartments.[1] Most tumors affecting the skull base have their origin outside the skull base proper, mainly from the suprahyoid neck, and secondarily affect the skull base by direct or perineural extent. Primary and secondary bone tumors tend to be forgotten. The skull base division into anterior, central, and posterior, so useful in the differential diagnosis of extrinsic skull base lesions, does not apply when lesions originate from the fibrocartilaginous elements of the skull base proper as they are common to all skull base compartments.[1] Therefore, when facing a lesion arising from bone the same rules for the differential diagnosis of bone lesions seen elsewhere in the body should be applied.

Except for metastases, bone tumors of the skull base are overall rare and often a diagnostic dilemma. Benign tumors and bone dysplasias can behave aggressively, and some malignant tumors can look misleadingly benign.[2] Although imaging features can be quite helpful in the differential diagnosis, they are not very familiar to radiologists who do not routinely deal with skull base lesions and only a scant specific literature is available on this subject. Moreover, secondary/metastatic tumors account for the majority of bony skull base lesions, with primary skull base bone tumors being rather rare. To simplify the approach, it is useful to divide bone lesions of the skull base into three major groups: those related to developmental anomalies and embryonic remnants, primary and secondary

bone tumors, and diffuse or multifocal bone lesions (Table 15.1).

This chapter reviews the imaging technique and focuses on developmental lesions originating from embryonic remnants trapped within the skull base during embryonic development and diffuse bone lesions, including bone dysplasias and infection; the following chapter addresses primary and secondary bone tumors.

## IMAGING TECHNIQUE

Imaging of bone lesions in the skull base obeys the same principles applied to bone lesions elsewhere. To the exception of plain radiographs, which, in most centers, are no longer performed to investigate the skull base, and ultrasound imaging, with obvious limitations in the assessment of this anatomic region, the same imaging techniques (CT, MRI, bone scintigraphy, and fludeoxyglucose [FDG]-PET CT) are routinely used for diagnosing, staging, and follow-up of patients with skull base bone lesions.[3] Volumetric CT acquisition parallel to the skull base with axial, coronal, and sagittal thin, millimetric, reconstructions on both soft tissue and high-resolution bone algorithm should be obtained. Contrast-enhanced imaging is performed to assess the pattern of vascularization of a given lesion, as well as to determine its relationship with major adjacent vessels and assess their patency.[3] It provides a map of the bony anatomy, required for surgical planning, and allows three-dimensional (3D) reconstructions to help planning skull base reconstruction or grafting on the basis of 3D modeling and 3D printing. CT is the imaging technique with the highest sensitivity to depict calcification and ossification, critical in the assessment of bone or cartilage matrix-producing tumors and in depicting different types of

**TABLE 15.1**
**Skull Base Bone Lesions**

### DEVELOPMENTAL/EMBRYONIC REMNANTS

| | |
|---|---|
| Developmental | Arrested pneumatization of the sphenoid sinus |
| | Giant arachnoid granulations/arachnoidoceles |
| | Sphenoid wing dysplasia |
| | Petrous apex cephaloceles |
| | Basal cephaloceles |

Embryonic remnants

| | |
|---|---|
| Ectodermal | Epidermoid/dermoid cysts |
| Meningothelial | Arachnoid granulations |
| | Intradiploic arachnoid cysts |
| | Intradiploic/en plaque meningiomas |
| Notochord | Ecchordosis physalifora |
| | Chordoma |
| Pharyngohypophyseal canal | Persistent craniopharyngeal canal |
| | Rhatke pouch cyst |
| | Craniopharyngioma |
| | Intraosseous pituitary adenoma |

### BONE TUMORS

Primary

| | |
|---|---|
| Benign | Osteoma |
| | Osteoid osteoma |
| | Osteoblastoma |
| | Ossifying fibroma |
| | Enchondroma/osteochondroma |
| | Chondroblastoma |

| | |
|---|---|
| | Chondromyxoid fibroma |
| | Intraosseous hemangioma |
| | Aneurysmal bone cyst |
| | Giant cell tumor/osteoclastoma |
| | Brown tumor |
| | Eosinophilic granuloma |
| Malignant | Metastasis |
| | Plasmacytoma/multiple myeloma |
| | Lymphoma |
| | Chloroma/granulocytic sarcoma |
| | Ewing sarcoma |
| | Osteosarcoma |
| | Chondrosarcoma |

Secondary

| | |
|---|---|
| | Metastasis |
| | Lymphoma |
| | Leukemia (chloroma) |

### DIFFUSE BONE LESIONS

| |
|---|
| Fibrous dysplasia |
| Paget disease |
| Osteopetrosis |
| Osteopoikilosis |
| Melorheostosis |
| Infection (skull base osteomyelitis) |

### MULTIFOCAL BONE LESIONS

| |
|---|
| Metastases |
| Multiple myeloma |
| Brown tumors |
| Eosinophilic granulomas |

periosteal reaction.[4] The pattern of bone involvement and the evaluation of the transition zone, between tumor and normal bone, are also best depicted on CT. Still, for some authors, CT remains the most accurate technique in the diagnosis of fibroosseous lesions, which may show misleading imaging findings on other techniques, such as MR and bone scintigraphy. Moreover, as most bone lesions heal by ossification and sclerosis, CT is very useful to assess tumor response to treatment.[4]

MRI is the modality of choice to evaluate the full extent of a bone tumor, including the extent of bone marrow involvement, presence of soft tissue components, meningeal and intracranial extent, involvement of cranial nerves and vessels, and relationship with adjacent soft tissues of the supra-hyoid neck. T1-weighted (T1W) images show clearly abnormal replacement of the fatty bone marrow, whereas T2-weighted (T2W) and short-tau inversion recovery (STIR) images clearly depict tumor matrix and any associated bone marrow edema. Contrast-enhanced fat-suppressed T1W images evaluate tumor enhancement and can clearly differentiate enhancing lesions from the surrounding fatty marrow.[5] MR is also used to assess tumor response to chemo and radiation treatment by differentiating necrosis from viable tumor. This information can be derived from contrast-enhanced fat-suppressed T1W images, diffusion-weighted images (DWI), and dynamic contrast-enhanced perfusion-weighted images (DCE-PWI). DWI is very useful to support the diagnosis of small round cell tumors that tend to show low mean apparent diffusion coefficient (ADC) values and to differentiate bone malignancies from infection. Moreover, in the case of skull base osteomyelitis, it is routinely used to depict complications such as abscesses or subdural empyema, also featured by restricted diffusion.[3] Whole-body DWI can depict diffuse and multifocal abnormalities and is being increasingly used for staging multiple myeloma and metastatic bone disease.[6] MR angiography (MRA) and MR venography (MRV) may be required to assess the patency of any adjacent arteries and rule out dural sinus invasion or thrombosis, respectively. Bone scintigraphy using $^{99m}$Tc-MDP (methylene diphosphonate) and $^{18}$F-NaF PET-CT are very sensitive techniques in the detection of osteoblastic activity, whereas $^{18}$FDG-PET depicts tissues with high glucose metabolic rates.[7,8] These functional techniques have the advantage of imaging the entire skeleton and therefore are useful to detect diffuse and multiple lesions. $^{67}$Ga-single-photon emission CT (SPECT) and $^{99m}$Tc MDP-triphasic SPECT should be the choice for the early diagnosis and to monitor treatment response in patients with skull base osteomyelitis.[9,10]

Bone scans can be used to depict bone-forming tumors, including osteogenic primary tumors and sclerotic metastasis, as well as any bone healing process. Tumors causing rapid bone destruction with no compensatory bone formation are missed by this technique, with the most striking examples being multiple myeloma and bone metastases from thyroid cancer.[11] The flare phenomenon, a diffuse increase in $^{99m}$Tc-MDP uptake after treatment of bone metastases persisting until 6 months after treatment, is a well-known limitation in the assessment of tumor response and should not be mistaken for disease progression.[3]

Imaging is also widely used to direct biopsies to relevant tumor areas avoiding cystic/necrotic regions. In skull base lesions, most biopsies are performed endoscopically.[12]

## GENERAL IMAGING FEATURES OF BONE LESIONS HELPFUL IN THE DIFFERENTIAL DIAGNOSIS

Although, in most cases, the final diagnosis of a bone lesion requires a biopsy specimen, there are several lesions in which a biopsy may be misleading without appropriate radiologic-pathologic correlation. Well-known examples are fibroosseous lesions, such as fibrous dysplasia, often mistaken on pathology for a sarcoma.[13] Therefore, imaging plays an essential role in the diagnosis and further management of patients, particularly in an anatomic area occult to clinical inspection. Most general imaging features of bone tumors in the remainder of the skeletal system apply to the skull base, and one should bear in mind that the skull base is composed of flat bones originating from endochondral ossification.

One of the most important epidemiologic factors affecting the differential diagnosis of a bone tumor is age, with several tumors occurring only before the closure of growth plates and others showing specific incidence patterns.[14] Clinical presentation and setting can also be helpful: in a patient with a known primary cancer and a skull base lesion, a bone metastasis should be high on the differential list, whereas in an immunocompromised patient with a sinonasal or temporal bone infection, skull base osteomyelitis should be highly considered. Symptoms from bone lesions of the skull base are nonspecific and include headache, cranial nerve' dysfunction, sinonasal obstruction, and proptosis, just to mention the most common.[15]

The general patterns of bone lesions apply to the skull base and help limit the differential diagnosis. Bone lesions can be lytic, characterized by bone destruction or replacement; sclerotic, featured mainly by bone production with ossified or calcified matrix; or mixed, showing elements of both bone destruction and bone formation. Although single, focal lesions suggest a primary benign or malignant bone tumor, diffuse bone involvement is most often seen in fibroosseous dysplasias, Paget disease, renal osteodystrophy, metastatic bone involvement, infection, and lymphoma.[14] The presence of multiple focal bone lesions shortens the differential diagnosis to metastatic bone disease, multiple myeloma, Langerhans cell histiocytosis in pediatric age, brown tumors associated with hyperparathyroidism, and developmental/syndromic lesions such as multiple osteomas or enchondromas associated with osteopoikilosis, melorheostosis, and Maffuci and Ollier syndromes.[14] Patterns of tumor growth and their transition to normal adjacent bone correlate with tumor aggressiveness, with most benign lesions leading to bone expansion and remodeling with a sharp, geographic transition to normal adjacent bone and most malignant lesions showing a moth-eaten, permeative, or destructive pattern with cortical disruption, ill-defined borders, and a wide transition zone. The pattern of periosteal reaction is also useful to differentiate benign slow-growing tumors from aggressive, rapidly growing tumors. The former usually show a thick, laminated, onion-skin pattern of periosteal reaction, whereas the latter show periosteal rupture (Codman triangle), air-on-end, or a spiculated, sunburst pattern.[14,16,17] Tumors are further classified into bone forming, containing more or less mineralized osteoid matrix, which can show a ground-glass pattern in the case of fibroosseous lesions; cartilage producing, which often show a calcified matrix, containing chondroid-like calcifications; or neither bone nor cartilage forming, such as hematopoietic, vascular, fibrous, or giant-cell-related tumors.[17]

## Developmental Bone Lesions of the Skull Base

Developmental skull base lesions include arrested pneumatization of the skull base, giant and aberrant arachnoid granulations, sphenoid wing dysplasia, and basal cephaloceles.

**Arrested pneumatization of the skull base** is a common developmental variant. Right before the pneumatization of craniofacial bones, during the development of the sinonasal and otomastoid cavities, there is a conversion of the hematopoietic red bone marrow into fatty yellow marrow.[18] If pneumatization arrests, a lytic, nonexpansive area with fat density/signal intensity, with lobulated sclerotic borders and occasional calcifications, ensues and can be easily mistaken for a pathologic lesion. Frequent locations in the skull base are the clivus and greater sphenoid wing[19] (Fig. 15.1).

**Giant, aberrant arachnoid granulations or arachnoidoceles** are another common developmental anomaly seen in the skull base. Arachnoid or Pacchioni granulations are normal projections of arachnoid villi through the dura mater into the dural sinuses that allow cerebrospinal fluid (CSF) flow into the venous system. When over 10 mm in size, they are called giant and are responsible for irregularly shaped lytic lesions, often seen in and around dural venous sinuses, close to penetrating cortical veins. They show as filling defects on postcontrast CT and/or MR images and can mimic dural sinus thrombosis.[20] When these granulations fail to migrate into the venous sinuses, they are called

aberrant arachnoid granulations or arachnoidoceles and are most often seen in the floor of the middle cranial fossa and posterior aspect of the temporal bone.[21] These granulations contain trapped CSF, which does not communicate with the venous system, and may enlarge over time as a result of chronic transmission of CSF pulsations, leading to slowly growing lytic defects with sclerotic margins that follow CSF density/signal intensity on CT/MRI and may show faint enhancement of the adjacent dura[21] (Fig. 15.2). Adjacent bone erosion may ensue with secondary herniation of these giant granulations into the paranasal sinuses, temporal bone, or orbit, shown on imaging as meningeal outpouchings or pseudomeningoceles (Fig. 15.3). Although they are usually asymptomatic incidental findings, CSF leaks are a potential complication of these developmental lesions.[22] Aberrant arachnoid granulations can potentially be confused with other lytic skull base lesions on CT. On MRI, however, the diagnosis is usually straightforward, as the lesion follows the signal intensity of CSF in all pulse sequences and does not enhance. A signal intensity slightly above that of CSF on proton density weighted (PDW) and fluid-attenuated inversion recovery (FLAIR) images can be seen and reflects a slight increase in protein concentration inside the trapped fluid.

**Sphenoid wing dysplasia** is a developmental condition that can occur as an isolated finding or as a feature of neurofibromatosis type 1 (NF1) and is one of the six diagnostic criteria for this disease.[23] In isolated cases, it seems to result from defective ossification of the sphenoid bone, whereas in patients with NF1 it may be progressive and secondary to an underlying plexiform neurofibroma.[24] It can be asymptomatic or present clinically as pulsatile exophthalmos, enophthalmos, visual impairment, diplopia, or conjunctivitis. On imaging, it is featured by partial

Arrested pneumatization of the sphenoid sinus

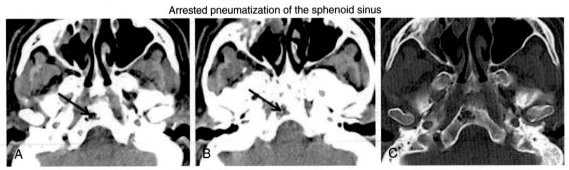

FIG. 15.1 CT section through the skull base on soft tissue (**A** and **B**) and bone (**C**) windows show a discrete lytic lesion, with a lobulated contour and thin sclerotic margin in the right lateral aspect of the clivus. The lesion shows fat density (*arrow* in **A** and **B**) and a few speckled calcifications. These features strongly suggest arrested pneumatization of the sphenoid sinus.

Clival arachnoidocele

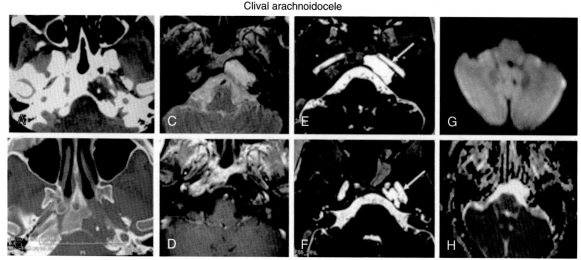

FIG. 15.2 CT of the skull base on soft tissue **(A)** and bone windows **(B)** demonstrates a lytic lesion with lobulated contour in the left petroclival region (*asterisk* in **A** and **B**) showing fluid-like density and without marginal sclerosis. On MRI, **(C)** axial T2-weighted, **(D)** contrast-enhanced T1-weighted, **(E** and **F)** constructive interference in steady state (CISS) and diffusion-weighted imaging (DWI), b1000 **(G)**, and ADC **(H)**, the lesion follows the signal intensity of cerebrospinal fluid, including on DWI, and shows no contrast enhancement. The absence of restricted diffusion on DWI excludes an epidermoid cyst, the main differential in this case. Axial CISS images clearly show that the lesion is separate from the petrous carotid artery (*arrow* in **E**) and from Meckel cave (*arrow* in **F**). These imaging features are typical for an arachnoidocele, an incidental finding in this particular patient.

Aberrant arachnoid granulations with an associated  pseudomeningocele

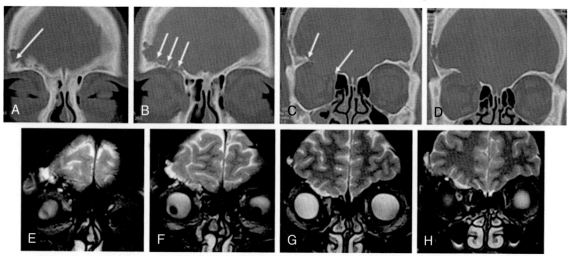

FIG. 15.3 Coronal CT sections on bone windows **(A–D)** show irregularly shaped lytic lesions in the right orbital plate of the frontal bone at the anterior skull base leading to bone erosion and to a wide bone defect in the outer table of the orbital roof (*arrows*). Coronal T2-weighted MR images **(E–H)** show intradiploic multicystic appearance and meningeal herniation of the arachnoid and subarachnoid space into the superior extraconal compartment of the orbit impinging upon the superior rectus/levator palpebrae complex. This patient complained of ptosis and limitation in upward gaze. Diagnosis: Aberrant arachnoid granulations with an associated pseudomeningocele.

Petrous apex pseudomeningocele

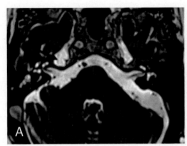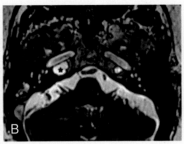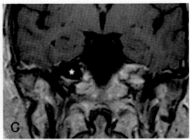

FIG. 15.4 MRI, axial constructive interference in steady state **(A and B)**, and coronal postgadolinium T1-weighted images show a strikingly asymmetric Meckel cave because of cystic enlargement on the right side (*asterisk* in **B** and **C**) and smooth remodeling of the anterior and superior petrous ridge, containing prolapse fibers of the trigeminal nerve (*black arrow* in **A**). These findings are pathognomonic for a petrous apex pseudomeningocele.

or total absence of the greater sphenoid wing and elevation of the lesser sphenoid wing, leading to widening of the superior orbital fissure, increased anteroposterior diameter of the middle cranial fossa, orbital enlargement, and the appearance of an empty orbit (bare orbit sign).[25] Other associated findings include a middle cranial fossa arachnoid cyst and potential meningeal or temporal pole herniation through the bony defect into the orbit causing secondary proptosis.

**Petrous apex cephalocele** is rare and represents a congenital or acquired cystic expansion and herniation of the posterolateral Meckel cave into the petrous apex secondary to the chronic transmission of CSF pulsations through a patent porus trigeminus combined with a congenitally thinned or dehiscent bone at the roof of the petrous apex[26] (Fig. 15.4). Acquired cases seem to be secondary to increased intracranial pressure, as there is a known association with an empty sella, pseudotumor cerebri, and expansive intracranial lesions[27] (Fig. 15.5). On imaging, they are featured by a cystic enlargement of Meckel cave with smooth remodeling of the anterior aspect of the superior petrous ridge and, occasionally, containing prolapsed fibers of the trigeminal nerve. Although most cases are incidental and asymptomatic, some have been associated with trigeminal neuropathy, CSF otorrhea, recurrent meningitis, and pulsatile tinnitus, as they may erode posteriorly into the otic capsule and/or pneumatized petrous air cells.[26]

**Basal cephaloceles** represent herniation of intracranial contents through congenital or acquired skull base defects. There are two different pathophysiologic mechanisms to explain this developmental anomaly: failure of neural tube closure and developmental failure of ossification centers of the skull base.[28] Basal cephaloceles are named according to the anatomic location of the skull base defect as sphenopharyngeal (through the basisphenoid into the pharynx), sphenoorbital (through the superior orbital fissure), sphenoethmoidal (through the sphenoethmoid synchondrosis), transethmoidal (through the cribiform plate), and sphenomaxillary (into the maxillary sinus).[28] Transphenoidal cephaloceles are rare and may occur between the basisphenoid and the greater sphenoid wing, most often resulting from incomplete fusion of their ossification centers. This developmental anomaly, known as the lateral craniopharyngeal or Stenberg canal, provides a weak spot for the herniation of meninges and/or overlying temporal lobe into the lateral recess of the sphenoid sinus[29] (Fig. 15.6). A complete Stenberg canal is seen in 4% of adults, whereas persistent vestiges of this canal are much more common, seen in 30% of individuals.[30] The oval foramen is another potential weak spot for the herniation of intracranial contents into the masticator space[31] (Fig. 15.7).

## Lesions Originating From Embryonic Remnants

These comprise lesions related to **ectodermal remnants**, including epidermoid and dermoid cysts; those originating from **meningoendothelial remnants**, such as intradiploic arachnoid cysts and intradiploic or "en plaque" meningiomas; those arising from **remnants of the pharyngohypophyseal canal**, including Rathke pouch cysts, craniopharyngiomas and intraosseous pituitary adenomas, and, finally, those arising from **notochordal remnants**, ecchordosis physaliphora and chordoma.

Secondary bilateral petrous apex meningoceles

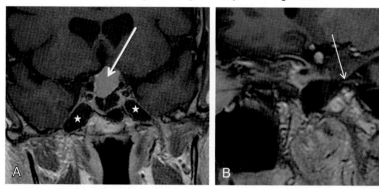

FIG. 15.5 Coronal **(A)** and sagittal **(B)** postgadolinium T1-weighted images show bilateral cystic enlargement of Meckel cave (*asterisks* in **A**) presumably secondary to increased intracranial pressure in this patient with a large suprasellar meningioma (*arrow* in **A**). Note, on the sagittal image, slight enlargement of the porus trigeminus with free cerebrospinal fluid flow into the cave (*arrow* in **B**). Presumed diagnosis: Bilateral petrous apex cephaloceles secondary to increased intracranial pressure.

Craniopharyngeal or Stenberg's canal meningoencephalocele

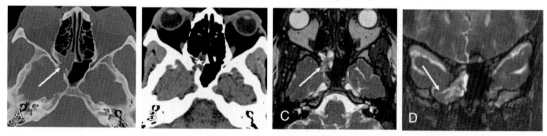

Courtesy from Dr. Vera Cruz e Silva

FIG. 15.6 CT axial images on bone **(A)** and soft tissue **(B)** windows demonstrate a bone defect in the lateral wall of the sphenoid body at the junction with the greater sphenoid wing (*arrow* in **A**) and associated opacification of the ipsilateral sphenoid sinus (*asterisk* in **B**). Corresponding MR on axial **(C)** and coronal **(D)** T2-weighted images show herniation of meninges and of the mesial temporal lobe (*arrows* in **C** and **D**) into the sphenoid sinus through the bony defect. Diagnosis: Stenberg canal meningoencephalocele. (Case courtesy from Dr. Mariana Horta.)

**Epidermoid cysts** originate from remnants of the ectoderm that become entrapped within the bony skull base during embryonic development. When located in the petrous apex, they are also called congenital cholesteatomas. On imaging, they appear as cystic lesions with a lobulated contour, insinuating along the crevices of adjacent structures and remodeling adjacent bone.[32] As opposed to arachnoid cysts, they often show internal architecture that can be best appreciated on PD, T2W, or 3D heavily T2W MR images and on DWI, restricted diffusion, with high signal intensity on high "b" values

and low signal intensity on ADC maps. After gadolinium administration, faint, peripheral enhancement may be seen (Fig. 15.8). Dermoids are more common in the anterior skull base, in and around the crista galli process, and the main distinguishing feature from epidermoid cysts is the presence of mesodermal derivates such as fat globules or skin appendages.[33] Fat globules are featured on MRI as intracystic target-like nodular structures resembling a "sac of marbles."

Lesions arising from meningoendothelial remnants include arachnoid cysts and intradiploic or

Transphenoidalmeningoencephalocele

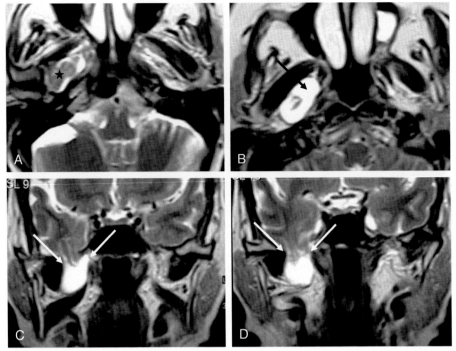

FIG. 15.7 Axial T2-weighted (T2W) MR images **(A** and **B)** demonstrate a mixed partially solid (*asterisk* in **A**) and partially cystic (*arrow* in **B**) lesion in the upper masticator space close to the skull base at the level of foramen ovale. Coronal T2W images **(C** and **D)** depict herniation of both meninges and the inferior temporal gyrus through the bone defect pushing the pterygoid muscles caudally. Diagnosis: Transphenoidal meningoencephalocele through an enlarged foramen ovale (*arrows* in **C** and **D**).

Petrous apex cholesteatoma/ epidermoid cyst

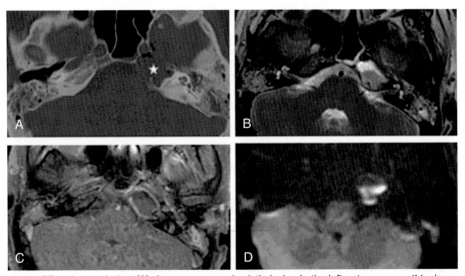

FIG. 15.8 CT on bone window **(A)** shows an expansive lytic lesion in the left petrous apex, thinning and remodeling cortical bone (*asterisk*). The lesion shows heterogeneous signal intensity on the axial T2-weighted image **(B)** with some internal architecture on its posterior aspect, faint peripheral enhancement on the axial postgadolinium T1-weighted image **(C),** and restricted diffusion shown as high signal intensity on the b1000 image **(D)**. Diagnosis: Petrous apex cholesteatoma or epidermoid cyst.

en plaque meningiomas. **Intradiploic arachnoid cysts** can be secondary to the growth of giant arachnoid granulations into the skull base, to the entrapment of meningocytes or cap arachnoid cells within skull base sutures during embryonic development, to trauma or molding of the head during birth, or to meningeal differentiation of multipotent mesenchymal cells. These cysts present on imaging as irregularly shaped osteolytic lesions of fluid density/signal intensity with only mild or no bone expansion. Meningeal remnants trapped within skull base sutures can also give rise to primary intraosseous meningiomas, known as **intradiploic, en plaque meningiomas**. These tumors result from growth of meningeal cells along the Haversian canals of trabecular bone, eliciting a dramatic hyperostotic reaction from which the name hyperostotic meningiomas derived.[34] The sphenoid ridge and sphenoid wing are the most common locations for these rare

tumors, representing only 2%–9% of all meningiomas, also known as sphenoorbital or pterional meningiomas[35] (Fig. 15.9). The presence of a thin layer of dural infiltration distinguishes primary from secondary intradiploic meningiomas, the later secondary to a dural-based meningioma that has grown into adjacent bone. CT best depicts the intraosseous component, showing the typical periosteal pattern of hyperostosis and the irregular contour on the surface of the hyperostotic bone.[34,36] On MRI the lesion follows the signal intensity of compact bone in all sequences, with very little or no enhancement after gadolinium administration.[34] These features can help in the differential diagnosis from other hyperostotic lesions such as osteoma, fibrous dysplasia, Paget disease, sclerotic bone metastases, and osteogenic osteosarcoma. A minority of intradiploic meningiomas may show an osteolytic or mixed lytic/sclerotic pattern.[34]

Intradiploic meningioma of the greater sphenoid wing

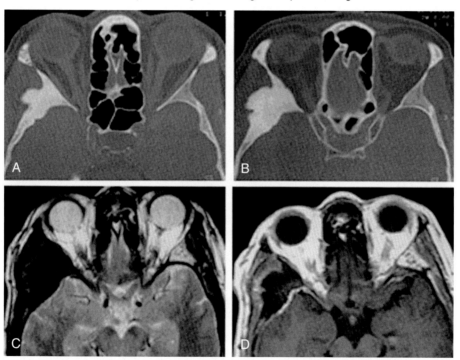

FIG. 15.9 CT axial images in bone windows **(A** and **B)** show an ill-defined, expansive sclerotic lesion centered in the sphenoid triangle in the lateral aspect of the greater sphenoid wing, with an ill-defined, air-on-end, lobulated contour. On corresponding MRI, the lesion shows low signal intensity on T2W image (C) and linear dural enhancement at the intracranial dural margin with no enhancement in the central core, on post-gadolinium T1W image (D). Diagnosis: Intradiploic meningioma.

Bony defects and tumors related to the craniopharyngeal canal or Rathke pouch include persistence of the pharyngohypophyseal canal, craniopharyngioma, and intraosseous pituitary adenoma. The **pharyngohypophyseal canal** is a remnant of the Rathke pouch that may persist in adult life as a vertical cleft in the sphenoid body at the site of fusion just posterior to the tuberculum sella extending superiorly from the sella to the nasopharyngeal roof inferiorly[37] (Figs. 15.10 and 15.11). These remnants may eventually give rise to benign cystic lesions, the so-called Rathke cleft pouch cyst or tumors, craniopharyngiomas. The difference between the two is simply the composition of the cystic wall. In Rathke cyst the wall is lined by cuboidal or columnar epithelium, which may be ciliated and may contain goblet cells, responsible for the production of mucin and accounting for the increased T1W signal intensity of these cysts, whereas craniopharyngiomas are lined by squamous or basal cell epithelium, which results from metaplasia of squamous epithelial remnants of the adenohypophysis or infundibulum or from

Persistent craniopharyngeal canal

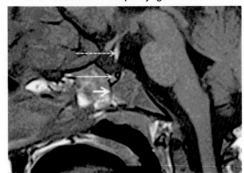

FIG. 15.10 MRI of the sella turcica, sagittal T1-weighted (T1W) image demonstrates a thin bony cleft extending from the roof of the nasopharynx to the floor of the sella (*short arrow*). Also note an ectopic neurohypophysis adjacent to the hypothalamus, recognized by its spontaneous bright signal on T1W images (*dashed arrow*), and vestigial pituitary tissue at the sellar floor (*arrow*). Diagnosis: Persistent craniopharyngeal canal with vestigial adenohypophysis and ectopic neurohypophysis in a 4-year-old boy with growth delay and panhypopituitarism.

Persistent craniopharyngeal canal with pituitary gland agenesis/ectopia

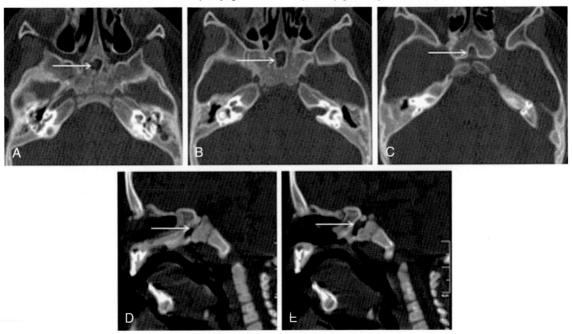

Courtesy from Dr. Isabel Amaral

FIG. 15.11 CT of the sella turcica on a 2-year-old girl with panhypopituitarism: Axial (**A–C**) and sagittal (**D** and **E**) images in bone window depict a large bony cleft in the body of the sphenoid extending from the nasopharynx to the floor of the sella (*arrows*), which is flattened. No pituitary tissue was noted inside the sella. Diagnosis: Persistent craniopharyngeal canal with pituitary aplasia/ectopia.

ectopic embryonic cell rests of enamel organs.[38] CT imaging can be useful on this distinction, as craniopharyngiomas tend to calcify, whereas Rathke cysts do not. Typical imaging features include the presence of cystic components (85%), calcifications (80%), and a solid nodular enhancing component in variable amounts.[39] These tumors, most often suprasellar (90%), may also develop within the sella or, on occasion, within the basisphenoid or at the roof of the nasopharynx.[39] Another potential bone lesion related to the embryonic development of the pituitary gland is the **intraosseous pituitary adenoma** (Fig. 15.12), a tumor arising from an ectopic intraosseous pituitary gland that fails to ascend to its normal position trapped by the development of the bony skull base.[40] This condition is distinct from an invasive pituitary macroadenoma, which originates from a eutopic pituitary gland and secondarily invades the underlying bone. Important features that suggest the diagnosis are the presence of an empty sella, deviation of the pituitary stalk, downward displacement

of the optic chiasm, and an ectopic neurohypophysis, easily recognized by its spontaneous high signal intensity on T1W images.[40]

Bone lesions associated with notochordal remnants include **ecchordosis physaliphora** and **chordomas**. In normal conditions, notochordal cells regress between 1 and 3 years of age. Persistence of notochordal remnants has been classified into benign notochordal rests, consisting of small conglomerates less than 1 cm in size, and giant notochordal rests, which may vary between 1 and 4 cm in size and may be mistaken for chordoma.[41] Like chordomas, they show an increased signal intensity on T2W images. However, they are asymptomatic incidental imaging findings, are not associated with bone destruction, do not change the configuration of bone, and should not grow on follow-up studies. On imaging, they present as small, smooth lytic defects nested in the clivus seldom with an associated soft tissue mass, bulging from the dorsal aspect of the clivus into the prepontine cistern[42] (Fig. 15.13). The signal intensity is usually more homogenous when compared with chordomas

Intra-osseous pituitary adenoma

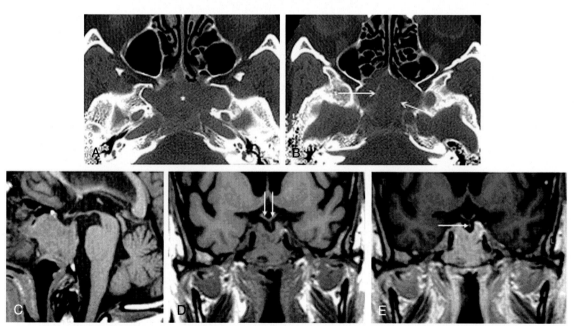

FIG. 15.12 Axial CT scan on bone windows **(A** and **B)** demonstrate a large lytic lesion of the central skull base involving the sphenoid body, sphenoid sinus, and clivus (*asterisk*), with some bony remnants within it (*arrows* in **B**). Corresponding MR, sagittal T1-weighted (T1W) **(C)**, and coronal pre- **(D)**, and postgadolinium **(E)** T1W images show a large soft tissue enhancing lesion replacing and expanding the clivus and partially filling the sphenoid sinus accompanied by downward deviation of the sellar floor with inferior retraction of the optic chiasm (*arrows* in **D**) and leftward deviation of the pituitary stalk (*arrow* in **E**). Diagnosis: Intraosseous pituitary macroadenoma.

Notochordal remants/ ecchordosis physaliphora

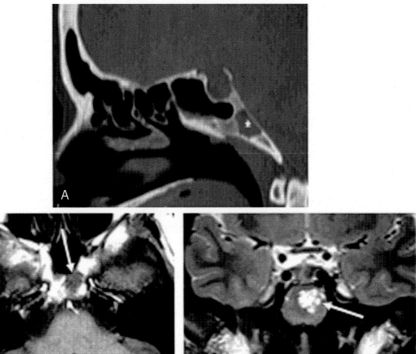

FIG. 15.13 CT sagittal section in bone window **(A)** shows a well-defined lytic lesion in the posterior aspect of the clivus (*asterisk*), without expansion or cortical disruption on the corresponding MRI, axial T1-weighted (T1W) **(B)** and coronal T2-weighted (T2W) image **(C)**. The lesion is hypointense on the T1W image and hyperintense on the coronal T2W image (*arrows*), showing a lobulated contour best appreciated on the T2W image. This lesion remained stable over long-term follow-up (over 5 years). A presumed diagnosis of ecchordosis physaliphora was made.

and the enhancement tends to be faint but may be variable.[42] **Chordomas** are rare malignant neoplasms arising from remnants of the cranial or caudal end of the primitive notochord. In the skull base, they are typically located in the basisphenoid, grossly midline in position, and show a lobulated contour.[43] On CT, they manifest as expansive, destructive lytic lesions and a moderately enhancing soft tissue mass, which may contain remnants of bone trabecula inside.[44] On MRI, the signal intensity can be quite heterogeneous, reflecting the variegated tumor components: myxoid, blood, and residues of bony trabecula of the clivus destroyed by the tumor. Most often, lesions tend to show intermediate to low signal intensity on T1W images, heterogeneously high signal intensity on T2W images, and a typical reticular, honeycomb pattern of contrast enhancement after gadolinium administration[44] (Fig. 15.14). According to

their exact location and pattern of spread clival chordomas are classified into upper, middle, and lower, with implications on surgical management.[45] Upper chordomas occur rostral to the trigeminal nerve in the region of the dorsum sella, middle chordomas between the emergence of the trigeminal and glossopharyngeal nerves, and lower chordomas below the emergence of cranial nerve IX. Extension is laterally to the petrous apex and cavernous sinus, anteriorly to the sphenoid sinus and roof of the nasopharynx, superiorly into the sella and parasellar region, posteriorly into the prepontine cistern and jugular foramen and, inferiorly, into the foramen magnum and cervical spinal canal, dorsally, and into the nasopharyngeal mucosal space and parapharyngeal space, ventrally.[45]

The main differential diagnosis is with petroclival chondrosarcoma, metastasis, plasmacytoma, direct

Clival chordoma

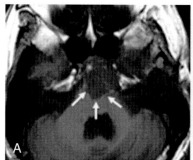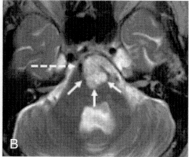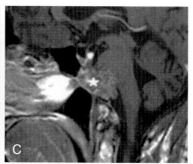

**FIG. 15.14** MR axial T1-weighted (T1W) **(A)** and T2-weighted (T2W) **(B)** images and sagittal gadolinium-enhanced T1W images (C) show an expansive and destructive lesion centered in the clivus, which protrudes into the prepontine cistern indenting the pons—"thumb sign" (*arrows*)—and pushing the basilar artery to the right side (*dashed arrow*). The lesion is hypointense on T1W and heterogeneously hyperintense on T2W and shows a typical honeycomb, reticular pattern, after gadolinium administration (*asterisk*). Diagnosis: Clival chordoma.

skull base invasion by nasopharyngeal carcinoma, squamous cell carcinoma of the sphenoid sinus, and invasive or intradiploic pituitary macroadenoma.[44]

Complete surgical excision is the best chance for disease control but may not be possible because of unacceptable morbidity. Proton beam radiation therapy has been used successfully to treat residual disease.[46]

### Diffuse Bone Lesions or Tumor-Like Conditions

This group of lesions is characterized by diffuse or multifocal nonneoplastic bone involvement, including disorders of endochondral ossification and infection. The former includes conditions such as fibrous dysplasia, Paget disease, osteopetrosis, and melorheostosis, just to mention the most common, and imaging plays an important role in this setting, as a biopsy without adequate radiologic correlation can be misleading, mimicking more aggressive neoplastic conditions such as osteosarcoma.[47] The latter most often results from aggressive infections in the setting of an immunocompromised patient, as in the case of malignant otitis externa in diabetic patients and invasive forms of fungal infection but may also be secondary to bacterial infections in children or neglected bacterial infections in immunocompetent adults, most often sinusitis, otitis, or petrous apicitis.[48]

**Fibrous dysplasia** is a developmental anomaly characterized by impaired osteoblastic differentiation and maturation leading to replacement of normal bone by vascularized fibrous tissue interspersed with islands of immature woven bone. It can affect only one

(monostotic) or multiple bones (polyostotic), can be limited to craniofacial bones (craniofacial fibrous dysplasia), or affect exclusively the maxilla and mandible (cherubism).[14] This is mainly a pediatric condition affecting children and young adults, with 55% of cases diagnosed before age 30 years and most polyostotic forms, before age 10 years.[14]

It can be isolated or part of a syndromic condition, such as McCune Albright and Mazabraud syndromes. Craniofacial fibrous dysplasia accounts for 50% of cases of polyostotic forms, and clinical presentation is often by craniofacial deformity, impingement upon neurovascular skull base foramina and canals secondary to bone expansion, or obstruction of sinonasal drainage pathways with mucocele formation.[49] The disease evolves following three different disease stages: predominantly lytic, mixed, and predominantly sclerotic.[14] These stages show different imaging features: the lytic or active phase is characterized by bone demineralization and expansion because of the presence of highly vascularized, nonmineralized, fibrous stroma and by strong contrast enhancement best appreciated on gadolinium-enhanced T1W images; the sclerotic phase is featured by a ground-glass pattern reflecting the presence of coarse and disorganized mineralized bone trabecula, which is best seen on CT; the mixed phase shows changes of both the lytic and sclerotic phases.[49]

Typical CT features include bone marrow expansion with preservation of the cortical lining, geographic interface with adjacent normal bone, absent periosteal reaction unless complicated by fracture, and a lytic,

Fibrous dysplasia

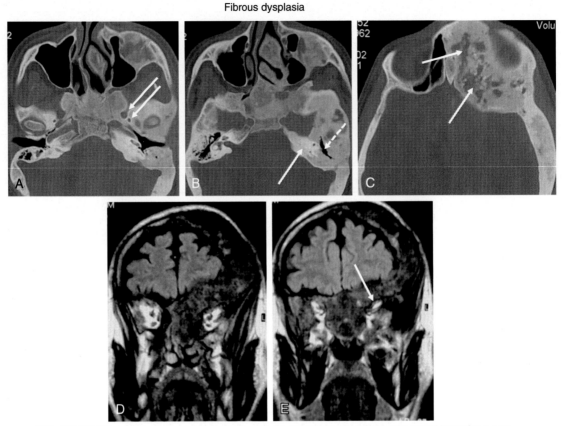

FIG. 15.15 CT axial sections on bone window **(A–C)** and MR coronal fluid-attenuated inversion recovery (FLAIR) **(D** and **E)** images on a 19-year-old boy with limitation on upward gaze on the left demonstrate diffuse thickening and expansion of the craniofacial bones with extensive skull base involvement. Bones are predominantly sclerotic with a ground-glass appearance but show some cystic areas more evident in the frontoorbital region (*arrows* in **C**). Note that, in spite of this extensive bone involvement, foramen ovale and foramen spinosum are patent (*arrows* in **A**). Note, on the left, the involvement of the petrous bone and otic capsule (*arrow* in **B**) and the stenosis of the middle ear cavity (*dashed arrow* in **B**). MR images show the impact of the lesion over the optic canal (*arrow* in **E**) and orbital contents. On FLAIR, bone changes are mostly hypointense, with some foci of increased signal intensity corresponding to the small cystic areas on CT. Diagnosis: Craniofacial fibrous dysplasia, mixed/sclerotic phase.

ground-glass or sclerotic matrix depending on disease stage. MR appearance can be misleadingly aggressive during the active phase when the fatty marrow is replaced by fibrous tissue, which is of intermediate to low signal intensity on T1W, is heterogeneously hyperintense on T2W, and shows moderate to strong enhancement on postcontrast T1W images[50] (Fig. 15.15). The chronic, burned-out phase is characterized by low signal intensity on both T1 and T2W images with almost no contrast enhancement. STIR and contrast-enhanced MR images are used to monitor disease activity, which

affects patients' management. Moreover, MR is particularly well suited to demonstrate the effect of these lesions upon neurovascular structures.[50] The main differential diagnosis is with nonossifying fibroma, a more aggressive and limited form of fibrous dysplasia and Paget disease, a condition affecting older patients (see following discussion).

The most common complications are pathologic fractures (rare in the craniofacial region) and sarcomatous transformation (osteosarcoma, fibrosarcoma, malignant fibrous histiocytoma, or chondrosarcoma), which affects less than 1% of patients, is more often associated with polyostotic disease, and, apparently, is related to prior radiation therapy.[51,52]

As the natural history of the disease is often auto-limited, evolving to a burned-out nonactive phase after puberty, no treatment is required unless neurovascular or sinonasal impingements require decompressive surgery, particularly compression of the orbital nerve and orbital contents.[51]

**Paget disease or osteitis deformans** is a chronic bone disease most often diagnosed after the age of 65 years, with increasing prevalence thereafter. It ranks as the second most common bone disease of the elderly immediately after osteoporosis. The etiology is unknown, although some genetic and environmental predisposing factors have been identified, accounting for the well-known ethnic and geographic clustering of this condition.[53]

Paget disease is characterized by abnormal bone turnover, starting with increased osteoclastic activity and followed by compensatory osteoblastic activity producing disorganized, poorly mineralized trabecular bone, rich in vascular fibrous tissue. This bone, although thicker, is mechanically weaker than normal bone and is prone to deformity and fracture.[54] The disease is most often multifocal and affects predominantly the spine, pelvis, skull, and proximal long bones. Similar to fibrous dysplasia, three phases of the disease are recognized: a lytic or active phase featured by osteoclastic hyperactivity, a mixed phase of both osteoclastic and osteoblastic activity, and a sclerotic, predominantly inactive burned-out phase.[55] Clinically, over 70% of patients are asymptomatic, and the disease is found incidentally on imaging studies. The remaining 30% of patients present with pain, craniofacial deformity, hearing loss (due to compression of the vestibular cochlear nerve at the internal auditory canal or involvement of the ossicular chain by the disease), and signs and symptoms of neurovascular compression.[54]

Typical imaging features of the craniofacial bones, in the early lytic phase, include well-defined lytic areas involving both the diploë and inner and outer tables, the so-called osteoporosis circumscripta. On MRI, it manifests as areas of low signal intensity replacing the fatty bone marrow on T1W images and a heterogeneous speckled appearance on T2W, STIR, and contrast-enhanced T1W images, reflecting the presence of fibrovascular marrow changes.[56] The mixed phase is characterized by the so-called jigsaw or mosaic pattern featuring disorganized and thickened bone trabecula interspersed with lytic changes

and the cotton-wool appearance that reflects the presence of ill-defined fluffy patches of mineralized, sclerotic bone inside areas of osteolysis, best recognized on plain films and more often seen in the skull.[57] In the sclerotic, predominantly inactive phase, bone sclerosis predominates with a ground-glass pattern depicted on CT and low signal intensity on all MR sequences with little or no enhancement. Bone thickening and expansion, involving both the medullary cavity and cortical bone, is responsible for craniofacial deformity and impingement upon neurovascular foramina.[57] An important clue for the differential diagnosis with other conditions is the persistence of T1W hyperintensities in the medullary cavity reflecting the presence of fatty bone marrow. Skull base flattening secondary to bone softening is a common occurrence and may lead to basilar invagination. Another potential complication besides bone fracture is malignant degeneration to osteosarcoma, occurring in less than 1% of cases.[58]

Treatment can include decompressive surgery, when neurovascular impingement is an issue, or bisphosphonates to restrain osteoclastic activity, promote healing of osteolytic lesions, and ameliorate bone pain.[59]

**Osteopetrosis**, Albers-Schönberg disease, or marble bone disease is a rare hereditary disorder characterized by defective osteoclastic function with failure of proper resorption and remodeling of spongiotic bone resulting in thick, sclerotic, brittle bones. The infantile autosomal recessive type is usually fatal. The benign, autosomal dominant, adult type can be asymptomatic or manifest by recurrent fractures, mild anemia, and, occasionally, cranial nerve palsies caused by narrowing of neurovascular foramina and is consistent with a normal life expectancy. It is further subdivided into type 1, characterized by extensive osteosclerosis of the skull with compromise of cranial nerves, and type 2, featured by vertebral and pelvic girdle involvement with increased risk of fractures.

On CT imaging, type 1 disease shows diffuse sclerosis of the cranial vault and skull base, which is replaced by dense, thickened, amorphous, and structureless bones with obliteration of the normal trabecular pattern.[60] MRI also discloses thickened bone, homogeneously hypointense on both T1W and T2W images (black bone) because of loss of normal bone marrow signal intensity and of the corticomedullary discrimination (Fig. 15.16). Moreover, MR is the modality of choice to demonstrate the involvement of cranial nerves at the neurovascular foramina.[60]

Osteopetrosis

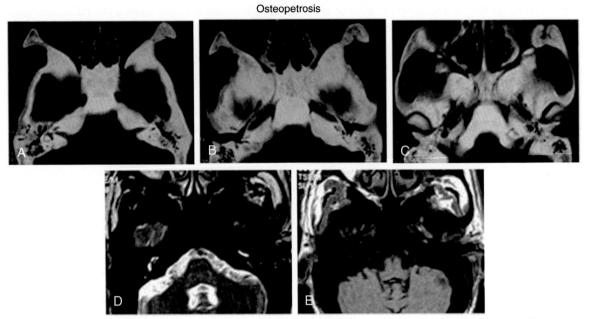

FIG. 15.16 CT, axial sections in bone window **(A–C)** disclose diffuse sclerosis of craniofacial bones and skull base, without significant bone expansion. There is complete loss of the corticomedullary differentiation, with structureless bones. Note that the bone density is similar and indistinct from that of the otic capsule. On MR, axial T2-weighted **(D)** and fluid-attenuated inversion recovery images **(E)**, note the very low signal intensity of all craniofacial bones ("black bones"), with loss of bone marrow cavity. Diagnosis: Osteopetrosis (adult type 1).

The main differential diagnosis is with fibrous dysplasia, renal osteodystrophy, melorheostosis, fluorosis, and pyknodysostosis.[47]

Bone marrow transplantation is the treatment of choice for normalizing bone marrow function and bone production.[61]

Other sclerosing bone dysplasias, such as **osteopoikilosis** and **melorheostosis**, only rarely affect the skull base. **Osteopoikilosis** is an autosomal dominant disorder characterized by multiple benign enostosis, which develop during childhood and do not regress thereafter. The condition is of no clinical significance, and the main concern is to avoid mistaking it for other pathologies such as sclerotic bone metastasis, in the appropriate clinical setting.[62] Osteopoikilosis is an incidental radiologic finding manifesting as multiple islands of dense cortical bone within the medullary cavity, which tend to cluster around joints.[63] On MRI, these discrete lesions of variable size, ranging from a few millimeters to 1 or 2 cm, follow the signal intensity of compact bone on all pulse sequences and, on bone scintigraphy, as opposed to sclerotic bone metastases, do not

show increased uptake.[64] **Melorheostosis** or Leri disease is a rare mesenchymal dysplasia characterized by areas of cortical bone sclerosis with a typical appearance of dripping or melting wax. This developmental condition is most often multifocal and may be found incidentally but, as opposed to osteopoikilosis, can be clinically significant, producing bone deformity, pain, and joint stiffness. In the craniofacial region, imaging features are atypical and often mistaken for fibrous dysplasia, showing expansive bone lesions with flowing bone trabecula lacking a ground-glass appearance.[65]

**Skull base osteomyelitis** should also be considered when facing diffuse involvement of the skull base in the adequate clinical setting. It is most often secondary to aggressive infections originating in the temporal bone or sinonasal region, and immunocompromised patients are particularly prone.[66] **Malignant or necrotizing otitis externa** is a *Pseudomonas aeruginosa* infection of the external auditory canal afflicting, most commonly, diabetic patients. If not properly treated, the infection can spread medially into the middle ear cavity (MEC), petrous apex, and central skull base and posteriorly into the posterior

Central skull base osteomyelitis secondary to a malignant otitis externa

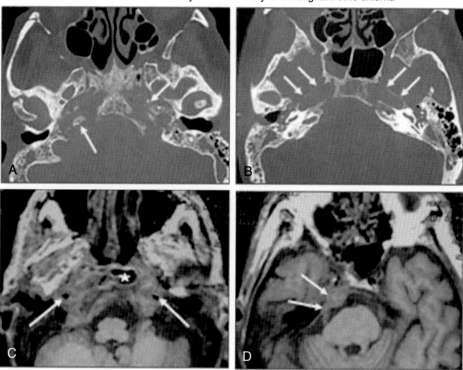

FIG. 15.17 A 73-year-old diabetic man severely sick with altered consciousness. CT, axial sections on bone window **(A** and **B)** show a permeative "moth-eaten" pattern of bone destruction affecting the petrous apices and central skull base, including the petrous carotid canal (*arrows* in **B**), with some remaining fragments of bone trabecula inside the areas of osteolysis (*arrows* in **A**). Opacification of the middle ear cavities and an air-fluid level in the right sphenoid sinus are also noted. Corresponding MR, axial T1-weighted images **(C** and **D)** show an infiltrating soft tissue mass encasing the petrous segments of the carotid artery with luminal stenosis (*arrows* in **C**). Also note a central area of low signal intensity in the clivus, suggesting necrosis (*asterisk* in **C**) and abnormal soft tissue filling Meckel cave and extending along the cisternal segment of the right trigeminal nerve (*arrows* in **D**). Diagnosis: Malignant otitis externa complicated with skull base osteomyelitis and carotid arteritis.

cranial fossa, affecting the jugular foramen and sigmoid and transverse sinuses[67] (Figs. 15.17 and 15.18). Potentially life-threatening complications include dural venous sinus thrombosis (most often the sigmoid, transverse, and cavernous sinuses), pachy or leptomeningitis, epidural or subdural empyema, brain abscess, encasement of the internal carotid artery, and infarcts.[68]

CT imaging discloses a lytic permeative pattern affecting the trabecular bone of the clivus and/or petrous temporal bone, and MRI shows replacement of the fatty bone marrow by an inflammatory enhancing mass. Bone necrosis, bone sequestra, and microabscesses may also be seen. Gallium scans can be quite helpful in the diagnosis and follow-up of the disease.[9]

**Invasive forms of fungal infections**, such as mucormycosis and aspergillosis, are another set of aggressive infections that may spread to the skull base, most often afflicting immunocompromised patients. Infection usually starts in the nose and paranasal sinuses, transgresses the sinonasal mucosa, and grows angiocentrically along vessel walls, leading to bone necrosis and transgression of sinus walls. Infection tends to spread into the orbit and into the intracranial compartment either via the cribiform plate, to the anterior cranial fossa, or via the superior orbital fissure into the middle cranial fossa and cavernous sinus. Involvement and encasement of the internal carotid artery is a life-threatening complication of this disease.[69] CT demonstrates a thick, irregular,

Skull base osteomyelitis secondary to a malignant otitis externa

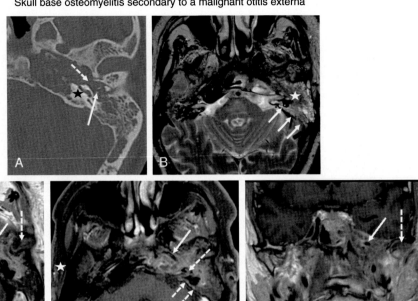

FIG. 15.18 CT axial section on bone window **(A)** shows complete opacification of the middle ear cavity, with permeative, lytic changes in adjacent bones, including the ossicles (*arrow*), anterior wall of the tympanic cavity (*dashed arrow*), petrous apex and petrous carotid canal, sparing the otic capsule (*asterisk*). Axial T2-weighted image of the corresponding MR **(B)** is relevant for the predominantly low signal intensity of the soft tissue mass (*asterisk*), which also fills the adjacent sigmoid sinus (*arrows* in **B**). Postcontrast axial **(C** and **D)** and coronal **(E)** T1-weighted images demonstrate strong enhancement of this infiltrating mass, which encases the petrous segment of the left carotid artery (*arrows* in **C**, **D**, and **E**) with stenosis and irregularity of its lumen. Note the necrotic, nonenhancing areas within the lesion reflecting necrosis. Also note the dural enhancement along the posterior petrous ridge, along the internal auditory canal, and labyrinthine enhancement more striking in the cochlea (*dashed arrows* in **D**). There is also involvement of the temporomandibular joint (TMJ) (*dashed arrows* in **C** and **D**) and infratemporal fossa (*dashed arrows* in **E**). Diagnosis: Malignant otitis externa, complicated with sigmoid sinus thrombosis, petrous carotid arteritis, labyrinthitis, and TMJ infectious arthritis.

sinonasal mucosal thickening often with spontaneously hyperdense components, reflecting the presence of fungal hyphae, areas of permeative bone erosion, and abnormal soft tissue outside the sinus walls. The orbit and periorbital fat, premaxillary soft tissues, pterygopalatine fossa, infratemporal fossa, orbital apex, inferior and superior orbital fissures, and neurovascular central skull base foramina should be carefully inspected when fungal infection is suspected. On MR, the most suggestive imaging findings include heterogeneous signal intensity of the inflammatory tissue with spontaneously high signal intensity on T1W and low signal intensity on T2W images, featuring the presence of manganese in the fungal hyphae, presence of necrotic nonenhancing tissue, bone marrow replacement, and cortical bone erosion.[48] When the infection reaches the internal carotid artery, encasement, luminal narrowing, and irregularity account for invasion of the arterial wall. Adjacent brain parenchyma of the temporal poles and frontobasal region should be carefully inspected to rule out vasogenic brain edema.[10] Postcontrast T1W images with fat suppression are useful to assess orbital involvement and perineural and perivascular spread of the disease, as well as to depict areas of avascular necrosis. MRV and MRA techniques are often added for better assessment of dural sinus thrombosis and carotid artery invasion and DWI to assist in the differential diagnosis of skull base malignancy[70] (Fig. 15.19).

Central skull base osteomyelitis secondary to invasive fungal infection

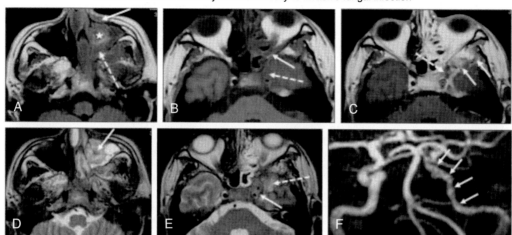

FIG. 15.19 MRI of the brain and paranasal sinuses on a 27-year-old HIV-positive man shows abnormal soft tissue in the nasoethmoid region and maxillary sinus on the left, which transgresses the bony walls of the sinus cavities and extends anteriorly, into the premaxillary soft tissues (*arrow* in **A**), posteriorly into the pterygopalatine fossa (*dashed arrow* in **A**) and into the inferior orbital fissure (*arrow* in **B**), the cavernous sinus (*dashed arrow* in **B** and *arrows* in **E**) and into the middle cranial fossa, best appreciated on the T2-weighted (T2W) images with accompanying vasogenic edema (*dashed arrow* in **E**) and enhancement of the temporal pole (*arrows* in **C**). The mass is heterogeneous in signal intensity owing to areas of high signal intensity on T1-weighted (*asterisk* in **A**), low signal intensity on T2W (*arrow* in **D**), and strong contrast enhancement after gadolinium with nonenhancing areas in the cavernous sinus reflecting thrombus (*dashed arrow* in **C**). Note the encasement of the cavernous and petrous carotid artery best appreciated on the corresponding MR angiography (*arrows* in **E**). Diagnosis: Invasive mucormycosis in an immunocompromised patient best appreciated on the corresponding MR angiography (arrows in **F**).

## SUMMARY

Bone lesions of the skull base encompass a wide variety of differential diagnoses. Clinical and epidemiologic features are largely insufficient to orient patient's management, particularly because the skull base is hidden to clinical inspection and obtaining tissue for pathologic diagnosis is not always easy. Therefore, imaging plays a major role in refining the diagnosis and, particularly, in fully characterizing bone lesions of the skull base. CT, MRI, bone scintigraphy, and FDG-PET-CT often have a complementary role in this regard. Although imaging patterns of most bone diseases affecting the skull base reproduce those in other areas of the skeletal system, there are several specificities in this anatomic region that make diagnosis and patient's management quite challenging. Of particular note are developmental lesions related to embryonic remnants unique to the skull base, which require a basic knowledge on the embryonic development of the skull base and related neighboring structures. Moreover, bone dysplasias and other tumor-like conditions offer additional challenges in patient's management related to potential local complications

related to the involvement of sinonasal cavities, orbit, cranial nerves, dural venous sinuses, major intracranial vessels, and brain parenchyma. Also of note are the limitations of pathologic diagnosis, particularly in fibroosseous lesions, requiring radiologic correlation to reach an accurate final diagnosis.

## REFERENCES

1. Borges A. Imaging of the central skull base. *Neuroimaging Clin N Am.* 2009;19(4):669–696.
2. Borges A. Skull base tumours Part II. Central skull base tumours and intrinsic tumours of the bony skull base. *Eur J Radiol.* 2008;66(3):348–362.
3. Mintz DN, Hwang S. Bone tumor imaging, then and now: review article. *HSS J.* 2014;10(3):230–239.
4. Computed Tomography of bone tumors. Withehouse, Richard W. In: Imaging bone tumours and tumor-like conditions. Davies A Mark, Sundaram Murali, James Steven J. (Eds). NJ: Springer, 2009.
5. Hwang, Sinchun. Imaging techniques: Magnetic Resonance Imaging. In: Imaging bone tumours and tumor-like conditions. Davies A Mark, Sundaram Murali, James Steven J. (Eds). NJ: Springer, 2009.

6. Padhani AR, Koh DM, Collins DJ. Whole-body diffusion-weighted MR imaging in cancer: current status and research directions. *Radiology*. 2011;261(3):700–718.

7. Green, Ruth A. R. Nuclear Medicine. In: Imaging bone tumours and tumor-like conditions. Davies A Mark, Sundaram Murali, James Steven J. (Eds). NJ: Springer, 2009.

8. Miwa S, Otsuka T. Practical use of imaging technique for management of bone and soft tissue tumors. *J Orthop Sci*. 2017;22(3):391–400.

9. Chakraborty D, Bhattacharya A, Gupta AK, Panda NK, Das A, Mittal BR. Skull base osteomyelitis in otitis externa: the utility of triphasic and single photon emission computed tomography/computed tomography bone scintigraphy. *Indian J Nucl Med*. 2013;28(2):65–69.

10. Chang PC, Fischbein NJ, Holliday RA. Central skull base osteomyelitis in patients without otitis externa: imaging findings. *AJNR Am J Neuroradiol*. 2003;24(7):1310–1316.

11. Love C, Din AS, Tomas MB, Kalapparambath TP, Palestro CJ. Radionuclide bone imaging: an illustrative review. *Radiographics*. 2003;23(2):341–358.

12. Efune G, Perez CL, Tong L, Rihani J, Batra PS. Paranasal sinus and skull base fibro-osseous lesions: when is biopsy indicated for diagnosis? *Int Forum Allergy Rhinol*. 2012;2(2):160–165.

13. Riddle ND, Bui MM. Fibrous dysplasia. *Arch Pathol Lab Med*. 2013;137(1):134–138.

14. Helms C. *Fundamentals of Skeletal Radiology*. 3rd ed. Philadelphia, Pennsylvania: Elsevier, Saunders; 2005.

15. Kelly HR, Curtin HD. Imaging of skull base lesions. *Handb Clin Neurol*. 2016;135:637–657.

16. Osborne RL. The differential radiologic diagnosis of bone tumors. *CA Cancer J Clin*. 1974;24(4):194–211.

17. Franchi A. Epidemiology and classification of bone tumors. *Clin Cases Miner Bone Metab*. 2012;9(2):92–95.

18. Welker KM, DeLone DR, Lane JI, Gilbertson JR. Arrested pneumatization of the skull base: imaging characteristics. *AJR Am J Roentgenol*. 2008;190(6):1691–1696.

19. Kuntzler S, Jankowski R. Arrested pneumatization: witness of paranasal sinuses development? *Eur Ann Otorhinolaryngol Head Neck Dis*. 2014;131(3):167–170.

20. Trimble CR, Harnsberger HR, Castillo M, Brant-Zawadzki M, Osborn AG. "Giant" arachnoid granulations just like CSF?: NOT!!. *AJNR Am J Neuroradiol*. 2010;31(9):1724–1728.

21. Thiebaut S, Romanet P, Duvillard C, Farah W, Folia M. Sphenoid arachnoidocele: report of one case. *Rev Laryngol Otol Rhinol*. 2010;131(4–5):317–320.

22. Datouassi Y, Mllila Touati M, Chihani M, Aknaddar A, Ammar H, Bouaity B. Spontaneous cerebrospinal fluid leak of the sphenoid sinus mimicking allergic rhinitis, and managed successfully by a ventriculoperitoneal shunt: a case report. *J Med Case Rep*. 2016;10(1):308.

23. Ferner RE, Huson SM, Thomas N, et al. Guidelines for the diagnosis and management of individuals with neurofibromatosis 1. *J Med Genet*. 2007;44(2):81–88.

24. Lotfy M, Xu R, McGirt M, Sakr S, Ayoub B, Bydon A. Reconstruction of skull base defects in sphenoid wing dysplasia associated with neurofibromatosis I with titanium mesh. *Clin Neurol Neurosurg*. 2010;112(10):909–914.

25. Sherwani P, Faizi NA, Anand R, Narula MK. Bare orbit sign: classical sign in cranio-orbital-temporal neurofibromatosis 1. *Indian J Pediatr*. 2015;82(2):203–204.

26. Moore KR, Fischbein NJ, Harnsberger HR, et al. Petrous apex cephaloceles. *AJNR Am J Neuroradiol*. 2001;22(10):1867–1871.

27. Achilli V, Danesi G, Caverni L, Richichi M. Petrous apex arachnoid cyst: a case report and review of the literature. *Acta otorhinolaryngol Ital*. 2005;25(5):296–300.

28. Harada N, Nemoto M, Miyazaki C, et al. Basal encephalocele in an adult patient presenting with minor anomalies: a case report. *J Med Case Rep*. 2014;8:24.

29. Baranano CF, Cure J, Palmer JN, Woodworth BA. Sternberg's canal: fact or fiction? *Am J Rhinol Allergy*. 2009;23(2):167–171.

30. Bendersky DC, Landriel FA, Ajler PM, Hem SM, Carrizo AG. Sternberg's canal as a cause of encephalocele within the lateral recess of the sphenoid sinus: a report of two cases. *Surg Neurol Int*. 2011;2:171.

31. Shafa B, Arle J, Kotapka M. Unusual presentations of middle fossa encephaloceles: report of two cases. *Skull Base Surg*. 1999;9(4):289–294.

32. Chowdhury FH, Haque MR, Sarker MH. Intracranial epidermoid tumor; microneurosurgical management: an experience of 23 cases. *Asian J Neurosurg*. 2013;8(1):21–28.

33. Ray MJ, Barnett DW, Snipes GJ, Layton KF, Opatowsky MJ. Ruptured intracranial dermoid cyst. *Proceedings*. 2012;25(1):23–25.

34. Tokgoz N, Oner YA, Kaymaz M, Ucar M, Yilmaz G, Tali TE. Primary intraosseous meningioma: CT and MRI appearance. *AJNR Am J Neuroradiol*. 2005;26(8):2053–2056.

35. Hussaini SM, Dziurzynski K, Fratkin JD, Jordan JR, Hussain SA, Khan M. Intraosseous meningioma of the sphenoid bone. *Radiol Case Rep*. 2010;5(1):357.

36. Agrawal V, Ludwig N, Agrawal A, Bulsara KR. Intraosseous intracranial meningioma. *AJNR Am J Neuroradiol*. 2007;28(2):314–315.

37. Abele TA, Salzman KL, Harnsberger HR, Glastonbury CM. Craniopharyngeal canal and its spectrum of pathology. *AJNR Am J Neuroradiol*. 2014;35(4):772–777.

38. Byun WM, Kim OL, Kim D. MR imaging findings of Rathke's cleft cysts: significance of intracystic nodules. *AJNR Am J Neuroradiol*. 2000;21(3):485–488.

39. Zoicas F, Schofl C. Craniopharyngioma in adults. *Front Endocrinol*. 2012;3:46.

40. Kaushik C, Ramakrishnaiah R, Angtuaco EJ. Ectopic pituitary adenoma in persistent craniopharyngeal canal: case report and literature review. *J Comput Assist Tomogr*. 2010;34(4):612–614.

41. Mehnert F, Beschorner R, Kuker W, Hahn U, Nagele T. Retroclival ecchordosis physaliphora: MR imaging and review of the literature. *AJNR Am J Neuroradiol*. 2004;25(10):1851–1855.

42. Chihara C, Korogi Y, Kakeda S, et al. Ecchordosis physaliphora and its variants: proposed new classification based on high-resolution fast MR imaging employing steady-state acquisition. *Eur Radiol.* 2013;23(10):2854–2860.

43. Erdem E, Angtuaco EC, Van Hemert R, Park JS, Al-Mefty O. Comprehensive review of intracranial chordoma. *Radiographics.* 2003;23(4):995–1009.

44. Gehanne C, Delpierre I, Damry N, Devroede B, Brihaye P, Christophe C. Skull base chordoma: CT and MRI features. *JBR-BTR.* 2005;88(6):325–327.

45. Chugh R, Tawbi H, Lucas DR, Biermann JS, Schuetze SM, Baker LH. Chordoma: the nonsarcoma primary bone tumor. *Oncologist.* 2007;12(11):1344–1350.

46. Ferraresi V, Nuzzo C, Zoccali C, et al. Chordoma: clinical characteristics, management and prognosis of a case series of 25 patients. *BMC Cancer.* 2010;10:22.

47. Ihde LL, Forrester DM, Gottsegen CJ, et al. Sclerosing bone dysplasias: review and differentiation from other causes of osteosclerosis. *Radiographics.* 2011;31(7):1865–1882.

48. Blyth CC, Gomes L, Sorrell TC, da Cruz M, Sud A, Chen SC. Skull-base osteomyelitis: fungal vs. bacterial infection. *Clin Microbiol Infect.* 2011;17(2):306–311.

49. Chong VF, Khoo JB, Fan YF. Fibrous dysplasia involving the base of the skull. *AJR Am J Roentgenol.* 2002;178(3):717–720.

50. Atalar MH, Salk I, Savas R, Uysal IO, Egilmez H. CT and MR imaging in a large series of patients with craniofacial fibrous dysplasia. *Pol J Radiol.* 2015;80:232–240.

51. Lee JS, FitzGibbon EJ, Chen YR, et al. Clinical guidelines for the management of craniofacial fibrous dysplasia. *Orphanet J Rare Dis.* 2012;7(suppl 1):S2.

52. Mardekian SK, Tuluc M. Malignant sarcomatous transformation of fibrous dysplasia. *Head Neck Pathol.* 2015;9(1):100–103.

53. Hullar TE, Lustig LR. Paget's disease and fibrous dysplasia. *Otolaryngol Clin N Am.* 2003;36(4):707–732.

54. Shaker JL. Paget's disease of bone: a review of epidemiology, pathophysiology and management. *Ther Adv Musculoskelet Dis.* 2009;1(2):107–125.

55. Seton M. Paget's disease: epidemiology and pathophysiology. *Curr Osteoporos Rep.* 2008;6(4):125–129.

56. Theodorou DJ, Theodorou SJ, Kakitsubata Y. Imaging of Paget disease of bone and its musculoskeletal complications: self-assessment module. *AJR Am J Roentgenol.* 2011;196(suppl 6):WS53–WS56.

57. Smith SE, Murphey MD, Motamedi K, Mulligan ME, Resnik CS, Gannon FH. From the archives of the AFIP. Radiologic spectrum of Paget disease of bone and its complications with pathologic correlation. *Radiographics.* 2002;22(5):1191–1216.

58. Wermers RA, Tiegs RD, Atkinson EJ, Achenbach SJ, Melton 3rd LJ. Morbidity and mortality associated with Paget's disease of bone: a population-based study. *J Bone Miner Res.* 2008;23(6):819–825.

59. Josse RG, Hanley DA, Kendler D, Ste Marie LG, Adachi JD, Brown J. Diagnosis and treatment of Paget's disease of bone. *Clin Invest Med.* 2007;30(5):E210–E223.

60. Cure JK, Key LL, Goltra DD, VanTassel P. Cranial MR imaging of osteopetrosis. *AJNR Am J Neuroradiol.* 2000;21(6):1110–1115.

61. Wilson CJ, Vellodi A. Autosomal recessive osteopetrosis: diagnosis, management, and outcome. *Arch Dis Child.* 2000;83(5):449–452.

62. Panda A, Gamanagatti S, Jana M, Gupta AK. Skeletal dysplasias: a radiographic approach and review of common non-lethal skeletal dysplasias. *World J Radiol.* 2014;6(10):808–825.

63. Lew PP, Ngai SS, Hamidi R, et al. Imaging of disorders affecting the bone and skin. *Radiographics.* 2014;34(1):197–216.

64. Negi RS, Manchanda KL, Sanga S, Chand S, Goswami G. Osteopoikilosis – spotted bone disease. *Med J Armed Forces India.* 2013;69(2):196–198.

65. McDermott M, Branstetter BF, Seethala RR. Craniofacial melorheostosis. *J Comput Assist Tomogr.* 2008;32(5):825–827.

66. Clark MP, Pretorius PM, Byren I, Milford CA. Central or atypical skull base osteomyelitis: diagnosis and treatment. *Skull Base.* 2009;19(4):247–254.

67. Illing E, Zolotar M, Ross E, Olaleye O, Molony N. Malignant otitis externa with skull base osteomyelitis. *J Surg Case Rep.* 2011;2011(5):6.

68. Miyabe H, Uno A, Nakajima T, et al. A case of skull base osteomyelitis with multiple cerebral infarction. *Case Rep Otolaryngol.* 2016;2016:9252361.

69. Chan LL, Singh S, Jones D, Diaz Jr EM, Ginsberg LE. Imaging of mucormycosis skull base osteomyelitis. *AJNR Am J Neuroradiol.* 2000;21(5):828–831.

70. Ozgen B, Oguz KK, Cila A. Diffusion MR imaging features of skull base osteomyelitis compared with skull base malignancy. *AJNR Am J Neuroradiol.* 2011;32(1):179–184.

# CHAPTER 16

# Skull Base Bone Lesions II: Benign and Malignant Tumors

ALEXANDRA BORGES, MD

## INTRODUCTION

Most tumors affecting the skull base result from hematogenous spread of primary malignancies outside the skull base (hematogenous bone metastases) or from direct invasion or perineural spread of neoplasms arising from neighboring structures of the suprahyoid neck. As the skull base provides a frontier between the intracranial compartment and the extracranial head and neck, the first and most important issue in the differential diagnosis of a skull base lesion is to decide its site of origin: the bone elements of the skull base proper, the intracranial compartment, or the suprahyoid neck.[1]

With the exception of metastases, bone tumors of the skull base are overall rare and can be a diagnostic dilemma. When facing a bone tumor in the skull base, the same rules used for the differential diagnosis of skeletal tumors elsewhere in the body should be applied, taking into account the specificities of this anatomic location regarding tumor extent and treatment planning. Although imaging features can be quite helpful in the differential diagnosis, they are not very familiar to radiologists who do not routinely deal with skull base lesions and only a scant specific literature is available on this subject. This chapter specifically focuses on primary and secondary skull base bone tumors. For the imaging technique, general rules for the differential diagnosis, and developmental and diffuse skull base lesions, please refer to the previous chapter (Table 16.1).

## BONE TUMORS

Primary bone tumors encompass a variety of benign and malignant neoplasms. With the exception of osteomas and intraosseous hemangiomas in the benign category and metastases and multiple myeloma on the malignant side, other tumors are quite rare in the skull base. The imaging features of these primary and secondary bone tumors are similar to those of bone tumors arising in other sites of the skeleton, although the treatment and implications on patient's management derive from the specificities of this particular location. The imaging features of these lesions in the skull base are reviewed.

### Benign Tumors

These can be divided into bone-forming lesions, characterized by the presence of a variable amount of ossified osteoid matrix (such as osteoma, osteoid osteoma, osteoblastoma, and ossifying fibroma); cartilage-producing tumors characterized by a variable amount of chondroid matrix and, commonly, by the presence of chondroid-like calcifications (such as enchondroma, chondroma, chondroblastoma, and chondromyxoid fibroma); and bone tumors that produce neither osteoid nor chondroid matrix, although they may contain fragments of remaining trabecular bone inside.[2] The cellular component of these tumors is variable: osteoclast-like multinucleated giant cells, such as in giant cell lesions (giant cell tumor and brown tumors secondary to hyperparathyroidism); blood vessels and blood, such as in hemangiomas and in aneurysmal bone cysts; or abnormal proliferations of histiocytic cells, such as in eosinophilic granuloma.[3] In this last category, most lesions present as lytic, punched-out, bubbly lesions with variable matrix depending on their cell of origin.

### Bone-forming tumors

Although **osteomas** are rare, they are the most common benign primary skull base tumors, with an estimated prevalence of 0.4%–1%.[4] Most cases are sporadic, but the association with Gardner syndrome is well documented. They can arise from any bone, although they are most often encountered in the anterior skull base arising in or around the sinonasal cavities.[5] Their pathophysiology remains controversial. According to the embryologic theory, the most widely accepted, they

**TABLE 16.1**
**Simplified Classification of Bone Lesions of the Skull Base**

| BONE TUMORS | | | | |
|---|---|---|---|---|
| Primary | | | Osteosarcoma | |
| Benign | Osteoma | | Chondrosarcoma | |
| | Osteoid osteoma | Secondary | | |
| | Osteoblastoma | | Metastasis | |
| | Ossifying fibroma | | Lymphoma | |
| | Enchondroma/osteochondroma | | Leukemia (chloroma) | |
| | Chondroblastoma | **DIFFUSE BONE LESIONS** | | |
| | Chondromyxoid fibroma | | Fibrous dysplasia | |
| | Intraosseous hemangioma | | Paget disease | |
| | Aneurysmal bone cyst | | Osteopetrosis | |
| | Giant cell tumor/osteoclastoma | | Osteopoikilosis | |
| | Brown tumor | | Melorheostosis | |
| | Eosinophilic granuloma | | Infection (skull base osteomyelitis) | |
| Malignant | Metastasis | **MULTIFOCAL BONE LESIONS** | | |
| | Plasmacytoma/multiple myeloma | | Metastases | |
| | Lymphoma | | Multiple myeloma | |
| | Chloroma/granulocytic sarcoma | | Brown tumors | |
| | Ewing sarcoma | | Eosinophilic granulomas | |

arise from cartilaginous remnants in the junctional zone around the ethmoid labyrinth.[4]

These osteogenic tumors can be of cancellous or compact bone, the latter also called ivory osteomas.[6] They are often small lesions of no clinical significance, except for the potential obstruction of sinus ostia or infundibula with secondary development of mucoceles. Rarely, they can attain large dimensions, above 3 cm in size, and are then named giant osteomas.[6] These lesions can become large enough to protrude into the anterior cranial fossa or orbital contents and become symptomatic, requiring surgical correction.[5] On imaging, they are well-defined, sessile or pedunculated, sclerotic lesions, of compact or trabecular bone density/signal intensity (Figs. 16.1 and 16.2).

**Osteoid osteomas** are also exceedingly rare in the skull base with only a few cases reported in the literature, most affecting the anterior skull base, in or around the frontal or ethmoid sinuses.[7] Radiographically, these benign, slow-growing tumors are characterized by the presence of a radiolucent nidus, which may contain mineralized matrix, surrounded by reactive sclerosis. Large lesions, above 1.5 cm in size, are called giant osteoid osteoma or osteoblastoma and are featured by an increasing number of osteoclasts, a richly vascularized stroma, hemorrhage, and multinucleated giant cells responsible for a more heterogeneous imaging appearance with blood degradation products and enhancing septa.[8] When prominent, the sclerotic component of an osteoid osteoma may obscure the radiolucent nidus and hamper the diagnosis. In these circumstances the main differential diagnosis is with sclerosing forms of osteomyelitis (Brodie abscess), ossifying fibroma, fibrous dysplasia, and osteogenic osteosarcoma.[9] On bone scintigraphy (99mTc single-photon emission CT) the nidus of the lesion can be clearly identified as a "hot" zone, important information for surgery planning.[10]

These tumors are usually seen in the second and third decades and are more common in males. Small lesions in the skull base are often asymptomatic, as pain is not a prominent feature in this particular location. Clinical symptoms most often result from compression

Osteoma

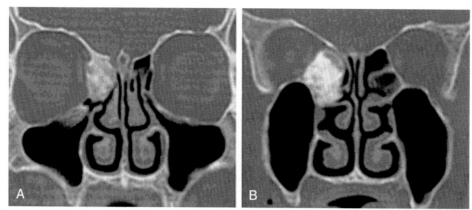

FIG. 16.1 Coronal CT images of the paranasal sinuses in bone windows (**A** and **B**) show a sclerotic lesion in the right ethmoid with a broad base in the medial wall of the orbit, obstructing the ethmoid air cells. The density of the lesion is similar to that of trabecular bone. Diagnosis: Osteoma of cancellous or spongiotic bone.

"Ivory" osteoma

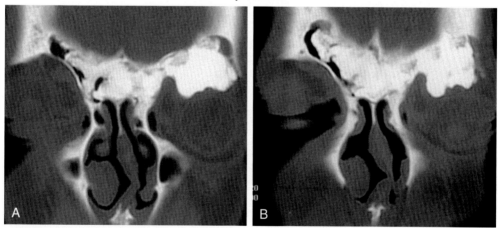

FIG. 16.2 CT of the paranasal sinus, coronal images on bone windows (**A** and **B**), show a lobulated sclerotic mass originating from the orbital plate of the frontal bone, filling in most of the frontal sinuses. On the left, the lesion protrudes into the superior orbital compartment, leading to downward displacement of the globe. The density of the lesion is similar to that of compact bone. Diagnosis: "Ivory" osteoma or osteoma of compact bone.

or displacement of adjacent structures, depending on their primary location within the skull base.

**Osteoblastoma** is a benign, osteoid-forming neoplasm, rich in osteoclasts, with a higher incidence in males, 90% occurring before 30 years of age and of rare occurrence in the skull base.[11] They are considered osteoid osteomas larger than 1.5 cm in size presenting, on imaging, as expansive, sharply circumscribed lesions, predominantly lytic but often with a mixed lytic-sclerotic pattern reflecting different degrees of osteoid production and matrix mineralization. Postcontrast images typically show enhancement of the tumor stroma as multiple enhancing septa. The growth pattern is geographic, with a peripheral sclerotic rim resembling an egg shell and remodeling adjacent bone[12] (Fig. 16.3). The association with aneurysmal bone cysts is a common occurrence featured by cystic areas with fluid-fluid levels.[12] Moreover, when large, areas of cortical disruption may ensue. Pathologically, two different forms of osteoblastoma have been recognized: benign and aggressive.[13] The latter is an exceedingly rare, locally aggressive, and destructive tumor with intermediate histologic features between benign osteoblastoma and osteosarcoma. A review of 71 skull base osteoblastomas has shown that the most common location is the temporal bone (36%), followed by the frontal bone (18%).[14] In this review, recurrence rates after surgery were 10% and 33% for gross total and subtotal resection, respectively, and higher, with an average of 57%, for the malignant counterpart.[14] However, gross total resection may be difficult for large skull base lesions and is associated with high morbidity.

**Ossifying fibroma** is a benign, locally aggressive bone-forming tumor of young children, most commonly seen under age 10 years (juvenile ossifying fibroma). These tumors belong to the spectrum of fibroosseous lesions, which range from nonossifying fibromas (fibrous cortical defect) to fibrous dysplasia.[15] Classification and nomenclature are confusing and a matter of controversy, including cementifying or cementoossifying fibroma, psammomatoid or juvenile ossifying fibroma, and ossifying fibromyxoid tumor.[16] Some authors consider these as separate entities, whereas others believe they are variants of the same entity. To further complicate the matter, there are hybrid fibroosseous lesions containing elements of aneurysmal bone cyst, ossifying fibroma, and cementifying fibroma.[15]

Osteoblatoma

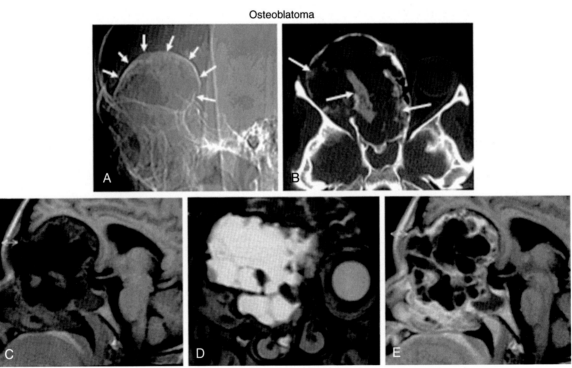

FIG. 16.3 CT images, sagittal topogram **(A)** and axial section in bone window **(B)** show an expansive, sharply circumscribed, predominantly lytic lesion, containing scattered areas of mineralized osteoid matrix (*arrows* in **B**) and a peripheral sclerotic rim resembling an "egg shell" (*arrows* in **A**). On MR, the lesion is heterogeneous in signal intensity, mostly hypointense on T1-weighted (T1W) images **(C)** and strikingly hyperintense on T2-weighted images **(D)**, with thin septa and hypointense flecks inside corresponding to the mineralized matrix on CT. After gadolinium administration (sagittal postcontrast T1W image) **(E)** there is marginal enhancement as well as enhancement of the internal septa. There is bone expansion and smooth remodeling featuring a slow-growing process. The lesion is centered in the anterior skull base involving the nasoethmoidal and orbital region extending posteriorly into the body of the sphenoid bone. Note the inferior displacement of the orbital contents and the mass effect upon the basal frontal lobe, without vasogenic brain edema. Diagnosis: Skull base osteoblastoma.

The conventional ossifying fibroma is a solitary, slow-growing lesion, which tends to be more aggressive in children.[17] The jaws, skull base, and temporal bone are the most common locations in the craniofacial region. Lesions in the pediatric age group are subdivided into psammomatoid and trabecular ossifying fibromas, the former featured by the presence of psammoma body islands (juvenile psammomatoid ossifying fibroma) and the latter by a clinically aggressive behavior (juvenile active ossifying fibroma).[17]

Clinical presentation depends on lesion location but is often by craniofacial deformity and compressive symptoms such as proptosis, nasal obstruction, and headache.

On plain films and CT imaging, ossifying fibroma presents as a well-circumscribed, often expansive, unilocular, osteolytic lesion with a sclerotic rim of variable thickness, reflecting an osteoblastic rimming, which may show a ground-glass appearance similar to fibrous dysplasia[18] (Figs. 16.4 and 16.5). On MRI, it shows low signal intensity on T1-weighted (T1W) images, intermediate to high signal intensity on T2-weighted (T2W) images, and moderate contrast enhancement. Differential diagnosis is mainly with fibrous dysplasia, osteoblastoma, aneurysmal bone cyst, giant cell tumor, and osteosarcoma. On pathology, tumors are composed of fibrocellular tissue and mineralized matrix in variable amounts.[15]

The best treatment option is wide, en bloc tumor resection, which is not always possible in the skull base. Recurrences are not uncommon, particularly after curettage or simple tumor enucleation.[17]

Ossifying fibroma

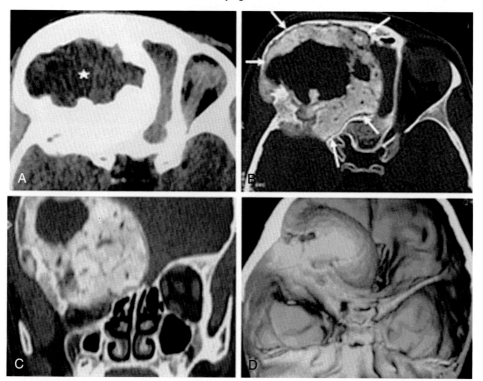

FIG. 16.4 CT of a 17-year-old boy with a rock hard supraorbital mass and proptosis: Axial sections in soft tissue **(A)**, axial **(B)** and coronal **(C)** sections in bone window, and 3D reconstruction **(E)** demonstrate an expansive lesion with a hypodense central core (*asterisk*) and a thick rim of ossified matrix, with a ground-glass appearance and geographic borders with adjacent bone (*arrows* in **B**). The lesion is centered in the anterior skull base at the orbital plate of the right frontal bone and lesser sphenoid wing and shows a striking mass effect upon the orbital contents **(C)** and in the floor of the anterior cranial fossa **(D)**. Diagnosis: Ossifying fibroma (juvenile ossifying fibroma).

Ossifying fibroma

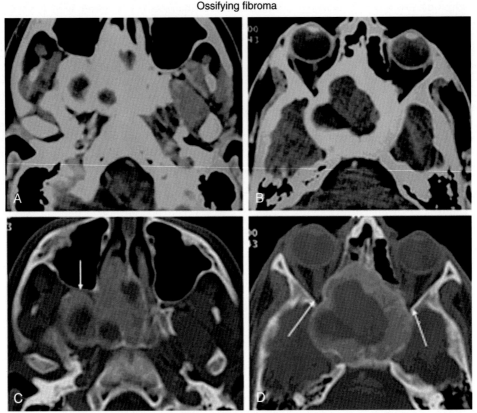

FIG. 16.5 CT scan in an 8-year-old boy with nasal obstruction. Axial soft tissue **(A and B)** and bone windows **(C and D)** show an expansive lesion located in the central skull base affecting the sphenoid body, pterygoid plates and posterior ethmoid complex, and nasal turbinates on the right side, with a central hypodense core and osteoblastic rimming with a ground-glass appearance. The lesion is well defined with geographic margins and causes a mass effect upon the pterygopalatine fossa on the right side (*arrow* in **C**) and orbital apex bilaterally (*arrows* in **D**). Diagnosis: Ossifying fibroma.

### Cartilage-forming tumors

**Chondroma, enchondroma, or osteochondroma** are relatively common benign cartilaginous neoplasms that may be sporadic or syndromic; the latter is associated with Ollier or Maffuci disease.[19] They are more commonly diagnosed in childhood and early adulthood, with a peak incidence between 10 and 30 years of age.[20] In the skull base, however, these tumors are exceedingly rare and may originate not only from chondrocytic cells in cranial sutures but also from the dura, brain parenchyma, ventricular system, and choroid plexus, resulting from chondroid metaplasia of immature embryonic cells.[20] From the few cases reported in the literature the most common location is the sphenoethmoid region and clivus, but they can occur in any bone originating from endochondral ossification.[21] In the skull base, they show a slight female predilection and are most often diagnosed in the third decade.[19] These slow-growing tumors are clinically silent and come to clinical attention only when they are large enough to produce neurologic symptoms, often related to cranial nerves' dysfunction or increased intracranial pressure. Biopsy is often misleading, as cytologic features suggest a more aggressive lesion (hypercellularity, anisocariosis, and nuclear hyperchromasia), and therefore, histologic analysis of the full specimen is mandatory to reach the final diagnosis.[22] On imaging, they are characterized by a narrow transition zone, well-defined scalloped margins, cortical expansion, presence of chondroid-type calcifications and absence of periosteal reaction, bone marrow or soft tissue edema, or soft tissue mass.[23]

Two different tumor types are recognized: type 1 is more homogeneous, isodense, or of mixed density with minimal to moderate enhancement and type 2 is characterized by the presence of a hypodense, cystic central core.[23] On MRI, lesions tend to be lobular and show intermediate to low signal intensity on T1W images and high to mixed signal intensity on T2W images depending on the variable amount of chondroid calcification. Occasionally, they may rupture the cortex and show an exophytic growth into the surrounding structures. Contrast enhancement is mainly peripheral and along the tumoral septa.[23] In the skull base the main differential diagnoses are with chondrosarcoma and other chondroid tumors, chordoma and meningioma.[19] On pathology, mature hyaline cartilage, variable amounts of calcifications, and a thick fibrous capsule are typical for this lesion. Immunostaining is positive for protein S100 and negative for cytokeratins and EMA (epithelial membrane antigen).

In the context of multiple enchondromatosis syndromes the diagnosis is usually straightforward and the risk of malignant degeneration into a chondrosarcoma is higher, particularly in Maffuci disease (25%–30% in Ollier disease and over 90% in Maffuci disease).[24] In other body locations, the presence of pain outside the context of a pathologic fracture is suspicious for malignant degeneration, but this rule is difficult to apply to the skull base.

**Chondroblastomas** are epiphyseal tumors of long bones, thought to arise from epiphyseal growth plates, subarticular in location and quite rare in the head and neck region.[2,25] In the skull base, the most common location is the temporal bone squamosa, accounting for its endochondral ossification. From there, tumors can grow into the middle cranial fossa, temporomandibular joint (TMJ), and middle ear cavity.[26] Clinical symptoms are often related to hearing and balance dysfunction, such as hearing loss, tinnitus, and otalgia, as well as swelling of the temporal fossa.[26] Seizures can also occur as a consequence of temporal lobe compression and cortical irritation. On imaging, these benign, locally aggressive tumors manifest as expansive lytic lesions, sharply delineated from the adjacent structures by a thin sclerotic rim, with a fuzzy and rarefied appearance, containing variable areas of calcification. On MRI, the tumor matrix tends to be hyperintense on T2W images, reflecting the presence of hyaline cartilage, with variable areas of low T1W and T2W signal intensity reflecting chondroid-like calcifications[27] (Fig. 16.6). Associated aneurysmal bone cysts are present in one-third of cases, shown as

expansive lytic areas with fluid-fluid levels. Adjacent synovitis with joint effusion in the adjacent TMJ, periosteal reaction, and bone marrow edema may also be seen.[28]

On imaging, the main differential diagnosis is with other expansive lytic lesions with a bubbly appearance, such as giant cell tumor, aneurysmal bone cyst, and hypervascular metastases, and with other lesions containing chondroid matrix, such as chondromyxoid fibroma and chondrosarcoma.[29] On pathology, chondroblastomas are composed of polyhedral chondroblasts, within a reticulin network showing pericellular calcifications in a typical "chicken wire" pattern.[30] Scattered osteoclast-like giant cells surround foci of chondroid matrix. Immunohistochemistry is mandatory for the differential diagnosis: chondroblastomas show immunopositivity for protein S100, whereas the main lesions to be considered in the differential, both on imaging and pathologic grounds, do not.[31] Although this is mainly a benign tumor, rare cases of malignant chondroblastomas have been reported.[32] In the skull base, radical excision with eventual bone grafting rather than curettage is the treatment of choice associated with a decreased incidence of tumor recurrence (43% in the former vs. 27% in the latter). In cases of incomplete resection, radiation therapy should be offered to these patients.[33]

**Chondromyxoid fibroma** is a rare, slow-growing, predominantly metaphyseal tumor, found in young adults in the second and third decades of life, being exceedingly rare in the craniofacial region, with only 67 cases described in the English literature.[34] Although this tumor is benign, it is often mistaken for a more aggressive lesion because of its infiltrative/destructive appearance, and it is prone to local recurrence when incompletely resected, a common occurrence in skull base lesions.[35] On CT, these tumors manifest as an osteolytic, lobulated, expansive lesion often surrounded by a sclerotic margin, occasionally with discrete calcification of the tumor matrix (seen in 25%–75% of cases), resembling a nonossifying fibroma.[34] On MR, they show low signal intensity on T1W and heterogenous contrast enhancement after gadolinium administration. When fibrous tissue predominates, lesions show low to intermediate signal intensity on T2W images, whereas when a chondroid or myxoid matrix is dominant, lesions are T2 hyperintense[36] (Fig. 16.7). The main differential diagnosis is with other myxoid tumors: chordoma, chondroid chordoma, and chondrosarcoma, which are much more commonly seen

Chondroblastoma

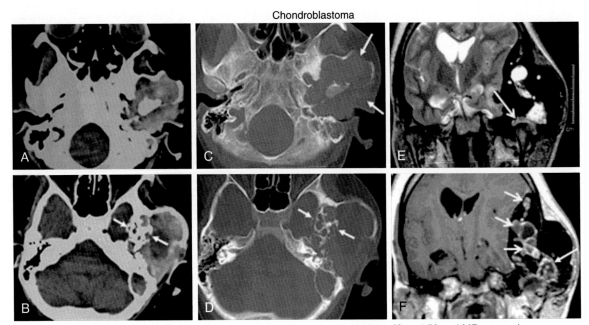

FIG. 16.6 CT axial sections in soft tissue (**A** and **B**) and bone windows (**C** and **D**) and MR, coronal T2-weighted image (**E**) and contrast-enhanced T1-weighted image show a large lesion with a lobulated contour, and a bubbly appearance, expanding and remodeling adjacent cortical bone. CT depicts areas of bone dehiscence (*arrows* in **B** and **C**) and, in the medial aspect, the lesion shows calcified matrix (*arrows* in **B** and **D**). On MR, there are multiple globular areas of high signal intensity inside the tumor mass reflecting foci of hyaline cartilage, with peripheral enhancement after gadolinium administration (*arrows* in **F**). Also note synovitis and effusion in the adjacent temporomandibular joint (*arrow* in **E**). The lesion is centered in the temporal bone and lateral aspect of the greater sphenoid wing, affecting the glenoid cavity of the temporomandibular joint, accounting for its subarticular origin. It extends medially into the middle ear cavity and mastoid and more anteriorly into the middle cranial fossa with an extensive mass effect upon the underlying temporal and frontal lobes, without signs of intradural invasion. Diagnosis: Chondroblastoma.

in the skull base.[37] Pathologically, chondromyxoid fibromas are characterized by the presence of lobules of spindle-shaped or stellate cells in a background of abundant myxoid or chondroid intercellular material, containing multinucleated giant cells.[35] Complete surgical resection is the treatment of choice, although often impossible in skull base tumors lying close to vital neurovascular structures. The benefit of postoperative radiation treatment for irresectable, residual, and recurrent disease is controversial.[37]

### *Tumors without osteoid or chondroid matrix*

**Intraosseous hemangiomas** are benign vascular lesions originating from the bone marrow. The most common locations are the vertebrae and calvaria, particularly the frontal and parietal bones, with skull base hemangiomas being exceedingly rare.[38] In the craniofacial

region, the maxilla, zygoma, vomer, and mandible are most commonly affected, and those lesions involving the orbital walls are called primary intraosseous orbital hemangiomas.[39] Hemangiomas have also been reported in the temporal bone, most often in the region of the geniculate fossa, and the main differential diagnosis is with facial nerve hemangiomas, which originate from the perineural vascular plexus rather than the petrous bone proper.[40] In the skull base, only 33 lesions have been reported so far, affecting the occipital condyle, sphenoorbital region, and greater sphenoid wing.[38]

Hemangiomas tend to be confined to the bone marrow cavity, with atypical or more aggressive hemangiomas having an associated soft tissue component. These are slow-growing, commonly asymptomatic lesions found incidentally on unrelated imaging

Chondromyxoid fibroma

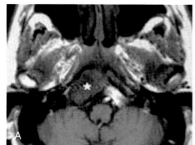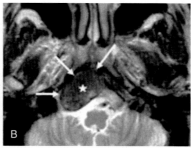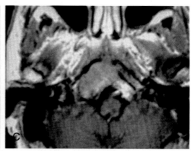

FIG. 16.7 MRI of the skull base, axial T1-weighted (T1W) **(A)**, T2-weighted (T2W) **(B)**, and postgadolinium T1W **(C)** images show an expansive lesion (*asterisks* in **A** and **B**) centered in the clivus with a sclerotic margin that is more prominent in the ventral aspect of the lesion (*arrows* in **B**). The lesion is hypointense on T1W and T2W images and shows moderate contrast enhancement. Diagnosis: Chondromyxoid fibroma with predominance of fibrous component (responsible for the low signal intensity on the T2W image).

studies, but occasionally, they can cause headaches and craniofacial symptoms secondary to compression of neighboring structures.[38] On CT imaging, they present as lytic lesions surrounded by a thin sclerotic rim. When these lesions contain coarse bony trabeculae, arranged from the center to the periphery, in a typical honeycomb/soap-bubble/sunburst pattern, they are called ossifying hemangiomas.[41] Hemangiomas can become large enough to expand and remodel cortical bone and lead to areas of dehiscence with associated soft tissue components. However, as opposed to osteogenic osteosarcomas, the periosteal lining tends to remain intact and the soft tissue component does not invade adjacent structures.[41] On MR, lesions are mottled in appearance, with variable signal intensity on T1W, often hyperintense on T2W and showing delayed, centripetal contrast-enhancement after gadolinium administration.[42] Areas of high signal intensity on T1W images reflect the presence of fatty marrow or fresh thrombus.[41]

In the skull base, they are often misdiagnosed for other more common lesions, and therefore the diagnosis is frequently made during exploratory surgery.

On pathology, depending on the type of vascular network, they are classified into capillary, cavernous, or venous hemangiomas and are composed of a tangle of endothelially lined vessels together with variable amounts of thrombus, fat, fibrous tissue, and smooth muscle.[43]

Treatment is required only for symptomatic lesions leading to mass effect or bleeding and includes embolization, sclerotherapy, surgical excision, and/or radiation therapy.[43]

**Aneurysmal bone cyst** is a lesion of uncertain etiology, composed of numerous blood-filled spaces without endothelial lining, separated by bone trabeculae, connective tissue, osteoid, and osteoclasts.[44] These lesions can be primary or secondary to other bone lesions such as osteoblastoma, chondroblastoma, fibrous dysplasia, giant cell tumor, and osteosarcoma and, therefore, they are often considered reactive lesions[12,45] (Fig. 16.3). Primary lesions are most often seen in young adults, around 80% before age 20 years. These lesions are rare in the craniofacial region; the most common location is the basisphenoid and paranasal sinuses. On imaging, the hallmark of this lesion is the presence of fluid-fluid levels, best appreciated on MRI owing to the sedimentation effect of blood degradation products, showing variable signal intensity. Lesions display a hemosiderin peripheral rim, hyperintense on both T1W and T2W images, with susceptibility artifact on T2* or susceptibility weighted imaging, and internal septa, which may enhance after gadolinium administration.[46] On CT, they present as a well-delineated, expansive, soap-bubbly multicystic lesion, with thin sclerotic margins without periosteal reaction unless complicated by fracture.[46] It should be noted, however, that many other lesions may show fluid-fluid levels, such as giant cell tumors, osteoblastoma, chondroblastoma, and osteosarcoma (particularly the telangiectatic subtype), just to mention the most common.[47] Treatment is by curettage or complete surgical resection when possible. Preoperative embolization may help reduce tumor size and decrease surgical bleeding.[48]

**Giant cell tumors or osteoclastomas** originate from nonosteogenic stromal cells within the bone marrow cavity. They are part of the spectrum of giant cell lesions that also include giant cell granulomas and brown tumors and result from an overproliferation of osteoclasts.[49] This is a tumor of adulthood more commonly seen between 20 and 50 years of age, after growth plate closure. In long bones, they are typically epiphyseal, are subarticular in location, and present clinically with pain and local swelling.[49] The most common locations in the skull base are the sphenoid and temporal bones. Associated symptoms result from direct involvement or compression of adjacent structures and therefore they depend on on the exact location of the lesion and its size.[50] Hearing loss and cranial nerve and TMJ dysfunction are among the most frequent symptoms. Pathologically, giant cell tumors are characterized by the presence of multinucleated giant cells, spindle-shaped mononuclear cells, cysts, and multiple vessels that are prone to hemorrhage, accounting for the presence of hemosiderin-laden macrophages responsible for the increased density of these lesions on plain CT scans.[51]

On imaging studies, giant cell tumors, appear as sharply marginated, scalloped, lytic lesions, expanding and remodeling cortical bone, sometimes leading to areas of bony dehiscence, without sclerotic rim and mineralized or calcified matrix. MR features are variable depending on the degree of hemorrhage and presence of aneurysmal bone cyst component, which can be clearly differentiated on contrast-enhanced T1W images: solid tumor components enhance strongly, whereas the cystic components show only faint peripheral enhancement after gadolinium administration. Spontaneously T1W hyperintensities may be seen and reflect the presence of subacute bleeding. T2W images can also be used to differentiate hyperintense cystic components, often with fluid-fluid levels from intermediate to hypointense solid tumor components.[51] A hypointense rim of hemosiderin is the rule blending with the cortical margin of the lesion (Fig. 16.8).

**Brown tumors** are indistinguishable, both histologically and on imaging, from other giant cell tumors.[52]

Giant cell tumor /osteoclastoma with an associated ABC

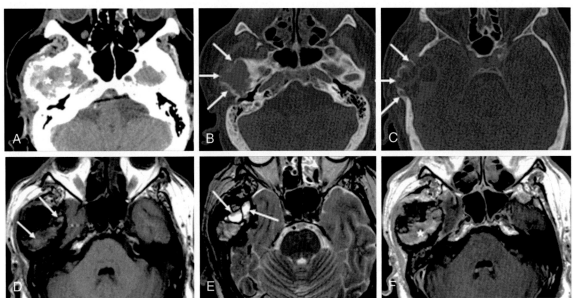

FIG. 16.8 CT axial sections in soft tissue **(A)** and bone window **(B and C)** show a lytic punched-out bone lesion (*asterisk* in **A**), with smooth lobulated remodeling of the cortical bone (*arrows* in **B** and **C**), centered in the lateral aspect of the greater sphenoid wing, lateral to the foramen ovale and temporal bone squamosa. The lesion is spontaneously hyperdense on CT and shows no mineralized matrix; on MRI, axial T1-weighted (T1W) **(D)**, T2-weighted (T2W) **(E)**, and postgadolinium T1W **(F)** images show variable signal intensity: predominantly hypointense on T1W showing foci of high signal intensity (*arrow* in **D**), with bright cystic areas on T2W with fluid-fluid levels suggesting aneurysmal bone cyst component (*arrows* in **E**) and areas of very low signal intensity at the tumor periphery, and demonstrating strong contrast enhancement after gadolinium administration (*asterisk* in **F**). Diagnosis: Giant cell tumor (osteoclastoma), with associated aneurysmal bone cyst.

Therefore, the diagnosis is based on serologic testing (serum levels of calcium and of parathyroid hormone). Imaging features are exactly the same as those described for giant cell tumors. Therefore, the hypothesis of brown tumors of hyperparathyroidism should always be a consideration, in particular, when multiple bone lesions are present. Further investigation of the neck, ideally by means of ultrasound imaging, may also be required to rule out a parathyroid adenoma (Fig. 16.9).

**Eosinophilic granulomas** are part of the spectrum of Langerhans histiocytosis and are the more localized form of the disease. These are benign proliferations of Langerhans cells that occur in the pediatric age, with a peak incidence between 2 and 4 years and exceedingly rare after age 30 years of age.[53] Involvement of the cranial vault and skull base account for over 50% of cases, with bilateral temporal bone lesions being a common presentation.[54] Local pain, swelling, and compressive symptoms of adjacent structures are the most common clinical presentations and depend on

lesion location. On CT imaging, the lesion manifests as a lytic punched-out lesion with serrated or beveled edges, without marginal sclerosis, associated with a spontaneously hyperdense, strongly enhancing soft tissue mass[54] (Fig. 16.10). On MR, lesions tend to be iso- to hypointense to muscle and slightly T2 hyperintense and demonstrate vivid contrast enhancement. The main differential diagnoses in this age group include rhabdomyosarcoma, leukemic infiltrates (chloroma), lymphoma, and metastatic neuroblastoma.[55] Pathology discloses the presence of Langerhans cells associated with an exuberant inflammatory infiltrate with eosinophilic predominance. The presence of Birbeck granules is virtually diagnostic and may be supported by protein S100 and CD1a antigen detection by immunohistochemistry.[54] For single localized lesions the best treatment option is complete surgical excision or radiation therapy. Local recurrence is not uncommon and tends to occur within 2 years after treatment. Therefore, long-term follow-up is advised to these patients.[56]

Brown tumor of hyperparathyroidism

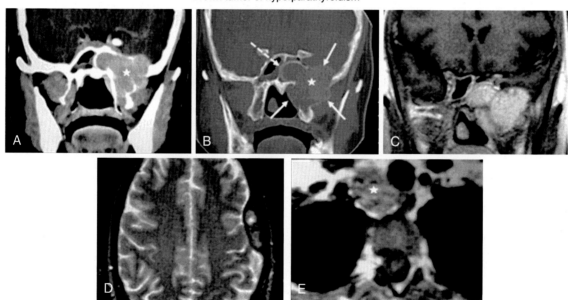

FIG. 16.9 CT and MR scan of a 52-year-old woman presenting with paresthesia of the right face. Coronal CT sections, contrast-enhanced soft tissue **(A)** and bone window demonstrate an expansive bone lesion centered at the base of the pterygoid plates, body of the sphenoid, and medial aspect of the greater sphenoid wing (*asterisks* in **A** and **B**), protruding medially into the sphenoid sinus (*dashed arrow* in **B**) with scalloped geographic margins and areas of cortical dehiscence (*arrows* in **B**) with no surrounding sclerosis or calcified matrix. Corresponding MR, contrast-enhanced coronal T1-weighted (T1W) **(C)** shows strong, homogeneous enhancement and axial T2-weighted **(D)** image discloses a second similar lesion in the left parietal calvarium. Axial T1W image through the infrahyoid neck **(E)** showed a well-defined oval-shaped enhancing lesion in the right paratracheal groove, posterior and inferior to the right thyroid lobe (*asterisk* in **E**). Diagnosis: Brown tumors secondary to a right inferior parathyroid adenoma (primary hyperparathyroidism).

Eosinophilic granuloma

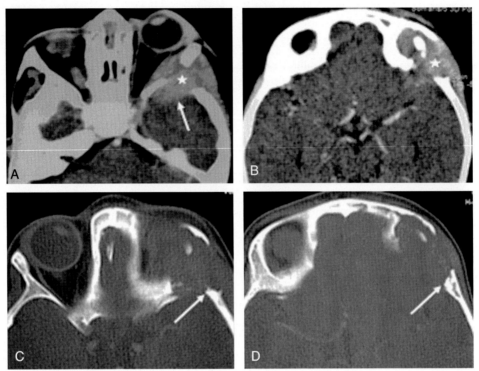

FIG. 16.10 CT on a 5-year-old girl with left-sided proptosis: axial section in soft tissue **(A** and **B)** and bone window **(C** and **D)** demonstrate a lytic punched-out lesion with beveled edges (*arrows* in **C** and **D**) with a strongly enhancing soft tissue component (*asterisks* in **A** and **B**). The lesion is centered at the sphenoid triangle and extends medially into the lateral extraconal orbital compartment, laterally into the temporal fossa and posteriorly into the middle cranial fossa, pushing the left temporal pole posteriorly (*arrow* in **A**). Diagnosis: Eosinophilic granuloma.

## Malignant Bone Tumors (Primary and Secondary)

Primary bone malignancies of the skull base are rare and include osteosarcoma, chondrosarcoma, and Ewing sarcoma. Plasmacytoma/multiple myeloma, lymphoma, leukemia (granulocytic sarcoma or chloroma), and hemangiosarcoma are only rarely primary to the skull base, with secondary involvement being far more common.[57] Metastatic disease from the hematogenous spread of a systemic primary cancer is, however, the most common skull base malignancy. Skull base involvement by direct invasion from nasopharyngeal cancer or perineural spread is beyond the scope of this chapter.

**Skull base metastasis** is the first cause of an aggressive tumoral lesion in the skull base. The most common primary tumors, in order of decreasing frequency, are the lung, breast, and prostate, although any other malignant histologies can metastasize to the skull base.[58] As metastatic bone disease results from hematogenous spread, marrow-rich bones, such as the clivus, petrous apex, and occipital condyles are primarily affected.[58] A skull base metastasis is only rarely the first sign of a systemic malignancy with the majority of patients already diagnosed with a primary tumor. Overall, skull base metastases are present in 4% of patients with cancer and skull metastasis in 15%–25%.[58] Over 90% of patients have skeletal metastases elsewhere. In the rare occasion of a solitary skull base metastasis, the most common primary tumors are renal cell and follicular thyroid cancer.[59] Clinical presentation is often by headache or cranial nerve deficits caused by involvement of neurovascular canals or foramina.

On imaging, skull base metastases can be lytic, sclerotic, or mixed. Morphologically, they can be further classified into focal, diffuse, or expansive (punched

Sclerotic metastasis from prostate cancer

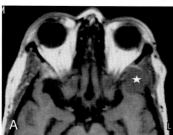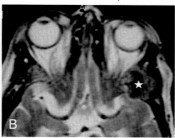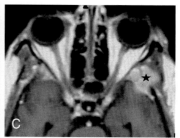

FIG. 16.11 A 67-year-old patient with prostate cancer. MRI of the brain demonstrates an irregularly shaped, expansive lesion centered at the right sphenoid triangle (*asterisks*) with low to intermediate signal intensity on T1-weighted (T1W) **(A)** and T2-weighted **(B)** images and with vivid, homogeneous enhancement on postgadolinium T1W images **(C)**. Diagnosis: Sclerotic bone metastasis from prostate cancer. The main differential diagnosis is with intradiploic meningioma and osteogenic osteosarcoma.

out). **Sclerotic metastases** are primarily associated with prostate and breast cancer, transitional cell carcinoma, carcinoid, medulloblastoma, neuroblastoma, mucinous colorectal adenocarcinoma, and lymphoma.[60] The sclerotic morphology can be secondary to reactive bone formation incited by the presence of the tumor mass or to bone formation inside the tumor stroma itself.

On CT, they present as ill-defined sclerotic lesions that may be confined to the trabecular bone or affect both trabecular and cortical bone. When large, they tend expand and transgress the cortical margins and may show an associated soft tissue mass. On MR, they are characterized by low signal intensity on T1W images, variable but predominantly low signal intensity on T2W images, and enhancement after gadolinium administration[61] (Fig. 16.11). They are fludeoxyglucose (FDG) avid on FDG-PET and show increased activity on bone scintigraphy. These imaging features, in the appropriate clinical setting, are often diagnostic of metastatic bone disease.[62] The main differential diagnosis of sclerotic bone metastasis includes sclerotic bone dysplasias, Paget disease, intradiploic meningiomas, osteogenic osteosarcoma, bone infarcts, and chronic osteomyelitis. **Osteolytic metastases** manifest by ill-defined discrete lytic lesions that may be limited to the trabecular bone or by larger lesions eroding the cortical bone. Cortical disruption, bone expansion, and associated soft tissue mass may all be present (Fig. 16.12). This morphology is the most common and is secondary to enzymatic bone destruction or caused by activation of osteoclasts incited by the tumor mass. Owing to the lack of osteoblastic activity, lytic metastases do not show an increased activity on bone scintigraphy.[60] On MRI, they are often hypointense

on T1W images and hyperintense on T2W images and STIR and show contrast enhancement with a tendency to follow the signal characteristics of the primary tumor (Fig. 16.13). Differential diagnosis is mainly with multiple myeloma/plasmacytoma and, when centered in the clivus or petroclival region, chordoma and chondrosarcoma.[61] Of particular note are hypervascular metastases, which tend to present as lytic, expansive, punched-out lesions, often containing vascular flow voids and enhancing vividly after gadolinium administration.[58] Differential diagnosis is with other hypervascular lesions. Depending on the location they may be mistaken for a paraganglioma, hemangiopericytoma, or a juvenile nasopharyngeal angiofibroma. The most common primaries are the thyroid, renal cell cancer, pheochromocytoma, Wilm tumor, melanoma, Ewing sarcoma, gastrointestinal and gynecologic cancers, and squamous cell cancer. **Mixed metastasis** shows features of both lytic and sclerotic metastasis, and the most common primaries are the breast, lung, cervix, and testicular carcinoma and prostate cancer.

An important clue in the differential diagnosis, particularly with osteosarcoma, is the absence of periosteal reaction outside the setting of a pathologic fracture. The few metastases that may elicit periosteal reaction are from prostate cancer, medulloblastoma, and retinoblastoma.[58]

The second most common malignant skull base lesion in adults is **multiple myeloma**. These lesions are composed of monoclonal proliferations of immunoglobulin-secreting plasma cells originating from the bone marrow, are more common in older patients, and have a male predominance.[63] When solitary, they are called **plasmacytoma**. These lesions, together with lymphoma, chloroma, Ewing

Osteolytic metastasis from colon cancer

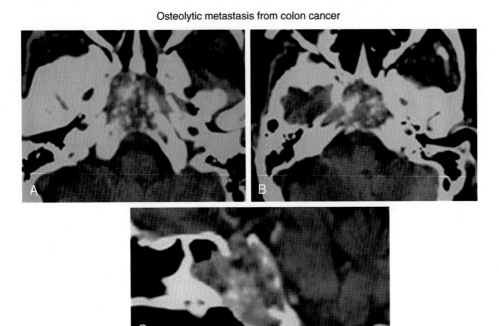

FIG. 16.12 Axial CT sections **(A** and **B)** and sagittal reconstruction **(C)** demonstrate a lytic lesion of the clivus and petrous apices, with an aggressive, permeative pattern of bone destruction showing fragments of trabecular bone inside, in a 54-year-old patient presenting with headache and VI nerve palsy. In this case, this single lytic metastasis was the first presentation of a colon cancer and the main differential considerations include clival chordoma, chondrosarcoma, and plasmacytoma/multiple myeloma.

Osteolytic metastasis from testicular choriocarcinoma

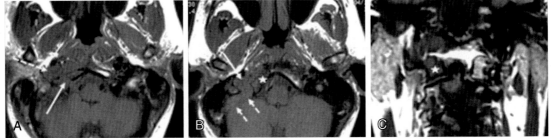

FIG. 16.13 MR axial **(A** and **B)** and coronal **(C)** T1-weighted images in a 23-year-old man with choriocarcinoma presenting with lower cranial nerve palsy (Collet-Sicard syndrome) show an ill-defined lesion in the right side of the clivus and lateral mass of C1 (*asterisks* in **B** and **C**), involving the jugular foramen (*arrow* in **B**), condylar canal (*arrow* in **A**), and sigmoid sinus (*dashed arrows* in **B**). The fatty bone marrow is replaced by a soft tissue mass of intermediate signal intensity, and there are areas of cortical bone erosion and associated soft tissue mass filling in the sigmoid sinus and extending, inferiorly, along the retrostyloid parapharyngeal space (*dashed arrow* in **A**). Diagnosis: Skull base metastasis from choriocarcinoma.

sarcoma, and metastatic neuroblastoma, belong to the category of small round cell tumors featured by hypercellularity, scant cytoplasm, and large nuclei, accounting for spontaneous hyperdensity on plain CT images, intermediate signal intensity on T1W images, intermediate to low signal intensity on T2W images, and restricted diffusion on diffusion-weighted imaging (DWI), with mean apparent diffusion coefficient values under $1.0 \times 10^{-3}\,\text{mm}^2/\text{s}$. The typical imaging appearance is that of a lytic punched-out lesion with

Skull base plasmacytoma

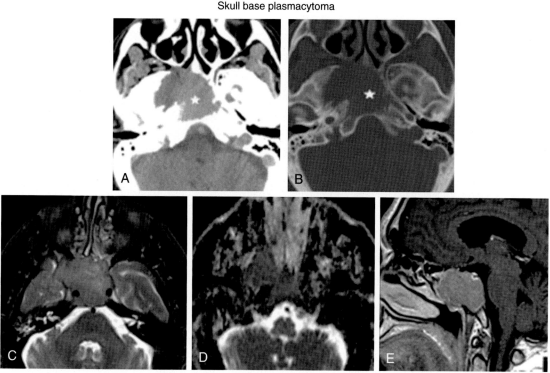

FIG. 16.14 CT of the skull base, axial sections in soft tissue **(A)** and bone windows **(B)** show a large punched-out lytic lesion (*asterisks* in **A** and **B**), homogeneous and spontaneously hyperdense on the plain soft tissue image (isodense with the blood inside the basilar artery and jugular foramen), centered in the clivus and greater sphenoid wing. On the corresponding MR, the lesion is hypointense on the T2-weighted image **(C)** and shows restricted diffusion with low signal intensity on the apparent diffusion coefficient map **(D)** and strong homogenous contrast enhancement on the postgadolinium sagittal T1-weighted image **(E)**. Diagnosis: Plasmacytoma.

no surrounding sclerosis. Moderate to intense homogeneous contrast enhancement is seen on both CT and MRI[64] (Fig. 16.14). On bone scintigraphy, these lesions are photopenic.[65] Treatment is with radiation therapy, with surgical resection reserved for lesions causing neurologic compromise. Close follow-up is needed, as local recurrences occur in 10% and progression to multiple myeloma occurs in 10%–30% of patients.[64]

Primary bone involvement of the skull base by **lymphoma** is exceedingly rare, accounting for 1%–2% of all skull base tumors and with only 30 cases described in the literature.[66] Most often, skull base involvement is secondary to direct invasion by a neighboring primary lesion, arising from the nasopharynx, sinonasal region, or orbit (Fig. 16.15), or associated with disseminated lymphoma, the latter more commonly seen in children.[67] The diagnosis

of **primary bone lymphoma** requires isolated focal or multifocal bone involvement without systemic disease at least until 6 months after the initial diagnosis.[68] Diffuse large B-cell lymphoma is the most common subtype. On imaging, bone involvement by lymphoma has no specific features and may show lytic, sclerotic, or mixed lesions. However, the most common imaging appearance is that of an ill-defined lytic lesion, with a permeative pattern of bone destruction, a wide transition zone to normal bone, cortical breaching, and associated soft tissue mass.[66] On MR, there is replacement of the fatty bone marrow by an expansive soft tissue mass of intermediate signal intensity on T1W images, low to intermediate signal intensity on T2W images, avid homogenous contrast enhancement, and restricted diffusion on DWI. The main differential diagnosis depends on the exact location but is mainly with eosinophilic

Non-hodgkin lymphoma

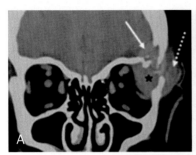 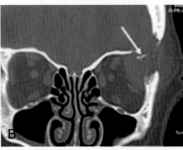 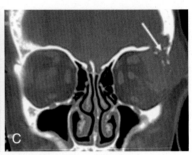

FIG. 16.15 CT of the orbits, plain coronal section in soft tissue **(A)** and bone windows **(B** and **C)** show a spontaneously hyperdense soft tissue mass (*asterisk* in **A**) involving the lacrimal gland fossa at the superolateral compartment of the left orbit with a permeative pattern of bone destruction and with fragments of bone engulfed in the lesion, featuring a rapidly growing mass (*arrows* in **B** and **C**). Superiorly the lesion extends into the anterior cranial fossa (*arrow* in **A**) and laterally into the temporal fossa (*dashed arrow* in **A**). Diagnosis: Lymphoma.

granuloma, Ewing sarcoma, chordoma, and metastatic neuroblastoma.[69] Treatment is with R-CHOP and proton beam radiation therapy.

**Chloroma**, granulocytic sarcoma, or extramedullary myeloblastoma of the skull base is uncommon. These tumors are composed of immature granulocytic cell precursors called myeloblasts and, most often, are associated with acute or chronic myeloid leukemia or other myeloproliferative disorders. The skin and bone are the most common locations, and bone involvement most often affects the skull, face, orbit, and paranasal sinuses. On imaging, they present as homogeneous soft tissue masses with features that are similar to other round cell tumors. In the clinical setting the diagnosis is usually straightforward[70] (Fig. 16.16).

**Osteosarcoma** is the second most frequent primary bone tumor in adults, after multiple myeloma, and the most common in children. A bimodal peak incidence is seen at the second and sixth decades, reflecting two different types of osteosarcomas: primary osteosarcomas, most often seen in children and young adults, between 10 and 20 years of age, and secondary osteosarcomas, seen in older patients and associated with malignant degeneration of Paget disease, extensive bone infarcts, or radiation therapy of a previous lesion.[71] Those occurring in the skull base are most often secondary either to Paget disease or to prior radiation treatment.

These bone-forming tumors show a variably ossified/calcified osteoid tumor matrix, which affects their imaging appearance: lytic, sclerotic, or mixed. On CT,

they manifest as aggressive permeative lesions with medullary and cortical bone destruction and a malignant type of periosteal reaction, often sunburst, air-on-end, or Codman triangle.[72] Extensively sclerotic neoplasms may mimic an intradiploic meningioma or a sclerotic bone metastasis (Fig. 16.17). MRI is the modality of choice to evaluate the full extent of lesions and shows variegated heterogeneous signal intensities reflecting the presence of ossified and nonossified tumor matrix, hemorrhages, calcifications, and peritumoral edema[72] (Fig. 16.18). Treatment is ideally with wide surgical excision. Radiation therapy is recommended for residual disease.

**Primary Ewing sarcoma** of the skull base is exceedingly rare, with metastatic disease to the skull base being much more common.[73] It is the second most common primary bone malignancy in children after osteosarcoma, with 95% of tumors diagnosed between 4 and 25 years of age. It is part of the spectrum of the primitive neuroectodermal tumors, hypercellular lesions composed of small blue round cells, originating from the medullary cavity and spreading along the Haversian canals. Only 2% of lesions occur in the craniofacial bones. On CT, they show as permeative, destructive, ill-defined lytic lesions, often with large soft tissue components lacking bone matrix. Periosteal reaction is often present with variable appearance: thick, laminated, or onion skin; Codman triangle; or a spiculated, sunburst, aggressive pattern.[74] When affecting flat bones, 30% are sclerotic. On MRI, lesions show low signal intensity on T1W images and prominent heterogeneous

Granulocytic sarcoma/ chloroma

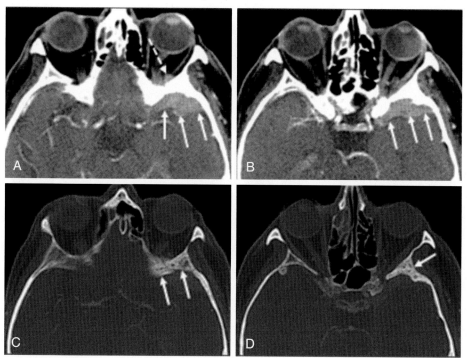

FIG. 16.16 A 19-year-old boy with chronic myelocytic leukemia. CT scan, postcontrast axial sections on soft tissue **(A** and **B)** and bone windows **(C** and **D)** show a homogeneous soft tissue mass centered at the sphenoid triangle with a small component in the posterior extraconal compartment of the orbit (*dashed arrow* in **A**) and a larger component in the middle cranial fossa indenting the anterior temporal pole (*arrows* in **A** and **B**). Bone windows show associated mixed lytic sclerotic changes in the sphenoid triangle (*arrows* in **C** and **D**). Diagnosis: Chloroma (granulocytic sarcoma).

Osteogenic osteosarcoma

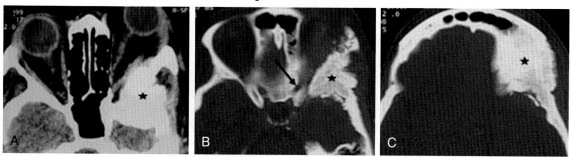

FIG. 16.17 CT of the skull base on a 15-year-old boy with left-sided proptosis and decreased vision. Axial sections on soft tissue **(A)** and bone windows **(B** and **C)** show a large expansive, ill-defined, sclerotic lesion centered in the sphenoid triangle, with an air-on-end, sunburst pattern of periosteal reaction (*asterisks*). The lesion affects the lateral and superior orbital walls and the lateral aspect of the greater sphenoid wing and extends posteriorly to the orbital apex (*arrow* in **B**). Marked proptosis is also seen. Diagnosis: Primary osteogenic osteosarcoma.

Chondroblastic osteosarcoma

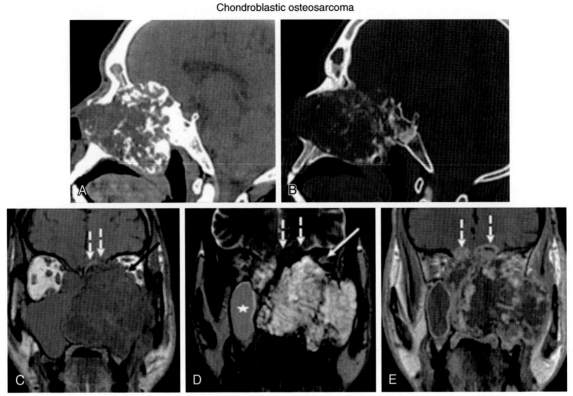

FIG. 16.18 CT of the paranasal sinuses and skull base in a 23-year-old man, sagittal reconstructions on soft tissue **(A)** and bone window **(B)** demonstrate a large expansive lesion in the sinonasal region involving the anterior and central skull base, invading the left orbit (*arrows* in **C** and **D**) and the anterior cranial fossa with no evidence of dural transgression (*dashed arrows* in **C**, **D**, and **E**). The lesion shows mineralized osteoid matrix and multiple coarse, chondroid-like calcifications. On MRI, coronal T1-weighted (T1W) **(C)**, T2-weighted (T2W) **(D)**, and postgadolinium T1W images, the lesion is markedly heterogeneous, showing low to intermediate signal intensity on T1W with areas of high signal intensity and high signal intensity on T2W, with irregular areas of signal void and inhomogeneous contrast enhancement, predominantly at the periphery and surrounding the mineralized foci. T2W images clearly discriminate the tumor from the postobstructive changes in the right maxillary sinus (*asterisk* in **D**). Diagnosis: Chondroblastic osteosarcoma.

enhancement and heterogenous signal intensity on T2W images, often with linear bands of low signal intensity providing a striated pattern[74]. Metastatic disease is primarily to bone and lungs. Treatment with adjuvant systemic chemotherapy and radiation therapy after surgical excision has improved the prognosis of these patients.[75]

**Chondrosarcoma** is a malignant tumor of the hyaline cartilage. In the skull base, these tumors originate from skull base synchondrosis, 75% from the petroclival and 20% from the spheno-vomerian synchondrosis.[76] Most often they are sporadic, but a few cases are secondary to Ollier and Maffuci syndromes. On MRI, they manifest as expansive lesions with a lobulated contour, with low signal intensity on T1W images and very bright signal intensity on T2W images, often higher than that of cerebrospinal fluid, accounting for the presence of hyaline cartilage. Focal punctate areas of signal void can be seen is 50% of cases, reflecting the presence of chondroid-like calcifications, which are best depicted on CT and are an important hallmark of this tumor[77] (Fig. 16.19). The paramedian location is useful in the differential diagnosis with chordoma, which is typically midline in location.[77] Petroclival

Petro-clival chondrosarcoma

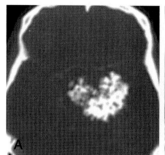
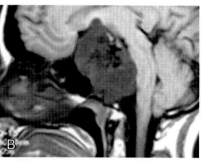
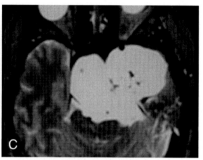

FIG. 16.19 CT of the brain, axial section in bone window **(A)** shows an expansive lesion in the left parasagittal central skull base with a lobulated contour and extensive coarse chondroid-like calcifications. On corresponding MR, sagittal T1-weighted image **(B)** the lesion shows low signal intensity with speckled areas of low and high signal intensity, and on the axial T2-weighted image **(C)** the lesion is strikingly hyperintense, more so than cerebrospinal fluid, with speckled areas of signal void, corresponding to the chondroid calcifications, obscured by the bright signal reflecting hyaline cartilage. Diagnosis: Large petro-clival chondrosarcoma.

chondrosarcomas often present with cranial nerve V and VI palsies because of involvement of Dorello canal and Meckel cave, respectively.[1] Wide surgical resection is the treatment modality of choice, as these slow-growing lesions are not very sensitive to radiation therapy.

Malignant vascular tumors of the skull base are a rarity, with a single report of an angiosarcoma (high-grade hemangioendotheliomas) in the English literature. This lesion, described in a 12-month-old child, was located in the basisphenoid and showed extensive bone destruction on CT and vivid arterial-like enhancement after gadolinium administration on MRI, with no other distinctive features.[78]

## SUMMARY

Bone lesions of the skull base encompass a wide variety of benign and malignant lesions. CT and MR have a complementary role in refining the diagnosis and, particularly, in fully characterizing bony skull base lesions. Most frequently the skull base is affected by secondary bone lesions. Primary bone tumors of the skull base are rare, and their imaging features are, overall, similar to those seen elsewhere in the skeleton. Even when benign, tumors may recur when not completely removed. Remember that benign lesions can have an aggressive appearance and that malignant lesions can look misleadingly benign. Therefore, radiologic-pathologic correlation is often mandatory to reach a final diagnosis.

## REFERENCES

1. Borges A. Skull base tumours part II. Central skull base tumours and intrinsic tumours of the bony skull base. *Eur J Radiol.* 2008;66(3):348–362.
2. Helms C. *Fundamentals of skeletal radiology.* 3rd ed. Philadelphia, Pennsylvania: Elsevier, Saunders; 2005.
3. Mintz DN, Hwang S. Bone tumor imaging, then and now: review article. *HSS J.* 2014;10(3):230–239.
4. Georgalas C, Goudakos J, Fokkens WJ. Osteoma of the skull base and sinuses. *Otolaryngol Clin N Am.* 2011;44(4). 875–890, vii.
5. McHugh JB, Mukherji SK, Lucas DR. Sino-orbital osteoma: a clinicopathologic study of 45 surgically treated cases with emphasis on tumors with osteoblastoma-like features. *Arch Pathol Lab Med.* 2009;133(10):1587–1593.
6. Adeleye AO. A giant, complex fronto-ethmoidal ivory osteoma: surgical technique in a resource-limited practice. *Surg Neurol Int.* 2010;1:97.
7. Grayeli AB, Redondo A, Sterkers O. Anterior skull base osteoid osteoma: case report. *Br J Neurosurg.* 1998;12(2): 173–175.
8. Musluman AM, Oba E, Yilmaz A, Kabukcuoglu F, Uysal E. Giant osteoid osteoma of the ethmoid bone with unusual large nidus. *J Neurosci Rural Pract.* 2012;3(3):383–385.
9. Chai JW, Hong SH, Choi JY, et al. Radiologic diagnosis of osteoid osteoma: from simple to challenging findings. *Radiographics.* 2010;30(3):737–749.
10. Murari SB, Sujith N, Ranadheer M, Sekhar PC, Kumari PA, Rao VP. Nidus localization in osteod osteoma by SPECT skeletal scintigraphy: aid to diagnosis and surgical approach. *Indian J Nucl Med.* 2010;25(1):16–19.

11. Pelargos PE, Nagasawa DT, Ung N, et al. Clinical characteristics and diagnostic imaging of cranial osteoblastoma. *J Clin Neurosci.* 2015;22(3):445–449.

12. Wang YC, Huang JS, Wu CJ, Jeng CM, Fan JK, Resnick D. A huge osteoblastoma with aneurysmal bone cyst in skull base. *Clin Imaging.* 2001;25(4):247–250.

13. Lucas DR. Osteoblastoma. *Arch Pathol Lab Med.* 2010; 134(10):1460–1466.

14. Pelargos PE, Nagasawa DT, Ung N, et al. A systematic review of skull base osteoblastoma: clinical features, treatment, and outcomes. *J Neurol Surg.* 2015. http://dx.doi.org/10.1055/s-0035-1546685.

15. Eversole R, Su L, ElMofty S. Benign fibro-osseous lesions of the craniofacial complex. A review. *Head Neck Pathol.* 2008;2(3):177–202.

16. Bohn OL, Kalmar JR, Allen CM, Kirsch C, Williams D, Leon ME. Trabecular and psammomatoid juvenile ossifying fibroma of the skull base mimicking psammomatoid meningioma. *Head Neck Pathol.* 2011;5(1):71–75.

17. Barrena Lopez C, Bollar Zabala A, Urculo Bareno E. Cranial juvenile psammomatoid ossifying fibroma: case report. *J Neurosurg Pediatr.* 2016;17(3):318–323.

18. Mohsenifar Z, Nouhi S, Abbas FM, Farhadi S, Abedin B. Ossifying fibroma of the ethmoid sinus: report of a rare case and review of literature. *J Res Med Sci.* 2011;16(6):841–847.

19. Hongo H, Oya S, Abe A, Matsui T. Solitary osteochondroma of the skull base: a case report and literature review. *J Neurol Surg Rep.* 2015;76(1):e13–e17.

20. Padhya TA, Athavale SM, Kathju S, Sarkar S, Mehta AR. Osteochondroma of the skull base. *Otolaryngol Head Neck Surg.* 2007;137(1):166–168.

21. Inwards CY. Update on cartilage forming tumors of the head and neck. *Head Neck Pathol.* 2007;1(1):67–74.

22. de Andrea CE, Kroon HM, Wolterbeek R, et al. Interobserver reliability in the histopathological diagnosis of cartilaginous tumors in patients with multiple osteochondromas. *Mod Pathol.* 2012;25(9):1275–1283.

23. Murphey MD, Choi JJ, Kransdorf MJ, Flemming DJ, Gannon FH. Imaging of osteochondroma: variants and complications with radiologic-pathologic correlation. *Radiographics.* 2000;20(5):1407–1434.

24. Burgetova A, Matejovsky Z, Zikan M, et al. The association of enchondromatosis with malignant transformed chondrosarcoma and ovarian juvenile granulosa cell tumor (Ollier disease). *Taiwan J Obstet Gynecol.* 2017;56(2):253–257.

25. Liu J, Ahmadpour A, Bewley AF, Lechpammer M, Bobinski M, Shahlaie K. Chondroblastoma of the clivus: case report and review. *J Neurol Surg Rep.* 2015;76(2):e258–e264.

26. Moorthy RK, Daniel RT, Rajshekhar V, Chacko G. Skull base chondroblastoma: a case report. *Neurol India.* 2002;50(4):534–536.

27. Douis H, Saifuddin A. The imaging of cartilaginous bone tumours. I. Benign lesions. *Skelet Radiol.* 2012;41(10):1195–1212.

28. Blancas C, Llauger J, Palmer J, Valverde S, Bague S. Imaging findings in chondroblastoma. *Radiologia.* 2008;50(5):416–423.

29. Lui YW, Dasari SB, Young RJ. Sphenoid masses in children: radiologic differential diagnosis with pathologic correlation. *AJNR Am J Neuroradiol.* 2011;32(4):617–626.

30. Eisenberg RL. Bubbly lesions of bone. *AJR Am J Roentgenol.* 2009;193(2):W79–W94.

31. Forest M, De Pinieux G. Chondroblastoma and its differential diagnosis. *Ann Pathol.* 2001;21(6):468–478.

32. Posl M, Werner M, Amling M, Ritzel H, Delling G. Malignant transformation of chondroblastoma. *Histopathology.* 1996;29(5):477–480.

33. Lin PP, Thenappan A, Deavers MT, Lewis VO, Yasko AW. Treatment and prognosis of chondroblastoma. *Clin Orthop Relat Res.* 2005;438:103–109.

34. Yaghi NK, DeMonte F. Chondromyxoid fibroma of the skull base and calvarium: surgical management and literature review. *J Neurol Surg Rep.* 2016;77(1):e023–e034.

35. D'Andrea G, Pesce A, Trasimeni G, et al. Chondromyxoid fibroma of the skull base: our experience with an elusive disease. *J Neurol Surg A Cent Eur Neurosurg.* 2017 Mar 2. http://dx.doi.org/10.1055/s-0037-1599137.

36. Crocker M, Corns R, Bodi I, Zrinzo A, Gleeson M, Thomas N. Chondromyxoid fibroma of the skull base invading the occipitocervical junction: report of a unique case and discussion. *Skull Base.* 2010;20(2):101–104.

37. Feuvret L, Noel G, Calugaru V, Terrier P, Habrand JL. Chondromyxoid fibroma of the skull base: differential diagnosis and radiotherapy: two case reports and a review of the literature. *Acta Oncol.* 2005;44(6):545–553.

38. Yang Y, Guan J, Ma W, et al. Primary intraosseous cavernous hemangioma in the skull. *Medicine.* 2016; 95(11):e3069.

39. Madge SN, Simon S, Abidin Z, et al. Primary orbital intraosseous hemangioma. *Ophthal Plast Reconstr Surg.* 2009;25(1):37–41.

40. Semaan MT, Slattery WH, Brackmann DE. Geniculate ganglion hemangiomas: clinical results and long-term follow-up. *Otol Neurotol.* 2010;31(4):665–670.

41. Politi M, Romeike BF, Papanagiotou P, et al. Intraosseous hemangioma of the skull with dural tail sign: radiologic features with pathologic correlation. *AJNR Am J Neuroradiol.* 2005;26(8):2049–2052.

42. Moore SL, Chun JK, Mitre SA, Som PM. Intraosseous hemangioma of the zygoma: CT and MR findings. *AJNR Am J Neuroradiol.* 2001;22(7):1383–1385.

43. George A, Mani V, Noufal A. Update on the classification of hemangioma. *J Oral Maxillofac Pathol.* 2014;18(suppl 1):S117–S120.

44. Goyal A, Rastogi S, Singh PP, Sharma S. Aneurysmal bone cyst at the base of the skull. *Ear Nose Throat J.* 2012;91(5):E7–E9.

45. Terkawi AS, Al-Qahtani KH, Baksh E, Soualmi L, Mohamed Ael B, Sabbagh AJ. Fibrous dysplasia and aneurysmal bone cyst of the skull base presenting with blindness: a report of a rare locally aggressive example. *Head Neck Oncol.* 2011;3:15.

46. Lin SP, Fang YC, Chu DC, Chang YC, Hsu CI. Characteristics of cranial aneurysmal bone cyst on computed tomography and magnetic resonance imaging. *J Formos Med Assoc.* 2007;106(3):255–259.

47. Nabavizadeh SA, Bilaniuk LT, Feygin T, Shekdar KV, Zimmerman RA, Vossough A. CT and MRI of pediatric skull lesions with fluid-fluid levels. *AJNR Am J Neuroradiol.* 2014;35(3):604–608.

48. Tsagozis P, Brosjo O. Current strategies for the treatment of aneurysmal bone cysts. *Orthop Rev.* 2015;7(4):6182.

49. Sobti A, Agrawal P, Agarwala S, Agarwal M. Giant cell tumor of bone – an overview. *Arch Bone Jt Surg.* 2016;4(1):2–9.

50. Wang Y, Honda K, Suzuki S, Ishikawa K. Giant cell tumor at the lateral skull base. *Am J Otolaryngol.* 2006;27(1):64–67.

51. Chakarun CJ, Forrester DM, Gottsegen CJ, Patel DB, White EA, Matcuk Jr GR. Giant cell tumor of bone: review, mimics, and new developments in treatment. *Radiographics.* 2013;33(1):197–211.

52. Al-Gahtany M, Cusimano M, Singer W, Bilbao J, Kovacs K, Marotta T. Brown tumors of the skull base. Case report and review of the literature. *J Neurosurg.* 2003;98(2):417–420.

53. Dalili H, Dalili Kajan Z. Eosinophilic granuloma of the skull base: patient with unique clinical moreover, radiographic presentation. *Acta Med Iran.* 2015;53(1):69–73.

54. Kaul R, Gupta N, Gupta S, Gupta M. Eosinophilic granuloma of skull bone. *J Cytol.* 2009;26(4):156–157.

55. D'Ambrosio N, Soohoo S, Warshall C, Johnson A, Karimi S. Craniofacial and intracranial manifestations of Langerhans cell histiocytosis: report of findings in 100 patients. *AJR Am J Roentgenol.* 2008;191(2):589–597.

56. Meyer A, Stark M, Karstens JH, Christiansen H, Bruns F. Langerhans cell histiocytosis of the cranial base: is low-dose radiotherapy effective? *Case Rep Oncol Med.* 2012;2012:789640.

57. Vrionis FD, Kienstra MA, Rivera M, Padhya TA. Malignant tumors of the anterior skull base. *Cancer Control.* 2004;11(3):144–151.

58. Laigle-Donadey F, Taillibert S, Martin-Duverneuil N, Hildebrand J, Delattre JY. Skull-base metastases. *J Neurooncol.* 2005;75(1):63–69.

59. Yeh HC, Yang SF, Ke HL, Lee KS, Huang CH, Wu WJ. Renal cell carcinoma presenting with skull metastasis: a case report and literature review. *Kaohsiung J Med Sci.* 2007;23(9):475–479.

60. Suva LJ, Washam C, Nicholas RW, Griffin RJ. Bone metastasis: mechanisms and therapeutic opportunities. *Nat Rev Endocrinol.* 2011;7(4):208–218.

61. O'Sullivan GJ, Carty FL, Cronin CG. Imaging of bone metastasis: an update. *World J Radiol.* 2015;7(8):202–211.

62. Koolen BB, Vegt E, Rutgers EJ, et al. FDG-avid sclerotic bone metastases in breast cancer patients: a PET/CT case series. *Ann Nucl Med.* 2012;26(1):86–91.

63. Joshi A, Jiang D, Singh P, Moffat D. Skull base presentation of multiple myeloma. *Ear Nose Throat J.* 2011;90(1):E6–E9.

64. Na'ara S, Amit M, Gil Z, Billan S. Plasmacytoma of the skull base: a meta-analysis. *J Neurol Surg B Skull Base.* 2016;77(1):61–65.

65. Derlin T, Bannas P. Imaging of multiple myeloma: current concepts. *World J Orthop.* 2014;5(3):272–282.

66. Hans FJ, Reinges MH, Nolte K, Reipke P, Krings T. Primary lymphoma of the skull base. *Neuroradiology.* 2005;47(7):539–542.

67. Dare AO, Datta RV, Loree TR, Hicks WL, Grand W. Sinonasal non-Hodgkin's lymphoma with skull base involvement. *Skull Base.* 2001;11(2):129–135.

68. Yang L, Li W, Chen M. Primary non-Hodgkin lymphoma of lateral skull base mimicking a trigeminal schwannoma: case report. *Int J Clin Exp Med.* 2015;8(6):10091–10094.

69. Choi HK, Cheon JE, Kim IO, et al. Central skull base lymphoma in children: MR and CT features. *Pediatr Radiol.* 2008;38(8):863–867.

70. Noh BW, Park SW, Chun JE, Kim JH, Kim HJ, Lim MK. Granulocytic sarcoma in the head and neck: CT and MR imaging findings. *Clin Exp Otorhinolaryngol.* 2009;2(2):66–71.

71. Ritter J, Bielack SS. Osteosarcoma. *Ann Oncol.* 2010;21(suppl 7). vii320–vii325.

72. Ahrari A, Labib M, Gravel D, Macdonald KI. Primary osteosarcoma of the skull base treated with endoscopic endonasal approach: a case report and literature review. *J Neurol Surg Rep.* 2015;76(2):e270–e274.

73. Cugati G, Singh M, Pande A, Symss NP, Chakravarthy VM, Ramamurthi R. Isolated skull base primary Ewing's sarcoma: an extremely rare location. *J Cancer Res Ther.* 2013;9(4):741–742.

74. Peersman B, Vanhoenacker FM, Heyman S, et al. Ewing's sarcoma: imaging features. *JBR-BTR.* 2007;90(5):368–376.

75. Bernstein M, Kovar H, Paulussen M, et al. Ewing's sarcoma family of tumors: current management. *Oncologist.* 2006;11(5):503–519.

76. Bloch O, Parsa AT. Skull base chondrosarcoma: evidence-based treatment paradigms. *Neurosurg Clin N Am.* 2013;24(1):89–96.

77. Almefty K, Pravdenkova S, Colli BO, Al-Mefty O, Gokden M. Chordoma and chondrosarcoma: similar, but quite different, skull base tumors. *Cancer.* 2007;110(11):2457–2467.

78. Renukaswamy GM, Boardman SJ, Sebire NJ, Hartley BE. Angiosarcoma of skull base in a 1-year-old child – a case report. *Int J Pediatr Otorhinolaryngol.* 2009;73(11):1598–1600.

# CHAPTER 17

# Neurointerventional Radiology for Skull Base Lesions

HON-MAN LIU, MD • YEN-HENG LIN MD, MS

In this chapter, we discuss the embolization of the most common hypervascular tumors and vascular lesions occurring at the skull base (i.e., the juvenile angiofibromas [JAFs], paragangliomas [PGLs], dural arteriovenous fistula [DAVF], and traumatic carotid-cavernous fistula [CCF]). Other rare diseases such as orbital arteriovenous malformation and aneurysm at the foramen magnum are not included. We provide an introduction to the pathogenesis of these diseases, the current methods of embolization, outcome assessment, and the controversies relating to the clinical management of these diseases.

## EMBOLIZATION OF HYPERVASCULAR TUMORS LOCATED AT THE SKULL BASE

The most common hypervascular tumors arising at the skull base are JAF and PGL (glomus tumor). Less common tumors include meningioma, hypervascular metastases, hemangiomas, and endolymphatic sac tumors.[1] Preoperative embolization is considered to be a relatively safe, minimally invasive, supplementary procedure. In the following sections, we discuss the goal of treatment, the functional anatomy, embolic materials, and methods of embolization and provide some details about the embolization of JAF and skull base glomus tumor.

## GOALS OF PREOPERATIVE EMBOLIZATION

The main goals of preoperative embolization of hypervascular tumors in the skull base are to shorten the operation time and decrease the intraoperative blood loss by obliterating the capillary bed and the proximal feeding arteries.[2,3] Other goals are to improve exposure of the tumor, enable a more radical removal of the tumor, and decrease recurrence rate. In comparing blood loss without and with preoperative embolization, one report found that blood loss was reduced from 750 to 400 mL on average,[4] but no cases with intracranial

extension were included in this assessment. Others[5,6] reported the mean intraoperative blood loss in patients with embolized tumors to be 770 mL compared with 1500 mL in patients with nonembolized tumors. We can speculate that a successful preoperative embolization could cut intraoperative blood loss in half.

Preoperative devascularization decreased recurrence rates from 11% to 7% and increased the absolute relapse-free rate from 56% to 73% in patients with JAF.[4] However, the contribution of preoperative arterial embolization to lowering JAF recurrence rates has been questioned.[7,8]

## FUNCTIONAL ANATOMY

The anatomy of vascular structures at the skull base is complex and variable. Most skull base structures draw their blood supply from the external carotid artery (ECA), but skull base tumors commonly receive blood from the internal carotid artery (ICA) and vertebral artery (VA), especially when the tumors extend intracranially. The extent of vascular anastomosis between the extracranial and intracranial vasculatures is another important issue to consider when selecting patients with skull base tumors for embolization. Dangerous anastomosis may exist between the ECA, ICA, VA, ophthalmic artery, ascending cervical artery, deep cervical artery, and spinal arteries.[9] Box 17.1 summarizes these dangerous anastomoses.

These dangerous anastomoses may not be revealed by preembolization diagnostic angiography and may appear suddenly as a result of the Venturi effect after partial embolization. Cerebral stroke is one of the major complications of embolization for skull base lesions and can occur when embolic material travels into the VA or ICA territories via existing anastomoses. Another concern during embolization of the skull base tumor is the blood supply to cranial nerves. Valavanis proposed the concept of "dangerous" and "safe" vessels for embolization. Arteries not supplying a cranial nerve were regarded as "safe," whereas arteries feeding a functional nerve were termed "dangerous."[10] The caliber of the tiny vasa nervorum is usually less than 60 μm. Devascularization of the vasa nervorum (a region of dangerous vessels) might cause cranial nerve palsy during embolization of the skull base tumor. To deal with dangerous vessels supplying both the tumor and cranial nerve, we have to use larger particles (>150 μm) and avoid liquid embolic agents.

## EMBOLIC MATERIALS

Embolic materials can be categorized as particles and liquids. See Box 17.2.

### Particulate Embolic Materials

Many different particles have been used for tumor embolization, and their further subdivision into polyvinyl alcohol (PVA), tris-acryl gelatin (embospheres), and polyzene F-coated hydrogel (embozenes) is based on the composition of the microsphere polymer matrix. PVA microspheres can be further subdivided into nonspherical PVA, spherical PVA, and acrylamido PVA.

The catheters required to inject these particles must have a larger inner diameter and be stiffer than those

---

**BOX 17.1**
**Extracranial-to-Intracranial Anastomoses**

1. Anterior or ophthalmic artery connections with facial and internal maxillary arteries;
2. Middle or petrocavernous internal carotid artery branches with internal maxillary and ascending pharyngeal branches;
3. Posterior or VB (Vertebrobasilar) connections with ascending pharyngeal, occipital, and subclavian artery branches, especially the ascending and deep cervical arteries.

---

**BOX 17.2**
**Common Embolic Materials Used for Devascularization in Head and Neck Tumor**

Particles
  Gelform
Polyvinyl alcohol (PVA)
  Tris-acryl gelatin (Embospheres)
  Polyzene-F hydrogel (Embozenes)
Liquid
  n-Butyl cyanoacrylate (NBCA)
  Ethylene vinyl alcohol copolymer (Onyx) (SQUID)

---

used for the delivery of liquid embolic agents. Catheters are wire guided and more difficult and hazardous to navigate through distal friable vessels than flow-guided catheters. All these restrictions make it difficult to optimize the particle size of embolic agents used to penetrate the capillary bed of the tumor without occluding the arterial pedicle or passing through the nidus into the venous system.

The size of the particles is important. Larger particle size (more than 150 μm) is believed to enable the efficient penetration of the tumor's capillary bed. Meanwhile, particle size more than 150 μm is also safe in cases of dangerous vessel embolization. The same is true for tris-acryl gelatin and polyzene-F hydrogel microspheres.

Tris-acryl gelatin and polyzene-F hydrogel microspheres do not aggregate and tend to lodge in vessels that are close in size to the particle diameter, and blood does not flow beyond the embolized region. They are less likely to clump and clog the microcatheter. By contrast, PVA particles aggregate in vessels larger than the particle's diameter, preventing blood flow into regions peripheral to the embolized region.[11] However, both methods produce only temporary occlusion.[12,13] Therefore, no more than 7 days between particle embolization and surgery is critical to ensure sufficient devascularization.[14] Seemingly, tris-acryl gelatin and polyzene-F hydrogel are superior to PVA for tumor penetration to achieve embolization. But one meta-analysis assessing five widely used embolic particles (three types of PVA particles, tris-acryl gelatin, and polyzene-F hydrogel) in uterine fibroid embolization found no evidence of the superiority of any embolic agent.[15]

### Liquid Embolic Materials

The two most widely used and most effective agents for embolizing vascular lesions are polymers: n-butyl cyanoacrylate (NBCA [Histoacryl], Braun, Melsungen, Germany, and Trufill, Cordis Neurovascular, Miami, FL) and ethylene-vinyl alcohol (EVA) (Onyx; EV3 Neurovascular, Irvine, CA) dissolved in the solvent base dimethyl sulfoxide (DMSO). Like Onyx, SQUID (Emboflu, Fribourg, Switzerland) is also an EVA dissolved in DMSO but it is available in different concentrations: 4.9% and 6.0%. Micronized tantalum powder is added to both Onyx and SQUID to provide radiopaque contrast. Both Onyx and SQUID must be vortexed (Vortex-Genie, Scientific Industries, Bohemia, NY) at least 20 min to ensure stable mixing of the tantalum with the polymer.

NBCA is a liquid monomer that polymerizes into an adhesive when in contact with an anionic solution (i.e., blood). It is radiolucent but becomes radiopaque when mixed with agents such as Lipiodol (Lipiodol Ultra Fluide, Guerbet, Solingen, France), Ethiodol (Savage Laboratories, Melville, NY), or Tantalum powder (American Elements, Los Angeles, CA). A small, flexible microcatheter is safely and gently navigated into the capillary bed of the tumor for NBCA delivery. A significant level of experience is needed to deliver NBCA appropriately. It is difficult to control the polymerization time of NBCA. In our institution, we usually mix NBCA with Lipiodol in a ratio of 1:2 to 1:3 to slow polymerization. The relationship between the NBCA to Lipiodol ratio and polymerization time is not linear. Gluing the microcatheter to the vessel wall is another risk. Delayed migration of the polymerized glue into the intracranial circulation 12 h after NBCA embolization has also been reported.[16]

The benefits of Onyx over NBCA have been well described.[3] Onyx polymerizes after contact with blood or any aqueous solution and with diffusion of the solvent DMSO. Onyx forms a spongy surface layer but remains liquid at its center. This characteristic causes it to flow like lava within blood vessels and to form a nonadherent plug without fragmentation during injection. During the Onyx injection, the operator can interrupt the procedure several times to allow assessment of the outcome of embolization and early recognition of dangerous intracranial anastomoses. SQUID (another EVA copolymer dissolved in DMSO polymer) has become available in Europe. It is less viscous (which facilitates vascular penetration), less dense, and contains 30% less tantalum, all of which may help visualize structures behind dense embolic casts under X-ray. The micronized tantalum particles in SQUID are smaller than those in Onyx and allegedly are dispersed into a more homogeneous suspension. SQUID has been successfully used for embolization of tumors without any complication.[17]

Particulate embolic agents are usually cheaper than liquid agents, but they have several disadvantages. The particles are radiolucent and require the addition of a contrast agent to indirectly determine the extent of tumor embolization. This adds to the embolic load, which should be a consideration when carrying out the procedure in young patients. The particles (especially PVA) tend to aggregate in and clog the microcatheters, necessitating recatheterization of the feeding arteries; this makes particulate embolization more time consuming than liquid embolization. The devascularization effect of particulate embolization is temporary,[12,13] and tumor resection should be performed within 7 days.

During surgical or endoscopic procedures, it is often very difficult to distinguish tumor tissue from the surrounding tissue. Onyx provides an additional advantage in that tumor tissue is readily distinguishable both visually and under X-ray examination, making it possible to determine intraoperatively whether residual tumor tissue exists and where it is located. The clear demarcation by Onyx of the tumor from its surroundings allows for complete tumor removal and may account for the much lower recurrence rates associated with Onyx use for embolization.[18]

Onyx and NBCA are associated with similar complications. However, Onyx use is also associated with trigeminocardiac reflex, a rare complication defined as the sudden onset of parasympathetic dysrhythmia, sympathetic hypotension, apnea, or gastric hypermotility during stimulation of any of the sensory branches of the trigeminal nerve.[19] Because Onyx use is more expensive and more time consuming than NBCA use, it should be reserved for selective cases.

## METHODS OF EMBOLIZATION
### Transarterial Embolization
Skull base tumors are often devascularized under general anesthesia. Some institutions monitor neurophysiologic activity (electroencephalography, somatosensory evoked potentials, and brainstem auditory evoked potentials) and maintain activated clotting times between 250 and 300 s during the procedure.[19,20] At our institution, we maneuver a 6Fr Envoy (Cordis; Miami Lakes, FL) guide catheter or 4Fr diagnostic catheter of 100 cm length (Vertebral, Glide catheter; Terumo, Tokyo, Japan) into the appropriate ECA and selectively catheterize the feeding vessels with either an SL-10 microcatheter (Stryker Neurovascular, Fremont, CA) or a 2.9F microcatheter (Progreat, Terumo) using the coaxial technique. Selective angiograms of those feeder arteries are performed to assess the portion of the tumor supplied by the artery, the degree of tumor pedicle vascularity, and the location of potentially dangerous extracranial/intracranial anastomoses (Fig. 17.1).

Particulate embolization of skull base tumors is performed by placing the microcatheter tip as close to the capillary bed of the tumor as possible under fluoroscopic guidance. The antegrade flow in the feeders carries the particles to the target tumor. We prefer to start with particles about 150–250 μm in diameter to penetrate the capillary bed of the tumor and then introduce particles 250–350 μm in diameter till contrast medium stasis is observed in the feeders (Fig. 17.2). Transarterial

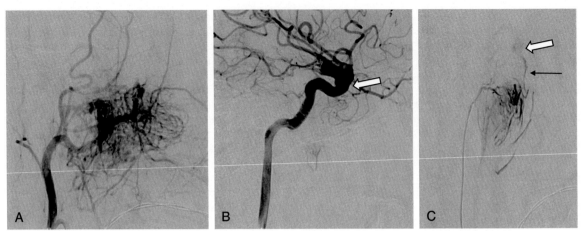

FIG. 17.1 A 15-year-old boy with juvenile angiofibroma suffered from repeated nasal bleeding and foreign body sensation in the throat for a long time. **(A)** An external carotid artery (ECA) lateral angiogram shows a hypervascular tumor in the nasopharynx and central skull base, which is supplied by multiple ECA branches, including the internal maxillary artery, accessory meningeal artery, ascending pharyngeal artery, and postauricular artery. **(B)** An internal carotid artery (ICA) lateral angiogram shows that multiple small branches from the petrous and cavernous ICA are also supplying the tumor. The clinoid ICA is slightly enlarged (*white arrow*). **(C)** A superselective angiogram of the ascending pharyngeal artery shows a direct communication (*black arrow*) between the tumor and the ICA (*white arrow*).

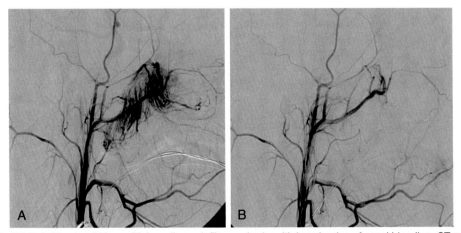

FIG. 17.2 A 15-year-old boy with juvenile angiofibroma had multiple episodes of nasal bleeding. CT and MR scan showed juvenile angiofibroma. **(A)** A preembolization external carotid artery (ECA) lateral angiogram shows mass lesion with profuse vascularity at the nasopharynx, upper oropharynx, and posterior nasal cavity. **(B)** An ECA lateral angiogram postembolization shows near total obliteration of the tumor vessels and tumor stain. Particulate embolization with polyvinyl alcohol was performed on this patient.

particulate embolization is performed under continuous fluoroscopic guidance until nearly complete stasis of the blood flow within each feeding pedicle is achieved. In some centers, nitroglycerine is administered intraarterially to prevent arterial spasm and to promote appropriate forward flow of particles.[20] Many authors prefer to block the main trunk with gelfoam pledgets (Gelfoam, Upjohn, Kalamazoo, MI) or platinum microcoils (Target Therapeutics, Fremont, CA) after obtaining cessation of flow. Sometimes, we use microcoils to occlude the branches supplying normal tissue to decrease the risk of damage to the normal tissue.

During NBCA embolization, the NBCA and Lipiodol are mixed in an appropriate ratio based on the flow dynamics and micro-angio-architecture depicted on the angiogram. The catheter is then prepared by flushing with 5% dextrose water. The NBCA-Lipiodol mixture is then injected slowly under guidance using a single-column method. Injection is stopped immediately if reflux or flow into dangerous vessels is found. After withdrawal under moderate negative pressure, the micro- and guide catheters are rapidly pulled away from the site of injection to prevent them from being glued in place. The technique is repeated as many times as necessary to achieve maximal devascularization of the neoplasm. Before the NBCA-Lipiodol injection for brain arteriovenous malformations, some authors prefer to have the patient under moderate hypotension or ask the anesthesiologist to apply a Valsalva maneuver to the patient during the injection because this increases venous pressure, preventing or reducing the movement of the NBCA-Lipiodol mixture into the draining vein.[21] We do not use this maneuver during devascularization of skull base tumors. The short polymerization time of NBCA limits the amount of embolic injected and always requires multiple injections. The injection of NBCA cannot be halted during the procedure to allow assessment of the degree of embolization and early recognition of dangerous anastomoses (Fig. 17.3).

Onyx polymerizes after contact with blood or any aqueous solution and with diffusion of the solvent DMSO. Compared with NBCA, Onyx is more easily controlled. However, all DMSO-compatible microcatheters are stiffer than the microcatheters used for injection of other agents, and DMSO can cause angionecrosis and vasospasm. Before injection, Onyx must be mixed for at least 20 min. Otherwise, visualization of the Onyx during injection could be suboptimal and sedimentation of the tantalum powder could block the microcatheter hub or shaft.

Onyx is available in two concentrations and viscosities: Onyx-18, with a polymer to solvent ratio of 6% and a viscosity of 18 cP and Onyx-34, with a polymer to solvent ratio of 8% and a viscosity of 34 cP. The impact of viscosity on intraparenchymal penetration is theoretically an important consideration.[22] In devascularization of skull base tumors, Onyx-18 is preferred.

Before embolization, removal of microcatheter redundancy should be done under fluoroscopic guidance. The contrast material in the microcatheter is cleared by flushing with saline. Then, DMSO is injected into the catheter to fill dead space in the microcatheter. Onyx injection is conducted under blank road map fluoroscopy over a 90-s period to replace the DMSO in the dead space, thereby eliminating the angionecrotic potential of DMSO.[23] Onyx infusion is stopped when reflux around the catheter tip is detected. After several minutes, a new blank road map is created and injection is resumed. Ideally, antegrade flow is reestablished, and the Onyx enters other compartments. This procedure (the plug and push technique) is repeated until the desired effect is obtained or a normal branching vessel can be occluded. After multiple rounds of injection, reflux, and waiting, the reflux may extend 1.0–1.5 cm from the tip of the microcatheter. Finally a plug may form around the tip completely blocking blood flow and changing pressure gradients within the tumor's capillary bed until Onyx penetrates the tumor more deeply. Unlike NBCA, Onyx requires that the microcatheter be pulled straight before retracting it with gradually increased force and then either snapping it out of the Onyx cast or slowly pulling it out. We use postembolization ECA angiograms to assess the degree of devascularization.

## Embolization by Direct Puncture

Many centers suggest direct intratumoral puncture as the first-choice devascularization technique for head and neck tumors. In our institution, the rationale for using direct puncture for skull base tumor devascularization is reserved for the following conditions: impossible superselective catheterization of the feeding arteries because of their small size and tortuosity, high possibility of reflux into a dangerous intracranial anastomosis, and persistence of leakage after transarterial embolization. Using the transarterial approach, optimal intraparenchymal tumor penetration with liquid agents is difficult to achieve unless the microcatheter is situated within 2 cm of the tumor.[3]

A single dose of preoperative antibiotics is administered because of the theoretical but low risk of infection from oral or nasal flora. A detailed angiographic evaluation of the degree of lesion is obtained, and the tumor extent is confirmed by CT or MR examination. Depending on the location of the tumor and the important adjacent neurovascular structures, needles can be placed directly into the tumor via the transzygomatic, transnasal, transoral, transbuccal, transpalatal, transorbital, or percutaneous route. Which approach is selected depends on proximity to the tumor and appropriate margins needed to protect vital neurovascular structures.[18,20] An 18- or 20-gauge needle is used to puncture the tumor under angiographic and fluoroscopic guidance and subsequently advanced to the center of the lesion under fluoroscopic road map guidance. An intratumoral angiogram is performed to confirm the position of the

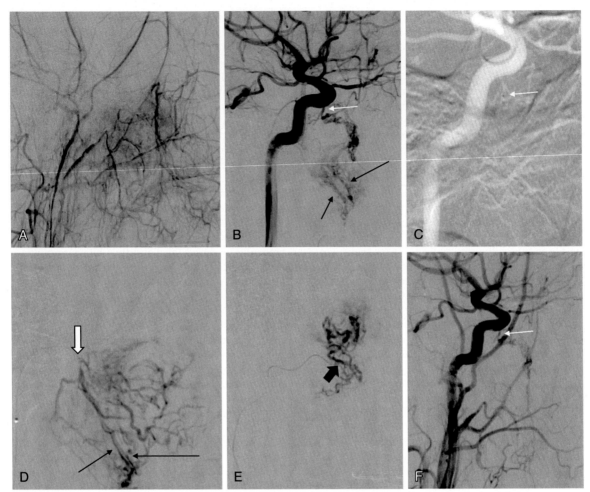

FIG. 17.3 A 14-year-old boy had multiple attacks of massive nasal bleeding, headache, and nasal obstruction for a long time with final diagnosis of juvenile angiofibroma. **(A)** An external carotid artery lateral late-phase angiogram shows diffuse tumor stain in the area of the nasopharynx, oropharynx, skull base, and nasal cavity. **(B)** An internal carotid artery (ICA) lateral angiogram shows that the tumor is also supplied by the inferior lateral trunk (*white arrow*) from the cavernous ICA, and small branches from the petrous ICA are associated with an obvious tumor stain (*black arrows*). **(C)** An ICA lateral road map shows the progress of the microcatheter tip (*white arrow*) as it passes into the inferior lateral trunk to the site of embolization with NBCA. A superselective angiogram shows the microcatheter in the ascending pharyngeal artery (**D**, *white arrow*) and internal maxillary artery branch (possible sphenopalatine artery, *black arrow*) (**E**). Please note that the inferior part of the tumor stain (*black arrow*) on **(D)** is similar to that shown in **(B)**. After multiple NBCA embolizations, the final postembolization CCA lateral angiogram **(F)** shows more than 95% of the tumor vessels are obliterated and the blood flow from the inferior lateral trunk (*white arrow*) is also decreased.

needle within the tumor, assess the microvasculature of the tumor, determine the venous drainage pattern, and identify dangerous intracranial anastomoses. Then the hub of the puncture needle is connected to a 10-cm Luer Lock extension tube. The dead space is slowly filled with DMSO (when Onyx is the embolic agent) or 5% dextrose water (when NBCA is the embolic agent) using a 1-mL Luer Lock syringe as needed. Embolization of the tumor is performed under subtracted road map guidance. In large heavily vascularized tumors, the needle can be redirected under road map guidance to a different compartment of the tumor to allow a more thorough penetration of embolic agents. Intermittent ECA and ICA angiography is needed to assess the degree of devascularization and detect hemodynamic changes such as recruitment of short arterial feeders from the ICA or VA after partial embolization. If this happens, placement of a temporal balloon at the origin of these arteries in the ICA or VA may theoretically be helpful in preventing nontarget embolization during further intratumoral injection of a liquid embolic agent. However, this increases the complexity of the procedure and may subject the patient to the additional risk of dissection or a thromboembolic event. Feeders from the ophthalmic artery are a relative contraindication for direct puncture embolization with a liquid embolic agent.[24,25] Embolization is continued until the desired degree of tumor penetration is achieved.

## COMPLICATIONS

Regardless of the method or materials used in the devascularization of skull base tumors, the most common complication is migration of the embolic agent to the ophthalmic artery or intracranial system. Inadvertent ocular embolization of the central retinal artery occurs via the middle meningeal artery in up to 3% of the population not identified by the preembolization study.[25] This can also happen when embolization of the recurrent meningeal artery, meningoophthalmic trunk, and normal vessel variants is performed.[26] Besides the common intracranial-extracranial anastomoses mentioned earlier, arteries such as the deep temporal, infraorbital, sphenopalatine, greater palatine, and ascending pharyngeal arteries and artery of the vidian canal have the potential for forming intracranial-extracranial anastomotic collateral networks[27] and may be the culprit vessels involved in cerebral stroke occurrence after extracranial embolization.

## JUVENILE ANGIOFIBROMA

JAFs account for approximately 0.05% of all head and neck neoplasms.[28] Surgical removal is widely accepted as the primary mode of JAF therapy. JAFs are highly vascular lesions, and their excision is frequently accompanied by significant intraoperative blood loss. Preoperative tumor devascularization is a supplementary treatment to minimize intraoperative blood loss.[29,30] All the treatments mentioned in the earlier sections can be applied to JAFs.

The blood supplied to JAFs is usually from internal maxillary artery branches, such as the sphenopalatine arteries, anterior ascending pharyngeal artery, and accessory meningeal artery. As the tumor grows, it receives blood from facial artery branches such as the

> ### BOX 17.3
> ### Classification System of Juvenile Angiofibromas (JAFs) Proposed by Yi et al.
>
> Type I: JAFs fundamentally localized to the nasal cavity, paranasal sinus, nasopharynx, or pterygopalatine fossa.
>
> Type II: JAF extending into the infratemporal fossa, cheek region, or orbital cavity, with anterior and/or minimal middle cranial fossa extension but intact dura mater.
>
> Type III: Calabash-like massive tumor lobe in the middle cranial fossa.

ascending palatine artery, ethmoidal branches of the ophthalmic artery, and ICA branches, such as the mandibulovidian/pterygovaginal artery, inferolateral trunk, meningohypophyseal trunk, and other petrous ICA segment branches.[31] JAF blood supply is often bilateral (in up to 30%–40% of cases).[32]

During surgery, the flow through the sphenopalatine artery is considered to be the source of profuse bleeding during removal of the tumor (Fig. 17.3). Preoperative occlusion of this artery can thus shorten the operative time, increase the safety of the operation, and help reduce the total perioperative blood loss.[33]

Many classifications have been proposed for the staging of JAFs.[34–40] A detailed discussion of these classifications is not within the scope of this chapter. Yet they are used for surgical planning and treatment. A concise easier-to-use staging system for deciding whether to perform devascularization in JAF (see Box 17.3) was proposed by Yi et al.[41] We propose that transarterial embolization (particles or liquid) can be used to devascularize type I lesions and direct puncture and/or the transarterial approach may be needed for type II lesions. In type III lesions, both the transarterial and direct puncture approaches are associated with a high risk of bleeding from the ICA and its branches and also from preexisting intracranial-extracranial anastomotic collaterals.

In comparison with the transarterial approach, direct puncture is associated with a shorter operation time. But current studies did not have sufficient power to show a statistically significant difference in estimated blood loss during subsequent tumor resection between the two methods.[42,43] Careful embolization via either direct tumor injection or a transarterial route is safe and effective in presurgical management of JAFs. Occasionally, direct percutaneous embolization with liquid agents in conjunction with standard endovascular embolization techniques may be a good alternative.[21]

## TYMPANOJUGULAR PARAGANGLIOMAS

Head and neck PGLs are rare tumors,[44] and they are classified by the sites of origin as carotid body tumors (at the bifurcation of the common carotid artery); jugular PGLs (close to the jugular bulb) and tympanic PGLs (in the middle ear), usually considered together (tympanojugular PGLs, TJPGLs); and vagal PGLs (along the vagus nerve). In a large reported series of 204 PGLs, 57% were carotid body tumors and 30% were TJPGLs.[45] PGLs have their origin in the paraganglia of the chemoreceptor system. TJPGLs arise from a small group of cells in the adventitia of the jugular bulb.

The natural history of PGLs is variable. Approximately 38%–60% of PGLs are slow growing, with the tumor's doubling time varying widely (0.6–21.5 years; mean growth range 0.2–1 mm/year).[46,47] In a study of 47 patients with PGL, 42% had stable tumors and 20% had tumors that decreased in size.[47]

Despite their benign origin, TJPGLs are locally aggressive, destructive neoplastic lesions and frequently invade the middle ear, temporal bone, and upper neck, with extension through the jugular foramen into the posterior cranial fossa. Based on their location, size, and extent, they have been classified by Fisch into four categories (see Box 17.4).[48]

Optimal management is multifactorial and highly dependent on the tumor (location, size, involvement of neurovascular structures, malignancy, and hormone production), the patient (age, comorbidities, and symptoms), and the genetic status (implying potential for recurrence, malignancy, or multicentric tumors).[49] Treatment of TJPGL remains controversial. Observation alone has been recommended, especially in the elderly and/or asymptomatic patients.[50] The main treatment modalities for TJPGL include surgery and radiotherapy. Overall, gross total resection is achievable in 78.2%–86% of the cases and is associated with a low surgical mortality rate (0%–2.7%),[49,51] but the success rate is generally lower in Fisch C and D class TJPGLs, and it decreases to 41% in class D tumors or 35% if the tumors have a large intradural extension. Surgery is associated with hemorrhagic, cerebrovascular, and neurologic risks (paresis of the lower cranial nerves leading to swallowing and speech problems, aspiration, feeding tube or tracheostomy dependence, facial palsy, and hearing loss).[49] The recurrence rate was 18.8% in one report with 112 months follow-up.[52] Surgery for large TJP-GLs is challenging because of their high vascularity and close relationship with delicate neurovascular structures.[53–55] However, favorable long-term results

---

> **BOX 17.4**
> **Adapted Fisch Classification of Tympanojugular Paragangliomas**
>
> Class A tumors are located along the tympanic plexus on the promontory
>
> Class B tumors invade the hypotympanum but do not erode the jugular bulb
>
> Class C tumors
>
>   C1 tumors destruction of the jugular bulb/foramen
>
>   C2 tumors invasion of the vertical carotid canal
>
>   C3 tumors invasion of the horizontal carotid canal
>
>   C4 tumors invasion of the cavernous sinus
>
> Class D: Besides the various degrees of invasion described for class C, intracranial extradural or intradural extension occurs
>
>   De1 intracranial and extradural invasion of up to 2 cm
>
>   De2 intracranial and extradural invasion of more than 2 cm
>
>   Di1 intracranial and intradural extension of up to 2 cm
>
>   Di2 intracranial and intradural extension of between 2 and 4 cm
>
>   Di3 intracranial and intradural extension of more than 4 cm

---

can be achieved by involving a multidisciplinary team in the planning and execution of surgery. Radiosurgery as the primary treatment revealed high rates of tumor growth control and relatively low morbidity in a series.[49] Owing to the relatively benign natural history of TJPGLs, a long follow-up duration is needed before a correct conclusion can be drawn about the efficacy of any treatment.

The primary arteries supplying blood to TJPGLs are the ascending pharyngeal artery, posterior auricular artery, and occipital artery (Fig. 17.4). The clival meningeal branches of the carotid artery and the meningeal branches of the VA supply the intracranial component in patients with Fisch class D TJPGL, and the posterior inferior cerebellar artery and the anterior inferior cerebellar artery supply the posterior intradural TJPGLs.[56,57] Preoperative embolization and interdisciplinary microsurgical resection of TJPGLs are the preferred treatment for selected patients because of their association with high tumor control rates and good long-term results.[58] Preoperative embolization can dramatically reduce tumor vascularity, operative times, blood loss, and surgical complications.

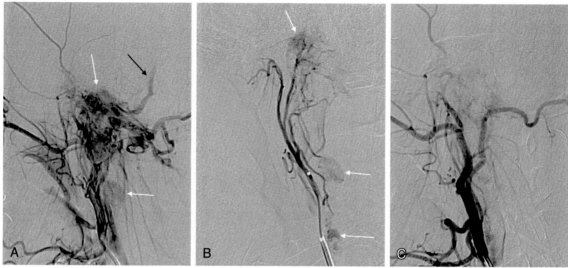

FIG. 17.4 A 45-year-old man complained of chronic headache and multiple palpable neck masses, which were confirmed to be paraganglioma. Swallowing was difficult in last few weeks. **(A)** An external carotid artery (ECA) lateral angiogram shows at least two hypervascular tumors in the upper neck and skull base. The large one (*white arrow*) is mainly supplied by the ascending pharyngeal artery, posterior auricular artery, middle meningeal artery, and occipital artery. An early drainage vein extends to the sigmoid sinus (*black arrow*), with obstruction of the internal jugular vein outlet. Another small hypervascular tumor (*lower white arrow*) is located in the middle neck near the central carotid artery bifurcation. **(B)** An ascending pharyngeal artery superselective lateral angiogram shows three hypervascular tumors (*white arrow*) at the jugular fossa, middle neck, and lower neck. **(C)** An ECA lateral angiogram postembolization with particles shows a marked decrease in the tumor blush and tumor stain of all three tumors.

In instances in which the ICA is encased, balloon occlusion is used to assess whether carotid sacrifice would be possible during surgery.[59] An alternative to sacrifice of the ICA is preoperative stenting.[60] This prevents the risk of the carotid rupture during surgery and obviates the need for balloon occlusion or bypass procedures.

However, the intimate anatomic relationship and overlapping blood supply between these tumors and cranial nerves (see Box 17.5) may contribute to a high incidence of cranial neuropathy (approximately 18%) after liquid agent embolization.[61]

Warren et al.[62] reported that postoperative new cranial neuropathy occurred less frequently when preoperative TJPGL devascularization was carried out by a combination of two procedures (embolization of the inferior petrous sinus and transarterial embolization) than by transarterial embolization alone (38% vs. 80%). However, the materials used in these procedures and postembolization outcome were not reported. So, further investigation is warranted.

The recently reported use of dual-lumen balloon catheter injection for preoperative Onyx embolization

| BOX 17.5 Dangerous Arteries During Embolization of Tympanojugular Paragangliomas | |
| --- | --- |
| Facial nerve | Petrosal branch of middle meningeal artery |
| | Stylomastoid branch of postauricular artery or occipital artery |
| Glossopharyngeal nerve, vagus nerve, and spinal accessory nerve | Jugular branch of neuromeningeal trunk of the ascending pharyngeal artery |
| Hypoglossal nerve | Hypoglossal branch of neuromeningeal trunk of the ascending pharyngeal artery |

of skull base PGLs in five patients showed promising results.[63] However, this has not yet been confirmed in a large series, and we still consider that liquid agents pose a higher risk of permanent cranial neuropathy.[64] A single embolization can be regarded as merely palliative

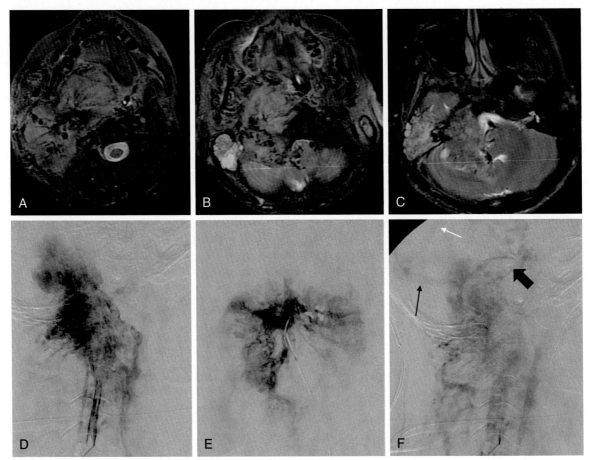

FIG. 17.5 A 65-year-old man had a huge head and neck paraganglioma for a long time. **(A–C)** Axial T2-weighted images show the huge tumor with mixed signal intensity and flow in the right neck, nasopharynx, skull base, temporal bone, and posterior fossa, with compression of the brain stem and cerebellum. **(D)** An external carotid artery (ECA) lateral angiogram and **(E)** ascending pharyngeal artery superselective frontal angiogram show a superabundance of tumor vessels and tumor stain extending from the lower neck to the intracranial region. **(F)** The early venous phase of the ECA lateral angiogram shows arteriovenous shunting with reflux into the transverse sinus (*small black arrow*) and inferior petrous sinus (*large black arrow*) and then to the cortical veins and straight sinus (*white arrow*). In patients with such advanced paragangliomas, palliative embolization or radiotherapy is the treatment of choice.

owing to the high revascularization rate,[57,65] although good short-term outcome has been reported in a small series.[66] We consider embolization to be the sole treatment for recurrent or inoperable TJPGLs (Fig 17.5)

## EMBOLIZATION FOR VASCULAR LESIONS IN THE SKULL BASE

In this section, we shall discuss the treatment of the two most common vascular lesions occurring in the skull base: DAVF and traumatic CCF.

### Dural Arteriovenous Fistula

Intracranial DAVF is a disease in which blood flow from the meningeal artery is shunted directly into the cerebral drainage venous system in the dura or associated osseous structure. It is considered an acquired disease, accounts for 10%–15% of intracranial vascular anomalies, and can occur anywhere in the pachymeninges.[67] Because intracranial DAVF varies in location and severity, it can vary in clinical manifestations and natural history. The pathophysiology is not yet completely understood, but cerebral venous thrombosis

**TABLE 17.1**
**Three Classification Systems of Intracranial DAVF Based on Angiographic Findings**

| DJINDIAN & MERLAND[5] | | COGNARD[1] | | BORDEN[6] | |
|---|---|---|---|---|---|
| Type I | Drainage into a sinus or a meningeal vein | Type I | Antegrade drainage into a sinus or meningeal vein | Type I | Drainage directly into dural venous sinuses or meningeal veins |
| Type II | Sinus drainage with reflux into a vein discharging into the sinus | Type IIa | As type I but with retrograde flow | Type II | Drainage into dural sinuses or meningeal veins with retrograde drainage into subarachnoid veins |
| Type III | Drainage solely into cortical veins | Type IIb | Reflux into cortical veins | Type III | Drainage into subarachnoid veins without dural sinus or meningeal venous drainage |
| Type IV | With supra- or infratentorial venous lake | Type IIa+b | Reflux into both sinus and cortical veins | | |
| | | Type III | Direct cortical venous drainage without venous ectasia | | |
| | | Type IV | Direct cortical venous drainage with venous ectasia | | |
| | | Type V | Spinal venous drainage | | |

and hypertension may play an important role. Many conditions are associated with its occurrence, such as trauma and hypercoagulation. A common hypothesis is that DAVFs form in three stages.[68,69] It begins with a thrombotic event in a compromised sinus, followed by formation of a fistula extending from the site of arterial occlusion to the vasa vasorum of the sinus wall, and ends with partial recanalization of the thrombosed segment, reflecting the complex nature of locoregional vasogenesis.

In more than 70% of cases, the disease occurs predominantly in the skull base region, including the cavernous sinus and transverse-sigmoid sinus. Other less frequent locations in the skull base include the anterior cranial base, superior sagittal sinus (SSS), tentorial incisura, hypoglossal canal, and foramen magnum, making it the most common neurovascular disease affecting the skull base.[70]

### Classification, clinical presentation, and diagnosis

Proper description of the disease is essential for subsequent management. A good way to describe these diseases is to separate them by location. This is still the most essential element of the classification of this entity. Subsequent classification systems added clinical implications, mainly based on natural history. There

are many different classification systems for this disease. The effort began with Djinjian and Merland.[5] Currently, the Cognard[67] and Borden[71] systems are the most popular and widely used. The three classification systems are listed in Table 17.1. We suggest readers become familiar with all three. Cognard classified the disease into types I through V, with two subtypes IIa and IIb, representing retrograde sinus flow and retrograde flow into the cortical vein, respectively. Borden classified the disease into types I–III. Type II is equivalent to Cognard type IIb, and type III is equivalent to Cognard type III or IV. Both systems call attention to corticovenous reflux, which is associated with aggressive clinical presentation and outcome.[72–74] Borden type I is considered benign, whereas type II and type III are considered aggressive. In a 7-year follow-up study, the aggressive type was associated with 8.1% of hemorrhagic events and 6.9% of nonhemorrhagic neurologic events.[72]

Clinical symptoms and signs of DAVF result from cerebral venous stasis and hypertension. Depending on the affected region, these manifestations are variable, reflecting the anatomic relation with adjacent venous structures. Overall, the most common clinical manifestation of intracranial DAVFs, especially transverse-sigmoid sinus DAVF, is pulsatile tinnitus and bruit due to their location at the skull base.[75] Cavernous sinus DAVF

(CSDAVF) commonly presents with eye symptoms. Hemorrhage is a dreaded manifestation and is associated with a mortality rate of 20%. Overall, intracranial DAVF is responsible for 6.4% of intracerebral hemorrhage secondary to vascular lesions. Some risk factors are associated with hemorrhagic complications (such as corticovenous reflux) and location (such as anterior fossa and tentorium cerebelli).[75,76] Other aggressive manifestations such as focal neurologic deficit, rapid progression dementia, seizure, and consciousness disturbance are also possible and associated with malignant disease course.[77]

Proper identification is crucial but sometimes time consuming. Because of its variable clinical manifestations, intracranial DAVF can be encountered by different specialists, such as otolaryngologists, ophthalmologists, neurologists, and neurosurgeons. In clinically suspicious conditions, imaging plays a major role in the diagnosis and risk stratification of the disease. CT and MR can be considered in clinically suspicious patients.[78] In noninvasive sectional images, feeding arteries, early shunting of the venous structure, and associated brain parenchymal change may be apparent. For example, enlargement of the meningeal arteries, early enhancement or abnormal flow-related signals in the dural sinuses, brain edema, and hemorrhage are the most common imaging signs. Duplex ultrasound is also useful for screening purposes.[79] The abnormally decreased resistance of feeding branches of the external carotid can be detected by duplex ultrasound. Currently, catheter angiography is still considered the golden standard diagnostic tool in this assessment and is still reserved for indeterminate conditions.

## Principles of endovascular treatment

Neurointerventional radiology is currently the most effective way to treat intracranial DAVF.[77] The treatment goals include curing the disease, changing its natural history to avoid a malignant course, and relieving the clinical symptoms to improve quality of life. There is still no solid evidence to suggest when treatment should be offered, but most interventionists treat patients with aggressive symptoms.[80] For patients with a benign course, there is no consensus on the strategy, and patients' preferences are important.

Aggressive disease impairs normal cerebral venous drainage, resulting in cerebral dysfunction and associated complications. The disease can cause cerebral venous dysfunction in two ways. First, the abnormally increased arterial flow from the fistula is often higher than the normal cerebral venous flow, thus increasing arterial pressure and impairing the normal cerebral venous drainage as the fistula increases in size. Second, the draining dural sinuses are commonly stenotic and even occluded in a fashion not yet completely understood, which may worsen the condition. Therefore, the treatment strategy is to reduce abnormal inflow and maintain normal cerebral drainage.

The fistula can be cured theoretically by obliterating either all the feeders or all the drainage routes. To be practical, removing the feeders is difficult because of the numerous anastomoses between different meningeal branches. The potential obliteration of the drainage route is more practical. If the latter strategy is to be followed, evaluating the potential drainage route is crucial to achieve satisfactory results and to avoid complications. If the venous outflow of the DAVF contributes to normal cerebral drainage, sacrifice of the venous outflow may impair this drainage and worsen venous hypertension. Even worse, incomplete fistula obliteration can result in suddenly increased flow and pressure in some cerebral veins, causing regional venous hypertension and even hemorrhage.

The principle of DAVF treatment briefly mentioned earlier emphasizes the importance of the target treatment site, whereby embolization is used as the main method of endovascular treatment and stenting of a stenosed sinus is sometimes required as an alternative or adjunct method.

### Transarterial and transvenous embolization

As mentioned earlier, all venous outflows must be obliterated to angiographically cure a DAVF. Both the transarterial and transvenous approaches can be used to achieve the goal of venous outflow closure. The choice depends mainly on the availability of approach routes, the availability of embolic agent, and the experience of the operator. Nevertheless, these approaches are not mutually exclusive and combining them is common.

The transarterial approach seems intuitive. However, because a DAVF can have many feeding arteries and recruit collateral vessels after partial treatment, complete embolization via limited arterial pedicles, especially using particulate embolic agents, is infrequent. Arterial delivery of embolic agents also carries a higher risk of nontarget embolization. With the introduction of liquid embolic agents, the success rate has increased.[81,82] For sigmoid sinus/transverse sinus (SS-TS) disease, especially Borden type III or Cognard type III and IV disease, because venous approach is sometimes difficult, the transarterial approach is often the only available choice. For SSS disease, transarterial approach is often chosen for symptoms palliation. Despite the success of the transarterial approach for treating disease in the anterior fossa or tentorial incisura, surgery is often considered to be the primary choice.[83,84]

The success of the transvenous approach is usually more likely in cases of easy venous access to the fistula. Complete embolization via the transvenous approach is reported in 71%–87.5% of cases.[85,86] As mentioned earlier, the objective of embolization is to obliterate all venous outflow from the fistula and to preserve the normal drainage outflow as much as possible. Angioarchitecture determines the endovascular approach. The transvenous approach is the rule for CSDAVF,[87] the preferred approach for SS-TS disease,[85,86,88] and a successful approach for anterior condylar or hypoglossal disease.[89] Sometimes, combined treatment is necessary when no suitable route can be identified for a single approach and complete cure is impossible. Fig. 17.6 describes a case illustrating the use of transvenous embolization.

### Embolic agents

Different embolic agents with distinct properties and advantages are used to achieve the above goal, including particles, coils, and liquid agents. Many of them have been extensively discussed in earlier sections; here we focus on the characteristics in dealing with the arteriovenous fistula.

The particles used should be delivered by antegrade flow. Therefore, delivery is usually via the transarterial route. PVA is commonly used. Selecting the size of the particle is crucial. If too large, the particle will cause premature proximal occlusion; if too small, the particle will pass through the fistula and flow into the venous circulation. Therefore, particles are currently less frequently used and often reserved for lesions through which blood flow is slow and for palliative treatment. In our clinical practice, we used particles only to consolidate incomplete responses to transvenous treatment.

Coils are another embolic agent. They are commonly used to occlude venous outflow and can achieve reasonably good outcomes.[90] Dense compaction is needed for effectiveness. Detachable coils can be deployed more controllably, making it easier to avoid unwanted venous occlusion. But nondetachable coils are also an option. Optimal catheterization is the key to successful coil embolization. Careful selection of the entry point and coil deployment sequence is crucial when multiple venous outflow channels need to be closed. Using coils is more time consuming and can be more expensive.

Liquid embolic agents, namely, Onyx and NBCA, are also popular choices.[91] Liquid embolic agents are usually delivered via arteries. NBCA has been used in the endovascular therapy of DAVF for decades.[92] It is an adhesive, and its injection requires fine adjustment of the concentration. Onyx is a nonadhesive and allows prolonged injection, which increases the likelihood of complete obliteration by injection through a limited number of arterial pedicles.[82,93] The plug-and-push technique has gained popularity in the past decade and is often used in Onyx embolization because all arterial feeders can be embolized with Onyx via injection from a single or a few pedicles.[94-96] However, its flow is not always predictable. The key features of different embolic agents are found in Box 17.6. Multiple ancillary techniques are available to facilitate more complete embolization. Fig. 17.7 describes a case illustrating the use of transarterial Onyx embolization.

### Ancillary techniques and alternative approaches

The technical challenges posed by endovascular treatment are mainly catheterization and control of the embolic agent. If catheter insertion into the desired venous outflow is successful, the microcoil is probably the most suitable embolic agent given the great control of its deployment. This is the case for cavernous DAVFs because the venous approach via the inferior petrosal sinus or superior ophthalmic vein (through the facial vein or direct puncture) is often achievable. If venous outflow is difficult or even impossible to catheterize, other embolic agents are often considered. Even for the cavernous DAVF, liquid embolic agents are sometimes used in combination with coils in venous embolization to save time and reduce the number of coils required; however, adjunct use of balloon protection is advised.[97-99]

In many circumstances, there is no appropriate transvenous route; therefore, a transarterial approach is adopted and liquid embolic agents are used. As mentioned earlier, NBCA and Onyx have very different properties. The NBCA does not always pass through the fistula to the venous outflow, especially when the location of the microcatheter tip is suboptimal.[100] Moore et al. reported that simultaneous injection of dextrose water via a guiding catheter facilitates NBCA delivery.[101] Onyx has a shorter history of use for DAVF treatment, and control of the flow of Onyx is slightly easier. As mentioned previously, the plug-and-push technique is used in Onyx embolization to achieve complete occlusion via injection from a single or a few pedicles. In our experience, this mostly occurred in Cognard type IV lesions of SS-TS with injection from a branch of the middle meningeal artery. For disease at other locations

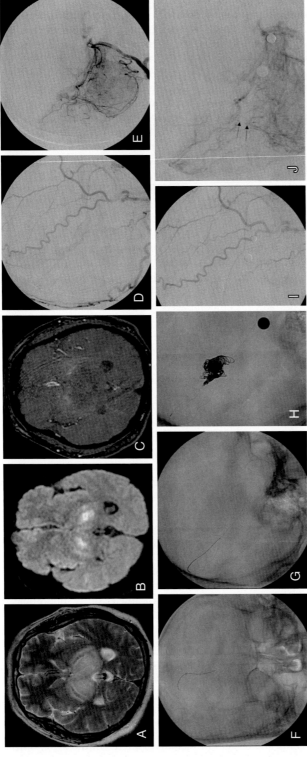

FIG. 17.6 A 43-year-old man with falcotentorial dural arteriovenous fistula (DAVF) underwent coil embolization to vein of Galen. The man had end-stage renal disease with hemodialysis for one and one-half years. Drowsiness, decreased verbal output, and malaise were noted for about a week. His consciousness deteriorated to a comatose state. Laboratory tests excluded central nervous system infection and demyelinating disease. **(A)** Axial T2-weighted MRI shows hyperintensities with positive mass effect over the bilateral thalami. **(B)** Axial diffusion-weighted image shows focal high signal within the thalami. **(C)** Axial time-of-flight images reveal clustered high-signal-intensity abnormalities at the vein of Galen (VOG; at the vein of Galen) as well as dilated bilateral superficial temporal arteries and occipital arteries. **(D)** A left lateral external carotid artery (ECA) angiogram shows early opacification of the VOG with retrograde flow, suggestive of DAVF. The straight sinus is not opacified. **(E)** The lateral left vertebral artery (VA) angiogram, lateral arterial phase, also demonstrates the fistula and venous congestion pattern. The straight sinus is also not opacified. **(F and G)** The microcatheter was navigated through the fistula to the VOG via the parietal branch of the right middle meningeal artery. The frontal and lateral skull views reveal the pathway of microcatheter advance. **(H)** Multiple detachable coils were used to embolize the VOG until flow stasis. The stored fluoroscopic lateral skull view shows the distribution of the radio-paque detachable coils. **(I)** A left ECA angiogram taken after transarterial embolization (TAE) shows the obliteration of the DAVF. **(J)** A post-TAE left VA angiogram shows that the straight sinus was reopened immediately after embolization (*black arrows*). His consciousness gradually returned to full orientation about 2 weeks after the procedure.

or more extensive disease, Onyx was less likely to achieve complete obliteration. Therefore, many flow-control techniques have been invented to improve Onyx delivery.[102] The relevant techniques include balloon sinus protection and injection following coil deployment. Reports on balloon protection show its potential role.[103–105] Placement of a balloon catheter in the arterial pedicle can also help decrease antegrade flow, enhancing the possibility of cure by the arterial approach.[106] In the author's opinion, routine use of a balloon is not recommended because the flow pattern may change after balloon inflation, raising concerns

about incomplete embolization or incidental occlusion of the normal drainage vein.

Another important ancillary technique is sinus stenting. Stenting is used to keep open stenotic or occluded sinuses because simple angioplasty may not be enough.[107,108] This is somewhat tricky because sinus embolization is a common definitive treatment strategy. The use of stents is reserved for cases in which normal cerebral drainage is through tributary drainage veins. This is usually reserved for DAVFs at the SS-TS,[109] e.g., placement of a stent into a narrow sigmoid sinus with antegrade flow in the vein of Labbé. Sinus stents are sometimes used as a buttress to maintain patency and facilitate liquid embolic agent injection. Therefore they are often deployed early during the treatment of extensive disease. Embolic agents and embolization techniques are not always mutually exclusive but can be used in complementary ways to treat many complicated cases. For example, in patients with extensive Cognard type IIA + B disease, transvenous coil embolization is often combined with transarterial Onyx embolization. A case illustrating the deployment of a sinus stent is presented in Fig. 17.8.

There are other ancillary techniques. Direct puncture of the sinus is mentioned in the literature and often used in cavernous DAVF.[110,111] As mentioned earlier, the

---

**BOX 17.6**
**Embolic Agents Used in Embolization of Intracranial Dural Arteriovenous Fistula**

**Particle:** transarterial, with antegrade flow, temporary effect.
**Coil:** transarterial or transvenous, more controllable, time consuming, and usually expensive.
**NBCA:** transarterial route, adhesive, need experience, permanent, risk of neuropathy.
**Onyx:** transarterial route, slow injection, deep penetration, permanent, risk of neuropathy or stroke.

---

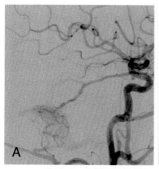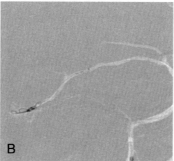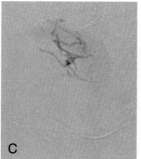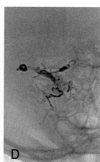

FIG. 17.7 A 41-year-old man with left transverse-sigmoid sinus dural arteriovenous fistula (DAVF) received transarterial embolization by Onyx. The patient had left-side pulsatile tinnitus for 1 year without other neurologic symptoms. The symptoms worsened and recently became unbearable. **(A)** A left lateral common carotid artery angiogram shows early opacification of the transverse-sigmoid sinus, suggestive of DAVF, Cognard type I. The arterial feeders are from the middle meningeal artery and occipital artery. No feeders from the internal carotid artery and no obvious corticovenous reflux are evident. **(B)** The microcatheter was navigated through the fistula into the sinus channel via the petrosquamous branch of the middle meningeal artery. Two detachable coils were used. **(C)** The dimethyl sulfoxide-compatible microcatheter was then navigated through the occipital artery as far as possible. This superselective lateral angiogram was performed via the microcatheter. Onyx was then injected slowly to obliterate the remaining fistula and feeders. **(D)** A stored lateral fluoroscopic view shows the distribution of the radiopaque Onyx and the previously deployed coils. **(E)** The posttransarterial embolization angiogram via the left external carotid artery shows total obliteration of the DAVF. The patient recovered well from the procedure, with no symptomatic recurrence noted after 1 year of follow-up.

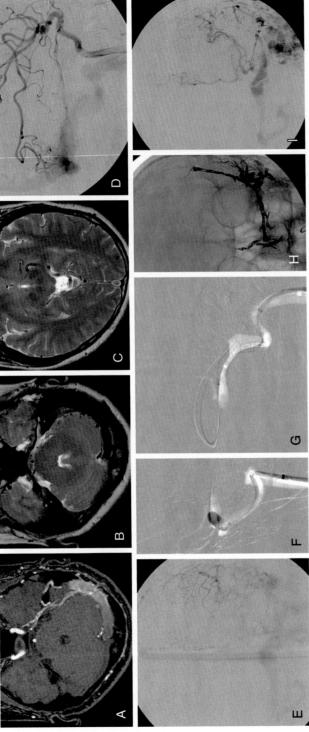

FIG. 17.8 A 33-year-old woman who had a left transverse-sigmoid sinus dural arteriovenous fistula (DAVF) and associated sinus stenosis received combined sinus stenting and endovascular embolization. The woman had left-side pulsatile tinnitus for 3 years and developed headache and seizure activity recently. **(A)** Time-of-flight MR angiography, axial view, reveals abnormal flow-related signal in the left transverse and sigmoid sinus, as well as dilated left external carotid artery branches and left marginal tentorial artery from the meningohypophyseal trunk, suggestive of DAVF. **(B and C)** An axial T2-weighted image shows a dilated left basal vein of Rosenthal with flow voids and some clustered flow voids within the left cerebellar surface pial vein. The picture is suggestive of a dangerous drainage pattern and aggressive clinical course. **(D)** A lateral left common carotid artery angiogram confirmed the diagnosis of left-side transverse-sigmoid DAVF. **(E)** A frontal internal carotid artery angiogram of the late arterial phase reveals retrograde flow from the left transverse sinus up to the superior sagittal sinus and contralateral transverse sinus, which is associated with the cortical vein in the left cerebrum and focal stenosis at the right transverse-sigmoid junction. **(F)** A stored fluoroscopic view shows the balloon angioplasty to the stenotic site at the right transverse-sigmoid junction via an approach from the right internal jugular vein. **(G)** A lateral stored fluoroscopic view demonstrates the subsequent stent placement (Precise) after angioplasty. **(H)** After stent placement, careful sequential coil embolization to the left cortical outflow and sinus tract was performed via an approach from the left internal jugular vein. A stored frontal skull view shows the distribution of the coils. **(I)** The posttransarterial embolization angiography shows a residual Cognard type IIA DAVF, but the retrograde flow to the superior sagittal sinus and cortical vein is not visible. The focal stenosis at the right transverse-sigmoid junction also improved after stenting. After the procedure, pulsatile tinnitus persisted but improved slightly. The headaches improved and the seizures disappeared. She was doing well after 1 year of follow-up and ready for pregnancy.

transvenous approach is the rule for CSDAVF. The most common route is the inferior petrous sinus, but it is not always feasible. Direct puncture and even surgical exposure are reasonable alternatives to the cavernous sinus approach. In our experience, this is less often required because the more flexible catheter may allow a transvenous approach via the facial vein. On the other hand, direct puncture to treat an SSS lesion is sometimes required because the other available approaches may not be possible, especially when treating large lesions. At other institutions, neurosurgical craniectomy to create a direct transverse or SSS approach may be feasible when other alternatives are not available.

### Postprocedural care and follow-up

Endovascular treatment is usually performed under general anesthesia; therefore, optimal airway and hemodynamic care are required immediately after the procedure. Patients are expected to stay in intensive care for at least 1 day to monitor the neurologic status. Local wound care is essential, especially for arterial puncture sites. For CSDAVF, transient cranial nerve palsy is possible, and giving appropriate reassurance is important. Headache, nausea, and vomiting are common complaints and often improve gradually. When postprocedural angiograms demonstrate venous stasis, anticoagulant may be needed. When an intracranial stent is deployed, continued dual antiplatelet agent use is essential to keep the vessel patent.

Clinical symptomatic improvement can be achieved when the presenting symptoms are pulsatile tinnitus or eye chemosis. For more aggressive symptoms caused by venous hypertension, such as consciousness disturbance or dementia, the likelihood of symptom relief is still possible but may take a longer time. During clinical follow-up, no further imaging is required if initial angiographic cure is achieved and clinical symptoms are stable. In clinically stable patients, there is no consensus regarding the length of follow-up, but in the author's opinion, disease progression after treatment is not common and usually occurs within 1 year. Any new neurologic symptom should prompt further evaluation, preferably by MRI.

### Outcome of endovascular treatment

In an earlier meta-analysis by Lucas,[112] the efficacy of only endovascular treatment ranged from 25% for cases of tentorial disease to 80% for cases of convexity/SSS disease. However, there have been advancements in technique and embolic agents over the past 2 decades. As mentioned earlier, the challenges of treatment depend on the disease location. For cavernous

sinus disease, the endovascular transvenous approach is reported to have a cure rate of about 70% and a permanent neurologic deficit rate of 2%–7%.[113,114] For transverse sinus disease, the transvenous approach can achieve an anatomic cure rate of 55%–70% and a permanent neurologic deficit rate of 5%–7%.[20,114] When the outcome was defined as improvement of clinical symptoms, then the treatment success rate was 90%–96%.[85,86,88] The author believes that this can be improved. Reports suggest that transarterial treatment has improved anatomic cure by NBCA and Onyx, up to 84%.[81,82] Endovascular therapy is still considered the primary method of intracranial DAVF treatment.[77,115]

### Alternative treatments

Although we mainly discuss the endovascular approach, other alternatives exist. In patients without aggressive clinical and radiographic features, conservative treatment is a reasonable choice, namely, observation and manual compression.[116] Up to 76% of CSDAVFs regress completely or partially, justifying the strategy.[117,118] Optimal ophthalmologic care is necessary to improve patient comfort. For other locations, the chance of spontaneous regression is unknown and periodic imaging evaluation is needed.

As mentioned earlier, a meta-analysis concluded that a combined surgical approach offers the best opportunity for anatomic cure of transverse sinus disease.[112] Multidisciplinary communication between the neurosurgeon and other interventionists is needed. A combined approach is preferable as a primary treatment option for disease in some locations, such as the anterior fossa and tentorial incisura.[112,119-121] DAVFs in these locations tend to be aggressive, but endovascular treatment is often difficult to perform and results in a low cure rate. For lesions in the SSS, skeletonization of the diseased sinus is feasible for complete cure. Surgery may also be used as adjunct therapy along with endovascular therapies, such as tract creation through direct puncture for cavernous sinus or SS-TS lesions.[122]

Radiosurgery is yet another choice for DAVF treatment. It is less invasive and better tolerated by poor candidates for general anesthesia.[123,124] The obliteration rate can be up to 80% for cavernous sinus disease. Other anatomic locations such as the transverse sinus and SSSs are also targets for treatment.[124-126] The reported outcome is arteriovenous fistula obliteration or regression after 2 years of follow-up in up to 92% of patients, 68% of whom achieve angiographic cure. Hemorrhage occurred in about 2% of patients. It is therefore considered less effective than endovascular therapy. The delayed efficacy of up to a few months also raises concerns for symptomatic patients prone to hemorrhage or permanent neurologic deficit.

## Traumatic Carotid-Cavernous Fistula

In this section, we prefer to use the abbreviation CCF when referring to direct carotid-cavernous fistula or traumatic carotid-cavernous fistula, in contrast to the DAVF that occurs at the cavernous sinus. This may be confusing to the reader, because CCF is classified as a DAVF subtype according to Barrow's classification.[127] The disease is actually very different from cavernous DAVF with respect to pathophysiology, natural history, and treatment. In the following section, we will briefly discuss those points.

### Clinical features and diagnosis

CCF is due to direct perforation of the cavernous segment of the ICA. About 80% of CCF is caused by traumatic insult, and the remaining 20% develop spontaneously, usually associated with an underlying connective tissue disorder or ruptured cavernous aneurysm. In traumatic CCF, the traumatic insults are high-energy, such as those that occur in traffic accidents, and commonly associated with other craniofacial injury. The diagnosis is commonly delayed because initial management is focused on intracranial or cervical vertebral injury, especially when moderate to severe brain injury and consciousness disturbance are involved. The disease can occur under other traumatic circumstances, usually iatrogenic, such as those that occur during endovascular or surgical treatment.[128] The disease is usually progressive, and the symptoms appear later. Traumatic CCF and its indirect DAVF counterpart have some overlapping presenting symptoms, such as bruit, visual blurring, diplopia, headache, and pain. The classic manifestation is "pulsatile exophthalmos." Because eye symptoms are common at presentation, an ophthalmologist is often the clinician to alert regarding the diagnosis.[129]

The diagnosis is usually suspected clinically from an appropriate clinical history and usually confirmed by computed tomography angiography (CTA) and magnetic resonance angiography (MRA).[130,131] Catheter angiography can detect shunting and flow steal if the ICA defect is large. CTA and MRA usually reveal early enhancement of the cavernous sinus and dilation of the superior ophthalmic vein as well. However, the ICA is usually abnormal and the perforated side is sometimes detected by CTA and MRA. CCFs and cavernous DAVFs are usually differentiated on CTA or MRA if carefully examined. CCFs also often show indirect evidence of associated cranial injury and morphologic change to the ICA.

### Principle of treatment

There are two goals of treatment. The first is to preserve the ICA as much as possible. The second is to obliterate the fistula to prevent further venous reflux and venous hypertension. However, CCF and cavernous DAVF are quite different because the condition of the ICA is quite different. One needs to remember that the ICA wall is torn in CCF. Therefore, the first goal (to preserve the ICA as much as possible) is sometimes not always achievable because of the difficulty of repair. Fortunately, severely damaged ICAs usually contribute little to cerebral perfusion because of excessive steal, justifying a strategy of permanent occlusion. Balloon occlusion test can be considered if there is any suspicion that the patient cannot tolerate permanent loss of the ICA. The second goal is more important, and every effort should be made to determine whether endovascular or surgical treatment would achieve it.

The optimal timing of treatment is a multidisciplinary decision. Usually the disease is progressive, and unlike its CSDAVF counterpart, the chance of spontaneous cure is very low.[132] Without treatment, visual loss is expected and can occur in up to 26% of cases if left untreated.[133] Therefore, treatment is warranted once diagnosis is established because of its aggressive natural history. Nevertheless, immediate treatment after diagnosis may not be possible or convenient because of concomitant craniofacial and other associated injury. On the other hand, the abnormal cortical venous reflux can worsen, causing venous congestion and complicating treatment. We propose treating the patient after stabilization of other neurologic conditions but not delaying treatment more than 3 months. If acute vision loss or other neurologic deficit is present, urgent treatment is warranted.

### Endovascular methods

The first embolization technique was developed in 1931 by Brooks who used a muscle embolus to occlude the ICA.[134] After the introduction of detachable balloons, Debrun developed the balloon technology for endovascular treatment in the 1970s.[135] Endovascular treatment has become the principal treatment for CCF since then. To achieve the goals mentioned earlier, either a transarterial or transvenous approach can be used, depending on the available routes and embolic agents.

Detachable balloons and microcoils are the preferred embolic agents.[136] Detachable balloons have

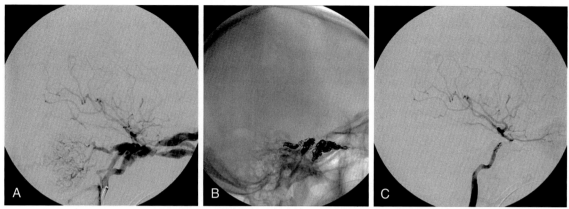

FIG. 17.9 A 19-year-old woman with left carotid-cavernous fistula (CCF) received transvenous coil embolization. The patient was a victim of a traffic accident resulting in a major head injury. Multiple intracranial hemorrhages and skull fractures occurred, and she was admitted to a neurologic intensive care unit. Traumatic CCF was diagnosed on CT angiography 50 days after the accident. **(A)** A lateral view of the early arterial phase on selective left internal carotid artery (ICA) catheter angiography shows the early opacification of the cavernous sinus with drainage into the superior and inferior ophthalmic veins, inferior petrous sinus, and superior petrosal sinus and associated medullary vein in the cerebellum. **(B)** A transvenous approach via the inferior petrosal sinus was used, and the venous outflow routes were closed sequentially. The spot skull lateral views demonstrate the distribution of the detachable coils in the venous outflows and cavernous sinus. **(C)** Posttransarterial embolization angiography shows the obliteration of the fistula after embolization and good preservation of the ICA. The postprocedure course was smooth, and neurologic status was stabilized. Her eye symptom gradually improved.

a longer history of clinical use (since the 1980s) and remain popular in some countries because of their lower cost. When using detachable balloons, the delivery system is navigated through the fistula to the cavernous sinus via a transarterial approach. Usually the device can be directed by flow, but problems may occur because of the difficult vascular architecture. Ancillary techniques such as the double-balloon technique can be used to facilitate balloon navigation.[137] The balloon is detached after its proper position is confirmed. Absolute bed rest for days is advised. The success rate is reported to be up to 95%, with morbidity and mortality rate up to 10%.[138] The treatment outcome is acceptable with a low recurrence rate during long-term follow-up.[139]

In the author's facility, we routinely use detachable coil embolization and think it is more controllable. A transvenous approach via the inferior petrosal sinus is the most preferred route. Although a transarterial approach is possible, it carries a high failure rate of up to 33% according to the literature.[140] The CCF transvenous approach is similar to its indirect DAVF counterpart, but it usually takes more coils and time to achieve a satisfactory effect because it is a high-flow lesion and the veins flowing from it are therefore more dilated

than in its indirect DAVF counterpart. The placement of coils near the fistula site is also preferred by interventionists to facilitate preservation of ICA integrity. However, care must be taken to avoid coil protrusion into the ICA. The key to successful transvenous embolization is closure of all possible venous outflows. Dense embolization is needed for the angiographic occlusion of existing outflow routes, including the inferior petrosal sinus, superior petrosal sinus, sphenoparietal sinus, superior ophthalmic vein, basilar plexus, and so on. Many detachable coils may be needed to ensure embolization. It is therefore more time consuming and expensive to perform than the detachable balloon technique. Nevertheless, transvenous coil embolization is a well-established method with a high successful rate if appropriately conducted.[141,142] Fig. 17.9 describes a case exemplifying the use of transvenous cavernous sinus embolization.

As for other ancillary techniques, additional use of push coil or liquid embolic agents in transvenous cavernous sinus embolization has been adopted by some authors.[75] Besides the above-mentioned mainstream therapy, intracranial stents are conceptually reasonable means of maintaining ICA patency or increasing the packing density near fistula sites. Stent graft use to occlude the perforated site[143-146] and stent-assisted coiling are also appealing.[147,148] However, these techniques are not always successful because the damage to the ICA is usually too extensive to repair, making the effort to preserve the ICA lumen unreliable. Furthermore, because these patients often have a recent history of intracranial hemorrhage, long-term antiplatelet use is contraindicated. A balloon-assisted coiling technique to preserve ICA can also be considered (Fig. 17.10).

In some cases, the securing of access to and embolization of all venous outflow routes may not be possible, especially if access to the approach route is limited.

Under such circumstances, permanent ICA occlusion can be used to achieve the treatment goal. Evaluation of the intracranial current flow status via complete angiography is suggested. Some authors propose routine use of the balloon occlusion test before permanent ICA sacrifice.[136] In our experience, occlusion of the parent artery seldom results in insufficient flow because the steal phenomenon reduces the contribution of the ICA to parenchymal perfusion. The procedure for ICA trapping is straightforward and can be done with detachable or pushable coils. However, careful evaluation of the perforation site is still needed. As mentioned before,

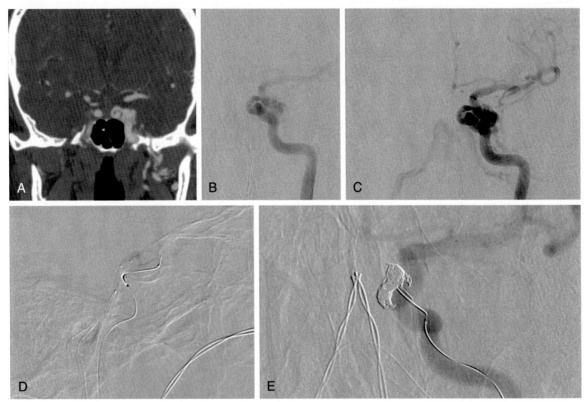

**FIG. 17.10** A 64-year-old man with left carotid-cavernous fistula received balloon-assisted coil embolization. The patient fell down 2 weeks before and struck his head on the ground. He complained of painful redness in his left eye. **(A)** Coronal CT angiography demonstrates the perforation site at the medial aspect of the cavernous internal carotid artery (ICA). **(B)** The early arterial phase of the frontal ICA angiogram confirms the diagnosis of direct cavernous carotid fistula. **(C)** The inferior petrous sinus was catheterized, and the microcatheter was navigated into the ICA through the perforation site. **(D)** The microcatheter was then retracted. Selective catheterization of the left ICA was performed, and a compliant balloon (Hyperglide) was inflated in the cavernous segment of the ICA for protection. The lateral stored fluoroscopic view demonstrates the position of the balloon and microcatheter. **(E)** Embolization was then performed using detachable coils via the venous catheter at the medial aspect of the cavernous sinus near the perforation site, under the protection of the balloon. The angiogram after transarterial embolization and deflation of the balloon shows no more opacification of the cavernous sinus. The symptoms were resolved after treatment. No recurrence was reported during the 1 year of follow-up.

sometimes the damage in the ICA extends beyond the angiographic borders of the lesion. In rare conditions, when the CCF occurs along with persistent primitive trigeminal artery, failure to recognize the congenital anomaly because of the steal phenomenon may result in inadequate treatment and persistent or even aggravated venous hypertension (Fig. 17.11).

### Postprocedural care and follow-up
After endovascular treatment, nausea and headache are possible because of change of intracranial flow pattern. Symptomatic treatment and encouragement of best rest are usually sufficient. Recuperation after detachable

balloon treatment requires absolute bed rest for at least 24 h. Symptomatic recurrence is possible because of balloon dislodgement or deflation. Retreatment is usually needed under such circumstances. When using detachable coils, transient cranial nerve palsy is not uncommon because of the mass effect of the coils in the cavernous sinus. Postprocedural neurologic deterioration is usually due to corticovenous reflux in association with incomplete treatment. Angiography is promptly needed for evaluation. MRI is also considered if there are no contraindications to evaluating parenchymal congestion. When an intracranial stent graft is inserted, use of antiplatelet drugs is crucial and

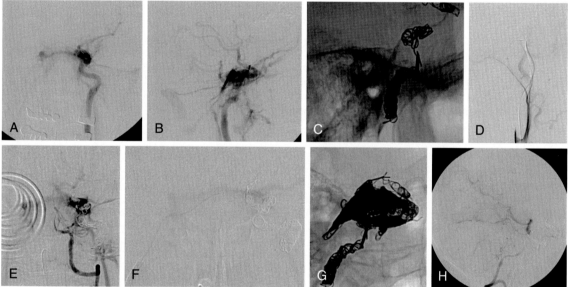

FIG. 17.11 A 61-year-old woman with persistent primitive trigeminal artery experienced initial failed carotid-cavernous fistula treatment by internal carotid artery (ICA) sacrifice. The patient had a motor vehicle accident resulting in major brain injury. Progressive left eye swelling with pupil dilatation was noted 2 days after the emergent neurosurgery. **(A)** A left frontal ICA angiography reveals the direct fistula between the left ICA and cavernous sinus, with very obvious steal phenomenon and poorly enhanced intracranial arteries. **(B)** A lateral ICA angiogram of the same study shows the presence of a persistent primitive trigeminal artery (PPTA). **(C)** Permanent occlusion of the left ICA was performed by deploying pushable coils. The stored fluoroscopy view shows the distribution of the coils. **(D)** A left common carotid artery angiogram after embolization shows complete flow stasis of the left ICA. However, the patient's consciousness deteriorated after the procedure on the same day. The patient adopted a decorticate posture on the right side and was returned to the neuroangiography suite. **(E)** A left vertebral artery (VA) angiogram shows persistent opacification of the cavernous sinus via the PPTA. The distal basilar artery (BA) is not clearly opacified. **(F)** Catheterization of the cavernous sinus was then performed via the right inferior petrosal sinus. The left cavernous sinus was then packed densely with detachable coils. **(G)** The lateral spot view demonstrates the distribution of the subsequently deployed coils. **(H)** A left VA angiography after embolization shows no residual opacification of the cavernous sinus. The BA and bilateral posterior cerebral arteries are clearly visible. The right-side muscle power improved to M5 status after the procedure. On the following days, the left temporooccipital lobe, right hippocampal, and right cerebellar infarcts, as well as some brainstem edema, were found on MRI (not shown). She was transferred to a rehabilitation facility after neurologic stabilization.

the efficacy should be checked. The appearance of new focal neurologic symptoms on the ipsilateral side is worrisome as a possible sign of thromboembolism and needs to be evaluated and treated immediately. Clinical follow-up after satisfactory treatment is suggested for at least 3–6 months. All symptomatic recurrences or new focal neurologic signs need further neuroimaging evaluation.

### Outcome

When detachable balloons are used, the cure rate is reported to be 85%–95%[149,150] and the ICA can be preserved in 60%–88% of cases.[117,135,149,150] When coils are used as embolic agents in the transarterial approach, the efficacy is even better.[151] As mentioned before, transvenous coil embolization is even more successful.[141,142]

### Alternative treatments

When endovascular treatment fails, usually because of a lack of an approach route, surgical procedures can be considered as salvage methods. Other possible choices for definite treatment include ICA ligation (which is an alternative to endovascular ICA trapping), surgical fistula trapping, transvenous packing, and intracranial-extracranial bypass (which can be used when parent artery occlusion is needed because of failed passage of balloon occlusion test). Intracranial-extracranial bypass is performed in a staged fashion along with endovascular trapping. The role of radiosurgery is limited in the treatment of direct CCFs because of their high-flow nature.

## REFERENCES

1. Jindal G, Miller T, Raghavan P, et al. Imaging evaluation and treatment of vascular lesions at the skull base. *Radiol Clin N Am.* 2017;55:151–166.
2. Gupta R, Thomas AJ, Horowitz M. Intracranial head and neck tumors: endovascular considerations, present and future. *Neurosurgery.* 2006;59(5 suppl):S251–S260.
3. Gore P, Theodore N, Brasiliense L, et al. The utility of onyx for preoperative embolization of cranial and spinal tumors. *Neurosurgery.* 2008;62:1204–1211.
4. Yang PW, Sheen TS, Ko JY, et al. Nasopharyngeal angiofibroma: a reappraisal of clinical features and treatment at National Taiwan University Hospital. *J Formos Med Assoc.* 1998,97:843–849. Erratum in: *J Formos Med Assoc* 1999;98:152.
5. Ardehali MM, Samimi Ardestani SH, Yazdani N, et al. Endoscopic approach for excision of juvenile nasopharyngeal angiofibroma: complications and outcomes. *Am J Otolaryngol.* 2010;31:343–349.
6. Paramasivam S, Niimi Y, Fifi J, et al. Onyx embolization using dual-lumen balloon catheter: initial experience and technical note. *J Neuroradiol.* 2013;40:294–302.
7. Lloyd G, Howard D, Lund VJ, et al. Imaging for juvenile angiofibroma. *J Laryngol Otol.* 2000;114:727–730.
8. Mann WJ, Jecker P, Amedee RG. Juvenile angiofibromas: changing surgical concept over the last 20 years. *Laryngoscope.* 2004;114:291–293.
9. Geibprasert S, Pongpech S, Armstrong D, et al. Dangerous extracranial-intracranial anastomoses and supply to the cranial nerves: vessels the neurointerventionalist needs to know. *AJNR Am J Neuroradiol.* 2009;30:1459–1468.
10. Valavanis A. Preoperative embolization of the head and neck: indications, patient selection, goals, and precautions. *Am J Neuroradiol.* 1986;7:943–952.
11. Yamamoto A, Imai S, Kobatake M, et al. Evaluation of trisacryl gelatin microsphere embolization with monochromatic X rays: comparison with polyvinyl alcohol particles. *J Vasc Interv Radiol.* 2006;17(11 Pt 1):1797–1802.
12. Sorimachi T, Koike T, Takeuchi S, et al. Embolization of cerebral arteriovenous malformations achieved with polyvinyl alcohol particles: angio- graphic reappearance and complications. *AJNR Am J Neuroradiol.* 1999;20:1323–1328.
13. Nichols DA, Rufenacht DA, Jack CR Jr, et al. Embolization of spinal dural arteriovenous fistula with polyvinyl alcohol particles: experience in 14 patients. *AJNR Am J Neuroradiol.* 1992;13:933–940.
14. Thibaut A, Collignon J. Embolization and surgical removal of nasopharyngeal angiofibroma. *Neuroradiology.* 1978;16:418–419.
15. Das R, Champaneria R, Daniels JP, et al. Comparison of embolic agents used in uterine artery embolisation: a systematic review and meta-analysis. *Cardiovasc Interv Radiol.* 2014;37:1179–1190.
16. Krishnamoorthy T, Gupta AK, Rajan JE, et al. Stroke from delayed embolization of polymerized glue following percutaneous direct injection of a carotid body tumor. *Korean J Radiol.* 2007;8:249–253.
17. Akmangit I, Daglioglu E, Kaya T, et al. Preliminary experience with squid: a new liquid embolizing agent for AVM, AV fistulas and tumors. *Turk Neurosurg.* 2014;24:565–570.
18. Lutz J, Holtmannspötter M, Flatz W, et al. Preoperative embolization to improve the surgical management and outcome of juvenile nasopharyngeal angiofibroma (JNA) in a single center: 10-year experience. *Clin Neuroradiol.* 2016;26:405–413.
19. Lv X, Li Y, Jiang C, et al. The incidence of trigeminocardiac reflex in endovascular treatment of dural arteriovenous fistula with Onyx. *Interv Neuroradiol.* 2010;16:59–63.
20. Chaloupka JC, Mangla S, Huddle DC, et al. Evolving experience with direct puncture therapeutic embolization for adjunctive and palliative management of head and neck hypervascular neoplasms. *Laryngoscope.* 1999;109:1864–1872.

21. Gemmete JJ, Chaudhary N, Pandey A, et al. Usefulness of percutaneously injected ethylene-vinyl alcohol copolymer in conjunction with standard endovascular embolization techniques for preoperative devascularization of hypervascular head and neck tumors: technique, initial experience, and correlation with surgical observations. *AJNR Am J Neuroradiol.* 2010;31:961–966.

22. Elhammady MS, Wolfe SQ, Ashour R, et al. Safety and efficacy of vascular tumor embolization using Onyx: is angiographic devascularization sufficient? *J Neurosurg.* 2010;112:1039–1045.

23. Murayama Y, Vinuela F, Ulhoa A, et al. Nonadhesive liquid embolic agent for cerebral arteriovenous mal-formations: preliminary histopathological studies in swine rete mirabile. *Neurosurgery.* 1998;43:1164–1175.

24. Casasco A, Houdart E, Biondi A, et al. Major complications of percutaneous embolization of skull-base tumors. *AJNR Am J Neuroradiol.* 1999;20:179–181.

25. Ramezani A, Haghighatkhah H, Moghadasi H, et al. A case of central retinal artery occlusion following embolization procedure for juvenile nasopharyngeal angiofibroma. *Indian J Ophthalmol.* 2010;58:419–421.

26. Wilms G, Peene P, Baert AL, et al. Pre-operative embolization of juvenile nasopharyngeal angiofibromas. *J Belge Radiol.* 1989;72:465–470.

27. Siddiqui AH, Chen PR. Intracranial collateral anastomoses: relevance to endovascular procedures. *Neurosurg Clin N Am.* 2009;20:279–296.

28. Gullane PJ, Davidson J, O'Dwyer T, et al. Juvenile angiofibroma: a review of the literature and a case series report. *Laryngoscope.* 1992;102:928–933.

29. Siniluoto TM, Luotonen JP, Tikkakoski TA, et al. Value of pre-operative embolization in surgery for nasopharyngeal angiofibroma. *J Laryngol Otol.* 1993;107:514–521.

30. Moulin G, Chagnaud C, Gras R, et al. Juvenile nasopharyngeal angiofibroma: comparison of blood loss during removal in embolized group versus nonembolized group. *Cardiovasc Interv Radiol.* 1995;18:158–161.

31. Davis KR. Embolization of epistaxis and juvenile nasopharyngeal angiofibromas. *AJR Am J Roentgenol.* 1987;148:209–218.

32. Wu AW, Mowry SE, Vinuela F, et al. Bilateral vascular supply in juvenile nasopharyngeal angiofibromas. *Laryngoscope.* 2011;121:639–643.

33. El Sharkawy AA. Endonasal endoscopic management of juvenile nasopharyngeal angiofibroma without angiographic embolization. *Eur Arch Otorhinolaryngol.* 2013;270:2051–2055.

34. Sessions RB, Bryan RN, Nacierin RM, et al. Radiographic staging of juvenile angiofibroma. *Head Neck Surg.* 1981;3:279–283.

35. Fisch U. The infratemporal fossa approach for nasopharyngeal tumors. *Laryngoscope.* 1983;93:36–44.

36. Chandler JR, Goulding R, Moskowitz L, et al. Nasopharyngeal angiofibroma: staging and management. *Ann Otol Rhinol Laryngol.* 1984;93:322–329.

37. Andrews JC, Fisch U, Valavanis A, et al. The surgical management of extensive nasopharyngeal angiofibroma with infratemporal fossa approach. *Laryngoscope.* 1989;99:429–437.

38. Radkowski D, McGill T, Healy G, et al. Angiofibroma: changes in staging and treatment. *Arch Otolaryngol Head Neck Surg.* 1996;122:122–129.

39. Onerci M, Oğretmenoğlu O, Yücel T. Juvenile nasopharyngeal angiofibroma: a revised staging system. *Rhinology.* 2006;44:39–45.

40. Snyderman CH, Pant H, Carrau RL, et al. A new endoscopic staging system for angiofibromas. *Arch Otolaryngol Head Neck Surg.* 2010;136:588–594.

41. Yi Z, Fang Z, Lin G, et al. Nasopharyngeal angiofibroma: a concise classification system and appropriate treatment options. *Am J Otolaryngol.* 2013;34:133–141.

42. Elhammady MS, Johnson JN, Peterson EC, et al. Preoperative embolization of juvenile nasopharyngeal angiofibromas: transarterial versus direct tumoral puncture. *World Neurosurg.* 2011;76:328–334.

43. Karmon Y, Siddiqui AH, Hopkins III LN. Juvenile nasopharyngeal angiofibroma—how should we embolize, if at all? *World Neurosurg.* 2011;76:263–265.

44. Lack EE, Cubilla AL, Woodruff JM, et al. Paragangliomas of the head and neck region: a clinical study of 69 patients. *Cancer.* 1977;39:397–409.

45. Erickson D, Kudva YC, Ebersold MJ, et al. Benign paragangliomas: clinical presentation and treatment outcomes in 236 patients. *J Clin Endocrinol Metab.* 2001;86:5210–5216.

46. Jansen JC, van den Berg R, Kuiper A, et al. Estimation of growth rate in patients with head and neck paragangliomas influences the treatment proposal. *Cancer.* 2000;88:2811–2816.

47. Langerman A, Athavale SM, Rangarajan SV, et al. Natural history of cervical paragangliomas: outcomes of observation of 43 patients. *Arch Otolaryngol Head Neck Surg.* 2012;138:341–345.

48. Fisch U, Mattox D. Infratemporal fossa approach type A. Classification of glomus temporale tumours. In: *Microsurgery of the Skull Base.* Stuttgart, Germany: Thieme; 1988:p136–p152.

49. Capatina C, Ntali G, Karavitaki N, et al. The management of head-and-neck paragangliomas. *Endocr Relat Cancer.* 2013;20:R291–R305.

50. Lieberson RE, Adler JR, Soltys SG, et al. Stereotactic radiosurgery as the primary treatment for new and recurrent paragangliomas: is open surgical resection still the treatment of choice? *World Neurosurg.* 2012;77:745–761.

51. Ivan ME, Sughrue ME, Clark AJ, et al. A meta-analysis of tumor control rates and treatment-related morbidity for patients with glomus jugulare tumors. *J Neurosurg.* 2011;114:1299–1305.

52. Papaspyrou K, Mann WJ, Amedee RG. Management of head and neck paragangliomas: review of 120 patients. *Head Neck.* 2009;31:381–387.

53. Al-Mefty O, Teixeira A. Complex tumors of the glomus jugulare: criteria, treatment, and outcome. *J Neurosurg.* 2002;97:1356–1366.

54. Liu JK, Sameshima T, Gottfried ON, et al. The combined transmastoid retro- and infralabyrinthine transjugular transcondylar transtubercular high cervical approach for resection of glomus jugulare tumors. *Neurosurgery.* 2006;59:115–125.

55. Sanna M, Shin SH, De Donato G, et al. Management of complex tympanojugular paragangliomas including endovascular intervention. *Laryngoscope.* 2011;121:1372–1382.

56. Moret J, Delvert JC, Bretonneau CH, et al. Vascularization of the ear: normal-variations-glomus tumors. *J Neuroradiol.* 1982;9:209–260.

57. White JB, Link MJ, Cloft HJ. Endovascular embolization of paragangliomas: a safe adjuvant to treatment. *J Vasc Interv Neurol.* 2008;1:37–41.

58. Harati A, Deitmer T, Rohde S, et al. Microsurgical treatment of large and giant tympanojugular paragangliomas. *Surg Neurol Int.* 2014;5:179.

59. Eckard DA, Purdy PD, Bonte FJ. Temporary balloon occlusion of the carotid artery combined with brain blood flow imaging as a test to predict tolerance prior to permanent carotid sacrifice. *AJNR Am J Neuroradiol.* 1992;13:1565–1569.

60. Piazza P, Di Lella F, Bacciu A, et al. Preoperative protective stenting of the internal carotid artery in the management of complex head and neck paragangliomas: long-term results. *Audiol Neurootol.* 2013;18:345–352.

61. Gaynor BG, Elhammady MS, Jethanamest D, et al. Incidence of cranial nerve palsy after preoperative embolization of glomus jugulare tumors using Onyx. *J Neurosurg.* 2014;120:377–381.

62. Warren III FM, McCool RR, Hunt JO, et al. Preoperative embolization of the inferior petrosal sinus in surgery for glomus jugulare tumors. *Otol Neurotol.* 2011;32:1538–1541.

63. Ladner TR, He L, Davis BJ, et al. Initial experience with dual-lumen balloon catheter injection for preoperative Onyx embolization of skull base paragangliomas. *J Neurosurg.* 2016;124:1813–1819.

64. Gartrell BC, Hansen MR, Gantz BJ, et al. Facial and lower cranial neuropathies after preoperative embolization of jugular foramen lesions with ethylene vinyl alcohol. *Otol Neurotol.* 2012;33:1270–1275.

65. Patel SJ, Sekhar LN, Cass SP, et al. Combined approaches for resection of extensive glomus jugulare tumors. A review of 12 cases. *J Neurosurg.* 1994;80:1026–1038.

66. Dalfino JC, Drazin D, Nair A, et al. Successful Onyx embolization of a giant glomus jugulare: case report and review of nonsurgical treatment options. *World Neurosurg* 2014;81. 842.e11-6.

67. Cognard C, Gobin YP, Pierot L, et al. Cerebral dural arteriovenous fistulas: clinical and angiographic correlation with a revised classification of venous drainage. *Radiology.* 1995;194:671–680.

68. Houser OW, Campbell JK, Campbell RJ, et al. Arteriovenous malformation affecting the transverse dural venous sinus–an acquired lesion. *Mayo Clin Proc.* 1979;54:651–661.

69. Mullan S. Reflections upon the nature and management of intracranial and intraspinal vascular malformations and fistulae. *J Neurosurg.* 1994;80:606–616.

70. Chaichana KL, Coon AL, Tamargo RJ, et al. Dural arteriovenous fistulas: epidemiology and clinical presentation. *Neurosurg Clin N Am.* 2012;23:7–13.

71. Borden JA, Wu JK, Shucart WA. A proposed classification for spinal and cranial dural arteriovenous fistulous malformations and implications for treatment. *J Neurosurg.* 1995;82:166–179.

72. van Dijk JM, terBrugge KG, Willinsky RA, et al. Clinical course of cranial dural arteriovenous fistulas with long-term persistent cortical venous reflux. *Stroke.* 2002;33:1233–1236.

73. Kobayashi A, Al-Shahi Salman R. Prognosis and treatment of intracranial dural arteriovenous fistulae: a systematic review and meta-analysis. *Int J Stroke.* 2014;9:670–677.

74. Söderman M, Pavic L, Edner G, et al. Natural history of dural arteriovenous shunts. *Stroke.* 2008;39:1735–1739.

75. Brown RD Jr, Wiebers DO, Nichols DA. Intracranial dural arteriovenous fistulae: angiographic predictors of intracranial hemorrhage and clinical outcome in nonsurgical patients. *J Neurosurg.* 1994;81:531–538.

76. Davies MA, Ter Brugge K, Willinsky R, et al. The natural history and management of intracranial dural arteriovenous fistulae. Part 2: aggressive lesions. *Interv Neuroradiol.* 1997;3:303–311.

77. Miller TR, Gandhi D. Intracranial dural arteriovenous fistulae: clinical presentation and management strategies. *Stroke.* 2015;46:2017–2025.

78. Lin YH, Lin HH, Liu HM, et al. Diagnostic performance of CT and MRI on the detection of symptomatic intracranial dural arteriovenous fistula: a meta-analysis with indirect comparison. *Neuroradiology.* 2016;58:753–763.

79. Tsai LK, Yeh SJ, Chen YC, et al. Screen for intracranial dural arteriovenous fistulae with carotid duplex sonography. *J Neurol Neurosurg Psychiatry.* 2009;80:1225–1229.

80. Lee S-K, Hetts SW, Halbach V, et al. Standard and guidelines: intracranial dural arteriovenous shunts. *J Neurointerv Surg.* November 27, 2015 (Epub ahead of print).

81. Kim DJ, Willinsky RA, Krings T, et al. Intracranial dural arteriovenous shunts: transarterial glue embolization-experience in 115 consecutive patients. *Radiology.* 2011;258:554–561.

82. Cognard C, Januel AC, Silva NA Jr, et al. Endovascular treatment of intracranial dural arteriovenous fistulas with cortical venous drainage: new management using Onyx. *AJNR Am J Neuroradiol.* 2008;29:235–241.

83. Liu S, Lee DC, Tanoura T. Tentorial dural arteriovenous fistula of the medial tentorial artery. *Radiol Case Rep.* 2016;11:242–244.

84. Kim H-J, Yang J-H, Lee H-J, et al. Tentorial dural arteriovenous fistula treated using transarterial onyx embolization. *J Korean Neurosurg Soc.* 2015;58:276–280.

85. Roy D, Raymond J. The role of transvenous embolization in the treatment of intracranial dural arteriovenous fistulas. *Neurosurgery.* 1997;40:1133–1141. Discussion 1141–1144.

86. Urtasun F, Biondi A, Casaco A, et al. Cerebral dural arteriovenous fistulas: percutaneous transvenous embolization. *Radiology.* 1996;199:209–217.

87. Yoshida K, Melake M, Oishi H, et al. Transvenous embolization of dural carotid cavernous fistulas: a series of 44 consecutive patients. *AJNR Am J Neuroradiol.* 2010;31:651–655.

88. Olteanu-Nerbe V, Uhl E, Steiger HJ, et al. Dural arteriovenous fistulas including the transverse and sigmoid sinuses: results of treatment in 30 cases. *Acta Neurochir.* 1997;139:307–318.

89. Hsu Y-H, Lee C-W, Liu H-M, et al. Endovascular treatment and computed imaging follow-up of 14 anterior condylar dural arteriovenous fistulas. *Interv Neuroradiol.* 2013;20:368–377.

90. Ng PP, Higashida RT, Cullen S, et al. Endovascular strategies for carotid cavernous and intracerebral dural arteriovenous fistulas. *Neurosurg Focus.* 2003;15:ECP1.

91. Narayanan S. Endovascular management of intracranial dural arteriovenous fistulas. *Neurol Clin.* 2010;28:899–911.

92. Guedin P, Gaillard S, Boulin A, et al. Therapeutic management of intracranial dural arteriovenous shunts with leptomeningeal venous drainage: report of 53 consecutive patients with emphasis on transarterial embolization with acrylic glue. *J Neurosurg.* 2010;112:603–610.

93. Nogueira RG, Dabus G, Rabinov JD, et al. Preliminary experience with onyx embolization for the treatment of intracranial dural arteriovenous fistulas. *AJNR Am J Neuroradiol.* 2008;29:91–97.

94. Saraf R, Shrivastava M, Kumar N, et al. Embolization of cranial dural arteriovenous fistulae with ONYX: indications, techniques, and outcomes. *Indian J Radiol Imaging.* 2010;20:26–33.

95. Hu YC, Newman CB, Dashti SR, et al. Cranial dural arteriovenous fistula: transarterial Onyx embolization experience and technical nuances. *J Neurointerv Surg.* 2011;3:5–13.

96. Natarajan SK, Ghodke B, Kim LJ, et al. Multimodality treatment of intracranial dural arteriovenous fistulas in the Onyx era: a single center experience. *World Neurosurg.* 2010;73:365–379.

97. Wakhloo AK, Perlow A, Linfante I, et al. Transvenous n-butyl-cyanoacrylate infusion for complex dural carotid cavernous fistulas: technical considerations and clinical outcome. *AJNR Am J Neuroradiol.* 2005;26:1888–1897.

98. Shaibani A, Rohany M, Parkinson R, et al. Primary treatment of an indirect carotid cavernous fistula by injection of N-butyl cyanoacrylate in the dural wall of the cavernous sinus. *Surg Neurol.* 2007;67:403–408. Discussion 408.

99. Suzuki S, Lee DW, Jahan R, et al. Transvenous treatment of spontaneous dural carotid-cavernous fistulas using a combination of detachable coils and Onyx. *AJNR Am J Neuroradiol.* 2006;27:1346–1349.

100. Miyamoto N, Naito I, Shimizu T, et al. Efficacy and limitations of transarterial acrylic glue embolization for intracranial dural arteriovenous fistulas. *Neurol Med Chir.* 2015;55:163–172.

101. Moore C, Murphy K, Gailloud P. Improved distal distribution of n-butyl cyanoacrylate glue by simultaneous injection of dextrose 5% through the guiding catheter: technical note. *Neuroradiology.* 2006;48:327–332.

102. Shi ZS, Loh Y, Gonzalez N, et al. Flow control techniques for Onyx embolization of intracranial dural arteriovenous fistulae. *J Neurointerv Surg.* 2013;5:311–316.

103. Shi ZS, Loh Y, Duckwiler GR, et al. Balloon-assisted transarterial embolization of intracranial dural arteriovenous fistulas. *J Neurosurg.* 2009;110:921–928.

104. Huo X, Li Y, Jiang C, Wu Z. Balloon-assisted endovascular treatment of intracranial dural arteriovenous fistulas. *Turk Neurosurg.* 2014;24:658–663.

105. Levrier O, Métellus P, Fuentes S, et al. Use of a self-expanding stent with balloon angioplasty in the treatment of dural arteriovenous fistulas involving the transverse and/or sigmoid sinus: functional and neuroimaging-based outcome in 10 patients. *J Neurosurg.* 2006;104:254–263.

106. Kim ST, Jeong HW, Seo J. Onyx embolization of dural arteriovenous fistula, using scepter C balloon catheter: a case report. *Neurointervention.* 2013;8:110–114.

107. Takada S, Isaka F, Nakakuki T, et al. Torcular dural arteriovenous fistula treated via stent placement and angioplasty in the affected straight and transverse sinuses: case report. *J Neurosurg.* 2015;122:1208–1213.

108. Murata T, Nagashima H, Ichinose S, et al. Successful stentings for bilateral jugular bulb stenosis/occlusion in a case of bilateral transverse sinuses dural arteriovenous fistulas: case report. *J Neuroendovasc Ther.* 2016;10:127–133.

109. Murphy KJ, Gailloud P, Venbrux A, et al. Endovascular treatment of a grade IV transverse sinus dural arteriovenous fistula by sinus recanalization, angioplasty, and stent placement: technical case report. *Neurosurgery.* 2000;46:497–500. Discussion 500–501.

110. White JB, Layton KF, Evans AJ, et al. Transorbital puncture for the treatment of cavernous sinus dural arteriovenous fistulas. *AJNR Am J Neuroradiol.* 2007;28:1415–1417.

111. Dashti SR, Fiorella D, Spetzler RF, et al. Transorbital endovascular embolization of dural carotid-cavernous fistula: access to cavernous sinus through direct puncture: case examples and technical report. *Neurosurgery.* 2011;68(1 suppl operative):75–83. Discussion 83.

112. Lucas CP, Zabramski JM, Spetzler RF, et al. Treatment for intracranial dural arteriovenous malformations: a meta-analysis from the English language literature. *Neurosurgery.* 1997;40:1119–1130. Discussion 1130–12.

113. Jung KH, Kwon BJ, Chu K, et al. Clinical and angiographic factors related to the prognosis of cavernous sinus dural arteriovenous fistula. *Neuroradiology*. 2011;53:983–992.

114. Halbach VV, Higashida RT, Hieshima GB, et al. Transvenous embolization of dural fistulas involving the cavernous sinus. *AJNR Am J Neuroradiol*. 1989;10:10377–10383.

115. Gandhi D, Chen J, Pearl M, et al. Intracranial dural arteriovenous fistulas: classification, imaging findings, and treatment. *AJNR Am J Neuroradiol*. 2012;33:1007–1013.

116. Kai Y, Morioka M, Yano S, et al. External manual carotid compression is effective in patients with cavernous sinus dural arteriovenous fistulae. *Interv Neuroradiol*. 2007;13(suppl 1):115–122.

117. Phelps CD, Thompson HS, Ossoinig KC. The diagnosis and prognosis of atypical carotid-cavernous fistula (red-eyed shunt syndrome). *Am J Ophthalmol*. 1982;93:423–436.

118. Sasaki H, Nukui H, Kaneko M, et al. Long-term observations in cases with spontaneous carotid-cavernous fistulas. *Acta Neurochir*. 1988;90:117–120.

119. Thompson BG, Doppman JL, Oldfield EH. Treatment of cranial dural arteriovenous fistulae by interruption of leptomeningeal venous drainage. *J Neurosurg*. 1994;80:617–623.

120. Tomak PR, Cloft HJ, Kaga A, et al. Evolution of the management of tentorial dural arteriovenous malformations. *Neurosurgery*. 2003;52:750–760. Discussion 760–762.

121. Zhou LF, Chen L, Song DL, et al. Tentorial dural arteriovenous fistulas. *Surg Neurol*. 2007;67:472–481. Discussion 481–482.

122. Pierot L, Visot A, Boulin A, et al. Combined neurosurgical and neuroradiological treatment of a complex superior sagittal sinus dural fistula: technical note. *Neurosurgery*. 1998;42:194–197.

123. Friedman JA, Pollock BE, Nichols DA, et al. Results of combined stereotactic radiosurgery and transarterial embolization for dural arteriovenous fistulas of the transverse and sigmoid sinuses. *J Neurosurg*. 2001;94:886–891.

124. O'Leary S, Hodgson TJ, Coley SC, et al. Intracranial dural arteriovenous malformations: results of stereotactic radiosurgery in 17 patients. *Clin Oncol*. 2002;14:97–102.

125. Maruyama K, Shin M, Kurita H, et al. Stereotactic radiosurgery for dural arteriovenous fistula involving the superior sagittal sinus. *J Neurosurg*. 2002;97(5 suppl):481–483.

126. Soderman M, Edner G, Ericson K, et al. Gamma knife surgery for dural arteriovenous shunts: 25 years of experience. *J Neurosurg*. 2006;104:867–875.

127. Barrow DL, Spector RH, Braun IF, et al. Classification and treatment of spontaneous carotid-cavernous sinus fistulas. *J Neurosurg*. 1985;62:248–256.

128. Park H-R, Yoon S-M, Shim J-J, et al. Iatrogenic carotid-cavernous fistula after stent assisted coil embolization of posterior communicating artery aneurysm. *J Cerebrovasc Endovasc Neurosurg*. 2015;17:43–48.

129. de Keizer R. Carotid-cavernous and orbital arteriovenous fistulas: ocular features, diagnostic and hemodynamic considerations in relation to visual impairment and morbidity. *Orbit*. 2003;22:121–142.

130. Coskun O, Hamon M, Catroux G, et al. Carotid-cavernous fistulas: diagnosis with spiral CT angiography. *Am J Neuroradiol*. 2000;21:712–716.

131. Chen CC, Chang PC, Shy CG, et al. CT angiography and MR angiography in the evaluation of carotid cavernous sinus fistula prior to embolization: a comparison of techniques. *Am J Neuroradiol*. 2005;26:2349–2356.

132. Higashida RT, Hieshima GB, Halbach VV, et al. Closure of carotid cavernous sinus fistulae by external compression of the carotid artery and jugular vein. *Acta Radiol Suppl*. 1986;369:580–583.

133. Palestine AG, Younge BR, Piepgras DG. Visual prognosis in carotid-cavernous fistula. *Arch Ophthalmol*. 1981;99:1600–1603.

134. Kupersmith MJ. *Neurovascular Neuropharmacology*. Berlin, Heidelberg: Springer; 1993.

135. Debrun G, Lacour P, Vinuela F, et al. Treatment of 54 traumatic carotid-cavernous fistulas. *J Neurosurg*. 1981;55:678–692.

136. Gemmete JJ, Ansari SA, Gandhi D. Endovascular treatment of carotid cavernous fistulas. *Neuroimaging Clin N Am*. 2009;19:241–255.

137. Teng MM, Chang CY, Chiang JH, et al. Double-balloon technique for embolization of carotid cavernous fistulas. *AJNR Am J Neuroradiol*. 2000;21:1753–1756.

138. Ducruet AF, Albuquerque FC, Crowley RW, et al. The evolution of endovascular treatment of carotid cavernous fistulas: a single-center experience. *World Neurosurg*. 2013;80:538–548.

139. Lewis AI, Tomsick TA, Tew JM Jr, et al. Long-term results in direct carotid-cavernous fistulas after treatment with detachable balloons. *J Neurosurg*. 1996;84:400–404.

140. Luo C-B, Teng MM-H, Chang F-C, et al. Transarterial detachable coil embolization of direct carotid-cavernous fistula: immediate and long-term outcomes. *J Chin Med Assoc*. 2013;76:31–36.

141. Nesbit GM, Barnwell SL. The use of electrolytically detachable coils in treating high-flow arteriovenous fistulas. *AJNR Am J Neuroradiol*. 1998;19:1565–1569.

142. Jansen O, Dorfler A, Forsting M, et al. Endovascular therapy of arteriovenous fistulae with electrolytically detachable coils. *Neuroradiology*. 1999;41:951–957.

143. Troffkin NA, Given II CA. Combined transarterial N-butyl cyanoacrylate and coil embolization of direct carotid-cavernous fistulas. Report of two cases. *J Neurosurg*. 2007;106:903–906.

144. Kocer N, Kizilkilic O, Albayram S, et al. Treatment of iatrogenic internal carotid artery laceration and carotid cavernous fistula with endovascular stent-graft placement. *AJNR Am J Neuroradiol*. 2002;23:442–446.

145. Gomez F, Escobar W, Gomez AM, et al. Treatment of carotid cavernous fistulas using covered stents: midterm results in seven patients. *AJNR Am J Neuroradiol*. 2007;28:1762–1768.

146. Zaidat OO, Lazzaro MA, Niu T, et al. Multimodal endovascular therapy of traumatic and spontaneous carotid cavernous fistula using coils, n-BCA, Onyx and stent graft. *J Neurointerv Surg.* 2011;3:255–262.
147. Moron FE, Klucznik RP, Mawad ME, et al. Endovascular treatment of high-flow carotid cavernous fistulas by stent-assisted coil placement. *AJNR Am J Neuroradiol.* 2005;26:1399–1404.
148. Lee CY, Yim MB, Kim IM, et al. Traumatic aneurysm of the supraclinoid internal carotid artery and an associated carotid-cavernous fistula: vascular reconstruction performed using intravascular implantation of stents and coils. Case report. *J Neurosurg.* 2004;100:115–119.
149. Goto K, Hieshima G, Higashida R, et al. Treatment of direct carotid cavernous sinus fistulae. Various therapeutic approaches and results in 148 cases. *Acta Radiol Suppl.* 1985;369:576–579.
150. Higashida RT, Halbach VV, Tsai FY, et al. Interventional neurovascular treatment of traumatic carotid and vertebral artery lesions: results in 234 cases. *AJR Am J Roentgenol.* 1989;153:577–582.
151. van Rooij WJ, Sluzewski M, Beute GN. Ruptured cavernous sinus aneurysms causing carotid cavernous fistula: incidence, clinical presentation, treatment, and outcome. *AJNR Am J Neuroradiol.* 2006;27:185–189.

# Index

---

*Note*: Page numbers followed by "f" indicate figures, "t" indicate tables and "b" indicate boxes.